Ready Reckoner in GYNECOLOGY

Ready Reckoner in

GYNECOLOGY

Editor

Ruchika Garg

MD MRCOG 1 FICOG FICMCH FIMS FMAS MAMS FIAOG (Gold Medalist)

Professor and Unit Head

Department of Obstetrics and Gynecology

SN Medical College

Agra, Uttar Pradesh, India

Editor-in-Chief, Journal of Midlife Health

Executive Editor, Journal of SAFOG

Forewords

Gangadhar Sahoo

Muralidhar V Pai

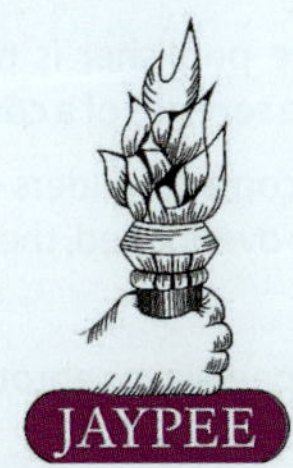

JAYPEE BROTHERS MEDICAL PUBLISHERS

The Health Sciences Publisher

New Delhi | London

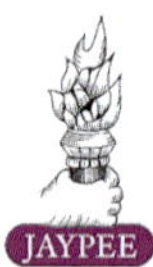

JAYPEE **Jaypee Brothers Medical Publishers (P) Ltd**

Headquarters
EMCA House, 23/23-B
Ansari Road, Daryaganj
New Delhi 110 002, India
Landline: +91-11-23272143, +91-11-23272703
+91-11-23282021, +91-11-23245672
e-mail: jaypee@jaypeebrothers.com

Corporate Office
4838/24, Ansari Road, Daryaganj
New Delhi 110 002, India
Phone: +91-11-43574357
Fax: +91-11-43574314
e-mail: jaypee@jaypeebrothers.com

Overseas Office
JP Medical Ltd.
83, Victoria Street, London
SW1H 0HW (UK)
Phone: +44-20 3170 8910
e-mail: info@jpmedpub.com

EU GPSR Authorised Representative
Logos Europe, 9 rue Nicolas Poussin
17000, La Rochelle, France
Phone: +33 (0) 6 67 93 73 78
e-mail: contact@logoseurope.eu

Website: www.jaypeebrothers.com
Website: www.jaypeedigital.com

Ready Reckoner in Gynecology

First Edition: **2026**

ISBN: 978-93-7545-962-0

Printed in India

Contributors

Abhipreet Bhattacharyya MBBS
Academic Junior Resident
Department of Obstetrics and Gynecology
All India Institute of Medical Sciences
Deoghar, Jharkhand, India

Afreen Mahaboob
MBBS MS (Obs & Gyne) MRCOG 1
Senior Resident
Department of Obstetrics and Gynecology
Ramaiah Medical College and Hospitals
Bengaluru, Karnataka, India

Akanksha Gupta MBBS MS
Associate Professor
Department of Gynecology
SN Medical College
Agra, Uttar Pradesh, India

Anu Chaudhary MBBS MS DNB
Senior Resident
Department of Obstetrics and Gynecology
Maharani Laxmi Bai Medical College
Jhansi, Uttar Pradesh, India

Anusha Singh MS FMAS
Senior Resident
Department of Obstetrics and Gynecology
SN Medical College
Agra, Uttar Pradesh, India

Deepa Chaudhary MBBS MS (Obs & Gyne) FMAS (Minimal Access Surgery) FARM (Reproductive Medicine) Diploma in Urogynaecology (Kiel University, Germany)
Professor
Department of Obstetrics and Gynecology
Sawai Man Singh Medical College
Jaipur, Rajasthan, India

Gaurav Desai MS FCPS FMAS
Assistant Professor
Department of Obstetrics and Gynecology
Seth Gordhandas Sunderdas Medical College
and King Memorial Hospital
Mumbai, Maharashtra, India

Jyothi GS
MBBS MD (Obs & Gyne) PGDMLE FICOG FICMCH
Professor and Head
Department of Obstetrics and Gynecology
Ramaiah Medical College and Hospitals
Bengaluru, Karnataka, India

Kavita Chaudhary MS FMAS
Senior Resident
Department of Obstetrics and Gynecology
SN Medical College
Agra, Uttar Pradesh, India

Kshama Nilesh Uplenchwar
DNB DGO MRCOG
Director, Women's Clinic
& IUI Centre, Pune
Honorary Consultant
Department of Obstetrics and Gynecology
Deenanath Mangeshkar Hospital and
Research Centre
Pune, Maharashtra, India

Mishu Mangla MBBS MS (Obs & Gyne) PDCC (Maternal & Fetal Medicine)
Associate Professor
Department of Obstetrics
and Gynecology
All India Institute of Medical Sciences
Yadadri Bhuvanagiri, Telangana, India

Neelansha Varshney MBBS MD
Senior Resident
Department of Gynecology
SN Medical College
Agra, Uttar Pradesh

Poojitha Kalyani Kanikaram
MBBS MS (Obs & Gyne)
Senior Resident
Department of Obstetrics and Gynecology
All India Institute of Medical Sciences
Yadadri Bhuvanagiri, Telangana, India

Preeti Nitsure Deshpande
MS MRCOG FICOG Fellowship Infertility
Advanced Endoscopy
Training IRCAD (France)
Consultant Obstetrician
and Gynecologist
SL Raheja-Fortis Hospital
Guru Nanak Hospital
KJ Somaiya Multispecialty Hospital
Surya Hospital, Chembur
Sambhav—Dr Preeti Deshpande's Clinic
Mumbai, Maharashtra, India

Priyanka Rai MBBS MS (Obs & Gyne)
Associate Professor
Department of Obstetrics and Gynecology
All India Institute of Medical Sciences
Deoghar, Jharkhand, India

Richa Bansal MBBS MS
Consultant Gynec-oncologist
Apollo Hospital
Navi Mumbai, Maharashtra, India

Ruchika Garg MD MRCOG 1 FICOG FICMCH FIMS FMAS MAMS FIAOG (Gold Medalist)
Professor and Unit Head
Department of Obstetrics and Gynecology
SN Medical College
Agra, Uttar Pradesh, India
Editor-in-Chief, Journal of Midlife Health
Executive Editor, Journal of SAFOG

Sachin Naiknaware MBBS MS (Obs & Gyne) FICLS FMAS Dip in Minimal Access Surgery Dip in IVF (UKSH Germany)
Associate Professor
Department of Obstetrics and Gynecology
Ideal Institute of Medical Sciences
Consultant Visiting Endoscopic Surgeon
Breach Candy Hospital, Wockhardt Hospital,
Parkview Hospital
Mumbai, Maharashtra, India

Sandeep Suhas Pophale MBBS MS Fellowship in Advanced Gyne Endoscopy Consultant, Endoscopic Surgeon, Infertility Specialist
Associate Professor
Department of Obstetrics and Gynecology
Government Grant Medical College
and Sir JJ Groups of Hospital
Mumbai, Maharashtra, India

Shaifali Singh MBBS MS
Resident
Department of Obstetrics and Gynecology
SN Medical College
Agra, Uttar Pradesh, India

Sharmeen Vazifdar MS DNB (Obs & Gyne)
Consultant
Department of Obstetrics and Gynecology
Vazifdar Clinic
Mumbai, Maharashtra, India

Shikha Singh MBBS MS
Professor and Head
Department of Gynecology
SN Medical College
Agra, Uttar Pradesh, India

Shivani Singh Bundela
MS (Obs & Gyne) FICMCH
Professor
Department of Obstetrics and Gynecology
Hind Institute of Medical Sciences
Lucknow, Uttar Pradesh, India

Shreedevi Tanksale DNB DGO Fellowship in Reproductive Medicine (India and UZ Leuven Belgium) FMAS DFP DE
Director
Department of Reproductive Medicine
Little Miracles Fertility Clinic
Mumbai, Maharashtra, India

Sumedha Sharad Pathade
MBBS MS DNB FMAS
Senior Resident
Department of Obstetrics and Gynecology
Lokmanya Tilak Municipal Medical College and General Hospital
Mumbai, Maharashtra, India

Tejal Poddar MS Fellowship in Reproductive Medicine (India and UZ Leuven Belgium) FMAS DFP DE BIMIE
Director
Department of Reproductive Medicine
Little Miracles Fertility Clinic
Mumbai, Maharashtra, India

Foreword

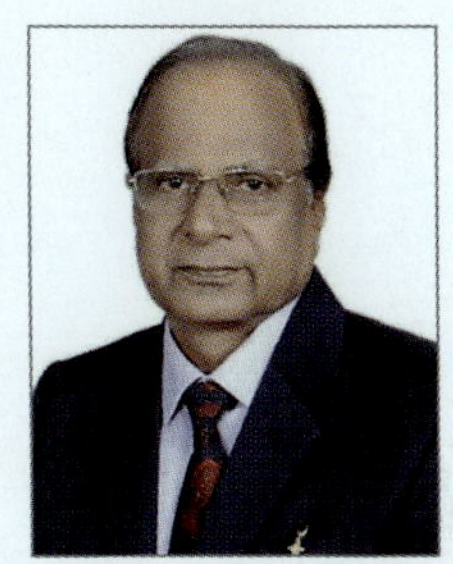

It gives me immense pleasure to present the book *Ready Reckoner in Gynecology*, meticulously compiled by *Professor Ruchika Garg*, a distinguished Academician and Clinician from the Department of Obstetrics and Gynecology, SN Medical College, Agra, Uttar Pradesh, India.

In the ever-evolving field of gynecology, postgraduate students, MBBS undergraduates, and aspirants preparing for competitive examinations like NEET-PG and DNB often grapple with vast syllabi, intricate guidelines, and the need for quick, reliable revision. This book serves as an indispensable companion—a concise yet comprehensive resource that distils essential concepts, high-yield facts, clinical algorithms, and exam-oriented points into an accessible format.

Her expertise, honed through years of teaching, research, and patient care, shines through in this work, making complex topics approachable and memorable. Designed for rapid reference during wards, clinics, or last-minute revisions, it empowers learners to excel academically and clinically.

I am confident that this ready-reckoner will become a trusted ally for generations of medical professionals.

Gangadhar Sahoo
MD (OBG)
Retired Professor and Head
Department of Obstetrics and Gynecology
VSS Medical College
Burla, Odisha, India
Dean, IMS and SUM Hospital, Bhubaneswar
Pro VC, SOA Deemed to be University, Bhubaneswar
President
Indian Society of Perinatology and
Reproductive Biology (ISOPARB) (2022–2023)

Foreword

It is with immense pleasure that I write this foreword for the *Ready Reckoner in Obstetrics*, expertly.

Obstetrics stands as one of the most dynamic and high-stakes branches of medicine. Rapidly evolving evidence from landmark trials, updated guidelines, and technological advancements demand that practitioners and students alike stay abreast of the latest knowledge.

This book masterfully addresses this need, serving as an essential companion for postgraduate students, MBBS students, FMGE aspirants preparing for NEET-PG, INI-CET, DNB examinations, and busy consultants who want to afresh their knowledge.

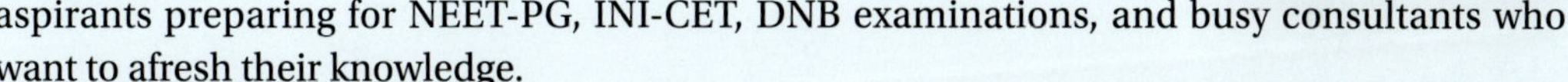

The *Ready Reckoner* distills vast obstetrics into concise, high-yield formats. Multiple algorithms for clinical decision-making have been added. Tables summarize critical comparisons aligned with 2025 WHO, FIGO, NICE, and ACOG guidelines. Multiple illustrations, including flowcharts, clarify complex scenarios visually.

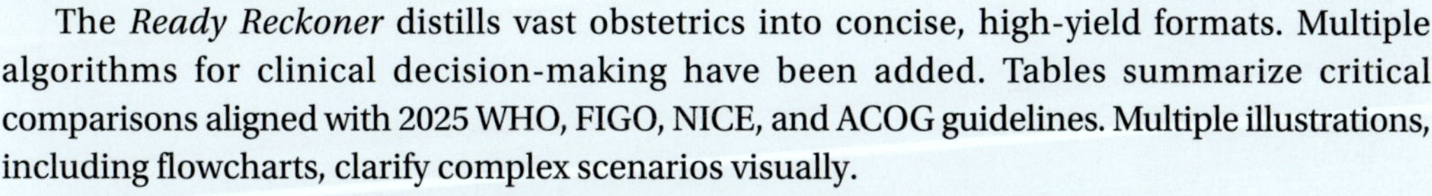

MCQs and high-yield facts tested in recent examinations have been added.

Editor (Professor) Ruchika Garg's meticulous curation ensures practicality to excel in wards, labor rooms, and theory examinations.

Whether tackling antepartum complications, intrapartum challenges, or puerperal issues, this book fosters confidence and competence.

In an era of information overload, it will be very helpful for quick revisions.

I wholeheartedly endorse it for all aspiring obstetricians, and I am confident it will elevate clinical practice and examination success alike.

Warm regards,

Muralidhar V Pai
MD FRCOG FICOG FKCOG FICMCH
Pro Vice Chancellor, Sikkim Manipal University
Dean, Sikkim Manipal Institute of Medical Sciences, Sikkim
Professor of Obstetrics and Gynecology

Preface

The field of obstetrics and gynecology demands a unique blend of theoretical knowledge, clinical acumen, and practical expertise. For postgraduate students pursuing MS or MD, mastering this specialty requires a comprehensive yet concise resource that bridges the gap between extensive textbooks and the time-sensitive needs of exam preparation. *Ready Reckoner in Gynecology* is crafted specifically for this purpose, offering a streamlined, high-yield guide tailored to the needs of postgraduate students preparing for both theory and practical examinations.

This book is designed with precision and clarity, presenting complex concepts in a structured, easy-to-digest format. It emphasizes tables, bullet points, and succinct explanations to facilitate quick revision and retention. The content is meticulously curated to cover the core topics of gynecology, including reproductive physiology, gynecological disorders, operative techniques, and recent advancements, aligning with the latest examination patterns and clinical guidelines. Each chapter integrates clinical evidence, management protocols, and practical tips to equip students with the tools needed to excel in written exams, viva voce, and clinical assessments. We thank our contributors who are all doyens in the subject. They have penned down their vast experiences in this book.

Without the love and support of our family members—husband Dr Prabhat Agrawal, children Pratham and Palakshi, parents Dr Anuradha and MC Agrawal, this Herculean task would not have seen the light of day. We express our gratitude to department faculty Professor Shikha Singh and Professor Richa Singh for their support and cooperation.

Our aim is to provide a reliable companion that not only aids in exam success but also fosters a deeper understanding of gynecological principles for future practice. We hope that this ready-reckoner serves as an indispensable resource for postgraduate students, empowering them to approach their examinations with confidence and competence. We thank Mr Jitendar P Vij (Group Chairman), Kritika Dua (Manager—Content Acquisition and Business Development), Ashish Kumar (Senior Business Manager), Aarti Kushwah (Development Editor), and Ruby Sharma (Business Manager) from M/s Jaypee Brothers Medical Publishers (P) Ltd, New Delhi, India, for their support and cooperation throughout the publication of this book.

Ruchika Garg
MD MRCOG 1 FICOG FICMCH FIMS FMAS MAMS FIAOG (Gold Medalist)
Professor and Unit Head
Department of Obstetrics and Gynecology
SN Medical College
Agra, Uttar Pradesh, India
Editor-in-Chief, Journal of Midlife Health
Executive Editor, Journal of SAFOG

Contents

SECTION 3 Gynecologic Oncology

SECTION 4 Contraception

SECTION 8 Viva

Basics and Developmental Gynecology

Physiology of Menstruation

Priyanka Rai, Abhipreet Bhattacharyya

INTRODUCTION

The menstrual cycle and ovulation are orchestrated by the hypothalamic–pituitary–ovarian (H–P–O) axis, a complex interplay of neuroendocrine signals regulating reproductive functions. Understanding this axis is crucial for managing gynecological disorders like infertility, abnormal uterine bleeding (AUB), and contraception.

HYPOTHALAMIC–PITUITARY–OVARIAN AXIS

The HPO axis integrates hypothalamic gonadotropin-releasing hormone (GnRH), pituitary gonadotropins (FSH, LH), and ovarian steroids (estrogen, progesterone) to regulate folliculogenesis, ovulation, and menstruation. Feedback mechanisms (positive and negative) finetune this process.

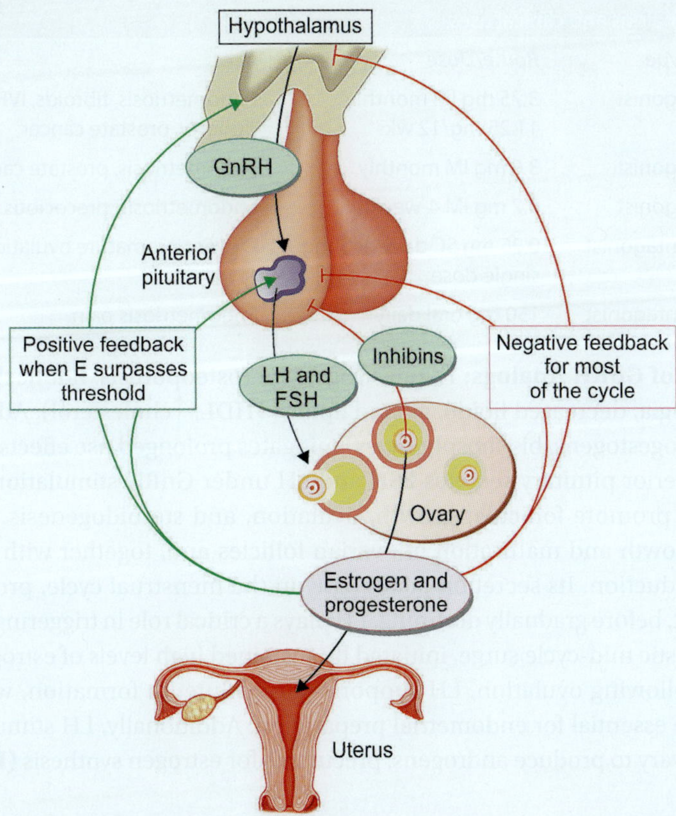

Hypothalamus

- **Location:** Base of the brain, below the thalamus, forming the tuber cinereum and pituitary stalk
- **Key Hormone:** GnRH (decapeptide, half-life 2–4 min), secreted by the arcuate nucleus in a pulsatile manner
    - **Pulsatility:**
        - Follicular phase: Every 60 min (high frequency, low amplitude).
        - Luteal phase: Every 180 min (low frequency, high amplitude).
    - **Actions:**
        - Pulsatile GnRH stimulates FSH/LH release, promoting ovulation.
        - Continuous GnRH causes pituitary downregulation, suppressing gonadotropins (used in IVF, endometriosis, fibroid management).
- **Regulation:**
    - Stimulated by estrogen, epinephrine, leptin.
    - Inhibited by dopamine, serotonin, opioids, gonadotropins.
    - External stimuli (stress, emotions) via cortical centers (e.g., temporal lobe) influence GnRH, affecting cycles.
- **Puberty Onset:** Triggered by leptin (adipocyte hormone), explaining earlier menarche in obese adolescents.
- **Other Secretions:** Prolactin-inhibiting factor (dopamine), thyrotropin-releasing factor, corticotropin-releasing factor.

TABLE 1: GnRH analogs and clinical uses.

Drug	*Type*	*Route/Dose*	*Uses*
Leuprolide	Agonist	3.75 mg IM monthly, 11.25 mg/12 wks	Endometriosis, fibroids, IVF, precocious puberty, prostate cancer
Goserelin	Agonist	3.6 mg IM monthly	Endometriosis, prostate cancer
Triptorelin	Agonist	3.7 mg IM 4-weekly	Endometriosis, precocious puberty
Cetrorelix	Antagonist	0.25 mg SC daily or 3 mg single dose	Prevent premature ovulation in IVF
Elagolix	Antagonist	150 mg oral daily	Endometriosis pain

- **Side Effects of GnRH Analogs:** Hypoestrogenism (osteoporosis, hot flashes), insomnia, nausea, myalgia, decreased libido, altered lipids (↓HDL, ↑cholesterol). Add-back therapy (estrogen, progestogens, bisphosphonates) mitigates prolonged use effects.

The anterior pituitary secretes FSH and LH under GnRH stimulation, which act on the ovary to promote follicular growth, ovulation, and steroidogenesis. FSH primarily drives the growth and maturation of ovarian follicles and, together with LH, stimulates estrogen production. Its secretion peaks early in the menstrual cycle, promoting follicle development, before gradually declining. LH plays a critical role in triggering ovulation with its characteristic mid-cycle surge, initiated by sustained high levels of estrogen via positive feedback. Following ovulation, LH supports corpus luteum formation, which produces progesterone essential for endometrial preparation. Additionally, LH stimulates the theca cells of the ovary to produce androgens, precursors for estrogen synthesis **(Fig. 1)**.

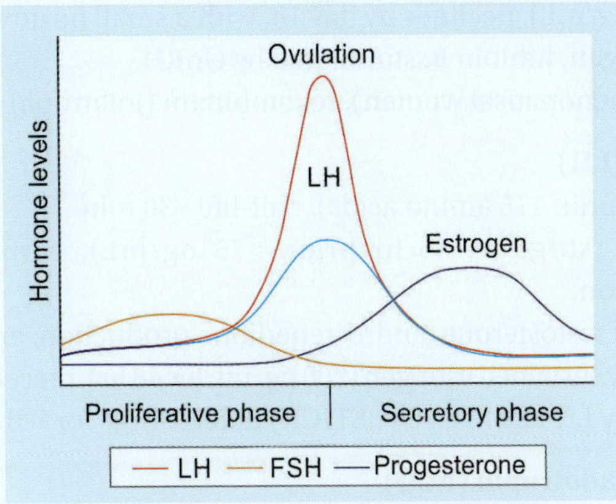

Fig. 1: Ovulation and relation with hormones.

Updates

- GnRH antagonists (e.g., Cetrorelix, Elagolix) are preferred in IVF for shorter cycles, fewer injections, and lower OHSS risk.
- Oral GnRH antagonists (e.g., Elagolix, Relugolix) are emerging for endometriosis and chronic pelvic pain, with ongoing evaluation for long-term safety.

Pituitary Gland

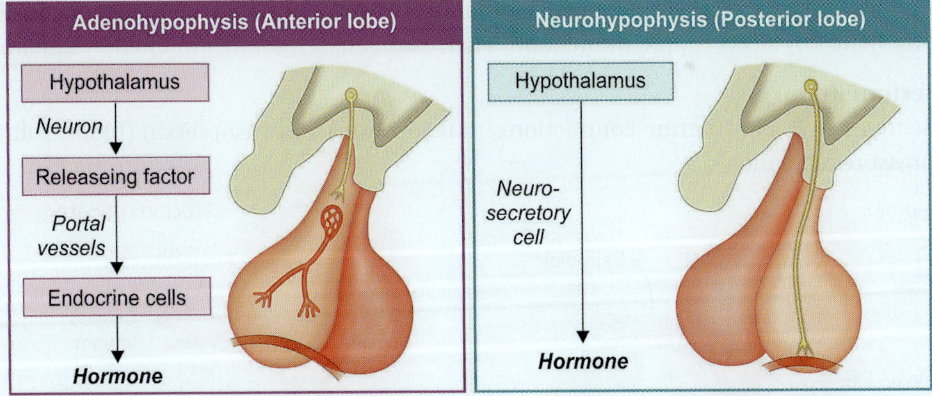

- **Location:** Sella turcica, comprises anterior (adenohypophysis) and posterior (neurohypophysis) lobes
- **Anterior Pituitary:**
  - Secretes FSH, LH, prolactin, TSH, ACTH via β-cells (basophils).
  - Hormones are glycoproteins with identical α-subunits (92 amino acids) and specific β-subunits.

Follicle-Stimulating Hormone (FSH)

- Glycoprotein (β-subunit: 115 amino acids), half-life ~4 hr.
- Stimulates primordial follicle growth, estrogen secretion, LH receptor development in granulosa cells.

- Peaks on day 7 (40 ng/mL), declines by day 18, with a small postovulatory peak.
- Suppressed by estrogen, inhibin B; stimulated by GnRH.
- **Sources:** Urinary (menopausal women), recombinant (follitropin α/β).

Luteinizing Hormone (LH)

- Glycoprotein (β-subunit: 115 amino acids), half-life ~30 min.
- Triggers ovulation (surge 24–36 hr prior, >75 ng/mL), corpus luteum formation, progesterone secretion.
- Stimulates theca cell testosterone/androstenedione production, aromatized to oestradiol.
- **LH Surge:** Induced by sustained estrogen (200 pg/mL for 48 hr), preceded by progesterone rise.
- **Clinical Use:** Urinary LH kits (e.g., OvuSTICK) detect surge for IUI/IVF timing.

Human Chorionic Gonadotropin (hCG)

- Secreted by syncytiotrophoblast, mimics LH (similar α-subunit, unique β-subunit).
- Supports corpus luteum in early pregnancy, used in anovulatory infertility, IVF, habitual abortion.
- **Sources:** Urinary (5,000/10,000 IU), recombinant (250 µg = 5,000 IU).
- **Detection:** Serum (1–2 mIU/mL), urine (20–50 mIU/mL).

Prolactin

- Polypeptide (198 amino acids), half-life ~ 30 min, secreted by α-cells.
- Normal: 8–25 ng/mL; >100 ng/mL suggests pituitary adenoma.
- Inhibits LH (not FSH), causing anovulation, amenorrhea, galactorrhea in hyperprolactinemia.
- Stimulated by sleep, nipple stimulation, TRH, estrogen, serotonin; inhibited by dopamine.

Posterior Pituitary

- Secretes oxytocin (uterine contractions, milk ejection) and vasopressin (blood volume/pressure regulation).

Ovary

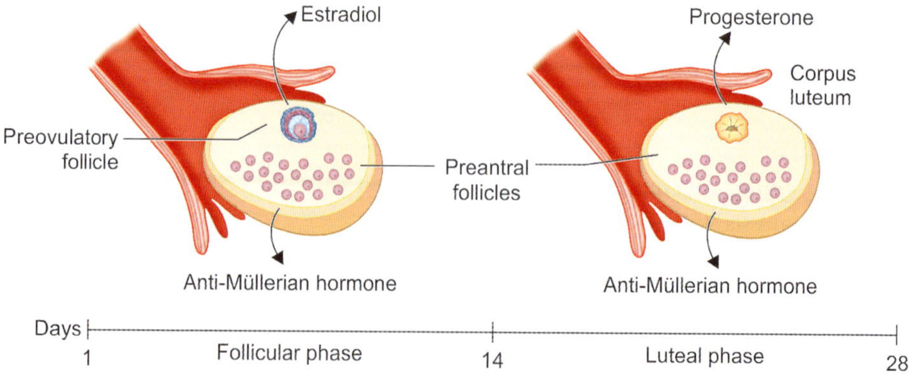

- **Steroidogenesis:** Produces estrogen, progesterone, androgens from cholesterol.

- **Estrogen:**
  - Secreted by theca/granulosa cells (follicular phase) and corpus luteum.
  - **Estradiol (E2):** Predominant, peaks 300–600 μ 48 hr pre-ovulation, 10× more potent than estrone (E1).
  - **Estrone:** Postmenopausal, from androstenedione aromatization.
  - **Estriol (E3):** Placental, pregnancy-specific.
  - **Binding:** 69% SHBG, 30% albumin, 1% free (active).
  - **Actions:**
    - Feminization (secondary sex characteristics).
    - Endometrial proliferation, uterine/cervical vascularity, myohyperplasia.
    - Breast ductal/parenchymal growth, areolar pigmentation.
    - Bone calcification, ↑HDL (cardioprotective), water/sodium retention.
    - Suppresses FSH, stimulates LH.
  - **Side Effects:** Thromboembolism, ↑SHBG, endometrial hyperplasia (unopposed).

Progesterone

- Secreted by corpus luteum (luteal phase, 20–40 mg/day), minor adrenal contribution (2–3 mg).
- Peaks mid-luteal (15 ng/mL), <15 ng/mL indicates luteal phase defect (LPD).
- **Binding:** 80% albumin, 20% corticosteroid-binding globulin.
- **Actions:**
  - Secretory endometrial hypertrophy, decidualization (pregnancy support).
  - Uterine myohyperplasia, reduced contraction frequency.
  - Cervical mucus tenacity, Fallopian tube peristalsis.
  - Breast acinar growth (with estrogen).
  - Thermogenic (↑0.5°C in luteal phase), water/sodium retention.
- **Side Effects:** Nausea, headache, breast tenderness, weight gain, virilization (some progestogens), ↓HDL, ↑LDL, thrombosis (3rd-gen progestogens).

Nonsteroidal Hormones

- **Inhibin:** Peptide (A and B), secreted by Graafian follicles, suppresses FSH, stimulates LH. High in PCOS, low postmenopause (<15 pg/mL).
- **Activin:** Stimulates FSH, enhances ovarian action.
- **Follistatin:** Suppresses FSH by inhibiting activin.
- **Anti-Müllerian Hormone (AMH)**:
  - Secreted by granulosa cells (preantral/antral follicles).
  - Normal: 1–6.8 ng/mL; <1 ng/mL (poor ovarian reserve), >10 ng/mL (PCOS, OHSS).
  - Used in ART for ovarian reserve assessment, gonadotropin dosing, donor egg decisions.
- **Relaxin:** Relaxes pelvic joints/muscles in pregnancy.

Androgens

- Testosterone (0.2–0.3 mg/day, 0.2–0.8 ng/mL), androstenedione, DHEA from ovarian stroma/adrenals.
- 80–85% bound to SHBG, 1–2% free (active, converted to DHT).
- High levels in PCOS cause anovulation, hirsutism, acne.

Menstrual Cycle

- **Duration:** ~28 days (21–35 days normal), bleeding 3–5 days, 50–200 mL blood loss.
- **Phases:**

Phases of the menstrual cycle

Cycle	Preovulation		Ovulation	Postovulation
Ovarian cycle	Follicular phase			Luteal phase
Uterine cycle	Period	Proliferative phase		Secretory phase

- **Follicular Phase (Days 1–12):**
    - FSH stimulates 5–15 primordial follicles; one dominant follicle matures.
    - Estradiol rises (50–600 μg), peaking 48 hr pre-ovulation, induces endometrial proliferation.
    - Inhibin B suppresses FSH, enhances LH surge.
- **Ovulation (Days 13–15):**
    - LH surge (>75 ng/mL, 24–36 hr prior) triggers follicular rupture, oocyte release.
    - Estradiol peak precedes LH surge; progesterone initiates 2 hr prior.
- **Luteal Phase (Days 16–28):**
    - Corpus luteum forms, secretes progesterone (15 ng/mL mid-luteal), induces secretory endometrium.
    - Progesterone inhibits LH; declining levels trigger menstruation.

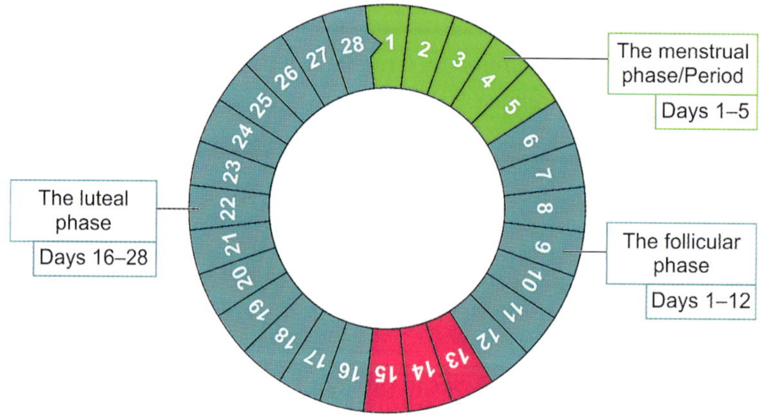

- **Endometrial Changes**

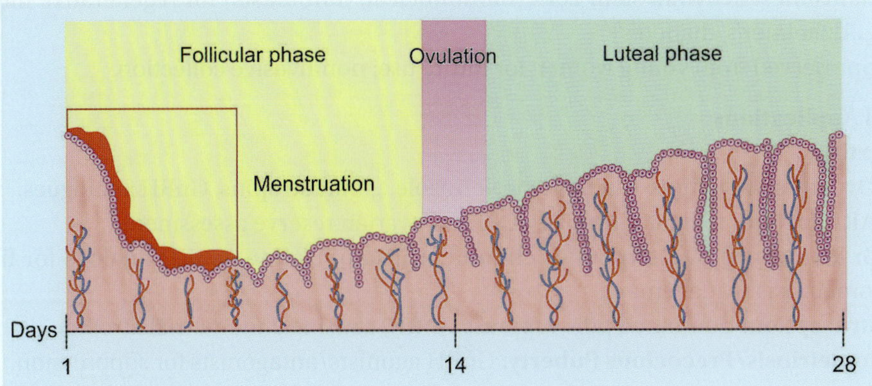

1. **Proliferative Phase:** Estrogen-driven epithelial, glandular, stromal growth; spiral arteries elongate.
2. **Secretory Phase:** Progesterone-induced glandular tortuosity, glycogen/mucus secretion.
3. **Menstruation:** Estrogen/progesterone decline causes vasoconstriction, ischemia, necrosis, and shedding of superficial endometrium.
4. **Prostaglandins:** PGE2 (vasodilatation, myocontraction), PGF2α (vasoconstriction, myocontraction) cause dysmenorrhea; PGI2 (vasodilatation) causes menorrhagia.

Feedback Mechanisms

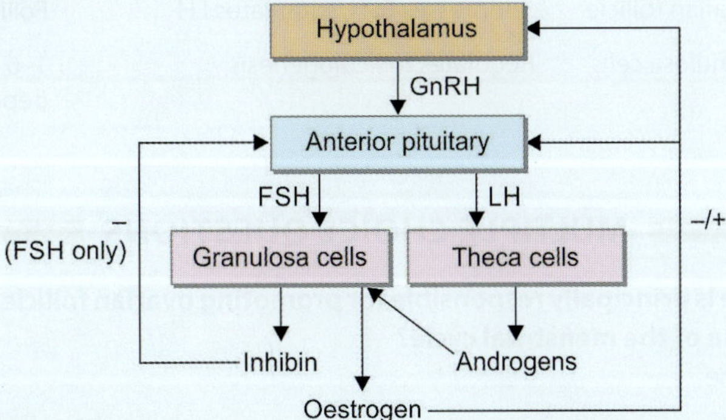

- **Long Loop:** Estrogen/progesterone feedback to hypothalamus/pituitary.
- **Short Loop:** Pituitary hormones (FSH/LH) feedback to hypothalamus.
- **Ultrashort Loop:** GnRH autoregulation within hypothalamus.

Leptin

- Adipocyte hormone stimulates GnRH at puberty, explaining earlier menarche in obesity.
- Low levels in anorexia nervosa cause amenorrhea via ↓LH.

Menstrual Fluid in Stem Cell Therapy

- Contains mesenchymal stem cells (mononuclear, fibroblasts) for regenerative medicine (e.g., Alzheimer's, diabetes).
- Cryopreserved from young women for future use; noninvasive collection.

Clinical Applications

- **Infertility:**
  - Ovulation induction: Clomiphene, letrozole, gonadotropins, GnRH analogues.
  - ART: hCG for follicular rupture, AMH for ovarian reserve assessment.
- **AUB:** Estrogen/progesterone for endometrial stabilization, GnRH analogs for fibroid/endometriosis management.
- **Contraception:** Combined pills suppress GnRH, causing endometrial atrophy.
- **Endometriosis/Precocious Puberty:** GnRH agonists/antagonists for suppression.

TABLE 2: Key hormones in menstrual cycle.

Hormone	*Source*	*Action*	*Peak*
GnRH	Hypothalamus	Stimulates FSH/LH	Pulsatile (60–180 min)
FSH	Anterior pituitary	Follicular growth, estrogen secretion	Day 7 (40 ng/mL)
LH	Anterior pituitary	Ovulation, progesterone secretion	Day 12–14 (>75 ng/mL)
Estradiol	Graafian follicle	Endometrial proliferation, LH surge	48 hr pre-ovulation (300–600 mcg)
Progesterone	Corpus luteum	Secretory endometrium, LH inhibition	Mid-luteal (15 ng/mL)
Inhibin B	Graafian follicle	Suppresses FSH, stimulates LH	Follicular phase
AMH	Granulosa cells	Regulates folliculogenesis	1–6.8 ng/mL (reproductive age)

MULTIPLE CHOICE QUESTIONS

Q1. What hormone is principally responsible for promoting ovarian follicle growth during the follicular phase of the menstrual cycle?

a. Progesterone
b. Estrogen
c. Follicle-stimulating hormone (FSH)
d. Luteinizing hormone (LH)

Ans. c. Follicle-stimulating hormone (FSH)

After the first recruitment, at the secondary follicle stage, FSH assumes responsibility for follicular development and differentiation, allowing a cohort of follicles to proceed with their differentiation. This process denotes the change from gonadotropin-independent to gonadotropin-dependent development.

Reference: Vermesh M, Kletzky OA. Longitudinal evaluation of the luteal phase and its transition into the follicular phase. J Clin Endocrinol Metab. 1987;65:653-8.

Q2. During which phase of the menstrual cycle does the endometrium reach its maximum thickness due to proliferation of glands and blood vessels?

a. Menstrual phase
b. Proliferative phase
c. Secretory phase
d. Luteal phase

Ans. b. Proliferative phase

The follicular phase of the menstrual cycle is when endometrial thickness increases, peaks before ovulation, plateaus in the early luteal phase, and finally decreases before menstruation. During the LH surge, the endometrial thickness can rise up to 12 mm.

Reference: Fleischer AC, Kalemeris GC, Entman SS. Sonographic depiction of the endometrium during normal cycles. Ultrasound Med Biol. 1986;12:271-7.

Q3. Which of the following is a characteristic of the luteal phase of the menstrual cycle?

a. Surge in LH release
b. Peak levels of estrogen
c. Increased progesterone secretion
d. Shedding of the endometrial lining

Ans. c. Increased progesterone secretion

Progesterone secretion causes eosinophilic secretory products to develop in the glandular lumen 48–72 hours after ovulation. The cellular effects of progesterone, in addition to estrogen, characterize the secretory phase of the menstrual cycle, in contrast to the proliferative period.

Reference: Ferenczy A, Bertrand G, Gelfand MM. Proliferation kinetics of human endometrium during the normal menstrual cycle. Am J Obstet Gynecol. 1979;133:859.

Q4. Which structure produces progesterone during the luteal phase of the menstrual cycle?

a. Corpus albicans
b. Corpus luteum
c. Graafian follicle
d. Theca interna cells

Ans. b. Corpus luteum

The corpus luteum, which is the main regulator of the luteal phase, emerges after ovulation from the remnant follicular shell. The structure gets its name from the yellow lutein pigment that is absorbed by the remaining membrane-bound granulosa cells in the follicle. As active secretory structures, these cells produce progesterone to keep the endometrium healthy during the luteal phase.

Reference: Anasti JN, Kalantaridou SN, Kimzey LM, et al. Human follicle fluid vascular endothelial growth factor concentrations are correlated with luteinization in spontaneously developing follicles. Hum Reprod. 1998;13:1144-7.

Q5. What is the primary function of human chorionic gonadotropin (hCG) during early pregnancy?

a. To prevent menstruation
b. To stimulate estrogen production
c. To maintain the corpus luteum
d. To induce ovulation

Ans. c. To maintain the corpus luteum

During early pregnancy, β-hCG after binding with the LH receptor on corpus luteum cells stimulate steroid hormone synthesis. Before placenta attains its full capability, the corpus luteum regulates the hormone synthesis which is critical for maintenance of pregnancy.

Reference: Zee J, Sammel MD, Chung K, et al. Ectopic pregnancy prediction in women with a pregnancy of unknown location: data beyond 48 h are necessary. Hum Reprod. 2014;29(3):441-7.

Q6. Which of the following accurately describes the role of prostaglandins in menstruation?

a. They cause vasoconstriction, reducing menstrual flow.
b. They promote the shedding of the endometrial lining.
c. They inhibit follicle growth during the menstrual cycle.
d. They stimulate progesterone production.

Ans. b. They promote the shedding of the endometrial lining.

A potent vasoconstrictor that can cause both arterial vasospasm and endometrial ischemia is prostaglandin F2α (PGF2α). Myometrial contractions caused by PGF2α may aid in the removal of sloughing endometrial tissue from the uterus and decrease the local blood supply to the uterine wall.

Reference: Kilic S, Yuksel B, Pinarli F, et al. Effect of stem cell application on Asherman syndrome, an experimental rat model. J Assist Reprod Genet. 2014;31:975-82.

Q7. In the absence of fertilization, which hormone levels decline, leading to the shedding of the endometrial lining?

a. Estrogen and progesterone
b. Luteinizing hormone (LH)
c. Human chorionic gonadotropin (hCG)
d. Follicle-stimulating hormone (FSH)

Ans. a. Estrogen and progesterone

The shedding is thought to be caused by the loss of the corpus luteum, which produces progesterone and estrogen. Endometrial ischemia is the result of a severe spiral artery vascular spasm that occurs after levels of steroidal hormones decline.

Reference: Kilic S, Yuksel B, Pinarli F, et al. Effect of stem cell application on Ashermansyndrome, an experimental rat model. J Assist Reprod Genet. 2014;31:975-82.

Q8. When does progesterone hormone synthesis begin during a normal menstrual cycle?

a. At the time of ovulation
b. 36 hours before ovulation
c. During early luteal phase
d. During late luteal phase

Ans. b. 36 hours before ovulation

The luteinized granulosa cells start producing a small amount of progesterone which is responsible for the FSH level surge and maintenance of LH surge

Reference: McNatty KP, Makris A, DeGrazia C, et al. The production of progesterone, androgens, and estrogens by granulosa cells, thecal tissue, and stromal tissue from human ovaries in vitro. J Clin Endocrinol Metab. 1979;49(5):687-99.

Q9. When does progesterone levels reach its peak during a menstrual cycle?

a. At the time of ovulation
b. Day 22 of menstrual cycle
c. Day 20 of menstrual cycle
d. 6 or 7 days after ovulation

Ans. d. 6 or 7 days after ovulation

By postovulatory day 6 or 7, the endometrium is most primed for blastocyst implantation and glandular secretory activity is typically at its peak.

Reference: Kilic S, Yuksel B, Pinarli F, et al. Effect of stem cell application on Asherman syndrome, an experimental rat model. J Assist Reprod Genet. 2014;31:975-82.

Q10. Which of the following is the correct hormonal status just before ovulation ?

a. High LH, high FSH
b. Low LH, high FSH
c. Low LH, low FSH
d. High LH, low FSH

Ans. a. High LH, high FSH

High estrogen levels of around 200 pg/mL for at least 48 hours are needed to initiate LH surge. The luteinized granulosa cells start producing a small amount of progesterone which is responsible for the FSH level surge and maintenance of LH surge. The FSH surge occurs in accordance with LH surge prior to ovulation.

Reference: Lemarchand-Béraud T, Zufferey MM, Reymond M, ct al. Maturation of the hypothalamo-pituitary-ovarian axis in adolescent girls. J Clin Endocrinol Metab. 1982;54(2):241-6.

LONG QUESTIONS

1. **Describe stages of follicular development during a normal menstrual cycle.**
(MS Obstetrics and Gynecology, 2010)

2. **Describe the phases of a normal menstrual cycle.**
(MS Obstetrics and Gynecology, 2019)

SHORT QUESTIONS

1. **Physiology of ovulation.** *(MS Obstetrics and Gynecology, 2017, 2022)*
2. **Two-cell two-gonadotropin theory of ovarian steroidogenesis.**
(MS Obstetrics and Gynecology, 2017)
3. **Explain the histologic alterations that occur in the endometrium at the various stages of the menstrual cycle.** *(MS Obstetrics and Gynecology, 2017)*
4. **Explain the changes in hormones that take place during a typical menstrual cycle.**
(MS Obstetrics and Gynecology, 20 Answers)

LONG ANSWERS

1. Follicular development, also known as folliculogenesis, refers to monthly recruitment of cohort of follicles, from which a single dominant follicle matures and is destined for ovulation.

The follicular development progresses through different stages **(Fig. 2)**:

- A. Preantral follicular stage includes:
  - i. Primordial follicles
  - ii. Primary follicles
  - iii. Secondary follicles
- Antral follicular stage includes:
  - i. Tertiary follicles

ii. Preovulatory or Graafian follicles

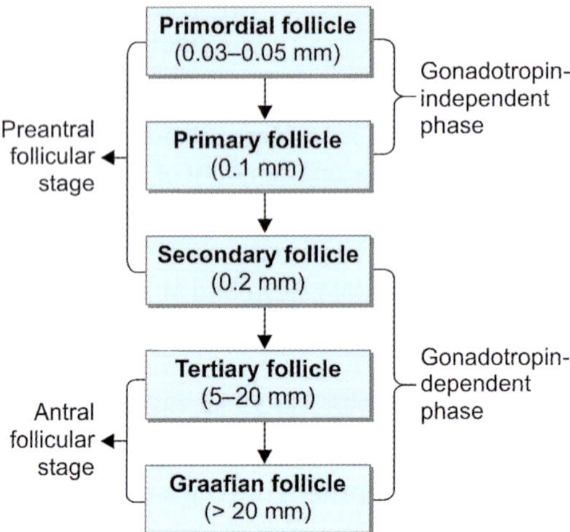

Fig. 2: Stages of follicular development.

A. Preantral Follicular Stage

i. *Primordial follicles:* These follicles have a single layer of flat epithelium -lined granulosa cells surrounding the primary oocyte which is arrested in meiosis I.[1] Their size ranges from 0.03 to 0.05 mm. Maintenance of constant numbers of primordial follicles ensures oocyte supply throughout reproductive years[2] **(Fig. 3)**.

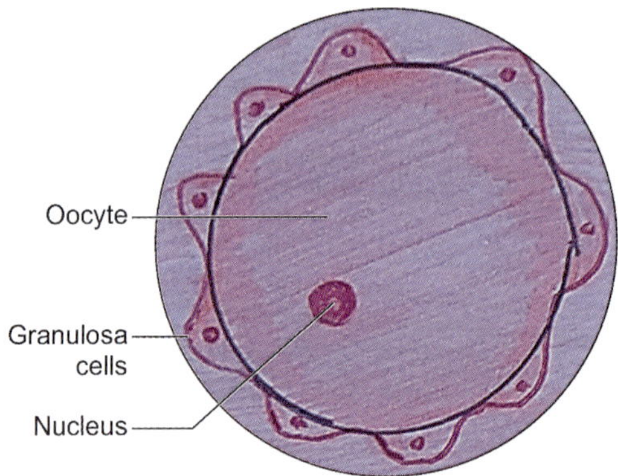

Fig. 3: Primordial follicle.

ii. *Primary follicles:* These follicles contain cuboidal epithelium-lined granulosa cells, which increase in number producing pseudostratification. The granulosa cells secrete protein-rich materials that form an extracellular capsule around the primary oocyte known as ZONA PELLUCIDA.[3] Intercellular gap junction forms between the granulosa cells and between granulosa cells and oocyte.[4] They are 0.1 mm in size. The granulosa cells express FSH receptors but there is no vascularization; hence, no endocrine effect is seen **(Fig. 4)**.

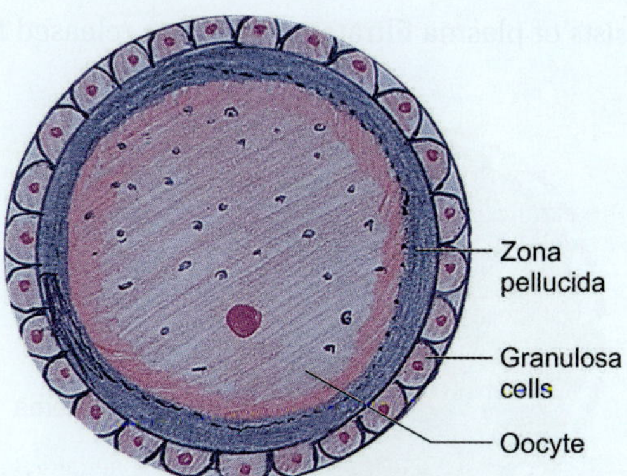

Fig. 4: Primary follicle.

Both primordial follicle and primary follicle stages are gonadotropin-independent stages of follicular development.

iii. *Secondary follicles:* Their size measures about 0.2 mm. The cuboidal granulosa cells become multilayered and the surrounding stromal cells differentiate to form theca cells. The granulosa cells express FSH receptors and theca cells express LH receptors along with neoangiogenesis. It is from this stage that gonadotropin dependency begins along with endocrine effect[1] **(Fig. 5)**.

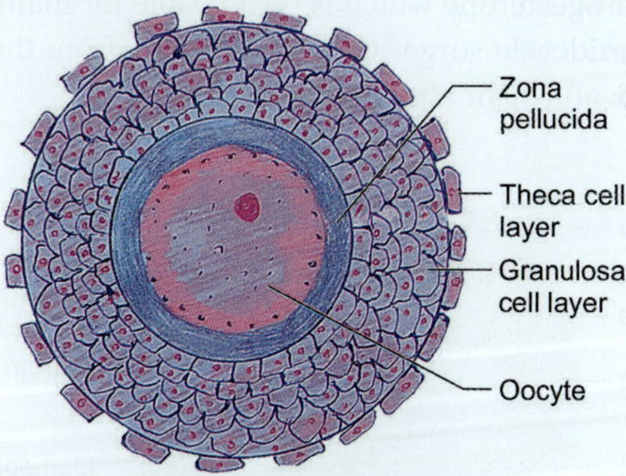

Fig. 5: Secondary follicle.

B. Antral Follicular Stage

i. *Tertiary follicles:* These follicles are characterized by formation of a fluid-filled cavity known as antral cavity. They are of two types: (1) Early tertiary follicles and (2) late tertiary follicles.

Early tertiary follicles size ranges from 0.5 to 5 mm. The theca cell layer differentiates into theca interna and theca externa.[5]

Late tertiary follicles ranges in size from 10 to 20 mm. The antral cavity functionally and histologically divides the granulosa cells into two groups. The granulosa cells which surround the oocyte are known as **cumulus oophorus** and granulosa cells which are surrounding the antral cavity form the mural granulosa or membrana granulosa . The antral cavity consists of plasma filtrates and factors released from the granulosa cells[6] **(Fig. 6)**.

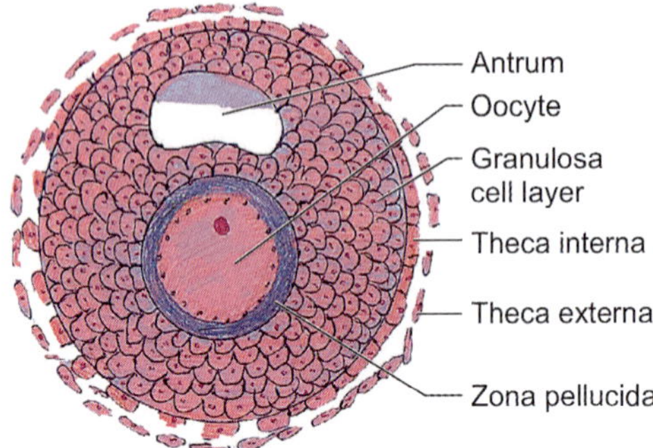

Fig. 6: Tertiary follicle.

ii. *Preovulatory follicles or graafian follicles:* The development of follicles ends at this point. It is roughly 20 mm in size. In this stage, the primary oocyte completes its first meiotic division, forms the secondary oocyte, and extrudes the first polar body just prior to ovulation.[1]

The granulosa cells release high amounts of estrogen, which will cause the LH surge to begin.[7] The elevated LH levels will lead to luteinization of granulosa cells leading to production of progesterone which is responsible for maintenance of LH surge and initiation of FSH midcycle surge.[8] Ovulation occurs from the mature graafian follicle 12 hr after LH peak and 36 hr after LH surge[9] **(Fig. 7)**.

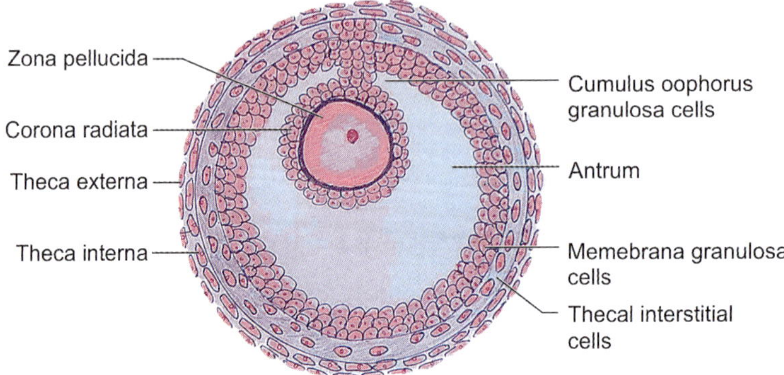

Fig. 7: Graafian follicle.

2. The reproductive system of women differs from that of men in that it regularly undergoes cyclic changes that, from a teleological standpoint, could be viewed as a periodic preparation for conception and pregnancy.[10]

Menstruation, or the shedding of uterine mucosa, is the most noticeable aspect of the menstrual cycle in humans and primates. This bleeding occurs periodically in the vagina.[11]

The average menstrual cycle lasts 28 +/– 7 days, with a menstrual flow lasting 4 +/– 2 days and a blood loss of approximately 20-60 mL.[12] It usually begins when a person is between the ages of 10 and 16 years and ends around the time they reach menopause, which is approximately 51 years.

It is divided in 4 phases:

1. Phase of menstruation
2. Proliferative phase
3. Phase of ovulation
4. Secretory phase

1. *Phase of menstruation:* With the declining levels of hormones at the end of secretory phase, the decidua functionalis of endometrium sheds off by a proccss known as menstruation.

    The menstrual cycle's first 5 days are dedicated to menstruation. During a menstrual cycle, only 25% of the blood is venous; the bulk of the blood is arterial. It contains a substantial amount of prostaglandins, tissue fragments, and fibrinolysin derived from uterine tissue.

    Because fibrinolysin lyses clots, menstrual blood often does not include clots until the flow is substantial. In healthy females, the average monthly blood loss ranges from 5 to 80 mL.

2. *Proliferative phase:* This phase begins after menstruation and lasts from day 6 to day 14 of menstrual cycle during which there is progressive mitotic growth of the decidua functionalis.

    Variations in the length of the follicular phase are the cause of the variability in the menstrual cycle duration. In this phase, estrogen is the primary hormone. During this phase, the endometrial glands become more tortuous. The endometrial thickness reaches up to 12 mm.[13]

3. *Phase of ovulation:* On day 14 of a typical 28-day cycle, or 14 days before menstruation, ovulation takes place. At the end of the proliferative cycle, follicular maturation and increased hormone synthesis result in high estrogen levels.

    Estrogen boosts both FSH and LH when it reaches a critical level of at least 200 pg/mL of plasma. The high levels of LH that happen during this time are known as the LH surge. As a result, the mature follicle divides, releasing an oocyte following the increase in LH.

    The concentration of both prostaglandins and proteolytic enzyme in the follicular wall are dramatically elevated by the midcycle LH surge.[14] These chemicals cause the follicular wall to gradually deteriorate, which eventually leads to the perforation of the wall and the development of the stigma, a superficial follicular protrusion that resembles a bleb.

    Ovulation is most likely characterized by the steady extrusion of the egg through this follicle gap, rather than a rupture of the follicular structure.[15] Despite the direct measurement of intrafollicular pressures, no explosive event was detected.

4. *Secretory phase:* In every cycle, this phase lasts from day 14 to day 28. The major hormone at this stage is progesterone, which also prepares the endometrium for possible implantation of fertilized eggs and maintains the corpus luteum.

    Eight days following ovulation is when progesterone levels peak. FSH and LH levels will decrease as a result of the anterior pituitary's negative feedback impact.

    During this phase, glycogen-rich subnuclear vacuoles appear which move from the base toward the lumen and the secretion process reaches its peak by postovulatory day 6.

SHORT ANSWERS

1. *Physiology of ovulation:* The ovary's dominant follicle bursts during ovulation, a physiological event. An egg is discharged into the abdominal cavity as a result. After then, it is absorbed by the fallopian tube's fimbriae, where it may fertilize.[16]

   High estrogen levels of around 200 pg/mL for at least 48 hours are needed to initiate LH surge.[7] The luteinized granulosa cells start producing a small amount of progesterone which is responsible for the FSH level surge and maintenance of LH surge.[17]

   The LH surge promotes the growth of cumulus cells, luteinization of granulosa cells, prostaglandin synthesis, and the restart of meiosis 1 in oocytes. 36–40 hours after the peak of LH, ovulation takes place.[18]

   The cumulus oophorus cells, or granulosa cells that surround the oocytes, do not express LH receptors; instead, they create tight connections with the oocytes, giving them a rough surface and a big size that aid in ovum pick by the fimbria.

   Collagenase and plasmin, which promote follicular wall weakening, are present in the antral follicular fluid.[19] Theca and granulosa cells will produce more tissue plasminogen activator in response to the gonadotropin surge.[20]

   Prostaglandins' production also reach a peak in the follicular fluid which are responsible for smooth muscle contraction of ovary and hence helps in ovulation.[15]

   After then, the follicular wall gradually deteriorates, leading to the wall's rupture and the development of the stigma—a superficial, bleb-like follicular protrusion.

   Instead of the follicular structure rupturing, ovulation is most likely defined by the egg's gradual ejection through the follicle gap. No explosive event was found, despite the intrafollicular pressures being directly measured.[15]

2. *Two-gonadotropin, two-cell theory:* The fundamental idea behind follicular development is the two-cell, two-gonadotropin theory.[21,22] This theory proposes that the synthesis of steroid hormones in growing follicles is compartmentalized and segregated. The majority of aromatase activity, which produces estrogen, is found in granulosa cells.[23]

   FSH stimulates some receptors on these cells, increasing aromatase activity.[24,25] Granulosa cells need androgens as a substrate for aromatization, but they lack a number of enzymes that are involved earlier in the steroidogenic process. The majority of LH receptors is present in the theca cells at this stage, and androgens are largely produced in response to stimulation by LH.[24,25]

   There is a synergistic relationship between theca cells and granulosa cells: Theca cells produce androgens (mostly androstenedione) in response to LH stimulation. These androgens are subsequently transported to granulosa cells where they undergo FSH-stimulated aromatization into estrogens. The follicle's environment is made favorable for ongoing growth and nourishment by these locally generated estrogens.[26]

   FSH and local estrogens also promote the synthesis and expression of FSH receptors, the proliferation and differentiation of granulosa cells, and the synthesis of estrogen. Androgens have two positive regulatory roles in follicular development. Androgens stimulate the growth of granulosa cells and their aromatase activity within the ovary.[27] The pituitary's release of gonadotropin is negatively impacted by an increase in peripheral estrogen levels.[28] At this point, increasing ovarian production of inhibin B further reduces FSH output.

A risk to the survival of follicular development arises from the decrease in FSH levels that occurs during the follicular phase. Follicles that possess an advantage in binding the decreasing FSH molecules, or those with an abundance of FSH receptors, are the only ones that can endure the ensuing adverse conditions.

The dominant follicle is therefore the one with the highest number of FSH receptors and the most estrogenic microenvironment.[29] FSH receptors increase in proportion to the population of granulosa cells since each one has a fixed and comparable amount of FSH receptors.[8,30]

The follicle continues to produce estrogen as it grows and develops, which lowers the amount of FSH in the blood and makes the environment more unfavorable for follicles that are in competition with it. This process keeps going until every member of the original cohort has developed atresia, except for the one dominant follicle.

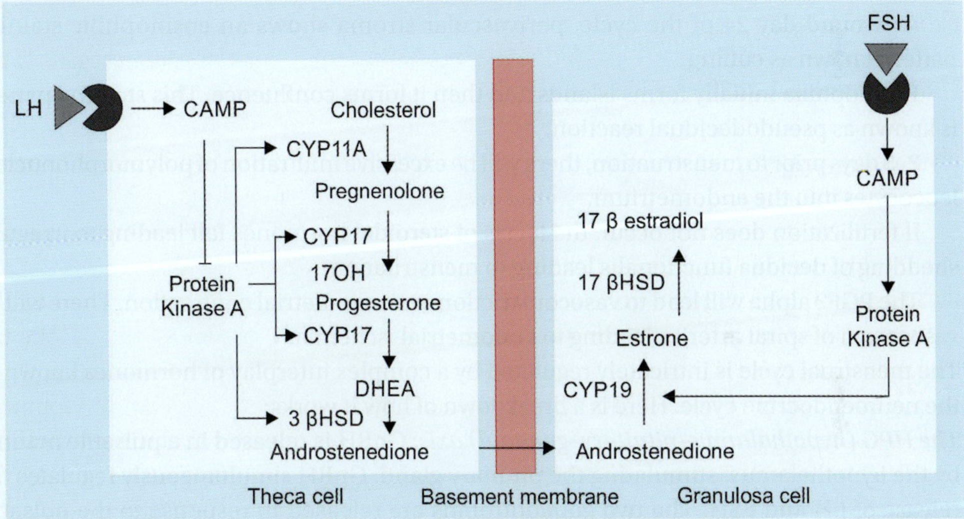

Two-cell, two-gonadotropin theory.

3. The histological changes seen in the different phases of menstruation are as follows:
Proliferative Phase: The decidua basalis is composed of primordial glands and thick, sparse stroma following the menstrual cycle. The decidua functionalis gradually develops into a mitotic spindle during the proliferative phase in response to rising levels of circulating estrogen, readying the embryo for implantation.[31]

When the proliferative phase begins, the endometrium is thin (1–2 mm). The primary change seen during this time is the endometrial glands' development into longer, twisted structures from their initial forms, which were straight, thin, and short[32]

The low columnar pattern of the lining epithelium of proliferating glands gives way to a pseudostratified appearance. During this time, the stroma stays dense and compact, and no apparent vascular structures are present.

Secretory Phase: On day 14, in a normal 28-day cycle, ovulation takes place 48–72 hours after ovulation progesterone secretion leads to appearance of eosinophilic secretory products within the glandular lumen. The cellular effects of progesterone, in addition to estrogen, characterize the secretory phase of the menstrual cycle, in contrast to the proliferative period.

The action of progesterone is antagonistic to estrogen and there is a gradual decrease in estrogen receptor concentration.[31]

There is a characteristic appearance of PAS-positive glycogen containing vacuoles.

Initially, the vacuoles appear in a subnuclear location which gradually move upward and gets secreted in an apocrine manner into glandular lumen.[33]

At around day 19 or 20 of cycle, the secretory activity reaches its peak which makes the endometrium ready for implantation.

The stroma initially remained unchanged but in the later phase at around the 7th postovulatory day, there is stromal edema.

During maximal stromal edema, the spiral arteries become clearly visible, which gradually lengthens and coils.

At around day 24 of the cycle, perivascular stroma shows an eosinophilic staining pattern known as cuffing.

Eosinophilia initially forms islands and then it forms confluence. This staining pattern is known as pseudodecidual reaction.

2–3 days prior to menstruation, there will be excessive infiltration of polymorphonuclear leucocytes into the endometrium.

If fertilization does not occur, the levels of steroidal hormones fall leading to irregular shedding of decidua functionalis leading to menstruation.

The PGF2 alpha will lead to vasoconstriction and myometrial contraction. There will be vasospasm of spiral arteries leading to endometrial ischemia.[34]

4. The menstrual cycle is intricately regulated by a complex interplay of hormones known as the neuroendocrine cycle. Here is a breakdown of how it works:
   The HPG (hypothalamus-pituitary-gonadal) axis: GnRH is released in a pulsatile manner by the hypothalamus, stimulating the pituitary gland. GnRH simultaneously regulates the release of LH and FSH. The two gonadotropins are released in response to the pulsatile release of GnRH, which makes it unique from other hormones in the body in that it requires pulsatile secretion to function.[35]

   GnRH secretion occurs in small amplitude, frequent pulses during the follicular phase. The frequency and amplitude of pulses increase in the late follicular phase. On the other hand, the time interval between pulses gradually lengthens during the luteal phase. Throughout the menstrual cycle, variations in LH and FSH are made possible by this fluctuation in pulse frequency of GnRH.[36]

   Pituitary gland: In response to GnRH, there is secretion of two key hormones:
   - *Follicle stimulating hormone:* It stimulates the growth of ovarian follicles in the ovary.
   - *Luteinizing hormone:* It causes the mature follicle to release an egg during ovulation and stimulates production of progesterone by the corpus luteum.

   Ovarian cycle:
   - *Follicular phase:* A cohort of developing follicles is recruited and during the early follicular phase FSH levels rise. As these follicles develop during the follicular period, they individually secrete progressively more estrogen.

Pituitary FSH secretion is negatively impacted by rising estrogen levels and by the middle of the follicular phase, it starts to decline. Furthermore, the developing follicles secrete inhibin B, which prevents the pituitary from secreting FSH.

Ovulation: On the other hand, LH first decreases in response to rising estradiol levels; however, a significant LH surge happens toward the end of the follicular phase (biphasic response).[14] The LH surge helps in resumption of meiosis 1 of oocytes, expansion of cumulus cells, luteinization of granulosa cells, and synthesis of prostaglandins. The ovulation occurs 36–40 after the LH surge.[18]

Luteal Phase: This is the luteal-secretory phase, which begins after ovulation.

During the early luteal phase, there is a fall in the estrogen levels, which is responsible for midcycle spotting.[37] After ovulation, follicle transforms into corpus luteum which produces progesterone, inhibin A, and estrogen.

Progesterone levels can be utilized as an indicator that ovulation has likely happened because they rise sharply following ovulation.

Gonadotropin release and the development of new follicles are centrally suppressed by progesterone, estrogen, and inhibin A. There is negative feedback effect by the steroidal hormones over the pituitary and hypothalamus. These steroidal hormones are raised during the corpus luteum's life and become lower when it dies, thus preparing the body for the next cycle.

Progesterone maintains the endometrium for potential implantation. If fertilization does not occur, the corpus luteum degenerates, leading to decreased progesterone and estrogen levels, which ultimately lead to onset of menses.

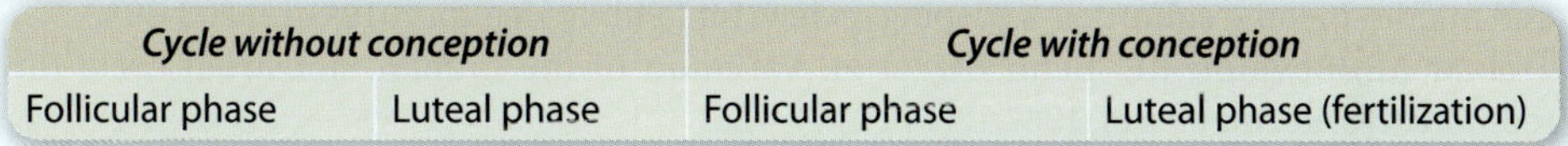

Cycle without conception		Cycle with conception	
Follicular phase	Luteal phase	Follicular phase	Luteal phase (fertilization)

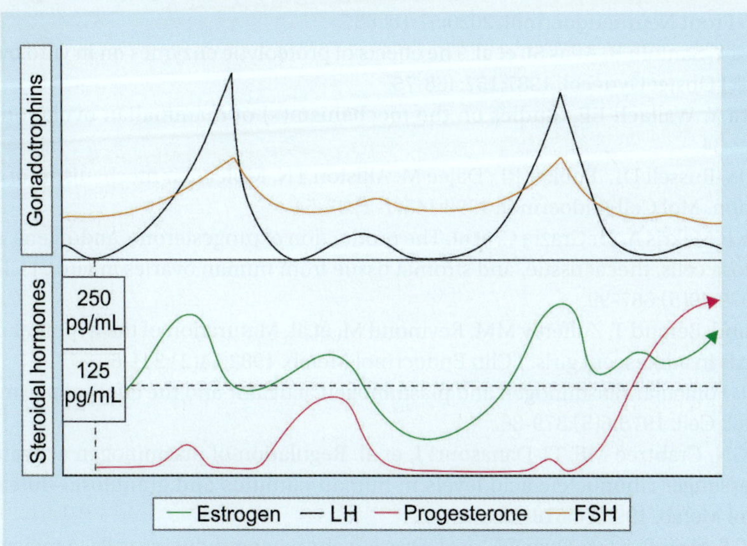

Hormonal changes during menstruation.

REFERENCES

1. Berek JS, Novak E. Physiology of menstruation. In: Berek JS (Ed). Berek and Novak's Gynecology, 16th edition. Philadelphia: Lippincott Williams & Wilkins; 2022.
2. Kim JY. Control of ovarian primordial follicle activation. Clin Exp Reprod Med. 2012;39(1):10-4.
3. Gupta SK. Role of zona pellucida glycoproteins during fertilization in humans. J Reprod Immunol. 2015;108:90-7.
4. Albertini DF, Anderson E. The appearance and structure of intercellular connections during the ontogeny of the rabbit ovarian follicle with particular reference to gap junctions. J Cell Biol. 1974;63(1):234-50.
5. Eppig JJ. A comparison between oocyte growth in coculture with granulosa cells and oocytes with granulosa cell-oocyte junctional contact maintained in vitro. J Exp Zool. 1979;209(2):345-53.
6. Asimakopoulos B, Köster F, Felberbaum R, et al. Cytokine and hormonal profile in blood serum and follicular fluids during ovarian stimulation with the multidose antagonist or the long agonist protocol. Hum Reprod. 2006;21(12):3091-5.
7. Young SR, Jaffe RB. Strength-duration characteristics of estrogen effects on gonadotropin response to gonadotropin-releasing hormone in women: II. Effects of varying concentrations of estradiol. J Clin Endocrinol Metab. 1976;42:432-42.
8. Reed BG, Carr BR. The normal menstrual cycle and the control of ovulation. [Updated 2015 May 22]. In: De Groot LJ, Chrousos G, Dungan K, et al. (Eds). Endotext [Internet]. South Dartmouth, MA:
9. Pauerstein CJ, Eddy CA, Croxatto HD, et al. Temporal relationship of estrogen, progesterone, luteinizing hormone levels to ovulation in women and infra-human primates. Am J Obstet Gynecol. 1978;130:876-86.
10. Rosner J, Samardzic T, Sarao MS. Physiology, Female Reproduction. StatPearls [Internet]. Treasure Island (FL): StatPearls Publishing; 2022.
11. Coast E, Lattof SR, Strong J. Puberty and menstruation knowledge among young adolescents in low- and middle-income countries: a scoping review. Int J Public Health. 2019;64(2):293-304.
12. Treloar AE, Boynton RE, Behn BG, et al. Variation of the human menstrual cycle through reproductive life. Int J Fertil. 1967;12(1 Pt 2):77-126.
13. Herbison AE. A simple model of estrous cycle negative and positive feedback regulation of GnRH secretion. Front Neuroendocrinol. 2020;57:100837.
14. Yoshimura Y, Santulli R, Atlas SJ, et al. The effects of proteolytic enzymes on in vitro ovulation in the rabbit. Am J Obstet Gynecol. 1987;157:468-75.
15. Yoshimura Y, Wallach EE. Studies on the mechanism(s) of mammalian ovulation. Fertil Steril. 1987;47:22-34.
16. Richards JS, Russell DL, Robker RL, Dajee M, Alliston TN. Molecular mechanisms of ovulation and luteinization. Mol Cell Endocrinol. 1998;145(1-2):47-54.
17. McNatty KP, Makris A, DeGrazia C, et al. The production of progesterone, androgens, and estrogens by granulosa cells, thecal tissue, and stromal tissue from human ovaries in vitro. J Clin Endocrinol Metab. 1979;49(5):687-99.
18. Lemarchand-Béraud T, Zufferey MM, Reymond M, et al. Maturation of the hypothalamo-pituitary-ovarian axis in adolescent girls. J Clin Endocrinol Metab. 1982;54(2):241-6.
19. Beers WH. Follicular plasminogen and plasminogen activator and the effect of plasmin on ovarian follicle wall. Cell. 1975;6(3):379-86.
20. Piquette GN, Crabtree ME, El-Danasouri I, et al. Regulation of plasminogen activator inhibitor-1 and-2 messenger ribonucleic acid levels in human cumulus and granulosa—luteal cells. J Clin Endocrinol Metab. 1993;76:518-52.
21. Erickson GF, Magoffin DA, Dyer CA, et al. Ovarian androgen producing cells: A review of structure/function relationships. Endocr Rev. 1985;6:371-99.

22. Erickson GF. An analysis of follicle development and ovum maturation. Semin Reprod Endocrinol. 1986;46:55-9.
23. Ryan KJ, Petro Z. Steroid biosynthesis of human ovarian granulosa and thecal cells. J Clin Endocrinol Metab. 1966;26:46-52.
24. Kobayashi M, Nakano R, Ooshima A. Immunohistochemical localization of pituitary gonadotropin and gonadal steroids confirms the two cells two gonadotropins hypothesis of steroidogenesis in the human ovary. J Endocrinol. 1990;126:483-8.
25. Yamoto M, Shima K, Nakano R. Gonadotropin receptors in human ovarian follicles and corpora lutea throughout the menstrual cycle. Horm Res. 1992;37(Suppl 1):5-11.
26. Hseuh AJ, Adashi EY, Jones PB, et al. Hormonal regulation of the differentiation of cultured ovarian granulosa cells. Endocr Rev. 1984;5:76-127.
27. Weil SJ, Vendola K, Zhou J, et al. Androgen receptor gene expression in the primate ovary: Cellular localization, regulation, and functional correlations. J Clin Endocrinol Metab. 1998;83:2479-85.
28. Chappel SC, Resko JA, Norman RL, et al. Studies on rhesus monkeys on the site where estrogen inhibits gonadotropins: Delivery of 17 β-estradiol to the hypothalamus and pituitary gland. J Clin Endocrinol Metab. 1981;52:1-8.
29. Chabab A, Hedon B, Arnal F, et al. Follicular steroids in relation to oocyte development in human ovarian stimulation protocols. Hum Reprod. 1986;1:449-54.
30. Amsterdam A, Rotmensch S. Structure-function relationships during granulosa cell differentiation. Endocr Rev. 1987;8(3):309-37.
31. Kilic S, Yuksel B, Pinarli F, et al. Effect of stem cell application on Asherman syndrome, an experimental rat model. J Assist Reprod Genet. 2014;31:975-82.
32. Ferenczy A, Bertrand G, Gelfand MM. Proliferation kinetics of human endometrium during the normal menstrual cycle. Am J Obstet Gynecol. 1979;133:859-67.
33. Schwarz BE. The production and biologic effects of uterine prostaglandins. Semin Reprod Endocrinol. 1983;1:189.
34. Noyes RW, Hertig AW, Rock J. Dating the endometrial biopsy. Fertil Steril. 1950;1:3-25.
35. Belchetz PE, Plant TM, Nakai Y, et al. Hypophyseal responses to continuous and 315 intermittent delivery of hypothalamic gonadotropin-releasing hormone. Science. 1978;202:631-3.
36. Yu B, Ruman J, Christman G. The role of peripheral gonadotropin-releasing hormone receptors in female reproduction. Fertil Steril. 2011;95:465-73.
37. Hoff JD, Quigley ME, Yen SS. Hormonal dynamics at midcycle: a reevaluation. J Clin Endocrinol Metab. 1983;57(4):792-6.

Anatomy and Physiology of Female Genital Tract

Ruchika Garg, Shaifali Singh

EXTERNAL GENITALIA (VULVA/PUDENDUM)

The vulva encompasses all visible external genital structures in the perineum, bounded anteriorly by the mons pubis, posteriorly by the rectum, and laterally by genitocrural folds. It is covered by keratinized stratified squamous epithelium.[1]

Components

- **Mons Pubis:** A subcutaneous adipose pad anterior to the pubis, covered with hair in adults (triangular escutcheon, base upward).
- **Labia Majora:** Paired skin folds with subcutaneous fat, pigmented externally with hair, and thin, hairless internally with sebaceous glands. Homologous to the male scrotum; supplied by venous plexuses prone to hematoma during childbirth.
- **Labia Minora:** Thin, fat-free skin folds within labia majora, dividing anteriorly to form the clitoral prepuce/frenulum and fusing posteriorly as the fourchette. Contain erectile tissue, vessels, and nerves; homologous to the penile urethra/skin.
- **Clitoris:** A 1.5–2 cm erectile structure with glans, body, and crura, attached to the symphysis pubis by the suspensory ligament. Richly innervated; homologous to the penis but separate from the urethra.
- **Vestibule:** A triangular space between the clitoris, fourchette, and labia minora, containing:
- **Urethral opening:** 1–1.5 cm below the pubic arch, with paraurethral (Skene's) ducts.
- **Vaginal orifice/hymen:** Partially closed by the hymen (crescentic in virgins, ruptured post-coitus/childbirth, forming carunculae myrtiformes).
- **Bartholin's ducts:** Open lateral to the hymen, secreting alkaline mucus during arousal; glands (pea-sized) lie in the superficial perineal pouch.
- **Skene's glands:** Largest paraurethral glands, homologous to the male prostate.

TABLE 1: Homology of external genitalia.

Female structure	*Male homologue*
Labia majora	Scrotum
Labia minora	Penile urethra/skin
Clitoris	Penis
Bartholin's glands	Bulbourethral glands
Skene's glands	Prostate
Vestibular bulbs	Corpus spongiosum

- **Vestibular Bulbs:** Bilateral erectile tissue masses beneath the vestibule, prone to hemorrhage during childbirth; homologous to the male corpus spongiosum.
- **Perineum:** Supports pelvic structures; detailed anatomy covered separately.

Blood Supply

- **Arteries:** Internal pudendal (labial, clitoral, vestibular bulb) and femoral (external pudendal).
- **Veins:** Drain to internal pudendal, vesical/vaginal plexuses, and long saphenous veins; varicosities common in pregnancy.

Lymphatics: Drain bilaterally to superficial inguinal, Cloquet's, and iliac nodes.

Nerve Supply

- *Anterosuperior:* Ilioinguinal, genitofemoral (L1, L2).
- *Posteroinferior:* Pudendal, posterior cutaneous nerve of thigh (S1–S4).

Development: Derived from ectodermal cloacal fossa (clitoris from genital tubercle, labia minora from genital folds, labia majora from labioscrotal swellings, vestibule from urogenital sinus).[2]

INTERNAL GENITALIA

The internal genitalia include the vagina, uterus, fallopian tubes, and ovaries, located within the pelvis and accessible via specialized instruments.[1]

Vagina

A fibromusculomembranous canal (7–9 cm) connecting the uterus to the vulva, serving as the excretory channel for menstrual blood, organ of copulation, and birth canal. It forms a 45° angle with the horizontal, parallel to the pelvic inlet.

Structure

- **Walls:** Anterior (7 cm), posterior (9 cm), and lateral; H-shaped in cross-section due to stiffer lateral walls.
- **Fornices:** Four vaginal vault clefts (anterior, posterior, two lateral) around the cervix; posterior fornix deepest.
- **Layers:**
  - *Mucosa:* Stratified squamous epithelium, acidic pH (4–5) due to Döderlein's bacilli producing lactic acid from glycogen.
  - *Submucosa:* Loose vascular tissue.
  - *Muscularis:* Inner circular, outer longitudinal smooth muscle.
  - *Fibrous coat:* Vascular endopelvic fascia.

Relations

- **Anterior:** Bladder (upper third), urethra (lower two-thirds).
- **Posterior:** Pouch of Douglas (upper third), rectum (middle third), anal canal/perineal body (lower third).
- **Lateral:** Pelvic cellular tissue/ureter/uterine artery (upper third), levator ani (middle third), bulbocavernosus/Bartholin's glands (lower third).

Blood Supply

- **Arteries:** Cervicovaginal (uterine), vaginal (internal iliac), middle rectal, internal pudendal; form anterior/posterior azygos arteries.
- **Veins:** Drain to internal iliac and pudendal veins.

Lymphatics

- Upper third: Internal iliac nodes.
- Middle third (to hymen): Internal iliac nodes.
- Below hymen: Superficial inguinal nodes.

Nerve Supply: Pelvic plexus (sympathetic/parasympathetic); lower part by pudendal nerve.

Development: Upper four-fifths (mucosa from sinovaginal bulbs, musculature from Müllerian ducts); lower one-fifth (urogenital sinus); orifice from genital fold ectoderm.[2]

Uterus

A hollow, pyriform muscular organ (8 cm long, 5 cm wide, 1.25 cm thick, 50–80 g) between the bladder and rectum, normally anteverted and anteflexed with dextrorotation.

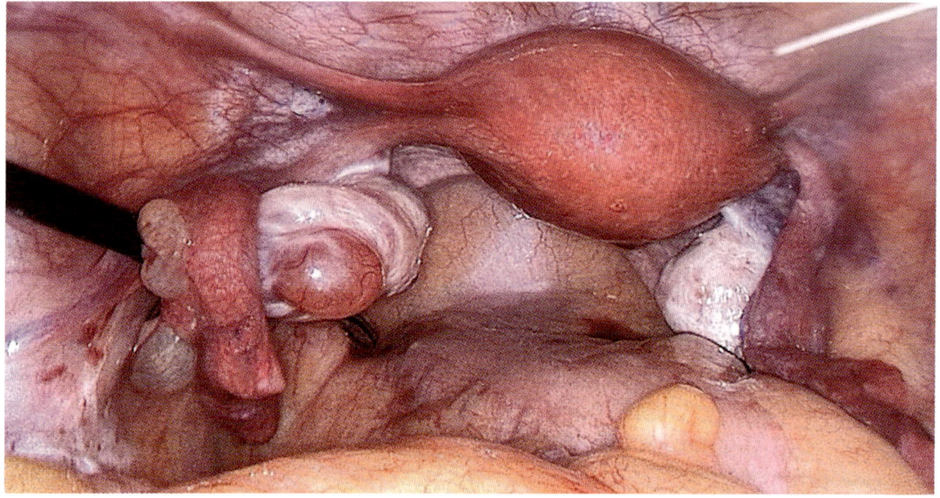

Figure showing uterus, ovary and epooophoron in fallopian tube.

Parts

- **Body/Corpus:** Includes fundus (above tubal openings) and body proper (triangular cavity, 3.5 cm).
- **Isthmus:** Constricted region (0.5 cm) between body and cervix.
- **Cervix:** Cylindrical (2.5 cm), with supravaginal and vaginal parts; cervical canal fusiform (2.5 cm).
  Cavity: Uterine cavity (6.5–7 cm) is triangular; cervical canal opens at external os.

Relations

- **Anterior:** Uterovesical pouch (above internal os), bladder (below internal os).

- **Posterior:** Pouch of Douglas (coils of intestine).
- **Lateral:** Broad ligament, Mackenrodt's ligament, uterine artery/ureter crossing.

Structure

- **Perimetrium:** Serosa (except lateral borders), adherent to myometrium.
- **Myometrium:** Smooth muscle (outer longitudinal, middle interlacing, inner circular during pregnancy).
- **Endometrium:** Ciliated columnar epithelium, stromal cells, tubular glands; transforms to decidua in pregnancy.
- **Cervix:** Fibrous connective tissue (10–15% smooth muscle); endocervix lined by columnar epithelium, vaginal cervix by stratified squamous epithelium.

Blood Supply

- **Arteries:** Uterine (internal iliac), ovarian, vaginal; extensive anastomosis. The blood supply is primarily derived from the **Internal Iliac Artery (Hypogastric Artery)**, which bifurcates into an anterior and posterior divisions. The uterine supply is a key part of this network.
  - ***Uterine Artery***
    - **Origin:** Arises from the **anterior division of the Internal Iliac Artery**.
    - **Course:** It runs medially within the base of the broad ligament (the cardinal ligament). Its iconic surgical path is where it **crosses over the ureter** superiorly ("water under the bridge") approximately 1.5–2 cm lateral to the cervix at the level of the internal os.
  - ***Branches and Supply***
    - **Ascending Branch:** Runs tortuously upward along the lateral margin of the uterus (within the broad ligament), anastomosing with the **Ovarian Artery**. It supplies the body and fundus of the uterus.
    - **Descending (Cervical) Branch:** Supplies the cervix and the upper part of the vagina.
    - **Vaginal Artery:** Often a branch of the uterine artery, contributing to the supply of the upper vagina.
  - ***Ovarian Artery***
    - **Origin:** Directly from the **Abdominal Aorta**, just below the renal arteries.
    - **Course:** Descends retroperitoneally, crossing the external iliac vessels to enter the suspensory ligament of the ovary. It runs through the mesovarium to reach the ovary.
    - **Supply:** The ovary, fallopian tube, and the cornu of the uterus. Its terminal branch anastomoses with the ascending branch of the Uterine Artery.
  - ***Other Major Pelvic Arteries (for context)***
    - **Internal Iliac Artery (Posterior Division):**
    - **Superior Gluteal Artery**
    - **Iliolumbar Artery**
    - **Lateral Sacral Arteries**
  - ***Internal Iliac Artery (Anterior Division)***
    - **Umbilical Artery:** Gives off the **Superior Vesical Arteries** to the bladder.
    - **Obturator Artery**

- **Internal Pudendal Artery:** Supplies the perineum, external genitalia, and lower vagina.
- **Inferior Vesical Artery** (in males)/**Vaginal Artery** (in females, often from uterine): Supplies the base of the bladder and vagina.
- **Middle Rectal Artery:** Supplies the rectum.
- **Superior Rectal Artery:** A continuation of the **Inferior Mesenteric Artery**, supplies the upper part of the rectum.

Venous Drainage

- The veins generally follow the arteries into the **Uterine Veins**, which empty into the **Internal Iliac Veins.**
- The **Ovarian Venous Plexus** forms the **Ovarian Veins**:
- The **right ovarian vein** drains directly into the **Inferior Vena Cava.**
- The **left ovarian vein** drains into the **Left Renal Vein.**

Lymphatics

- Fundus/upper body: Preaortic/lateral aortic nodes.
- Cornu: Superficial inguinal nodes (via round ligament).
- Lower body/cervix: External iliac, internal iliac, obturator, sacral nodes.

Nerve Supply: Sympathetic (T5–T6 motor, T10–L1 sensory), parasympathetic (S2–S4); cervix/uterus insensitive to touch/incision.

Development: Formed from fused Müllerian ducts.[2]

Fallopian Tubes

Paired, 10 cm tubes in the broad ligament, facilitating gamete transport and fertilization.

Parts

- **Intramural:** In uterine wall (1.25 cm, 1 mm diameter).
- **Isthmus:** Straight (3–4 cm, 2 mm diameter).
- **Ampulla:** Tortuous (5 cm), site of fertilization.
- **Infundibulum:** Wide (1.25 cm, 6 mm diameter), with fimbriae (ovarian fimbria attaches to ovary).

Structure

- **Serosa:** Peritoneum (except mesosalpinx attachment).
- **Muscularis:** Outer longitudinal, inner circular smooth muscle.
- **Mucosa:** Ciliated columnar (ovarian end), secretory columnar (isthmic end), peg cells; longitudinal folds.

Blood Supply: Uterine and ovarian arteries; veins to pampiniform plexus/ovarian veins.

Lymphatics: Drain to para-aortic nodes.

Nerve Supply: Uterine/ovarian nerves; sensitive to manipulation.

Development: Upper vertical Müllerian ducts (6–10 weeks).[2]

Ovaries

Paired, oval gonads (3 × 2 × 1 cm) for gamete maturation and steroidogenesis, located in the ovarian fossa.

Structure

- **Surface:** Cubical germinal epithelium.
- **Cortex:** Stromal cells, tunica albuginea, follicles (primordial, Graafian, corpus luteum), atretic structures.
- **Medulla:** Connective tissue, vessels, nerves, hilus cells (homologous to testicular interstitial cells).

Relations

- **Mesovarium:** Attaches to broad ligament, carrying vessels/nerves.
- **Posterior border:** Tubal ampulla, ureter, internal iliac artery.
- **Lateral surface:** Ovarian fossa (external iliac vein, obturator vessels/nerves).

Blood Supply

- **Arteries:** Ovarian (abdominal aorta).
- **Veins:** Pampiniform plexus to ovarian veins (right: inferior vena cava; left: renal vein).

Lymphatics: Para-aortic nodes.

Nerve Supply: Sympathetic (T10); sensitive to compression.

Development: Cortex of genital ridges (9th week), with germ cells from yolk sac.[2]

PHYSIOLOGY OF FEMALE GENITALIA IN PREGNANCY

Pregnancy induces profound anatomical and physiological changes in the genitalia and systemic physiology to support fetal development and parturition.[3]

Genital Changes

Uterus:

- **Size**: Increases from 50–80 g to ~1 kg; capacity from 10 mL to 5 L.
- **Dextrorotation:** Rotates rightward due to pelvic anatomy.
- **Braxton Hicks Contractions:** Irregular, painless contractions without cervical dilation.
- **Blood Flow:** Rises to 750 mL/min at term (~10% of cardiac output).
- **Vagina:** Increased vascularity, epithelial thickening, acidic pH maintained (4–5).
- **Cervix:** Softens (Hegar's sign), forms mucus plug.
- **Ovaries:** Corpus luteum supports early pregnancy; folliculogenesis suppressed.

Systemic Changes

Cardiovascular:

- Cardiac output: +40% (stroke volume +27%, heart rate +15–20%).
- Systemic vascular resistance: –21%; diastolic BP/MAP drops mid-pregnancy.
- Femoral venous pressure: Increased; hemodilution reduces hematocrit.

Hematological:

- Blood volume: +30–40% (plasma +40–50%, red cells +20–30%).
- Hypercoagulable state: Fibrinogen +50%, increased factors X, IX, VIII, VII, II, I; protein S decreased; 6-fold VTE risk.[4]

Respiratory:

- Tidal volume/minute ventilation: +40%.
- Residual volume: –20%; total lung capacity: –5%.
- PaO_2 increased, $PaCO_2$ decreased (facilitates fetal CO_2 transfer).

Metabolic:

- Hyperglycemia, hyperinsulinemia (insulin resistance due to human placental lactogen).
- Hyperlipidemia, positive nitrogen balance.
- Iron requirement: 1,000 mg (6–7 mg/day in second half); calcium: 1–1.5 g/day.
- **Skin:** Chloasma, linea nigra, striae gravidarum, pigmented nipples, palmar erythema.

Recent Advances

- 2023 studies highlight uterine vascular remodeling (spiral artery transformation) as critical for placentation, with AI-driven imaging improving detection of abnormal flow patterns.[5]
- Proteomic analysis of cervical mucus reveals biomarkers for preterm labor risk.

TABLE 2: Key physiological changes in pregnancy.

System	*Change*	*Clinical Impact*
Uterine blood flow	750 mL/min (term)	Supports fetal oxygenation
Cardiac output	+40%	Mimics cardiac disease; supports demand
Plasma volume	+40–50%	Hemodilution; reduced hematocrit
Fibrinogen	+50%	Hypercoagulability; VTE risk
Tidal volume	+40%	Enhances fetal CO_2 transfer
Iron requirement	1000 mg total	Prevents anemia; supports fetal growth

REFERENCES

1. Drake RL, Vogl AW, Mitchell AWM (Eds). Gray's Anatomy for Students, 5th edition. Philadelphia: Elsevier; 2023.
2. Sadler TW. Langman's Medical Embryology. Philadelphia: Wolters Kluwer; 2020.
3. Kalaitzopoulos DR, Panagopoulos A, Samant S, et al. Management of venous thromboembolism in pregnancy. Thromb Res. 2022;211:106-13.
4. Osol G, Mandala M. Maternal uterine vascular remodeling during pregnancy. Physiology (Bethesda). 2009;24:58-71.
5. Parry S, Leite R, Esplin MS, Bukowski R, Zhang H, Varner M, et al. Eunice Kennedy Shriver National Institute of Child Health and Human Development Genomic and Proteomic Network for Preterm Birth Research. Cervicovaginal fluid proteomic analysis to identify potential biomarkers for preterm birth. Am J Obstet Gynecol. 2020 May;222(5):493.e1-493.e13.

Disorders of Sex Development

Ruchika Garg

INTRODUCTION

Disorders of sex development (DSD) are congenital conditions characterized by atypical development of chromosomal, gonadal, or anatomical sex, leading to variations in reproductive organs and genitalia that deviate from typical male or female definitions. Phenotypic sex results from the differentiation of internal ducts and external genitalia under hormonal influence from differentiated gonads, driven by sex-determining genes.[1] The term "DSD" is preferred in medical contexts for its precision, avoiding overlap with concepts like transgender, gender dysphoria, or homosexuality, though the term "disorder" may carry stigma.[2] Incidence varies: 1 in 4,500–5,500 for specific DSD conditions, rising to 1 in 200–300 when including cryptorchidism and hypospadias.[3] Congenital adrenal hyperplasia (CAH) and mixed gonadal dysgenesis account for ~50% of genital ambiguity cases.[4]

Definitions

- **Disorders of Sex Development (DSD):** Congenital conditions with atypical chromosomal, gonadal, or anatomical sex development.[1] Examples: CAH, Androgen Insensitivity Syndrome (AIS), Turner syndrome, Klinefelter syndrome.
- **Intersex:** A social/identity term for individuals with sex characteristics not fitting binary male/female norms; less specific than DSD.[2]
- **Homosexuality:** Sexual orientation toward same-sex individuals; unrelated to DSD.[5]
- **Hermaphrodite:** An outdated term for organisms with both male and female reproductive organs; not used clinically for humans.[2]

Incidence

- **Overall:** 1:4,500–5,500 infants for specific DSD; 1:200–300 including cryptorchidism/hypospadias.[3]
- **46,XY DSD:** ~1:20,000 births.[4]
- **46,XX DSD:** ~1:14,000–15,000 (mostly CAH); varies geographically due to pathogenic allele frequency.[4]

Classification of DSD

DSDs are classified based on karyotype and underlying mechanisms.

TABLE 1: DSD Classification (ESPE/LWPES, 2020)[1,6]

Category	*Examples*	*Key features*
46,XX DSD	CAH, ovarian hyperandrogenism	Virilization, normal ovaries
46,XY DSD	AIS, 5α-reductase deficiency	Under masculinization, normal/dysfunctional testes
Sex chromosome DSD	Turner syndrome, Klinefelter syndrome	Mosaic karyotypes, gonadal dysgenesis
Ovotesticular DSD	Mixed gonadal dysgenesis	Mixed gonadal tissue, ambiguous genitalia

Citation in text: The ESPE/LWPES classification **(Table 1)** organizes DSD by karyotype, aiding diagnosis.[1,6]

Pathophysiology

Sexual differentiation involves molecular mechanisms directing the bipotential gonad (formed at 6–7 weeks' gestation) into testes or ovaries, driven by sex-determining genes.[7]

- **Bipotential Stage:** Gonadal ridge expresses genes (WT1, SF-1, DAX1, LHX9, WNT4). SF-1 regulates steroidogenesis; WT1 supports mesenchymal–epithelial interactions.[8]
- **Testis Development:**
  - **SRY Gene:** On Y chromosome, activates SOX9, promoting Sertoli cell differentiation and testicular organization.[9]
  - **Hormones:** AMH (Sertoli cells) regresses Müllerian ducts; testosterone and insulin-like factor-3 (Leydig cells) develop Wolffian ducts and external genitalia.[10]

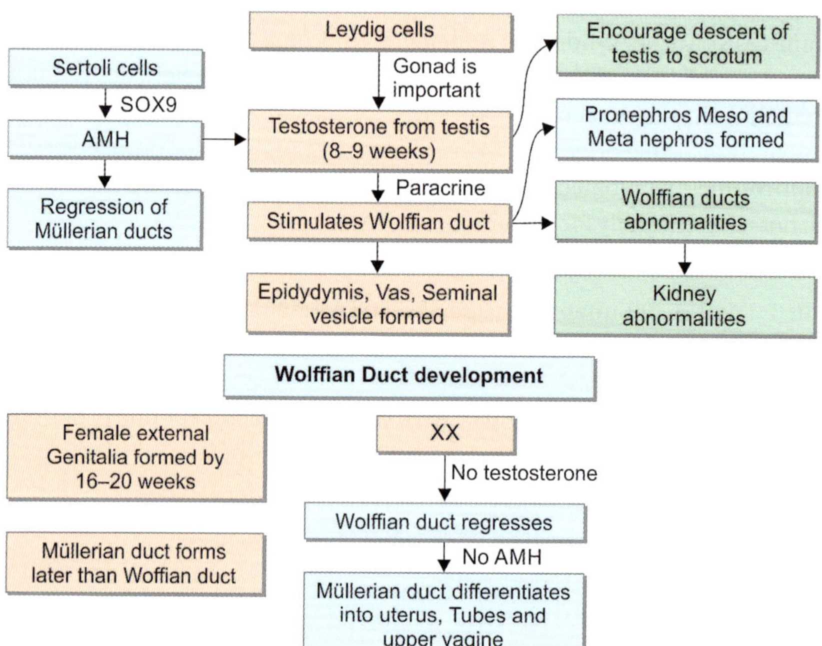

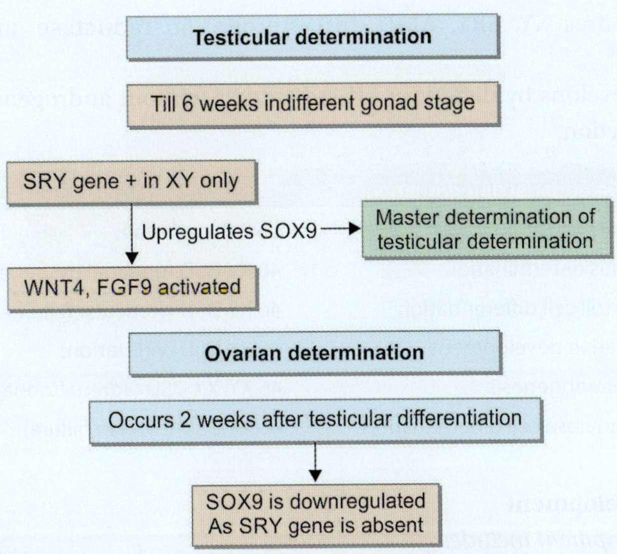

- **Ovary Development:** Absence of SRY allows WNT4, RSPO1, and FOXL2 to promote granulosa cell differentiation, inhibiting testicular pathways.[11]
- **External Genitalia:**

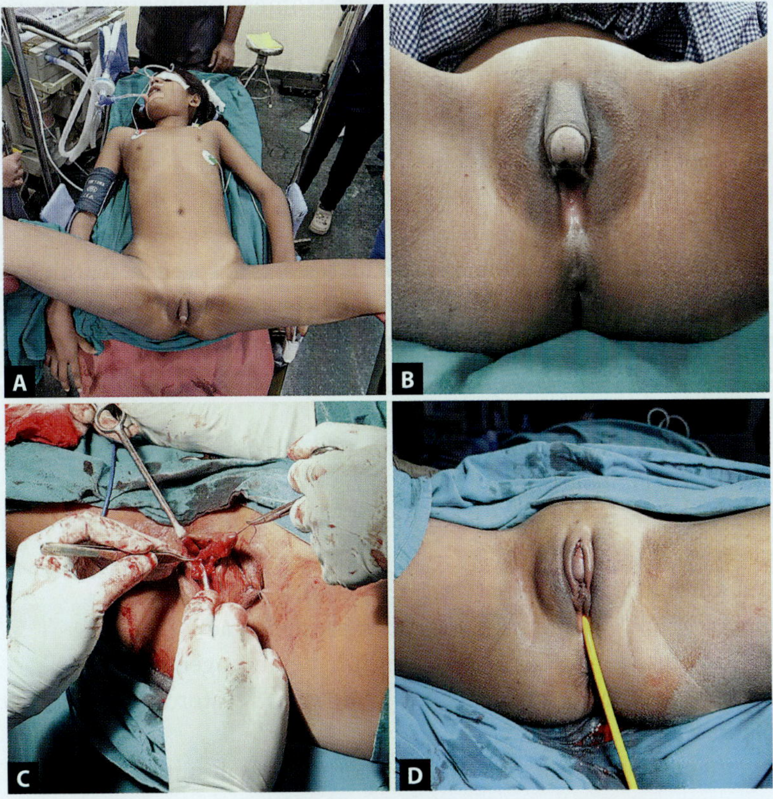

Courtesy: Yamini Ingale, DY Patil, Mumbai.

- **Male:** Requires XY, SRY, AMH, testosterone, 5α-reductase, and DHT receptor sensitivity.[10]
- **Female:** Develops by default in XX individuals without androgens; requires normal adrenal function.[11]

TABLE 2: Key genes in gonadal differentiation.[8,9,11]

Gene	*Role*	*DSD Association*
SRY	Testis determination	46,XY DSD (gonadal dysgenesis)
SOX9	Sertoli cell differentiation	46,XY DSD (testicular failure)
WNT4	Ovarian development	46,XX DSD (virilization)
SF-1	Steroidogenesis	46,XY/XX DSD (adrenal/gonadal defects)
FOXL2	Granulosa cell differentiation	46,XX DSD (ovarian failure)

Psychosexual Development

Psychosexual development includes:

- **Gender Identity:** Self-perception as male, female, or nonbinary.
- **Gender Role:** Sex-typical behaviors (e.g., toy preferences).
- **Sexual Orientation:** Attraction direction (heterosexual, bisexual, homosexual).[12]
- **Influences:** Prenatal androgens, sex chromosomes, brain structure, social/family dynamics.[12]
- **Gender Dysphoria:** Distress from mismatched assigned sex; more common in DSD but unpredictable.[13]

Common DSD Types

- **Klinefelter Syndrome (47,XXY; 1:500–1,000):**
  - **Etiology:** Extra X chromosome (classic/mosaic).
  - **Features:** Tall stature, gynecomastia, small testes, azoospermia, learning difficulties.
  - **Diagnosis:** High FSH/LH, low AMH/inhibin B, low testosterone (50–75%).
  - **Management:** Testosterone replacement; fertility rare.[14]
- **Turner Syndrome (45,X; 1:2,500)**:
  - **Etiology:** Monosomy X or mosaicism.
  - **Features:** Short stature, webbed neck, streak ovaries, cardiac anomalies.
  - **Diagnosis:** Prenatal ultrasound, high FSH/LH, delayed puberty.
  - **Management:** Estrogen/progesterone replacement, cardiovascular monitoring, gonadectomy if Y fragment.[15]
- **Congenital Adrenal Hyperplasia (CAH; 1:15,000):**
  - **Etiology:** CYP21A2 mutations (21-hydroxylase deficiency).
  - **Features:** Virilization (46,XX), salt-wasting, hyperandrogenemia.
  - **Diagnosis:** Newborn screening (17-hydroxyprogesterone), electrolytes, ACTH stimulation.
  - **Management:** Glucocorticoids, mineralocorticoids, salt supplementation.[16]

- **Androgen Insensitivity Syndrome (AIS; 46,XY):**
  - **Etiology:** X-linked AR gene mutations.
  - **Features:** Complete (CAIS): female phenotype; Partial (PAIS): ambiguous genitalia.
  - **Diagnosis:** Normal testosterone, high LH/FSH, absent Müllerian structures.
  - **Management:** Hormone replacement, gonadectomy (CAIS), psychological support (**Table 3**).[17]

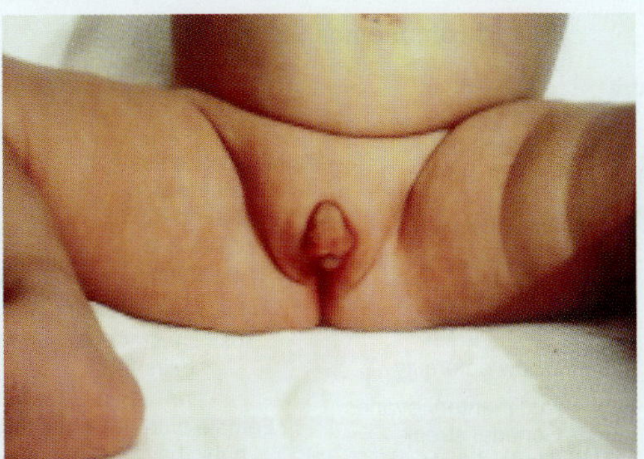

Ambiguous genitalia (clitoromegaly, bifid scrotum, rugated folds) due to classical 21-hydroxylase deficiency.

- **Cryptorchidism (2–4% term males):**
  - **Etiology:** Failure of testicular descent.
  - **Features:** Increased risk of hernia, torsion, malignancy.
  - **Management:** Orchidopexy by 12 months; hCG/GnRH therapy.[18]
- **Mixed Gonadal Dysgenesis**:
  - **Etiology:** Mosaic karyotypes (e.g., 45,X/46,XY).
  - **Features:** Asymmetrical gonads, ambiguous genitalia.
  - **Management:** Gonadectomy (malignancy risk), hormone replacement.[19]

TABLE 3: Differentiating CAH, 5α-Reductase deficiency, and AIS.[16,17,20]

Feature	*CAH (46,XX)*	*5α-Reductase Deficiency (46,XY)*	*AIS (46,XY)*
Genitalia	Virilized	Ambiguous, virilizes at puberty	Female/ambiguous
Gonads	Ovaries	Testes	Testes
Hormones	High androgens	Normal testosterone, low DHT	Normal testosterone
Management	Glucocorticoids	Gender assignment, surgery	Hormone, gonadectomy

CAH, 5α-reductase deficiency, and AIS require distinct management based on hormonal and anatomical profiles (**Table 3**).[16,17,20]

Investigations and Diagnostic Approach

(ESPE/LWPES Consensus, 2020)[6]

- Avoid gender assignment before expert evaluation.
- Use multidisciplinary teams (endocrinology, urology, genetics, psychology).
- Ensure gender assignment for all individuals.

- Promote open communication and shared decision-making.
- Maintain confidentiality.

Multidisciplinary Team

Includes pediatric endocrinology, surgery/urology, gynecology, genetics, psychology, neonatology, social work, and ethics.[6]

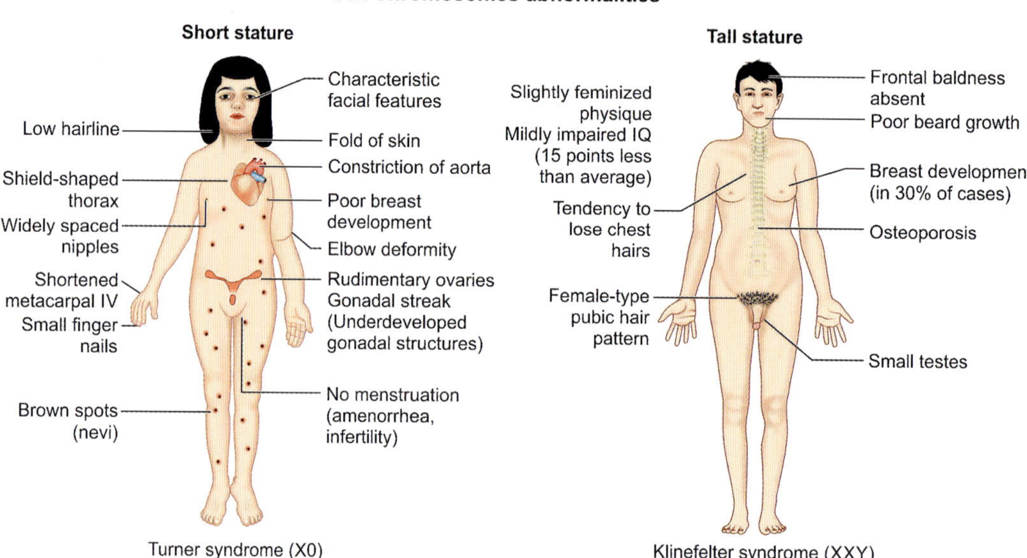

Diagnostic Evaluation

Molecular diagnosis is achieved in ~20% of DSD cases due to diagnostic gaps.[21] First-line tests (results within 48 hours):

- **Karyotyping:** X/Y-specific probes.
- **Imaging:** Abdominopelvic ultrasound.
- **Hormones:** 17-hydroxyprogesterone, testosterone, gonadotropins, AMH, electrolytes.
- **Stimulation Tests:** hCG (testicular function), ACTH (adrenal function).
- **Urine Steroid Analysis:** Gas chromatography-mass spectrometry.
- **Gonadal Biopsy:** For ambiguous cases.
- **Genetic Testing:** Next-generation sequencing, transcriptomics (ethical considerations).[22]

TABLE 4: Diagnostic tests for DSD.[21,22]

Test	*Purpose*
Karyotyping	Confirm chromosomal sex
Ultrasound	Assess internal genitalia/gonads
17-Hydroxyprogesterone	Screen for CAH
hCG Stimulation	Evaluate testicular function
Genetic Sequencing	Identify gene mutations

Citation in text: **Table 4** outlines essential diagnostic tests for DSD evaluation.[21,22]

Clinical Assessment

- **Vital Signs/General Exam:** Identify systemic features.
- **Perineal Exam:** Use Prader classification for genital ambiguity
- **History:** Prenatal exposures, family history of DSD.

Management

Gender Assignment:

- **Factors:** Diagnosis, genital appearance, surgical options, fertility potential, family/cultural context.[6]
- **Guidelines:**
  - *90% of 46,XX CAH and all 46,XY CAIS identify as female.*[23]
  - ~60% of 5α-reductase deficiency patients virilizing at puberty identify as male.[20]
  - Consider fertility potential in 5α-reductase/17β-HSD3 deficiencies.

Surgical Management

Surgical decisions are complex, balancing functional, psychological, and ethical considerations.[24]

Goals

- Normalize anatomy for function (urination, sexual activity).
- Preserve fertility where possible.
- Minimize psychological distress.

Procedures

- **Genital Reconstruction:**
  - **Clitoroplasty:** For severe virilization (Prader III–V) in CAH; preserves nerve supply.[24]
  - **Vaginoplasty:** For AIS or absent vagina; often delayed until puberty.[25]
  - **Hypospadias Repair:** For 46,XY DSD with urethral anomalies.
- **Gonadectomy:**
  - **Indications:** Malignancy risk (e.g., Y-chromosome in gonadal dysgenesis, CAIS).
  - **Timing:** Early childhood (Y-containing gonads in females); prepuberty for androgen biosynthesis defects.[26]
- **Urethral Reconstruction**: Ensures urinary function.
- **Fertility Preservation:** Laparoscopic utriculus excision, sperm banking in 46,XY DSD.[27]

Considerations

- **Timing:** Early surgery reduces parental distress but risks misalignment with future identity; delayed surgery allows patient autonomy.[24]
- **Techniques:** Nerve-sparing, minimally invasive (e.g., laparoscopic) approaches.[25]
- **Ethics:** Informed consent, avoid irreversible procedures in infancy.[6]

Sex Steroid Replacement

- **Indications:** Hypogonadism (gonadal dysgenesis, AIS).
- **Goals:** Mimic pubertal maturation, promote secondary sexual characteristics, bone health, psychosexual maturity.[28]

- **Regimens:**
  - **Males:** Intramuscular testosterone esters, oral/transdermal options.
  - **Females:** Estrogen/progesterone for Turner syndrome, CAIS.

Psychosocial Care

- **Role:** Essential for coping, gender identity, and quality of life.[29]
- **Components:**
  - Psychological screening for maladaptive coping.
  - Counseling on gender identity, sexual function, relationships.
  - Support groups for patients/families.
- **Challenges:** Sexual aversion, fear of rejection, low arousability.[29]

Emerging Trends and Guidelines

- **Genetic Diagnostics:** Multi-omics (transcriptomics, epigenomics) to bridge diagnostic gaps.[22]
- **Minimally Invasive Surgery:** Laparoscopic techniques reduce complications.[25]
- **Fertility Preservation:** Oocyte/sperm cryopreservation in DSD.[27]
- **WHO/ESPE Guidelines (2023):** Emphasize patient-centered care, deferred surgery, and psychosocial support.[1,6]

CONCLUSION

DSDs are complex conditions requiring multidisciplinary management to address medical, psychological, and ethical challenges. Accurate diagnosis, informed gender assignment, tailored surgical/hormonal interventions, and robust psychosocial support are critical. Advances in genetic diagnostics and minimally invasive techniques, coupled with patient-centered guidelines, enhance outcomes and quality of life.

KEY POINTS

- DSDs involve atypical sex development; incidence varies (1:4,500–5,500 specific, 1:200–300 overall).[3]
- SRY, WNT4, and SOX9 drive gonadal differentiation; mutations cause DSD.[9,11]
- Multidisciplinary teams ensure comprehensive care; avoid early gender assignment.[6]
- Surgical management balances function, fertility, and ethics; defer non-essential procedures.[24]
- Psychosocial support addresses gender dysphoria and quality of life.[29]

REFERENCES

1. Lee PA, Houk CP, Ahmed SF, et al. Consensus statement on management of intersex disorders. Pediatrics. 2016;137(6):e20160961.
2. Cools M, Nordenström A, Robeva R, et al. Caring for individuals with a difference of sex development (DSD): A consensus statement. Nat Rev Endocrinol. 2018;14(7):415-29.
3. Hughes IA, Houk C, Ahmed SF, et al. Incidence and prevalence of DSD: A global perspective. Horm Res Paediatr. 2019;91(3):145-53.

4. Arboleda VA, Sandberg DE, Vilain E. DSDs: Genetics, underlying pathologies and psychosexual differentiation. Nat Rev Endocrinol. 2017;13(10):578-89.
5. World Health Organization. Sexual orientation and gender identity: A human rights perspective. WHO, 2016.
6. European Society for Paediatric Endocrinology. Revised DSD management guidelines. ESPE, 2020.
7. Rey RA, Grinspon RP. Normal and abnormal sexual development. Best Pract Res Clin Endocrinol Metab. 2018;32(2):133-47.
8. Bashamboo A, McElreavey K. Gene mutations in disorders of sex development. Hum Genet. 2016;135(8):871-86.
9. Sekido R, Lovell-Badge R. Mechanisms of SRY and SOX9 in testicular differentiation. Development. 2017;144(10):1765-74.
10. Josso N, Rey RA, Picard JY. Anti-Müllerian hormone in DSD. Endocr Rev. 2019;40(4):911-29.
11. Nicol B, Yao HH. WNT4 and RSPO1 in ovarian development. Biol Reprod. 2018;99(1):45-53.
12. Hines M. Prenatal influences on psychosexual development in DSD. J Sex Res. 2017;54(4-5):526-36.
13. Sandberg DE, Gardner M, Cohen-Kettenis PT. Psychological aspects of DSD. Best Pract Res Clin Endocrinol Metab. 2019;33(3):101260.
14. Groth KA, Skakkebæk A, Høst C, et al. Klinefelter syndrome: A clinical update. J Clin Endocrinol Metab. 2018;103(1):15-24.
15. Gravholt CH, Andersen NH, Conway GS, et al. Clinical practice guidelines for Turner syndrome. Eur J Endocrinol. 2017;177(3):G1-G70.
16. Speiser PW, Arlt W, Auchus RJ, et al. Congenital adrenal hyperplasia: An Endocrine Society clinical practice guideline. J Clin Endocrinol Metab. 2018;103(11):4043-88.
17. Gottlieb B, Trifiro MA. Androgen insensitivity syndrome. GeneReviews. 2017.
18. Kolon TF, Herndon CDA, Baker LA, et al. Evaluation and treatment of cryptorchidism. J Urol. 2019;202(4):665-72.
19. Cools M, Wolffenbuttel KP, Hersmus R, et al. Mixed gonadal dysgenesis: A review. Horm Res Paediatr. 2018;89(5):359-68.
20. Maimoun L, Philibert P, Cammas B, et al. 5α-Reductase deficiency: Phenotype and management. J Clin Endocrinol Metab. 2017;102(6):1973-84.
21. Eggers S, Sadedin S, van den Bergen JA, et al. Genetic diagnostics in DSD: Current challenges. Hum Genet. 2016;135(9):1031-41.
22. Achermann JC, Domenice S, Bachega TASS, et al. Multi-omics approaches in DSD diagnostics. Nat Rev Endocrinol. 2020;16(6):295-306.
23. Dessens AB, Slijper FM, Drop SL. Gender dysphoria in DSD: A review. J Sex Res. 2017;54(4-5):537-47.
24. Wolffenbuttel KP, Hoebeke P. Surgical management of DSD: Current perspectives. J Pediatr Urol. 2018;14(5):401-8.
25. Creighton SM, Minto CL, Steele SJ. Feminizing genitoplasty in DSD. BJU Int. 2016;118(3):346-52.
26. Pleskacova J, Hersmus R, Oosterhuis JW, et al. Gonadal malignancy risk in DSD. J Clin Endocrinol Metab. 2017;102(7):2359-67.
27. Finlayson C, Johnson EK, Chen D, et al. Fertility preservation in DSD. Endocrinol Metab Clin North Am. 2019;48(4):795-811.
28. Bertelloni S, Baroncelli GI, Massart F. Hormone replacement in DSD. Horm Res Paediatr. 2018;90(2):77-87.
29. Ernst MM, Liao LM, Baratz AB, et al. Psychosocial care in DSD: Best practices. Horm Res Paediatr. 2020;93(3):145-56.

Adolescent Gynecology

Ruchika Garg, Anu Chaudhary

INTRODUCTION

Adolescence, defined by the World Health Organization (WHO) as the period between 10 and 19 years, is a phase of rapid physical, cognitive, and psychosocial growth.[1] Puberty, a critical component of adolescence, involves physical maturation leading to reproductive capability, while adolescence encompasses psychological and social maturity.[2] This chapter addresses key aspects of adolescent gynecology, including puberty, delayed puberty, primary amenorrhea, precocious puberty, puberty menorrhagia, Turner syndrome, and imperforate hymen, tailored for postgraduate medical education in low-resource settings.

Flowchart 1: Timeline of pubertal events in girls, highlighting thelarche, pubarche, growth spurt, and menarche.

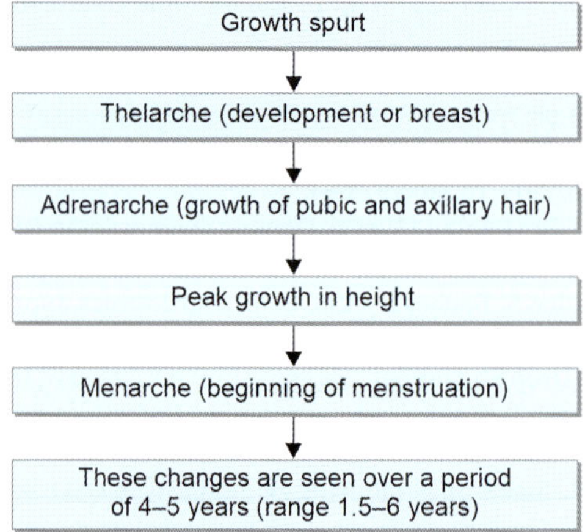

Q1. Define puberty and describe changes during puberty. *(20 Marks)*

Definition

Puberty is the process of physical maturation during which an adolescent develops secondary sexual characteristics and achieves reproductive capability.[2] It is distinct from adolescence, which includes psychological, social, and sexual maturity.[1]

Age of Onset

- **Girls:** Typically begins between 8 and 13 years, with menarche at 12–13 years.[2]
- **Boys:** Starts between 9 and 14 years.[2]

- **Variation:** Influenced by genetics, nutrition, environmental factors (e.g., endocrine disruptors), psychological stress, chronic illness, or excessive physical activity.[3]

Changes During Puberty

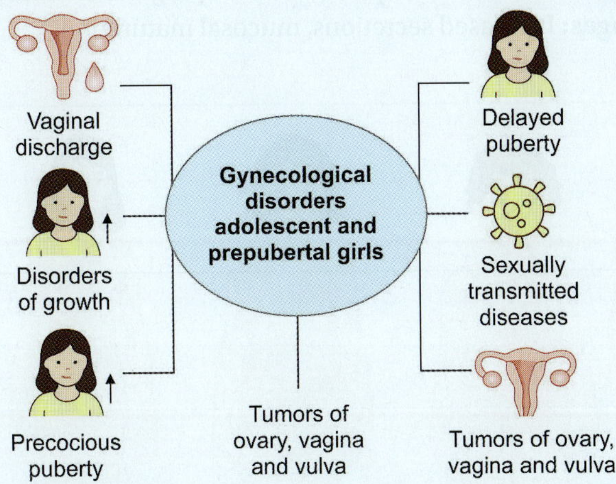

- **Endocrine Changes**
  - **Hypothalamic-Pituitary-Gonadal (HPG) Axis Activation:**
    - Pulsatile gonadotropin-releasing hormone (GnRH) release from the hypothalamus increases, initially during sleep, then continuously.[2]
    - GnRH stimulates the pituitary to secrete luteinizing hormone (LH) and follicle-stimulating hormone (FSH).[2]
  - **Ovarian Hormone Production:**
    - FSH promotes ovarian follicle growth; LH triggers ovulation and corpus luteum formation.[4]
    - **Estrogen (estradiol):** Drives breast development (thelarche), uterine growth, and menstrual cycle regulation.[4]
    - **Progesterone:** Prepares endometrium postovulation.[4]
    - **Adrenal Androgens (adrenarche):** Dehydroepiandrosterone (DHEA/DHEAS) from adrenal glands induces pubic/axillary hair and libido.[3]
    - **Growth Hormone (GH):** Estrogen enhances GH secretion, contributing to growth spurt.[3]
- **Physical Changes**
  - **Breast Development (Thelarche):**
    - First visible sign, starting at 8–13 years, driven by estrogen.[2]
    - Progresses through Tanner stages **(Table 1)**.[5]
  - **Pubic/Axillary Hair (Pubarche):**
    - Follows thelarche, driven by adrenal androgens; progresses through Tanner stages.[5]
    - Axillary hair appears later.[2]
  - **Growth Spurt:**
    - Peaks before menarche (9–14 years); driven by estrogen and GH.[3]
    - Requires adequate nutrition for optimal height gain.[3]

- **Menarche:**
    - Onset of menstruation (12–13 years), 2–3 years post-thelarche.[2]
    - Initial cycles often irregular; 50% anovulatory in first year.[6]
- **Body Composition:** Increased hip/thigh fat, shaping female contours.[2]
- **Vaginal Changes:** Increased secretions, mucosal maturation.[2]

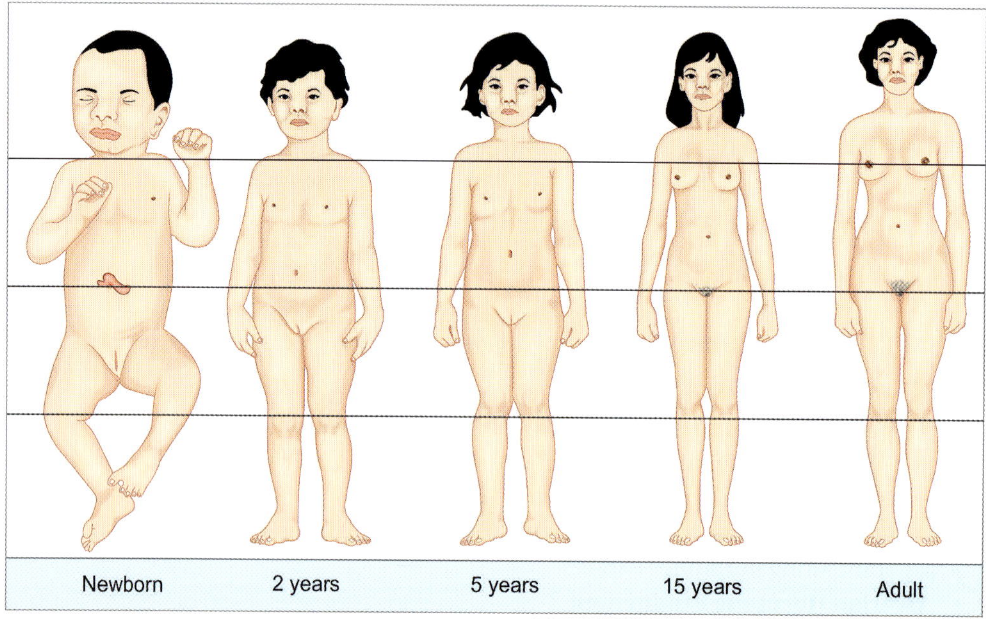

Vaginal changes in the female genitalia from newborn to adulthood.

- **Tanner Staging**

  Tanner staging classifies pubertal development **(Table 1)**.[5]
    - **Purpose:** Assesses normal progression, diagnoses precocious/delayed puberty, guides interventions.[5]

TABLE 1: Tanner staging for girls.

Stage	*Breast development (Thelarche)*	*Pubic hair (Pubarche)*
1.	Prepubertal: No glandular tissue, nipple raised	No pubic hair
2.	Breast bud: Small mound, areola enlarges	Sparse, lightly pigmented hair along labia
3.	Further breast/areola enlargement, no contour separation	Darker, coarser, curly hair over pubes
4.	Areola/nipple form secondary mound	Adult-type hair, smaller area, not on inner thighs
5.	Mature breast: Nipple raised, smooth contour	Adult quantity, extends to inner thighs

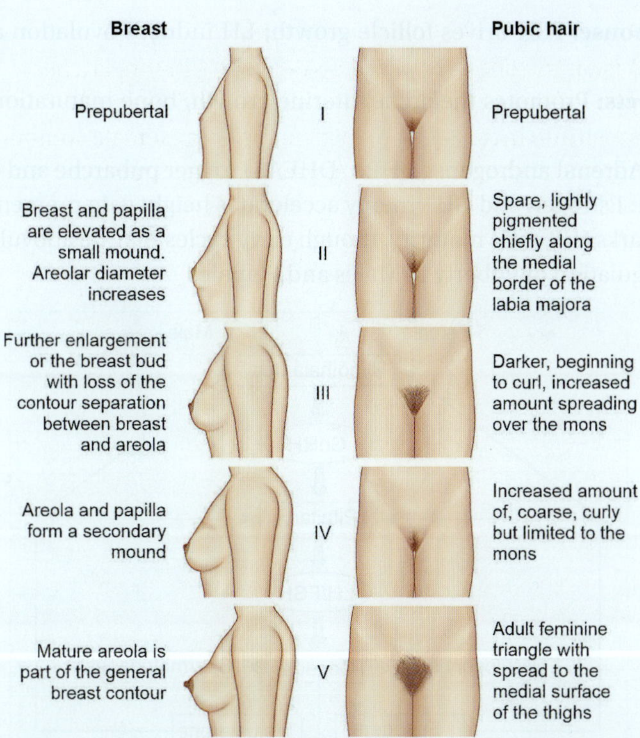

Tanner stages of female breast and pubic hair development.

- **Psychological Changes**
  - Enhanced cognitive abilities (abstract thinking).[7]
  - Emotional volatility, mood swings, identity development.[7]
  - Increased independence and personal values.[7]
- **Social Changes**
  - Peer relationships dominate; heightened social awareness.[7]
  - Exploration of romantic/sexual relationships influenced by hormonal changes.[7]
- **Abnormalities**
  - **Precocious Puberty:** Secondary sexual characteristics before age 8 (girls) or 9 (boys) years.[8]
  - **Central (GnRH-dependent):** HPG axis activation (e.g., hypothalamic tumors).
  - **Peripheral (GnRH-independent):** Exogenous hormones, adrenal/ovarian tumors.
  - **Isosexual/Heterosexual:** Consonant (normal sequence) or disconsonant (abnormal sequence, e.g., virilization in congenital adrenal hyperplasia).[8]
  - **Delayed Puberty:** No breast development by 13 or menarche by 15 years (girls); no testicular enlargement by 14 years (boys).[9]

Q2. Physiology of Puberty, Causes, and Management of Delayed Puberty. *(10 Marks)*

Physiology of Puberty

- **HPG Axis Activation:** Pulsatile GnRH release from the hypothalamus stimulates pituitary LH/FSH secretion, initially nocturnal and then continuous.[2]

- **Ovarian Response:** FSH drives follicle growth; LH induces ovulation and progesterone production.[4]
- **Estrogen Effects:** Promotes thelarche, uterine growth, bone maturation, and epiphyseal closure.[4]
- **Adrenarche:** Adrenal androgens (DHEA/DHEAS) trigger pubarche and libido.[3]
- **Growth Spurt:** Estrogen and GH synergy accelerates height gain premenarche.[3]
- **Menarche:** Marks HPG axis maturity, though early cycles may be anovulatory.[6]
Hormonal Regulation of Puberty in Males and Females

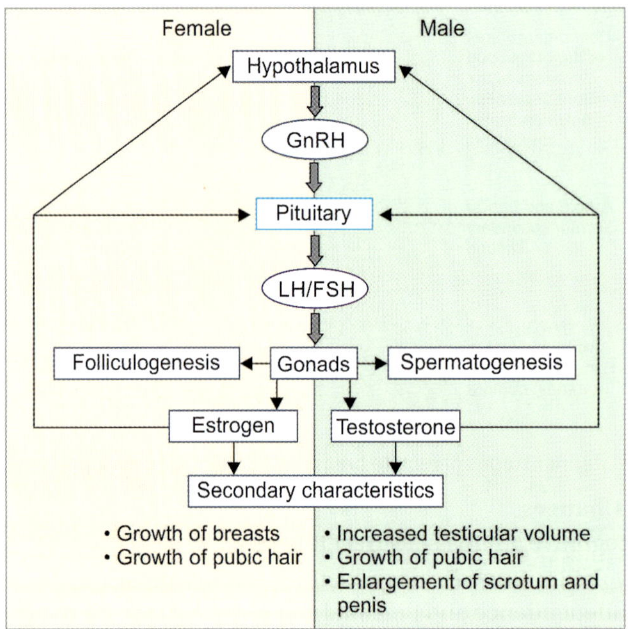

Causes of Delayed Puberty

Delayed puberty is the absence of secondary sexual characteristics by age 13 (girls) or 14 (boys) years.[9] Classified as:

- **Hypogonadotropic Hypogonadism (Central Causes, Low LH/FSH)**
  - **Constitutional Delay of Growth and Puberty (CDGP):** Most common, familial, temporary HPG axis delay.[9]
  - **Kallmann Syndrome:** GnRH deficiency with anosmia.[10]
  - **Prader-Willi Syndrome:** Obesity, delayed milestones, hypogonadism.[10]
  - **Chronic Illness:** Celiac disease, cystic fibrosis, inflammatory bowel disease.[11]
  - **Nutritional Deficiencies:** Malnutrition, anorexia nervosa.[11]
  - **Hypopituitarism:** Pituitary dysfunction (tumors, trauma).[10]
  - **Excessive Exercise:** Common in athletes.[11]
- **Hypergonadotropic Hypogonadism (Primary Gonadal Failure, High LH/FSH)**
  - **Turner Syndrome:** 45,X karyotype, ovarian failure.[12]
  - **Klinefelter Syndrome:** 47,XXY, testicular dysfunction (boys).[12]

- **Gonadal Dysgenesis:** Swyer syndrome (46,XY with female phenotype).[12]
- **Autoimmune Oophoritis/Orchitis:** Immune-mediated gonadal damage.[11]
- **Chemotherapy/Radiation:** Gonadal toxicity.[11]

TABLE 2: Causes of delayed puberty.

Category	*Examples*	*Mechanism*
Hypogonadotropic hypogonadism	CDGP, Kallmann syndrome, anorexia	Low GnRH/LH/FSH, HPG axis dysfunction
Hypergonadotropic hypogonadism	Turner syndrome, gonadal dysgenesis	Gonadal failure, high LH/FSH

Diagnostic Evaluation

- **History:** Pubertal milestones, chronic illness, exercise, stress, family history, anosmia, galactorrhea.[9]
- **Physical Exam:** Tanner staging, height/BMI, thyroid, Turner syndrome features (webbed neck, short stature).[9]
- **Investigations:**
  - **Hormonal Tests:** LH, FSH, estradiol/testosterone, TSH, prolactin, IGF-1.[9]
  - **Imaging:** Pelvic ultrasound (uterus/ovaries), MRI brain (pituitary), bone age X-ray.[9]
  - **Other:** CBC, ESR, Mantoux (TB), karyotyping (Turner/Klinefelter).[9]

Management

- **Observation:** For CDGP, monitor every 6 months; spontaneous puberty often occurs.[9]
- **Hormone Replacement Therapy (HRT):**
  - **Estrogen:** Initiate at 11–12 years for hypogonadism (e.g., Turner syndrome); transdermal estradiol (100 µg/day) or oral conjugated estrogen (0.625 mg/day), gradually increased.[13]
  - **Progesterone:** Add cyclic progestin (e.g., medroxyprogesterone) after 1–2 years or breakthrough bleeding to induce menses.[13]
  - **Monitoring:** Assess Tanner staging, bone density; supplement calcium (1,200 mg/day) and vitamin D (1,000 IU/day).[13]
- **Treat Underlying Cause:** Manage thyroid disorders, chronic illnesses, or hyperprolactinemia.[11]
- **Lifestyle:** Optimize nutrition, reduce exercise intensity, address eating disorders.[11]
- **Psychological Support:** Counseling, cognitive behavioral therapy (CBT) for emotional distress, low self-esteem.[14]

Q3. Define Primary Amenorrhea, Causes, Turner Syndrome, Investigations, and Management. *(10 Marks)*

Definition

Primary amenorrhea is the absence of menarche by age 15 years with normal secondary sexual characteristics or by age 13 years without secondary sexual characteristics.[15]

Causes

Requires intact hypothalamus, pituitary, ovaries, and genital outflow tract.[15] Classified by etiology:

- **Hypothalamic/Pituitary Disorders**
  - Functional hypothalamic amenorrhea (stress, exercise, anorexia).[15]
  - Tumors (prolactinomas, craniopharyngiomas), infiltrative diseases (TB, sarcoidosis).[15]
  - Kallmann syndrome, Prader-Willi syndrome.[10]
- **Ovarian Causes**
  - **Turner Syndrome:** 45,X, ovarian failure.[12]
  - **Gonadal Dysgenesis:** Swyer syndrome.[12]
  - **Androgen Insensitivity Syndrome (AIS):** 46,XY, female phenotype, absent uterus.[15]
  - **Chemotherapy/Radiation:** Ovarian damage.[11]
  - Autoimmune Oophoritis.[11]
- **Anatomic Abnormalities**
  - **Mayer-Rokitansky-Küster-Hauser (MRKH) Syndrome:** Absent/rudimentary uterus, normal ovaries.[16]
  - Imperforate Hymen, transverse vaginal septum, vaginal/cervical agenesis.[16]
  - AIS.[15]
- **Other**
  - **Endocrine:** Hypothyroidism, hyperthyroidism, PCOS, congenital adrenal hyperplasia.[15]
  - **Chronic Illness:** TB, celiac disease.[11]
  - **Systemic:** Malnutrition, extreme exercise.[11]

TABLE 3: Causes of primary amenorrhea.

Category	*Examples*	*Mechanism*
Hypothalamic/Pituitary	Kallmann syndrome, prolactinomas	Low GnRH/LH/FSH
Ovarian	Turner syndrome, gonadal dysgenesis	Ovarian failure, high LH/FSH
Anatomic	MRKH syndrome, imperforate hymen	Outflow tract obstruction
Endocrine/Systemic	PCOS, hypothyroidism, malnutrition	Hormonal imbalance, systemic stress

Turner Syndrome

- **Definition:** Chromosomal disorder (45,X or mosaicism) causing ovarian failure; incidence 1:2500 female births.[12]
- **Pathophysiology:** Loss of X chromosome (*SHOX* gene) disrupts growth and ovarian development, leading to streak gonads.[12]
  Clinical Features (shown in **Fig. 1**)
- **Physical:** Short stature, webbed neck, low hairline, cubitus valgus, broad chest, osteoporosis.[12]
- **Ovarian:** Primary amenorrhea, delayed puberty, infertility; mosaicism may allow spontaneous menarche.[12]

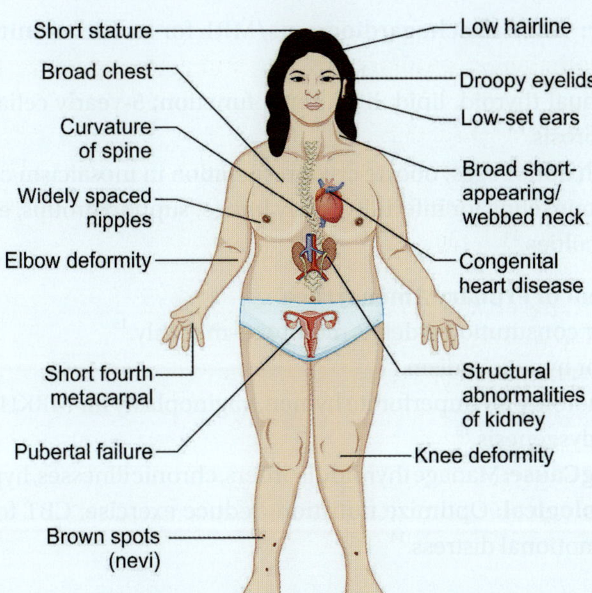

Fig. 1: Clinical features of Turner syndrome.

- **Cardiovascular:** Bicuspid aortic valve (30%), coarctation of aorta (12%), aortic dilation, hypertension.[12]
- **Renal:** Horseshoe kidney (30%), urinary tract infections.[12]
- **Other:** Lymphedema, hearing loss, autoimmune disorders (thyroiditis, celiac disease), learning difficulties (spatial reasoning).[12]

Investigations

- **Clinical:** Assess short stature, Tanner staging, Turner features.[12]
- **Hormonal:** High FSH/LH, low estradiol/AMH, thyroid function tests.[12]
- **Imaging:** Pelvic ultrasound (streak gonads), echocardiogram (heart defects), renal ultrasound.[12]
- **Karyotyping:** Confirms 45,X or mosaicism.[12]
- **Prenatal:** Diagnosed via chorionic villus sampling/amniocentesis for cystic hygroma, hydrops fetalis.[12]

Management

- **Growth Hormone (GH):** Recombinant GH from early childhood to improve adult height.[13]
- **Hormone Replacement Therapy (HRT):**
  - Estrogen (transdermal estradiol 100 µg/day) at 11–12 years to initiate puberty, uterine growth, bone health.[13]
  - Cyclic progesterone after 1–2 years or breakthrough bleeding.[13]
  - Early ethinyl estradiol (2 µg) at 8 years if delayed puberty confirmed.[17]

- **Cardiovascular:** Annual echocardiograms/MRI for aortic monitoring; surgery for coarctation.[12]
- **Monitoring:** Annual thyroid, lipid, liver, renal function; 5-yearly celiac screening; DEXA scans for osteoporosis.[17]
- **Fertility:** IVF with donor eggs; oocyte cryopreservation in mosaicism cases.[17]
- **Psychosocial:** Counseling for infertility, body image; support groups, educational support for learning difficulties.[14]

General Management of Primary Amenorrhea

- **Observation:** For constitutional delay, monitor 6-monthly.[15]
- **HRT:** As above for hypogonadism.[13]
- **Surgical:** Hymenotomy for imperforate hymen, vaginoplasty for MRKH/AIS, gonadectomy for AIS/gonadal dysgenesis.[16]
- **Treat Underlying Cause:** Manage thyroid disorders, chronic illnesses, hyperprolactinemia.[15]
- **Lifestyle/Psychological:** Optimize nutrition, reduce exercise, CBT for eating disorders, counseling for emotional distress.[14]

Flowchart 2: Primary amenorrhea evaluation and management.

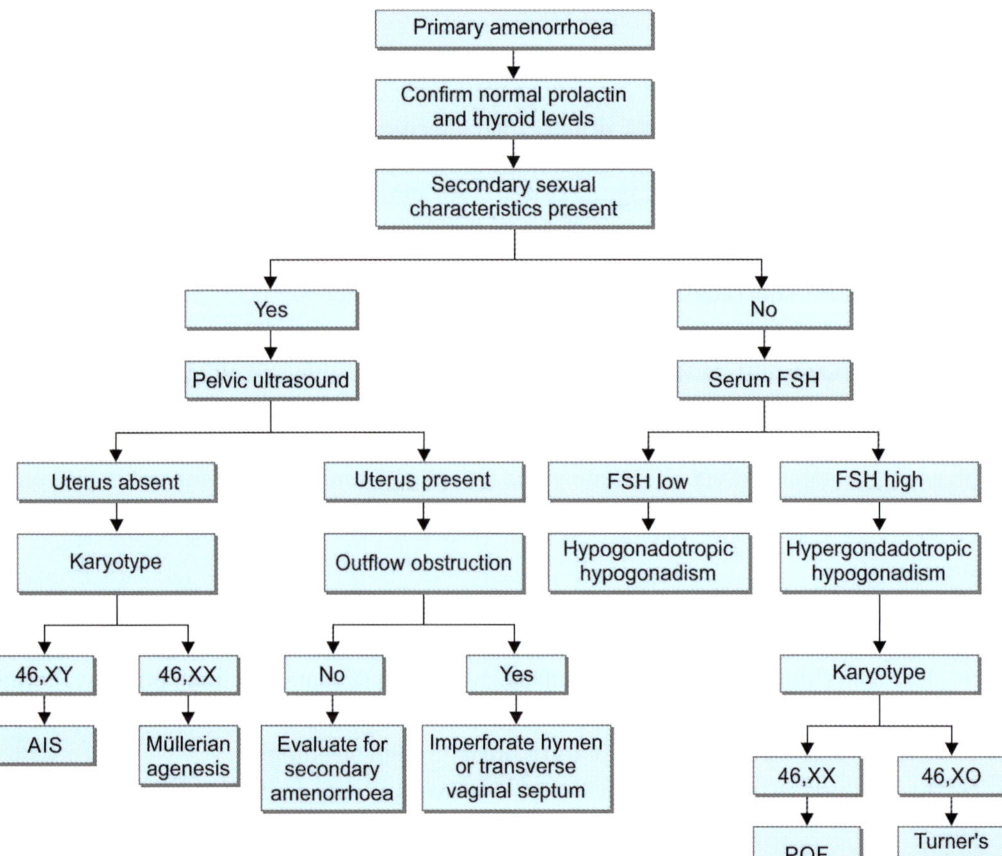

Q4. Precocious Puberty: Definition, Causes, and Management. *(10 Marks)*

Definition

Precocious puberty is the onset of secondary sexual characteristics before age 8 years in girls or 9 years in boys.[8]

Causes

- **Central Precocious Puberty (CPP, GnRH-dependent):**
  - Idiopathic (most common in girls).[8]
  - **CNS lesions:** Hypothalamic hamartomas, tumors, hydrocephalus.[8]
  - **CNS injury:** Trauma, radiation, infection.[8]
- **Peripheral Precocious Puberty (PPP, GnRH-independent):**
  - Ovarian/adrenal tumors (e.g., granulosa cell tumors, adrenal carcinoma).[8]
  - Congenital adrenal hyperplasia (CAH).[8]
  - Exogenous hormones (e.g., estrogen creams).[8]
  - **McCune–Albright syndrome:** Precocious puberty, café-au-lait spots, fibrous dysplasia.[8]
- **Types:** Isosexual (same-sex characteristics) or heterosexual (opposite-sex, e.g., virilization in CAH); consonant (normal sequence) or disconsonant.[8]

Management

- **Evaluation:**
  - **History/Exam:** Pubertal milestones, Tanner staging, neurological symptoms.[8]
  - **Hormonal Tests:** LH, FSH, estradiol, DHEA-S, 17-hydroxyprogesterone (CAH).[8]
  - **Imaging:** Pelvic ultrasound, MRI brain, bone age X-ray.[8]
  - **GnRH Stimulation Test:** Confirms CPP (LH rise).[8]
- **Treatment:**
  - **CPP:** GnRH agonists (leuprolide) to suppress HPG axis, delaying puberty until age-appropriate.[18]
  - **PPP:** Treat underlying cause (e.g., tumor resection, CAH management with glucocorticoids).[18]
  - **Psychosocial Support:** Counseling for emotional/social challenges.[14]

Q5. Puberty Menorrhagia: Definition, Etiology, Diagnosis, and Management. *(10 Marks)*

Definition

Puberty menorrhagia is excessive menstrual bleeding in adolescents that disrupts physical, social, emotional, or material quality of life.[19] Quantitatively, it involves bleeding >7 days or >80 mL/cycle.[19] Normal adolescent cycles: 21–45 days, 2–7 days duration, 30–40 mL loss.[19]

Etiology

- **Nonstructural:**
  - **Anovulation:** Most common, due to immature HPG axis; 50% cycles anovulatory in the first year postmenarche.[19]
  - **Coagulopathies:** Von Willebrand disease (VWD, 20% of cases), platelet disorders, factor deficiencies.[20]
  - **Endocrine:** Hypothyroidism, hyperthyroidism, PCOS, hyperprolactinemia.[19]
  - **Medications:** Anticoagulants, hormonal therapies.[19]

- **Structural:**
  - Uterine anomalies (polyps, fibroids, rare in adolescents).[19]
  - Pregnancy complications (miscarriage, retained products).[19]
  - Infections (TB, pelvic inflammatory disease, rare).[19]

TABLE 4: Etiology of puberty menorrhagia.

Category	*Examples*	*Prevalence*
Nonstructural	Anovulation, coagulopathies, endocrine	80–90%
Structural	Uterine anomalies, pregnancy complications	10–20%

Clinical Presentation

- Prolonged/heavy bleeding (>7 days, soaking pads hourly).[19]
- **Anemia symptoms:** Fatigue, pallor, dizziness.[19]
- Impact on school, sports, social life.[19]
- **Coagulopathy signs:** Epistaxis, petechiae, family history.[20]
- **Endocrine/infection symptoms:** Weight changes, fever, discharge.[19]

Diagnostic Approach

- **History:** Menstrual pattern, bleeding volume, anemia symptoms, sexual/contraception history, family history.[19]
- **Physical Exam:** Vitals, pallor, Tanner staging, pelvic exam (if structural/infectious cause suspected).[19]
- **Investigations:**
  - **Labs:** Urine pregnancy test, CBC, ferritin, coagulation profile (PT, aPTT, VWF), TSH, hormonal profile, ESR, Mantoux (TB), STI screening.[20]
  - **Imaging:** Pelvic ultrasound for structural causes.[19]

Management

- **Mild/Moderate Bleeding**:
  - **Non-Hormonal:**
    - NSAIDs (mefenamic acid, ibuprofen): Reduce blood loss via prostaglandin inhibition; avoid in coagulopathies.[19]
    - **Tranexamic acid:** Antifibrinolytic, reduces bleeding by 30–50%.[20]
  - **Hormonal:**
    - Combined oral contraceptives (COCs): Ethinyl estradiol (20–35 μg) with levonorgestrel; regularizes cycles, reduces flow.[21]
    - **Progestin-only:** Medroxyprogesterone (12+ days/cycle), levonorgestrel IUS (LNG-IUS).[21]
    - **Iron Therapy**: 60–120 mg/day for anemia.[19]
- **Severe Bleeding**:
  - **Hospitalization:** For hemodynamic instability (>1 pad/hour, hypotension).[21]
  - **IV Fluids**: Crystalloids for stabilization.
  - **IV Tranexamic Acid**: 1 g every 6–8 hours.
  - **COCs:** High-dose (30–50 μg ethinyl estradiol) every 6–8 hours until bleeding stops, then taper to one daily; avoid with tranexamic acid to reduce thrombosis risk.[21]

- **IV Conjugated Estrogen:** 25 mg every 4–6 hours (if available).[21]
- **Blood Transfusion:** For hemoglobin <10 g/dL or symptomatic anemia.[19]
- **Antiemetics:** For nausea with high-dose COCs.[21]
- **Surgical (Rare):** Suction evacuation, uterine balloon tamponade, or embolization for intractable bleeding.[19]
- **Underlying Causes**:
  - **Coagulopathies:** Desmopressin, factor replacement for VWD.[20]
  - **Endocrine:** Treat thyroid disorders, PCOS (metformin, COCs).[19]
  - **Psychosocial Support:** Counseling, family/school involvement.[14]

Flowchart 3: Algorithm for managing puberty menorrhagia.

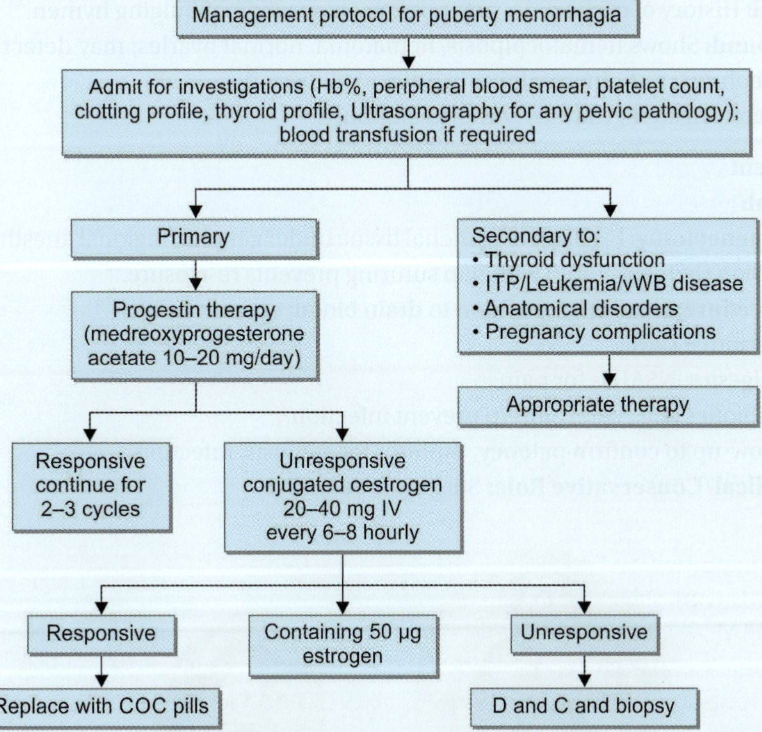

Q7–8. Imperforate Hymen: Definition, Clinical Features, Investigations, Management.

(10–20 Marks)

Definition

Imperforate hymen is a congenital anomaly where the hymen completely obstructs the vaginal opening, preventing menstrual flow.[22] Incidence is 1:1000–2000 females.[22]

Etiology and Pathogenesis

- **Embryology:** Vagina forms from urogenital sinus; sinovaginal bulbs fuse to create vaginal lumen, with hymen at the sinus-vaginal junction.[22] Failure of hymenal perforation during fetal life causes obstruction.[22]
- **Sporadic:** Not typically linked to other Müllerian or urinary anomalies.[22]

Clinical Features

- **Neonates/Infants:** Mucocolpos/hydrocolpos (vaginal secretions), bulging introitus.[22]
- **Adolescents:**
  - Primary amenorrhea, cyclic pelvic pain (hematocolposis).[22]
  - Palpable lower abdominal mass (hematometra).[23]
  - Urinary retention/difficulty due to pressure on bladder/ureter.[23]
  - Rarely, chronic cases lead to endometriosis, infertility, hydronephrosis.[23]
- **Physical Exam:** Bulging, bluish hymen; no visible vaginal opening; rectal exam reveals midline mass.[22]

Investigations

- **Clinical:** History of cyclic pain, amenorrhea; inspection of bulging hymen.[22]
- **Ultrasound:** Shows hematocolposis/hematoma, normal ovaries; may detect hydroureter/hydronephrosis or hematosalpinx in advanced cases.[22]
- **MRI:** Rarely needed, clarifies complex anatomy.

Management

- **Surgical:**
  - **Hymenectomy:** Excision of hymenal tissue under general/regional anesthesia; cruciate incision (hymenotomy) with flap suturing prevents re-closure.[22]
  - **Procedure:** Head-high position to drain blood; ensure sterility.[22]
- **Postoperative Care:**
  - Analgesics, NSAIDs for pain.
  - Antibiotics (e.g., cefazolin) to prevent infection.
  - Follow-up to confirm patency, monitor for stenosis, infection.
- **No Medical/Conservative Role:** Surgery is definitive.

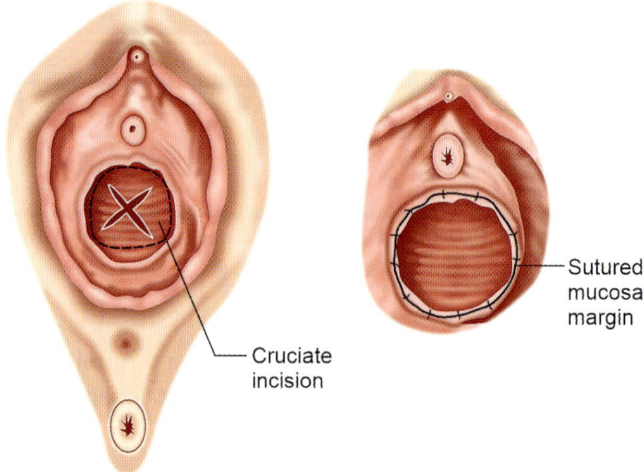

Fig. 2: Diagram of imperforate hymen and hymenectomy procedure.

Q9. Development of vagina and management of vaginal atresia/agenesis. *(20 Marks)*

Development of Vagina

- **Embryology:**
  - **6–12 Weeks Gestation:** Vagina forms from urogenital sinus and Müllerian ducts.[24]
  - **Urogenital Sinus:** Forms lower vagina; sinovaginal bulbs fuse to create vaginal plate, which canalizes to form lumen.[24]
  - **Müllerian Ducts:** Form upper vagina, cervix, uterus, fallopian tubes.[24]
  - **Hymen:** Junction of vaginal lumen and urogenital sinus; normally perforates perinatally.[22]
  - **Anomalies:** Vaginal atresia/agenesis results from Müllerian duct failure (e.g., MRKH syndrome) or incomplete canalization.[24]

Vaginal Atresia/Agenesis

- **Definition:** Partial (atresia) or complete (agenesis) absence of vaginal canal, often with uterine anomalies (MRKH).[16]
- **Prevalence:** MRKH affects 1:5000 females.[16]

Clinical Features

- Primary amenorrhea with normal puberty (ovaries intact).[16]
- Cyclic pelvic pain if hematometra (functional uterus).[16]
- Normal external genitalia, absent vaginal canal.[16]
- Associated anomalies: Renal (50%), skeletal (20%).[16]

Investigations

- **Clinical:** Normal Tanner staging, absent vaginal opening.[16]
- **Ultrasound:** Confirms absent/rudimentary uterus, normal ovaries; assesses renal anomalies.[16]
- **MRI:** Defines anatomy (vaginal/uterine absence, hematometra).[16]
- **Karyotype:** Confirms 46,XX in MRKH.[16]

Management

- **Nonsurgical:**
  - **Vaginal Dilators:** First-line for creating functional vagina; progressive dilation over months (Frank's method).[25] Success rate 85–90%. Noninvasive, patient-controlled.
  - **Counseling:** Address emotional impact, sexual function, infertility.
- **Surgical:**
  - **Vaginoplasty:** For dilator failure; techniques include McIndoe (skin graft), Davydov (peritoneal graft), or Vecchietti (traction-based).
    - **Success Rate:** 80–90% functional vagina.
    - **Complications:** Stenosis, infection.
  - **Uterine Considerations**: If functional uterus, preserve for potential fertility (surrogacy); otherwise, hysterectomy for hematometra.[16]
- **Psychosocial Support:** Counseling, support groups for body image, infertility.[14]
- **Fertility:** IVF with surrogacy or uterine transplantation (experimental).[17]

TABLE 5: Management options for vaginal atresia/agenesis.

Treatment	*Description*	*Success rate*	*Complications*
Vaginal dilators	Progressive dilation (Frank's method)	85–90%	Minimal, noninvasive
Vaginoplasty	Surgical creation of vaginal canal	80–90%	Stenosis, infection, fistula
IVF/Surrogacy	Fertility preservation, surrogacy	Varies	Ethical, access issues

REFERENCES

1. World Health Organization. Adolescent health. [online] Available from https://www.who.int/health-topics/adolescent-health. [Last accessed December, 2025].
2. Breehl L, Caban O. Physiology, puberty. StatPearls. 2023. [online] Available from https://www.ncbi.nlm.nih.gov/books/NBK534827/ [Last accessed December, 2025].
3. Klein DA, Emerick JE, Sylvester JE, Vogt KS. Disorders of puberty: diagnosis and management. Am Fam Physician. 2017;96(9):590-9.
4. Soliman AT, De Sanctis V. An approach to constitutional delay of growth and puberty. Indian J Endocrinol Metab. 2012;16(5):698-705.
5. Marshall WA, Tanner JM. Variations in pattern of female pubertal development of females. Arch Dis Child. 1969;44(235):291-303.
6. Munro MG, Balen AH, Cho SH, et al. FIGO ovulatory disorders classification system. Int J Gynaecol Obstet. 2022;159(1):1-20.
7. Blakemore SJ, Mills KL. Is adolescence a sensitive period for sociocultural processing? Annu Rev Psychol. 2014;65:187-207.
8. Latronico AC, Brito VN, Carel JC. Causes, diagnosis, and treatment of central precocious puberty. Lancet Diabetes Endocrinol. 2016;4(3):265-74.
9. Tang C, Gondal AZ, Damian M. Delayed Puberty. In: StatPearls [Internet]. Treasure Island (FL): StatPearls Publishing; 2023 Jul 31. Available from: https://www.ncbi.nlm.nih.gov/books/NBK544322/
10. Boehm U, Bouloux PM, Dattani MT, et al. Expert consensus document: European Consensus Statement on congenital hypogonadotropic hypogonadism—pathogenesis, diagnosis and treatment. Nat Rev Endocrinol. 2015;11(9):547-64.
11. Palmert MR, Dunkel L. Clinical practice. Delayed puberty. N Engl J Med. 2012;366(5):443-53.
12. Sharma L, Shankar Kikkeri N. Turner Syndrome. In: StatPearls [Internet]. Treasure Island (FL): StatPearls Publishing; 2023 (updated June 2025 in some records). Available from: https://www.ncbi.nlm.nih.gov/books/NBK554621/
13. Gravholt CH, Andersen NH, Conway GS, et al. Clinical practice guidelines for the care of girls and women with Turner syndrome: proceedings from the 2016 Cincinnati International Turner Syndrome Meeting. Eur J Endocrinol. 2017;177(3):G1-G70.
14. Klein DA, Paradise SL, Reeder RM. Amenorrhea: a systematic approach. Am Fam Physician. 2019;100(1):39-48.
15. Practice Committee of ASRM. Current evaluation of primary amenorrhea. Fertil Steril. 2019;42(2):219-25.
16. Oppelt P, et al. Clinical aspects of Mayer-Rokitansky-Kuester-Hauser syndrome: recommendations for clinical diagnosis and staging. Hum Reprod. 2006;21(3):792-7.
17. Herlin MK, et al. Mascarenhas M, Oliver J, Bhandari H. Routes to parenthood for women with Turner syndrome. The Obstetrician & Gynaecologist. 2019;21(1):43-50.
18. Eugster EA. Treatment of central precocious puberty. J Clin Endocrinol Metab. 2019;29(3):239-47.

19. Elmaogullari S, Aycan Z. Abnormal uterine bleeding in adolescents. J Clin Res Pediatr Endocrinol. 2018;10(3):191-7.
20. ACOG Committee Opinion No. 785. Screening and management of bleeding disorders in adolescents with heavy menstrual bleeding. Obstet Gynecol. 2019;134(3):e71-e83.
21. Walter SL, Channing S, Crouch NS. Heavy menstrual bleeding in adolescence. Obstet Gynaecol. 2024;25(1):45-52.
22. Abdelrahman HM, Jenkins SM, Feloney MP. Imperforate hymen. StatPearls. 2023. [online] Available from https://www.ncbi.nlm.nih.gov/books/NBK560576/ [Last accessed December, 2025]
23. Dietrich JE, Millar DM, Quint EH. Obstructive reproductive tract anomalies. J Pediatr Adolesc Gynecol. 2014;24(6):396-402.
24. Cunha GR, Robboy SJ, Kurita T, Isaacson D, Shen J, Cao M, Baskin LS. Development of the human female reproductive tract. Differentiation. 2018;103:46-65.
25. Edmonds DK. Management of vaginal agenesis. Curr Opin Obstet Gynecol. 2013 Oct;25(5):382-7.

Congenital Uterine Anomalies

Ruchika Garg

Definition: Congenital uterine anomalies (CUA) result from abnormal development or fusion of the Müllerian ducts, leading to structural variations in the uterus, cervix, and vagina. These anomalies are associated with reproductive and obstetric complications **(Fig. 1)**.

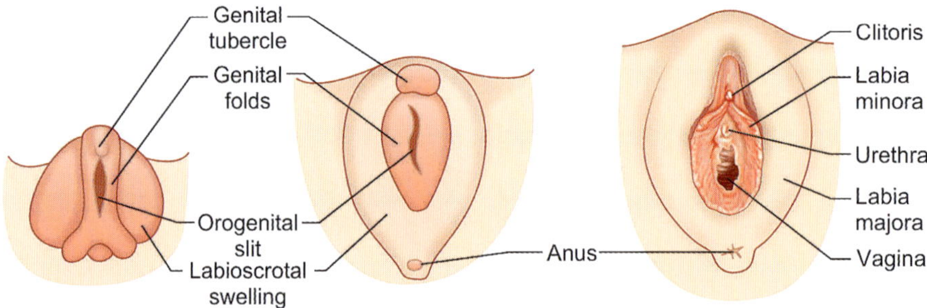

Fig. 1: Differentiation of female external genitalia.

Embryology

- Differentiation of Female Genital tract **(Fig. 1)**
- The development of the female genital tract is a complex process involving the sequential, coordinated differentiation of three primary embryonic structures: the **Mesonephric (Wolffian) ducts**, the **Paramesonephric (Müllerian) ducts**, and the **Urogenital Sinus**. This process is orchestrated by a cascade of genetic signals and hormonal influences, primarily the default pathway in the absence of anti-Müllerian hormone (AMH) and testosterone. Understanding this embryology is fundamental to diagnosing and managing congenital anomalies.

Timeline of Development

- **Embryonic Period (Weeks 4–10): The Foundation**
  - **Weeks 5–6:**
    - **Gonadal Indifferent Stage:** The gonads are bipotential. Two pairs of ducts are present: the **Mesonephric (Wolffian) ducts** and **Paramesonephric (Müllerian) ducts**.
    - Appearance **of Müllerian Ducts:** The Paramesonephric ducts begin to invaginate from the coelomic epithelium lateral to the cranial end of the Mesonephric ducts.
  - **Weeks 7–8:**
    - **Elongation and Guidance:** The Paramesonephric ducts elongate caudally. They use the Mesonephric ducts as "guide-wires", growing alongside them.

- Regression of Wolffian Ducts: In the absence of testosterone, the Mesonephric (Wolffian) ducts regress, leaving only vestigial structures (Gartner's duct cysts, epoophoron, paroophoron).

- **Weeks 9–10:**
  - **Fusion:** The caudal, vertical portions of the two Paramesonephric ducts meet in the midline and begin to fuse.
  - The fused ducts form a single Y-shaped tubular structure, the uterovaginal canal.

- **Transitional Period (Weeks 10-12): Organogenesis**
  - **Weeks 10–12:**
  - **Uterine Canalization:** The solid tip of the fused Müllerian ducts recanalizes to form the uterine cavity and the upper portion of the vagina.
  - **Absorption of the Septum:** The medial septum between the two fused ducts degenerates, forming a single, unified uterine cavity and cervical canal.
  - **Formation of the Vaginal Plate:** The endoderm of the Urogenital Sinus proliferates, forming two solid evaginations called the **Sinovaginal Bulbs**. These bulbs fuse to form the **Vaginal Plate**, which will give rise to the vaginal lumen.

- **Fetal Period (Week 12–Birth): Maturation and Differentiation**
  - **Weeks 12–20:**
    - **Vaginal Canalization:** The solid vaginal plate begins to canalize in a caudal-to-cranial direction, forming the vaginal lumen. The lumen remains separated from the urogenital sinus by the **Hymen**, which typically perforates perinatally.
    - **Definitive Epithelium:** The epithelium of the vagina and the ectocervix is derived from the endoderm of the urogenital sinus. The endometrial epithelium and the uterine tubes are derived from the mesoderm of the Paramesonephric ducts.
    - **Uterine Differentiation:** The uterine walls begin to organize into the distinct layers of the **endometrium** and **myometrium**. The broad and round ligaments are formed from the surrounding mesenchyme.
  - **Week 20–Term:**
    - **Cervical Development:** The cervix becomes distinct from the uterine corpus. The cervical glands develop, and the stroma becomes dense and fibrous.
    - **Formation of Fornices:** The cranial end of the vagina expands around the cervix, forming the vaginal fornices.
    - **Ovarian Descent:** The ovaries, which develop retroperitoneally in the abdomen, descend into the true pelvis, guided by the gubernaculum. The cranial part of the gubernaculum becomes the **ovarian ligament**, and the caudal part becomes the **round ligament of the uterus**.

- **Postnatal Period: Growth and Final Maturation**
  - **Birth:** The neonatal uterus is relatively large due to maternal estrogen exposure, with a prominent cervix (cervix-to-corpus ratio ~ 2:1). The endometrium may show a transient decidual reaction.
  - **Childhood:** The uterus becomes smaller, and the cervix-to-corpus ratio remains about 1:1.

- **Puberty:** With the onset of ovarian hormone production, the uterus grows rapidly, and the adult cervix-to-corpus ratio of 1:2 is established. The endometrium begins its cyclical proliferation and shedding.

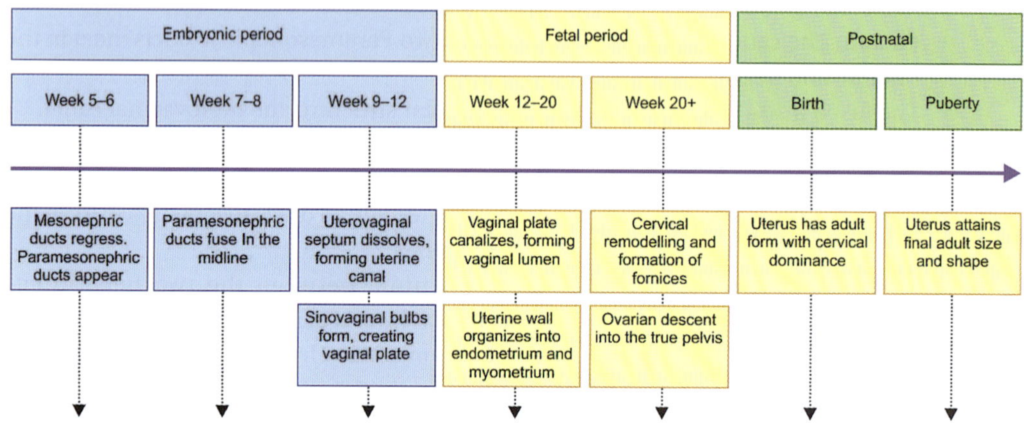

Female genital tract development timeline.

Clinical Correlates: Congenital Anomalies

- **Understanding** the embryological timeline explains the origin of common congenital uterine malformations,[1] classified by the ESHRE/ESGE system:
- **Failure of Formation:** (e.g., **U4—Hemi-uterus, U5—Aplastic uterus**)
  - **Cause:** Incomplete or failed development of one (U4) or both (U5) Paramesonephric ducts.
  - *Example:* **Unicornuate Uterus** results from complete or near-complete failure of one Müllerian duct to form.
- **Failure of Fusion:** (e.g., **U3—Bicorporeal Uterus, U2—Septate Uterus**)
  - **Cause:** Incomplete fusion of the caudal segments of the two Paramesonephric ducts.
  - *Example:* **Bicornuate Uterus** (U3) results from partial nonfusion, leading to a single cervix but a divided uterine body with an external fundal indentation.
- **Failure of Septum Resorption:** (e.g., **U2—Septate Uterus**)
  - **Cause:** Failure of the medial (uterovaginal) septum to dissolve after the ducts have fused.
  - *Example:* A **Septate Uterus** (U2) has a normal external contour but is divided internally by a fibrous septum, a major cause of recurrent pregnancy loss.
- **Müllerian Duct Development:**
  - Form at 5–6 weeks gestation from paramesonephric ducts.
  - Fuse midline to form uterus, cervix, and upper vagina by 10 weeks.
  - Canalization completes by 20 weeks, forming endometrial cavity and vaginal lumen.
  - Anomalies arise from failure of fusion, canalization, or resorption.

Classifications

Two primary classification systems are used: ESHRE/ESGE (2013) and ASRM MAC2021.

1. **ESHRE/ESGE Classification:**
   - **U0:** Normal uterus.
   - **U1:** Dysmorphic uterus (T-shaped, infantile, minor deformities).
   - **U2:** Septate uterus (partial or complete septum, normal external contour).
   - **U3:** Bicorporeal uterus (partial, complete, or septate, with fundal indentation).
   - **U4:** Hemi-uterus (unicornuate, with/without functional cavity).
   - **U5:** Aplastic uterus (absent uterus, with/without rudimentary cavity).
   - **U6:** Unclassified anomalies.
   - **Cervical Subclasses:** C0 (normal), C1 (septate), C2 (double), C3 (unilateral aplasia), C4 (aplasia).
   - **Vaginal Subclasses:** V0 (normal), V1 (nonobstructing septum), V2 (obstructing septum), V3 (transverse septum/imperforate hymen leading to hematocolpos and hematometra), V4 (aplasia).
   - **MRI** showing Hematocolpos

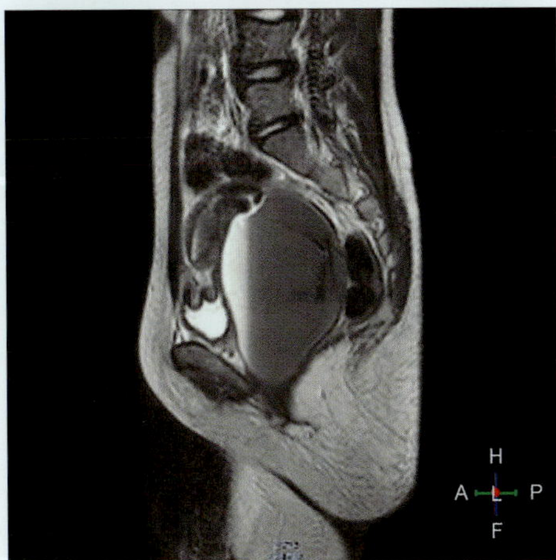

   - **Ultrasound** showing hematometra

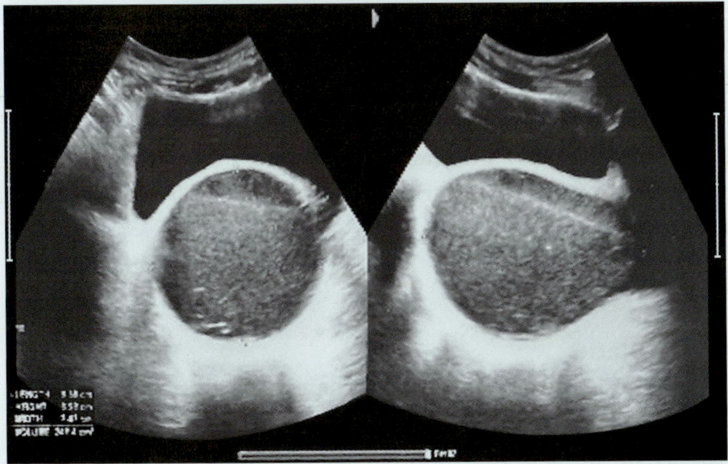

- **Cruciate** Incision to drain Hematometra

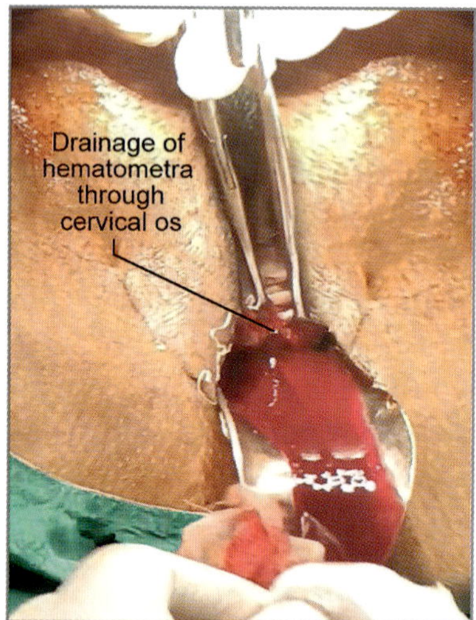

- **Unicornuate** uterus

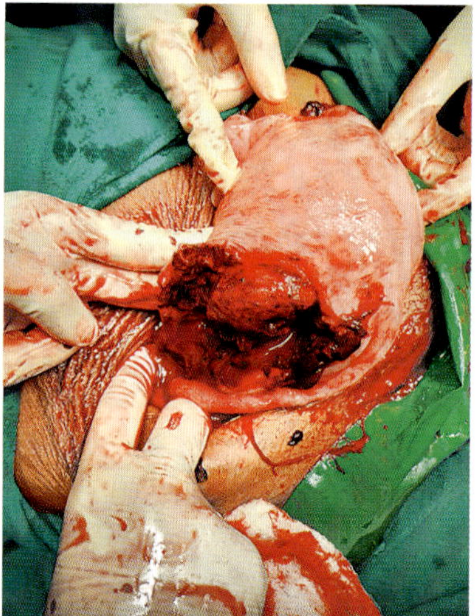

ESHRE/ESGE Classification (2023 Update—Current Standard)

This system offers a comprehensive, structured approach, classifying anomalies from the cervix to the uterine fundus.

Main Classes (U—Uterine):

- **U0: Normal Uterus**
- **U1: Dysmorphic Uterus**
  - **U1a: T-shaped** (Classically associated with in utero DES exposure)
  - **U1b: Infantile** (Uterine walls are thick, cavity is small)
  - **U1c: Others** (Any other dysmorphic cavity shape)

- **U2: Septate Uterus**
  - *Definition:* Normal fundal contour with an internal fibrous/muscular septum dividing the cavity.
  - **U2a: Partial Septum** (Septum does not reach the internal os)
  - **U2b: Complete Septum** (Septum extends to the internal/external os)
  - *Clinical Significance:* This is the anomaly most strongly associated with poor reproductive outcomes (recurrent pregnancy loss). Hysteroscopic septoplasty is the treatment of choice.[3]
- **U3: Bicorporeal Uterus**
  - *Definition:* Fundal indentation *affecting the external uterine contour*.
  - **U3a: Partial** (Fundal indentation is partial)
  - **U3b: Complete** (Fundal indentation extends to the internal os)
  - **U3c: Bicorporeal Septate** (A combination of external fundal indentation and an internal septum)
- **U4: Hemi-uterus**
  - *Definition:* Unilateral uterine development. The contralateral part can be either absent or rudimentary.
  - **U4a: With a Rudimentary Cavity** (Connected or not connected to the main cavity)
  - **U4b: Without a Rudimentary Cavity** (Contralateral horn is solid)
  - *Associated with:* High incidence of ipsilateral renal agenesis.
- **U5: Aplastic Uterus**
  - *Definition:* Absence of any recognizable uterine corpus.
  - **U5a: With Rudimentary Cavity** (e.g., Bilateral rudimentary cavities)
  - **U5b: Without any Rudimentary Cavity** (e.g., Uterine aplasia)
  - *Manifests as:* Mayer-Rokitansky-Küster-Hauser (MRKH) syndrome.

Associated Cervical (C) and Vaginal (V) Anomalies: The ESHRE/ESGE system separately classifies cervical (C0–C4) and vaginal (V0–V4) anomalies, providing a complete female genital tract description (e.g., U3bC2V0: Complete bicorporeal uterus with double cervix and normal vagina).

2. The ASRM (American Fertility Society) 2021 Classification

This system is also widely used and has been recently updated. It is more pictorial but less detailed in its subclassifications compared to ESHRE/ESGE.

Main Classes

- **Class I: Hypoplasia/Agenesis** (e.g., MRKH syndrome)
- **Class II: Unicornuate Uterus**
  - Communicating or noncommunicating rudimentary horn.
- **Class III: Didelphys Uterus**
  - Complete duplication of uterus and cervix (double uterus, double cervix).
- **Class IV: Bicornuate Uterus**
  - **Single** cervix with a fundal indentation >1 cm depth (equivalent to ESHRE/ESGE U3).
- **Class V: Septate Uterus**
  - **Normal** external contour with an internal septum (fundal indentation <1 cm depth).

- **Class VI: Arcuate Uterus**
  - Mild indentation of the fundal endometrium with a normal fundal contour. Now considered a normal variant by many.
- **Class VII: Diethylstilbestrol (DES)-related Anomalies**
  - T-shaped uterus and other structural changes.

Summary table: Key differentiating features

Malformation	*ESHRE/ESGE Class*	*ASRM Class*	*External Fundal Contour*	*Internal Division*
Normal	U0	–	Convex/Flat	None
Arcuate	(Part of U1c or normal)	VI	Convex/Flat	Mild fundal indentation
Septate	U2	V	Normal	Present (Fibromuscular)
Bicornuate/ Bicorporeal	U3	IV	Indented/Heart-shaped	Present (Myometrial)
Didelphys	U3b/C2	III	Two separate horns	Two completely separate cavities
Unicornuate	U4	II	Banana-shaped	Single cavity

Conclusion for Postgraduates

The **ESHRE/ESGE 2023 classification** is now considered the most detailed and clinically relevant system. The critical diagnostic step is differentiating a **septate uterus (U2)** from a **bicorporeal uterus (U3)**, as their management differs drastically. This distinction relies on 3D ultrasound or MRI to assess the *external fundal contour*.

Clinical Features

- **Symptoms:**
  - Often asymptomatic, diagnosed incidentally.
  - **Obstructive anomalies:** Primary amenorrhea, cryptomenorrhea, pelvic pain.
  - **Nonobstructive:** Dyspareunia (vaginal septum), infertility, recurrent miscarriage, preterm birth, malpresentation, postpartum hemorrhage, uterine rupture.
- **Associated Conditions:** Renal anomalies (e.g., agenesis, horseshoe kidney), endometriosis, endometrial carcinoma risk.[4]

Obstetric and gynecologic complications

Complication	*Associated Anomaly*
Recurrent miscarriage	Septate uterus, bicornuate uterus
Preterm birth	Bicornuate uterus, unicornuate uterus
Malpresentation	Bicornuate uterus, didelphys
Uterine rupture	Bicornuate uterus (poor lower segment)
Infertility	Septate uterus, unicornuate uterus
Cryptomenorrhea	Transverse vaginal septum, MRKH

Diagnosis

- **Noninvasive:**
  - **3D Ultrasound:** Gold standard, high sensitivity/specificity.
  - **MRI:** Comparable to 3D ultrasound, ideal for complex anomalies.
  - **Hysterosalpingography (HSG):** Limited accuracy, requires confirmation.
  - **Saline-Infusion Sonohysterography:** Visualizes endometrial contour.
- **Invasive:**
- **Hysteroscopy/Laparoscopy:** Definitive for complex anomalies.

Management

- **General Principles:**
  - Asymptomatic cases often require no intervention.
  - Treatment focuses on relieving obstruction, improving fertility, or preventing obstetric complications.
- **Specific Management:**
  - **Septate Uterus:**
    - Hysteroscopic septum resection for infertility or recurrent pregnancy loss.
    - **Techniques:** Cold scissors (preferred), unipolar/bipolar cautery, laser.
    - **Adjuncts:** Ultrasound/fluoroscopy guidance, postoperative Foley catheter, hyaluronic gel, or hormonal IUD to prevent adhesions.
    - **TRUST trial:** No significant benefit of resection versus expectant management in small sample.
  - **Bicornuate Uterus:**
    - Strassman metroplasty or laparoscopic unification for recurrent pregnancy loss (controversial, not prophylactic).
    - Avoid metroplasty in uterus didelphys (ESHRE guidelines).
  - **MRKH Syndrome:**
    - Neovagina creation (Vecchietti/Davydov methods).
    - Uterine transplantation for fertility (emerging).
  - **Pregnancy:**
    - High-risk monitoring.
    - Cervical length screening at 12 weeks, every 2–4 weeks from 16–24 weeks.
    - Cervical cerclage if cervical length ≤2.5 cm.

Bicornuate Uterus

- **Prevalence:** 0.4% of general population.
- **Features:**
  - Partial Müllerian duct fusion, fundal indentation >1 cm.
  - Associated with longitudinal vaginal septum (25%), renal anomalies.
- **Complications:** Menorrhagia, dysmenorrhea, preterm birth, recurrent miscarriage, malpresentation, uterine rupture, postpartum hemorrhage.
- **Diagnosis:** 3D ultrasound, MRI, or hysteroscopy/laparoscopy (differentiates from septate uterus).
- **Management:** Metroplasty for recurrent pregnancy loss; aggressive antenatal monitoring

Gartner's Duct Cyst

- A Gartner's duct cyst is a benign, fluid-filled swelling located in the anterolateral wall of the vagina. It arises from **vestigial remnants of the mesonephric (Wolffian) duct**, which normally regresses in female development. These cysts are typically small, asymptomatic, and discovered incidentally during pelvic examination. They are the most common cystic structure found in the vagina. When symptomatic due to size, they may cause dyspareunia, urinary symptoms, or a palpable vaginal mass, and can be managed with simple surgical excision or marsupialization

Imperforate Hymen and Cryptomenorrhea

- **Definition:** Imperforate hymen is the most common obstructive congenital anomaly of the female genital tract,[1] characterized by a failure of the hymenal membrane to canalize in utero. This results in a complete obstruction at the vaginal introitus
- **The** classic presentation, however, occurs in **adolescence** with primary amenorrhea.
- **The** obstruction prevents the egress of menstrual blood, leading to its accumulation within the vagina (hematocolpos), which can progressively extend into the uterus (hematometra) and even the fallopian tubes (hematosalpinx). This retrograde accumulation is a known cause of endometriosis.
- **Cryptomenorrhea:** This term (meaning "hidden flow") describes the condition where a patient experiences cyclical menstrual cycles and endometrial shedding, but the menstrual blood is trapped internally due to an outflow obstruction like an imperforate hymen. The patient has all the endocrine features of menstruation but exhibits primary amenorrhea.
- **Clinical Features:**
  - Primary amenorrhea in an otherwise well-developed adolescent with normal secondary sexual characteristics.
  - Cyclical pelvic pain and discomfort.
  - Bulging, bluish-tinted membrane at the vaginal introitus on inspection.
  - A palpable lower abdominal mass (due to hematocolpos).
  - Urinary retention or frequency due to pressure on the bladder.
- **Diagnosis:** Diagnosis is primarily clinical, based on inspection. Transperineal or transabdominal ultrasound confirms the diagnosis by revealing a distended vagina filled with fluid (hematocolpos).
- **Management:** Definitive treatment is a simple surgical procedure called **hymenectomy**, where a cruciate (cross-shaped) incision is made in the hymenal membrane to drain the retained blood. The excised edges are often sutured to prevent re-obstruction. The prognosis is excellent, with resolution of symptoms and normal future menstrual and reproductive function.

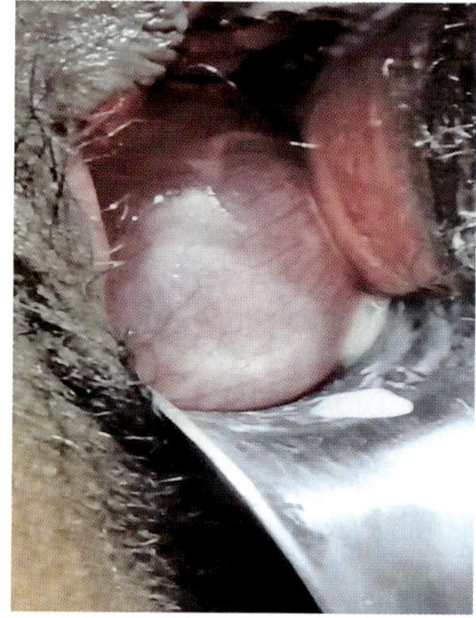

Gartner duct cyst remanent of wolffian duct.

MULTIPLE CHOICE QUESTIONS

Q1. What is the primary embryologic defect causing congenital uterine anomalies?

a. Failure of ovarian development
b. Abnormal fusion of Müllerian ducts
c. Incomplete descent of the uterus
d. Excessive endometrial proliferation

Ans. b. Abnormal fusion of Müllerian ducts

Explanation: CUA result from defective fusion, canalization, or resorption of Müllerian ducts during embryogenesis, leading to uterine, cervical, or vaginal anomalies.

Q2. Which classification system includes cervical and vaginal anomalies with uterine malformations?

a. Buttram and Gibbons (1979)
b. ASRM MAC2021
c. ESHRE/ESGE (2013)
d. AFS (1988)

Ans. c. ESHRE/ESGE (2013)

Explanation: ESHRE/ESGE classification uniquely incorporates uterine, cervical, and vaginal anomalies, unlike ASRM or earlier systems, which focus primarily on uterine defects.

Q3. A patient with a septate uterus has a septum extending to the internal os. How is this classified under ESHRE/ESGE?

a. U2a (partial septate)
b. U2b (complete septate)
c. U3a (partial bicorporeal)
d. U3b (complete bicorporeal)

Ans. b. U2b (complete septate)

Explanation: A septum extending to the internal os is classified as U2b (complete septate) under ESHRE/ESGE, as it fully divides the uterine cavity.

Q4. Which diagnostic modality is considered the gold standard for CUA?

a. Hysterosalpingography
b. 3D transvaginal ultrasound
c. CT scan
d. Plain X-ray

Ans. b. 3D transvaginal ultrasound

Explanation: 3D ultrasound is the gold standard due to its high sensitivity, specificity, and noninvasive nature for diagnosing CUA.

Q5. What is the most common obstetric complication associated with a bicornuate uterus?

a. Post-term pregnancy
b. Preterm birth
c. Macrosomia
d. Oligohydramnios

Ans. b. Preterm birth

Explanation: Bicornuate uterus is most commonly associated with preterm birth due to limited uterine capacity and abnormal lower segment development.

Q6. Which anomaly is most likely to present with primary amenorrhea and cryptomenorrhea?

a. Septate uterus
b. Transverse vaginal septum
c. Arcuate uterus
d. Bicornuate uterus

Ans. b. Transverse vaginal septum

Explanation: Transverse vaginal septum causes obstruction, leading to cryptomenorrhea and primary amenorrhea, unlike nonobstructive anomalies like septate uterus.

Q7. What is the preferred surgical technique for hysteroscopic septum resection?

a. Bipolar cautery
b. Cold scissors
c. Argon laser
d. Unipolar cautery

Ans. b. Cold scissors

Explanation: Cold scissors minimize collateral tissue damage during hysteroscopic septum resection, making them the preferred technique.

Q8. In MRKH syndrome, what is the primary fertility option currently emerging?

a. Ovarian transplantation
b. Uterine allotransplantation
c. Endometrial ablation
d. Hormonal therapy

Ans. b. Uterine allotransplantation

Explanation: Uterine transplantation is an emerging option for MRKH patients, enabling gestation of genetically related offspring, unlike other methods.

Q9. What cervical length threshold prompts consideration of cerclage in CUA pregnancies?

a. ≤1.5 cm
b. ≤2.5 cm
c. ≤3.5 cm
d. ≤4.5 cm

Ans. b. ≤2.5 cm

Explanation: Cervical cerclage is considered in CUA pregnancies when cervical length is ≤2.5 cm to prevent preterm labor.

Q10. Which anomaly is associated with a normal external uterine contour but a divided cavity?

a. Bicornuate uterus
b. Septate uterus
c. Unicornuate uterus
d. Uterus didelphys

Ans. b. Septate uterus

Explanation: Septate uterus has a normal external contour but a fibromuscular septum dividing the cavity, unlike bicornuate uterus (external indentation).

Q11. What is a common renal anomaly associated with uterus didelphys?

a. Polycystic kidney disease
b. Horseshoe kidney
c. Renal agenesis
d. Duplex kidney

Ans. c. Renal agenesis

Explanation: Renal agenesis is the most common renal anomaly associated with uterus didelphys due to shared embryologic origins of Müllerian and renal systems.

Q12. When is Strassman metroplasty indicated for a bicornuate uterus?

a. As a prophylactic measure
b. In asymptomatic cases
c. For recurrent pregnancy loss
d. For primary amenorrhea

Ans. c. For recurrent pregnancy loss

Explanation: Strassman metroplasty is indicated for bicornuate uterus in cases of recurrent pregnancy loss, not prophylactically or for other indications.

Q13. What is the main criticism of the ESHRE/ESGE classification?

a. Excludes vaginal anomalies
b. Overdiagnoses septate uterus
c. Lacks cervical subclassification
d. Ignores complex anomalies

Ans. b. Overdiagnoses septate uterus

Explanation: ESHRE/ESGE classification has been criticized for overdiagnosing septate uterus due to its objective criteria, compared to ASRM.

Q14. Which anomaly is characterized by complete absence of the uterus and upper vagina?

a. Uterus didelphys
b. MRKH syndrome
c. Septate uterus
d. T-shaped uterus

Ans. b. MRKH syndrome

Explanation: MRKH syndrome is characterized by congenital absence of the uterus and upper vagina, with normal ovaries and karyotype.

Q15. What is the recommended screening interval for cervical length in CUA pregnancies from 16 to 24 weeks?

a. Weekly
b. Every 2–4 weeks
c. Monthly
d. Once per trimester

Ans. b. Every 2–4 weeks

Explanation: Saving Babies' Lives Care Bundle recommends cervical length screening every 2–4 weeks from 16–24 weeks in CUA pregnancies to monitor preterm birth risk.

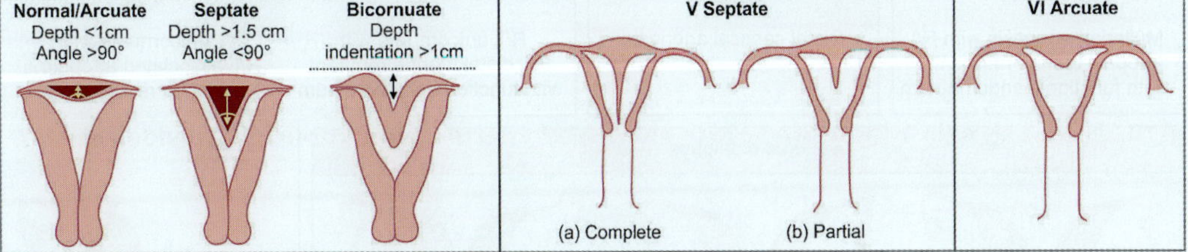

Fig. 2: ASRM classification 2016.

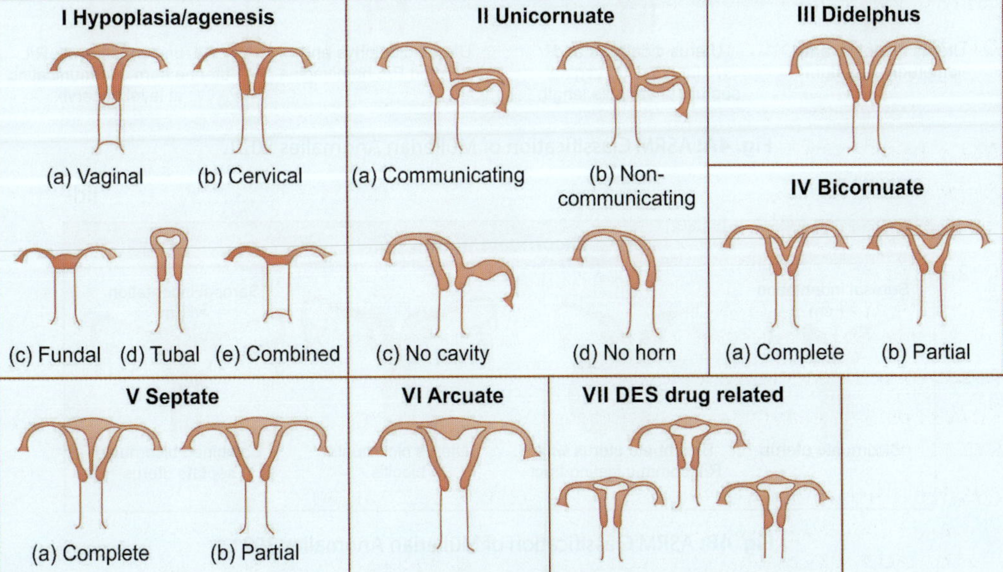

Fig. 3: ASRM classification.

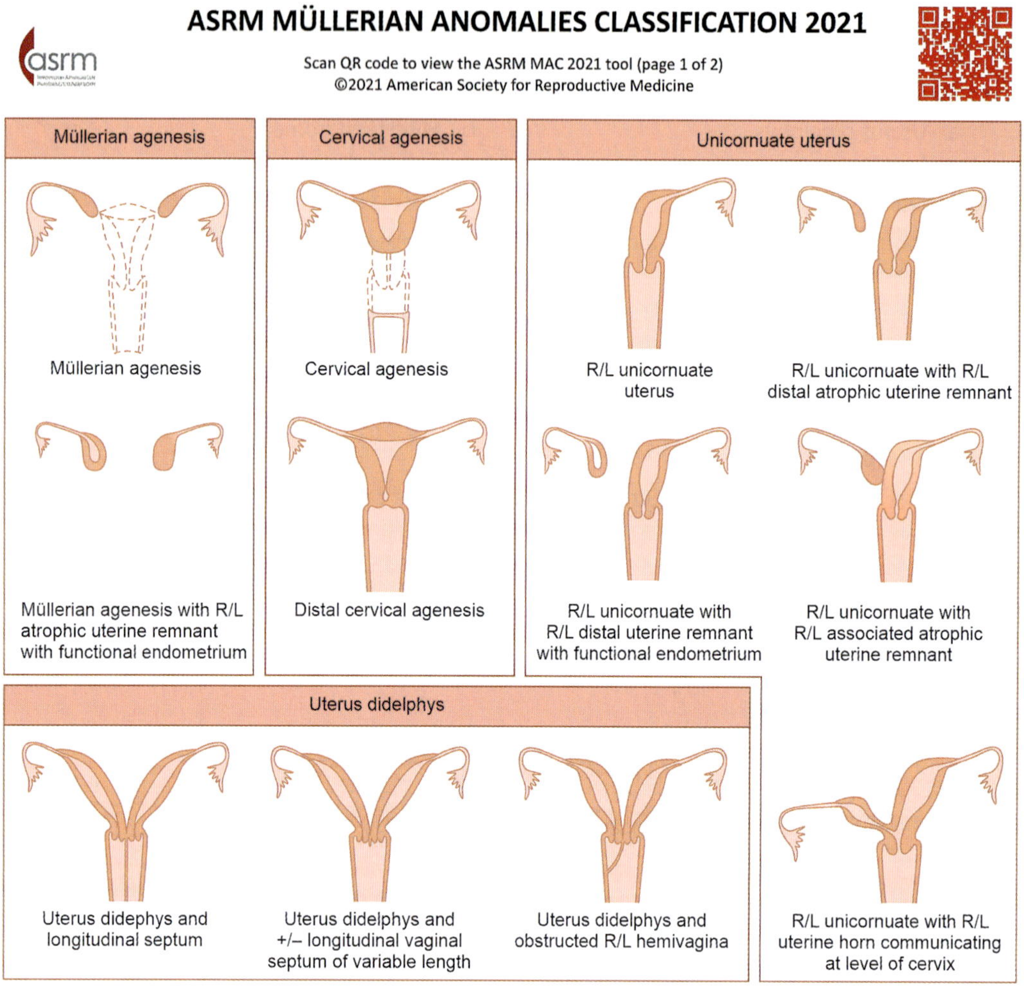

ASRM MÜLLERIAN ANOMALIES CLASSIFICATION 2021
asrm
Scan QR code to view the ASRM MAC 2021 tool (page 1 of 2)
©2021 American Society for Reproductive Medicine
Müllerian agenesis
Müllerian agenesis
Müllerian agenesis with R/L atrophic uterine remnant with functional endometrium
Cervical agenesis
Cervical agenesis
Distal cervical agenesis
Unicornuate uterus
R/L unicornuate uterus
R/L unicornuate with R/L distal atrophic uterine remnant
R/L unicornuate with R/L distal uterine remnant with functional endometrium
R/L unicornuate with R/L associated atrophic uterine remnant
R/L unicornuate with R/L uterine horn communicating at level of cervix
Uterus didelphys
Uterus didephys and longitudinal septum
Uterus didelphys and +/– longitudinal vaginal septum of variable length
Uterus didelphys and obstructed R/L hemivagina

Fig. 4A: ASRM Classification of Müllerian Anomalies 2021.

Bicornuate uterus
Serosal indentation >1 cm
Bicornuate uterus
Bicornuate uterus with R/L communicating tract
Uterus bicornuate bicollis
Serosal indentation >1 cm
Combined bicornuate septate uterus

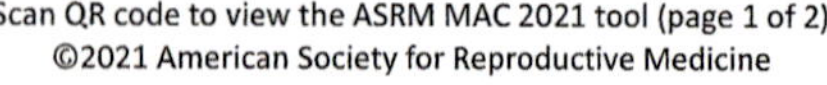

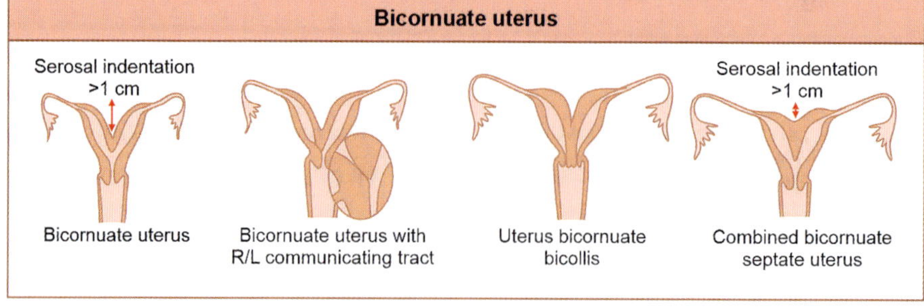

Fig. 4B: ASRM Classification of Müllerian Anomalies 2021.

Septate uterus
Transverse vaginal septum
Septum length >1 cm
Septum angle <90°
Arcuate/normal
Length ≤1cm angle >90°
Partial septate uterus
Normal/arcuate uterus
Robert's uterus
Mid vaginal septum
Complete septate uterus with duplicated cervices and longitudinal vaginal septum
Complete septate uterus with septate cervix and longitudinal vaginal septum
Complete septate uterus, duplicated cervices, and obstructed R/L hemivagina
Distal vaginal agenesis

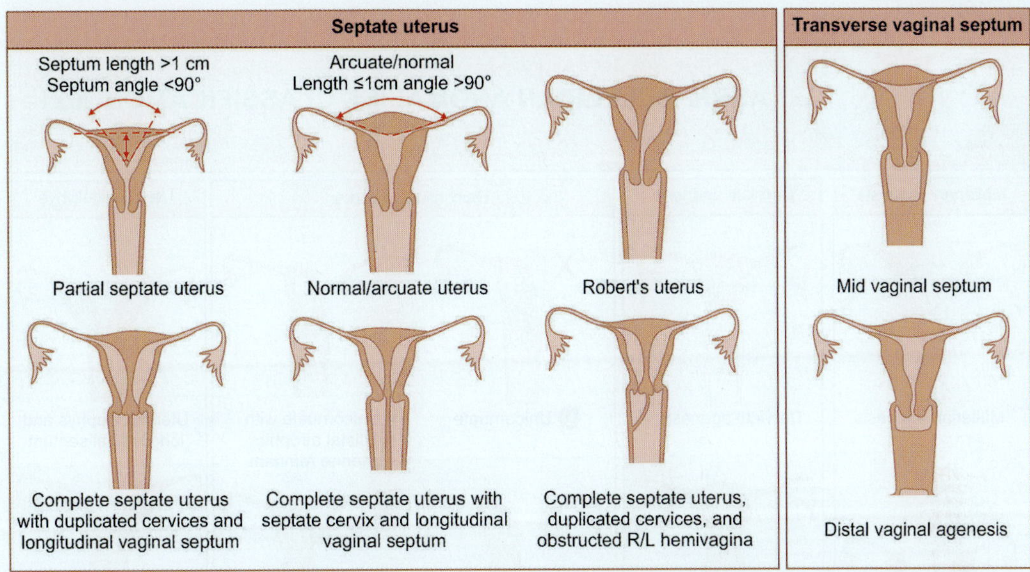

Fig. 4C: ASRM Classification of Müllerian Anomalies 2021.

Longitudinal vaginal septum
Complex anomalies
Longitudinal vaginal septum of variable length
Longitudinal vaginal septum of variable length and uterus didelphys
Bicornuate uterus with bilateral obstructed endometrial cavities
Uterus didelphys with communicating hemiuteri and unilateral r/l cervico-vaginal atresia
Obstructed R/L hemivagina and uterus didelphys
Longitudinal vaginal septum of variable length and complete septate uterus with duplicated cervix
Obstructed R/L hemivagina, hemiuterus and single cervix with separate contralateral R/L patent hemiuterus, cervix and vagina
Bicornuate uterus with R/L communicating tract and transverse vaginal septum
Obstructed R/L hemivagina and complete septate uterus with duplicated cervices
Scan QR code to view the ASRM MAC 2021 tool (page 2 of 2)
©2021 american society for reproductive medicine
Uterus isthmus agenesis

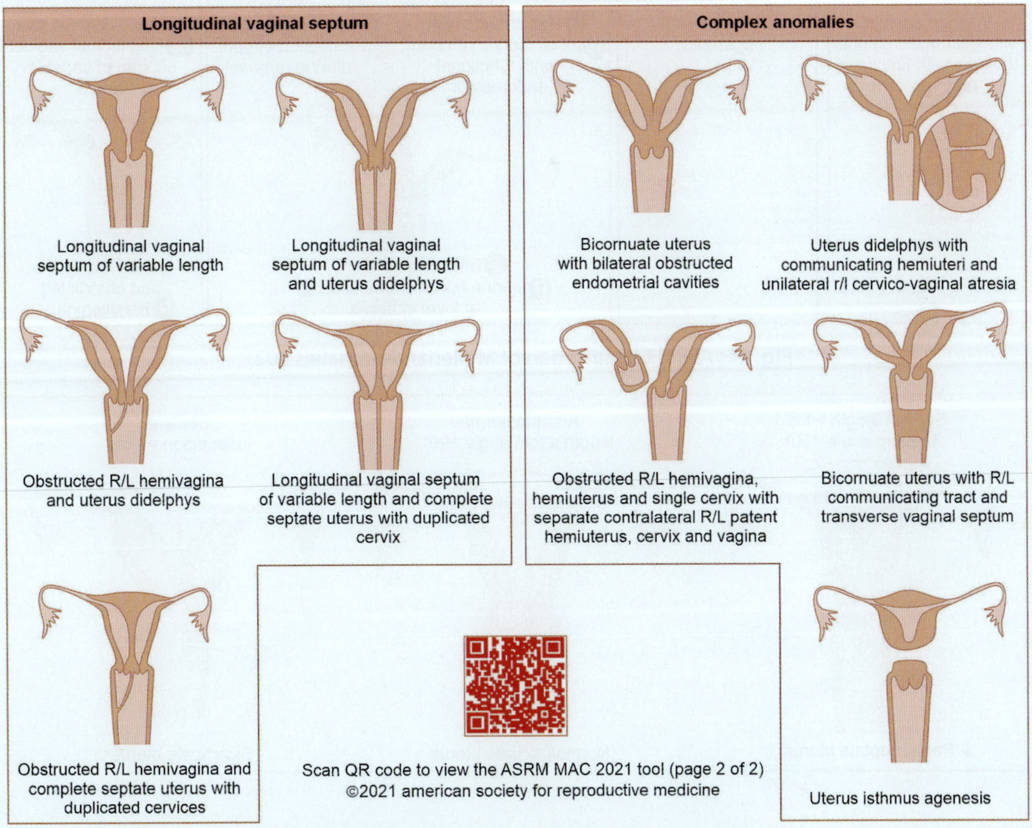

Fig. 4D: ASRM Classification of Müllerian Anomalies 2021.

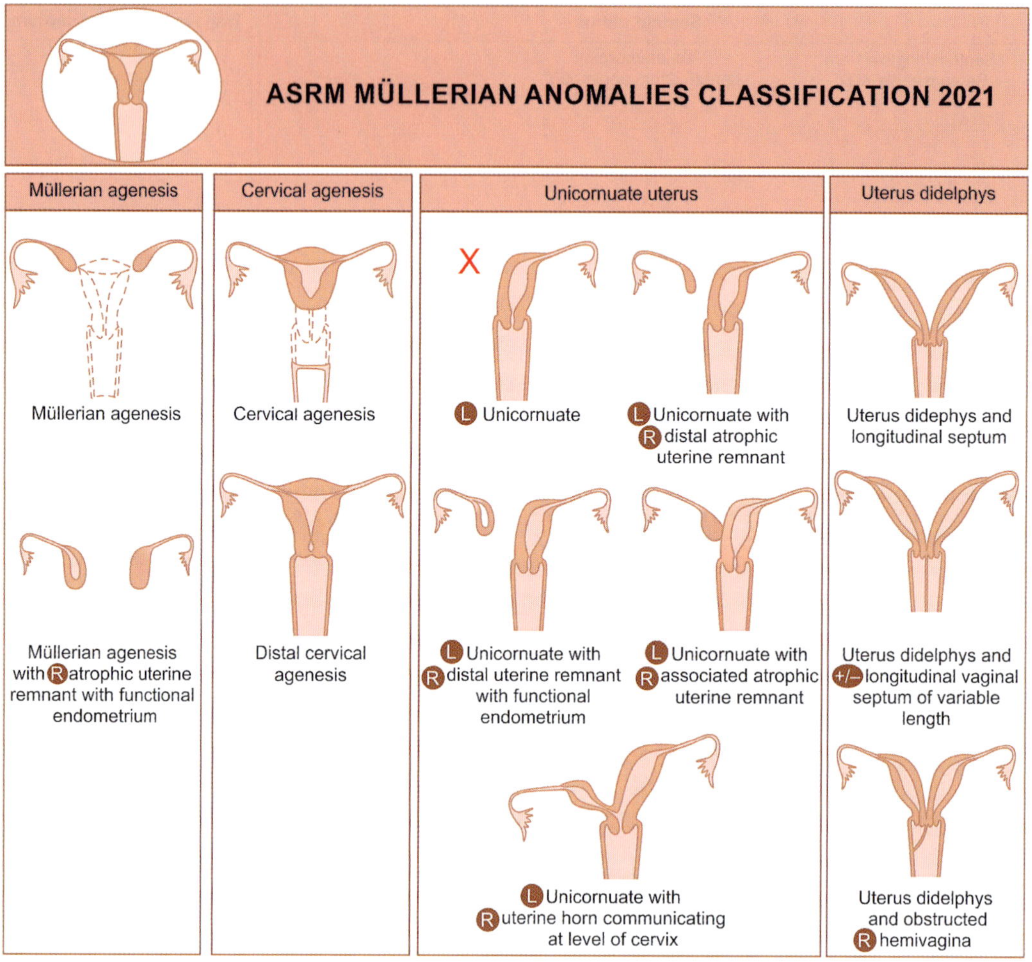

ASRM MÜLLERIAN ANOMALIES CLASSIFICATION 2021
Müllerian agenesis
Cervical agenesis
Unicornuate uterus
Uterus didelphys
X
Müllerian agenesis
Cervical agenesis
L Unicornuate
L Unicornuate with R distal atrophic uterine remnant
Uterus didephys and longitudinal septum
Müllerian agenesis with R atrophic uterine remnant with functional endometrium
Distal cervical agenesis
L Unicornuate with R distal uterine remnant with functional endometrium
L Unicornuate with R associated atrophic uterine remnant
Uterus didelphys and +/– longitudinal vaginal septum of variable length
L Unicornuate with R uterine horn communicating at level of cervix
Uterus didelphys and obstructed R hemivagina

Fig. 4E: ASRM Classification of Müllerian Anomalies 2021.

Septum length >1 cm
Septum angle <90°
Arcuate/normal
length ≤1cm angle >90°
Serosal
indentation >1 cm
Partial septate uterus
Normal/arcuate uterus
Bicornuate uterus

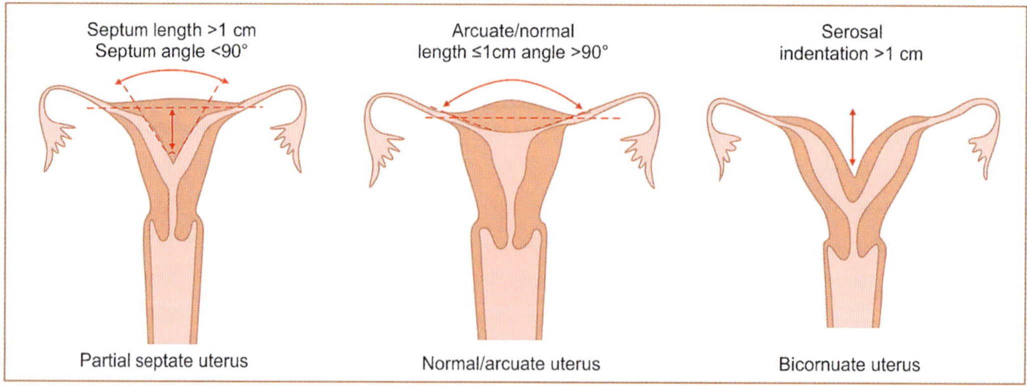

The ASRM Müllerian Anomalies Classification 2021 (MAC2021) classifies Müllerian anomalies into nine categories: Müllerian agenesis, Cervical agenesis, Unicornuate uterus, Uterus didelphys, Bicornuate uterus, Septate uterus, Longitudinal vaginal septum, Transverse vaginal septum, Complex uterine anomalies.[2]

REFERENCES

1. Theodoridis TD, Zepiridis L, Grimbizis GF. Bicorporeal uterus: Treatment options. In: Grimbizis G, Campo R, Tarlatzis B (Eds). Female Genital Tract Congenital Malformations. London: Springer; 2015.
2. Georgopapadakos N, Manoli A, Passia G, et al. Uterus Transplantation as a Therapy Method in Mayer-Rokitansky-Küster-Hauser Syndrome. Cureus. 2019;11(12):e6333.
3. Garzon S, Laganà AS, Di Spiezio Sardo A, et al. Hysteroscopic Metroplasty for T-Shaped Uterus: A Systematic Review and Meta-analysis of Reproductive Outcomes. Obstet Gynecol Surv. 2020;75(7):431-44.
4. Boehnke M, Zaretsky MV, Soranno DE, et al. Uterine didelphys with concomitant renal anomalies in both mother and fetus. J Pediatr Surg Case Rep. 2016;14:19-21

SECTION 2

Infertility

Hyperprolactinemia

Ruchika Garg, Preeti Nitsure Deshpande

Prolactin is a polypeptide hormone secreted by the anterior pituitary.

Its release is controlled by the hypothalamopituitary axis via dopaminergic inhibition. Dopamine acts as a prolactin-inhibitory factor.

There is a possible stimulatory effect with thyrotrophin-releasing hormone, gonadotropin-releasing hormone, and growth hormone-releasing hormone.

During pregnancy, secretion of prolactin increases under influence of estrogen and continues 6 months postpartum.

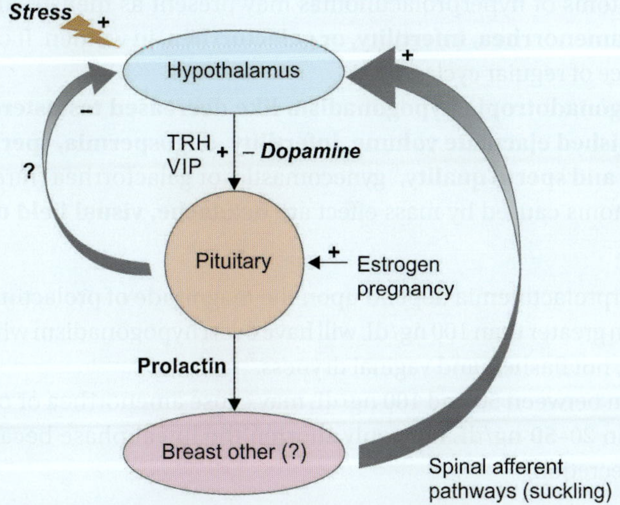

Regulation of prolactin secretion.

Prolactin is secreted as:

1. Monomeric form 80–90% which is the main active form
2. Dimeric form 8–20%
3. Polymeric form 1–5% which is called macroprolactin or big-big prolactin

Macroprolactin contains monomeric prolactin and antibody complex. Macroprolactinemia is biologically inactive and is associated with normal gonadal function. It does not cause symptoms.[1]

Serum PRL concentrations in normal adult males and females are less than 20 and 25 ng/mL respectively[2] (PRL conversion units: 1 μg/L = 21.2 mU/L [3]). Serum PRL is unaffected by food and a fasting sample is not necessary. However, diurnal variations occur and highest levels are seen in the morning.[3]

The NICE guideline recommends selective screening for patients with infertility only if there is anovulation, galactorrhea, or pituitary tumors.[4,5]

EFFECT OF PROLACTIN

High-level Prolactin inhibits ovulation secondary to inhibition LH release

It affects follicular development and function of the corpus luteum reducing progesterone levels. Prolactin may also suppress estrogen and progesterone secretion.

Moderate levels of Prolactin may or may not cause anovulation.[1]

SYMPTOMS

Hyperprolactinemia causes **galactorrhea-amenorrhea-infertility syndrome** in women as a mechanism that prolactin causes inhibition of gonadotropin-releasing hormone (GnRH) which leads to inhibition of luteinizing hormone (LH) and follicle-stimulating hormone (FSH) secretion.

Sign and symptoms of hyperprolactinomas may present as menstrual disturbances like **oligomenorrhea, amenorrhea, infertility, or galactorrhea**, in women. It can cause infertility even in the presence of regular cycles.

It causes **hypogonadotropic hypogonadism like decreased testosterone levels, libido, impotence, diminished ejaculate volume, infertility**, **oligospermia, spermatogenic arrest, impaired motility and sperm quality**,[6] gynecomastia, or galactorrhea (rare) in men.

Sign and symptoms caused by mass effect are **headache, visual field defect, or external ophthalmoplegia**.

Symptoms of hyperprolactinemia depend upon the magnitude of prolactin elevation as:

- Serum prolactin greater than 100 ng/dL will have overt hypogonadism with the presentation of amenorrhea, hot flashes, and vaginal dryness.[7]
- Serum prolactin between 50 and 100 ng/dL may cause amenorrhea or oligomenorrhea.
- Serum prolactin 20–50 ng/dL may only shorten the luteal phase because of insufficient progesterone secretion.

CAUSES OF HYPERPROLACTINEMIA

There are **physiological causes** for a rise in PRL such as **pregnancy, lactation, physical exertion or stress**. During pregnancy, PRL increases (80–400 ng/mL) in response to increasing estradiol.[2]

The causes of hyperprolactinemia are prolactin-secreting tumors which may be **Microprolactinoma or macroprolactinoma**. A microadenoma is described as having a maximum diameter of up to 10 mm (the maximal diameter of the normal pituitary gland), while a macroadenoma has a diameter larger than 10 mm.[1] **Giant adenomas** are defined as the presence of the largest diameter of the tumor being larger than 4 cm.[8]

A **microadenoma** is often visualized using MRI. Usually, the serum prolactin level is **below 200 ng/mL (4,000 mU/L)** in patients with microadenomas (less than 1 cm in size).

A **macroadenoma** that secretes prolactin is usually associated with a serum prolactin level of **more than 200 ng/mL (4,000 mU/L)**. If the macroadenoma is 1–2 cm in size, it secretes more than 200 to 1,000 ng/mL.

In **a macroadenoma more than 2 cm in size**, prolactin levels are **more than 1,000 ng/mL**.[9]

If the patient has a macroadenoma and a serum prolactin level of less than 200 ng/mL (4,000 mU/L), possibility of a nonfunctioning pituitary adenoma—pseudoprolactinoma, resulting from deprivation of some lactotrophs of dopaminergic inhibition, is there.

Also, hyperprolactinemia may be associated with other **pituitary diseases** like Acromegaly, Cushing's syndrome, infiltrative diseases like granulomas, sarcoidosis, Lymphocytic histiocytosis, and empty sella syndrome.[1]

Other causes include **hypothalamic disorders** like craniopharyngioma, suprasellar pituitary mass extension, **meningioma, dysgerminoma,** and **hypothalamic metastases weakening its inhibitory control over pituitary**. Also, **Tuberculosis and pituitary stalk section** may prevent inhibition of prolactin secretion.

Drugs causing hyperprolactinemia are antipsychotic drugs (dopamine receptor blocking agents) like risperidone, haloperidol, fluphenazine, etc., antiemetic (dopamine receptor antagonists) metoclopramide, domperidone, antihypertensive like Methyldopa, Tricyclic antidepressants, Cimetidine, Estrogens, and opiates.

Other conditions like **chronic renal failure, polycystic ovarian disease (PCOD), liver cirrhosis, primary hypothyroidism, Ectopic production of prolactin** in Bronchogenic carcinoma, hypernephromas, and ovarian germ cell tumors have been reported.[10]

PCOD is associated with raised LH and prolactin. It may be due to raised estrogen levels.[1]

Pseudocyesis may be associated with amenorrhea and elevated prolactin levels.[11]

INVESTIGATIONS

Prolactin Levels

Prolactin levels are checked after assessing the history.

Repeat blood test is needed to confirm raised levels and rule out macroprolactinemia.

Very high levels of prolactin found in macroadenomas can cause high dose hook effect where the prolactin-antibody complex formation leads to false readings. Hence, dilute and undiluted serum should be used.

Prolactin levels in disconnection hyperprolactinemia or nonfunctioning pituitary adenoma are rarely above 2,000 mIU/L 100 ng/mL).[12]

Higher levels are suggestive of prolactin-secreting tumors.

TSH levels can be done in case of hyperprolactinemia to detect hypothyroidism.

Diagnosis of Prolactinoma by Imaging

Accurate measurement of the size of the pituitary and of any tumor and its relationship to the optic chiasm and cavernous sinuses can be done by MR imaging. It can be used in cases where prolactin is **more than 1,000 mIU/L (50 ng/mL)**.[1] Cisternal herniation is also readily seen. If MRI is not available, CT scanning is also helpful but the resolution is less good, and it is less satisfactory for delineating the relationship of the diaphragm sellae (fold of dura mater) with the overlying optic chiasm. There is little place for routine skull X-ray other than for delineating bony structures.

Management

Prolactin is under predominant inhibitory control of hypothalamus through prolactin release inhibiting hormone (PRIH) which is dopamine that acts on pituitary lactotrophs D2 receptor.

Thus, **dopaminergic agonists** such as bromocriptine and cabergoline decrease plasma prolactin.

1. *Bromocriptine:* Bromocriptine is a synthetic ergot derivative which is a potent **dopamine agonist**. It has its greater action on D2 receptors and decreases prolactin release from pituitary, while at certain dopamine sites in the brain it acts as a partial agonist or antagonist of DI receptor.[13] It is also a weak adrenergic blocker.
   Additionally, it inhibits prolactin release from the anterior pituitary.[13]
   Bromocriptine is **preferred during pregnancy** because of more favorable data than cabergoline.

   Due to Inhibition of Prolactin, it restores ovulation in 80–90%, reduces size of prolactinoma in 70%, and results in pregnancy in 80–85%.[1]

   Side effects: Nausea, vomiting, constipation. Postural hypotension may be marked at initiation of therapy. Syncope may occur if starting dose is high. Hypotension is more likely in patients taking antihypertensive.

   Dosage: For initiation of therapy, dosage is 1.25–2.5 mg once a day. Dosage may be increased up to a dosage of 5 mg a day according to the patient's serum prolactin level.[13]
2. *Cabergoline:* Cabergoline is a D2 agonist which is more **potent and more selective for pituitary lactotrope D2 receptors**. It is the first-choice drug for treatment of hyperprolactinemia. Serum prolactin levels fall to the **normal range in 2–4 weeks** and in many women, it is found that they conceive within a year.

   Side effects: Same as bromocriptine but incidence is lower.

   Dosage: For initiation of therapy, dosage is 0.25 mg twice a week. Dosage may be increased up to a dosage of 1 mg twice a week according to the patient's serum prolactin level. The dose can be reduced from the typical dose of 0.25 mg twice a week to 0.25 mg once a week and then to 0.25 mg every other week before discontinuation. In patients with macroprolactinoma, it does not undermine tumor control.[14]
   It inhibits ovulation in 95% cases and causes reduction in tumor size in 80%.[1]

Side effects of DA therapy usually occur at the start of treatment and frequently disappear with continued therapy. If treatment is started with full doses or **increased** too quickly, **dizziness, nausea, and postural hypotension** may occur. To avoid such effects, DA must always be taken **during a meal**. Administration should be started at **night, with a snack, when the patient retires to bed**. Doses can be gradually increased afterward.

Cabergoline and pergolide are associated with a higher risk of **cardiac valvopathy in patients with Parkinson´s disease who receive a higher dose**.

- Before initiating treatment for hyperprolactinemia, **cardiovascular evaluation** should be performed and **echocardiography** should be considered to assess for valvular disease.

- **Dosage increases should not occur more rapidly than every 4 weeks**, so that the physician can assess the patient's response to each dosage level.
- If the patient does not respond adequately and no additional benefit is observed with higher doses, the **lowest dose that achieved maximal response** should be used and other therapeutic approaches considered.
- Patients receiving long-term treatment should undergo **periodic assessment of their cardiac status and echocardiography** should be done every 6–12 months for patients on long-term cabergoline.[1]
- Dopamine-agonist therapy is effective not only in patients with microadenomas but also in the majority of patients with **large prolactin-secreting tumors in reducing tumor size**. Moreover, emerging evidence points to the possibility of drug withdrawal after long-term treatment.

Role of Surgery may be required only in case of:
- Failed medical treatment
- Growing prolactinoma causing neurological and ophthalmic deficits
- Pituitary apoplexy where infarct or hemorrhage occurs into the prolactinoma causing visual disturbance[1]

Surgery is usually carried out through a trans-sphenoidal approach.

Radiation is rarely required in cases resistant to dopamine agonists and surgery.

Adverse effects of radiotherapy are hypopituitarism (70%), radiation necrosis (<1%), secondary neuropathy (1%), and secondary intracranial malignancy.[1]

SHORT NOTE

Q1. Management of hyperprolactinemia in infertility in females. *RGUHS (10 marks)*

Q2. Hyperprolactinemia. *MUHS (10 marks)*

MULTIPLE CHOICE QUESTIONS

Q1. What size of prolactinoma is defined as macroadenoma?

a. More than 5 mm in diameter
b. More than 10 mm in diameter
c. Less than 10 mm in diameter
d. More than 20 mm in diameter

Ans. b. More than 10 mm in diameter

Q2. All the following are physiological causes of hyperprolactinemia except:

a. Stress
b. Pregnancy
c. Lactation
d. PCOD

Ans. d. PCOD

Q3. Macroadenoma is best treated by

a. Dopamine agonist
b. Dopamine antagonist
c. Surgery
d. 5HT agonist

Ans. a. Dopamine agonist

Q4. Comparing Bromocriptine versus Cabergoline

a. Both belong to different groups so different side effects
b. Similar side effect as similar mechanism of action, Cabergoline is stronger and has more side effects
c. Similar side effects as similar mechanism of action, Bromocriptine is stronger and has more side effects
d. Similar side effects as similar mechanism of action, Cabergoline is stronger but has lesser side effects

Ans. d. Similar side effects as similar mechanism of action, Cabergoline is stronger but has lesser side effects

Q5. Which gland primarily secretes prolactin in females?

a. Hypothalamus
b. Anterior pituitary
c. Ovaries
c. Adrenal glands

Ans. b. Anterior pituitary

Q6. What is a common presentation of hyperprolactinemia in premenopausal females?

a. Weight loss
b. Galactorrhea
c. Hypertension
d. Galactorrhea, Amenorrhea, and Infertility

Ans. d. Galactorrhea, Amenorrhea, and Infertility

Q7. How does hyperprolactinemia typically affect the menstrual cycle?

a. Causes heavy, regular periods
b. Leads to amenorrhea or oligomenorrhea
c. Increases menstrual frequency
d. Has no effect on menstruation

Ans. b. Leads to amenorrhea or oligomenorrhea

Q8. Which of the following is the most common cause of pathological hyperprolactinemia?

a. Hypothyroidism
b. Pituitary prolactinoma
c. Chronic renal failure
d. Stress

Ans. b. Pituitary prolactinoma

Q9. Which medication class is a frequent cause of drug-induced hyperprolactinemia?

a. Antihypertensives
b. Antipsychotics
c. Antibiotics
d. Statins

Ans. b. Antipsychotics

Q10. What physiological condition can cause transient hyperprolactinemia?

a. Pregnancy
b. Menopause
c. Ovulation
d. Puberty

Ans. a. Pregnancy

Q11. Which hormone inhibits prolactin secretion under normal conditions?

a. Estrogen
b. Dopamine
c. Thyrotropin-releasing hormone (TRH)
d. Gonadotropin-releasing hormone (GnRH)

Ans. b. Dopamine

Q12. What imaging modality is preferred to evaluate a suspected pituitary prolactinoma?

a. Ultrasound of the pituitary
b. MRI of the brain
c. CT scan of the abdomen
d. X-ray of the skull

Ans. b. MRI of the brain

Q13. Which condition should be ruled out before diagnosing hyperprolactinemia?

a. Diabetes mellitus
b. Hypothyroidism
c. Hyperparathyroidism
d. Polycystic ovary syndrome (PCOS)

Ans. b. Hypothyroidism

Q14. What is the first-line treatment for most cases of hyperprolactinemia due to prolactinoma?

a. Surgical resection
b. Dopamine agonists
c. Estrogen replacement therapy
d. Radiation therapy

Ans. b. Dopamine agonists

Q15. Which dopamine agonist is commonly used to treat hyperprolactinemia?

a. Levothyroxine
b. Cabergoline
c. Metformin
d. Progesterone

Ans. b. Cabergoline

Q16. What is a potential side effect of dopamine agonist therapy for hyperprolactinemia?

a. Weight gain
b. Nausea
c. Hair growth
d. Hyperglycemia

Ans. b. Nausea

Q17. When is surgical intervention typically considered for hyperprolactinemia?

a. As first-line treatment for microprolactinomas
b. For large prolactinomas unresponsive to medical therapy
c. For all cases of hyperprolactinemia
d. For transient hyperprolactinemia during pregnancy

Ans. b. For large prolactinomas unresponsive to medical therapy

REFERENCES

1. Hamoda H, Khalaf Y, Carroll P. Hyperprolactinaemia and female reproductive function: what does the evidence say? Obstet Gynaecol. 2012;14(2):81-6.
2. Cleveland Clinic. [online] Available from https://myclevelandclinic.org/health/articles22429-prolactin [Last accessed December, 2025].
3. https://testguide.adhb.govt.nz/eguidemob/?gm=985&gs=3
4. NICE guideline. (2013). Fertility Problems: Assessment and treatment, CG156. [online] Available from https://www.nice.org.uk/guidance/cg156 [Last accessed December, 2025].
5. Gaillard S, Adeniran S, Villa C, et al. Outcome of giant pituitary tumors requiring surgery. Front Endocrinol. 2022;13:975560.
6. De Rosa M, Zarrilli S, Di Sarno A, et al. Hyperprolactinemia in men: Clinical and biochemical features and response to treatment. Endocrine. 2003;20:75-82.
7. Columbia Doctors. Hyperprolactinemia (prolaction disorder). [online] Available from https// www.columbiadoctors.org/treatments-conditions/hyperprolactinemia-prolaction-disorder [Last accessed December, 2025].

8. Solari D, Cavallo LM, Graziadio C, et al. Giant Nonfunctioning Pituitary Adenomas: Treatment Considerations. Brain Sci. 2022;12(9):1256.
9. Rajini Kanth R, Yatavelli KB. Prolactinoma. Treasure Island (FL): StatPearls Publishing; 2025 Jan-.
10. Dimitriadis GK, Wajman DS, Bidmead J, et al. Ectopic hyperprolactinaemia due to a malignant uterine tumor resembling ovarian sex cord tumours (UTROCST). Pituitary. 2020;23(6):641-7.
11. Tarin JJ, Hermeneglido C, Cano A, et al. Endocrinology and physiology of pseudocyesis. Reprod Biol Endocrinol. 2013;11:39.
12. Das A, Elafy O, Hayhurst C, et al. Disconnection hyperprolactinaemia and its correlation with tumour size: A study of 210 patients with histologically proven non-functioning pituitary macro-adenoma. [online] Available from https://www.endocrine-abstracts.org/ea/0070/ea0070aep700 [Last accessed December, 2025].
13. Ozery M, Wadhwa R. Bromocriptine. Treasure Island (FL): StatPearls Publishing; 2025 Jan-.. https://www.ncbi.nlm.nih.gov/books/NBK555948/
14. Paepegaey AC, Salanave S, Kamenicky P, et al. Cabergoline tapering is almost always successful in patients with macroprolactinoma. J Endocrinol Soc. 2017;1(3):221-30.

Ovulatory Factors and Infertility Assessment

Ruchika Garg, Shaifali Singh

Ovulatory issues cause 30–40% of female infertility. Menstrual history is key for ovulation prediction, with 18–20% of women experiencing menstrual dysfunction. Normal menstrual cycles range from 21 to 35 days (average 27–29 days), with variability mainly in the follicular phase; the luteal phase is typically fixed at 14 days. Regular cycles do not always guarantee ovulation, so documenting ovulation is crucial for conception.

Examination of Female Infertility

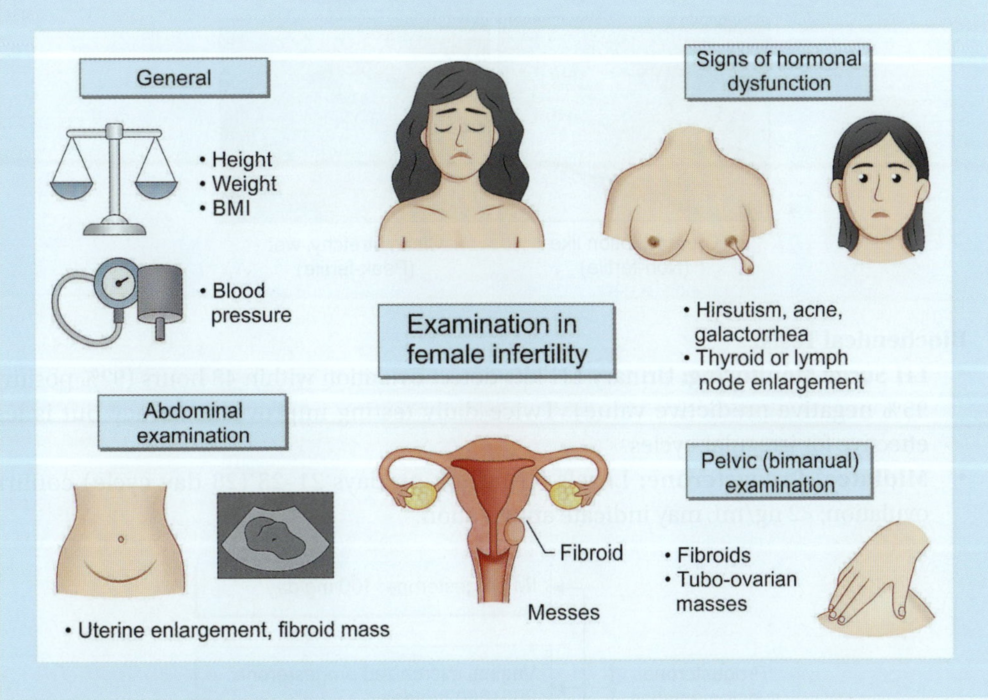

Methods to Document Ovulation

- **Clinical Methods:**
  - **Menstrual Cycle Charting:** Track menses for 3+ months; cycles of 21–35 days suggest ovulation.

- **Moliminal Symptoms:** Premenstrual symptoms (e.g., breast swelling, mood changes, midcycle cervical mucus) indicate ovulation.
- **Basal Body Temperature (BBT):** Postovulation progesterone raises BBT by 0.5–1°F for ~10 days, measured daily before activity. Smoking or irregular sleep can skew results.
- **Cervical Mucus:** Fertile mucus is clear, slippery, peaking 2–3 days before ovulation. Spinnbarkeit test assesses viscosity.

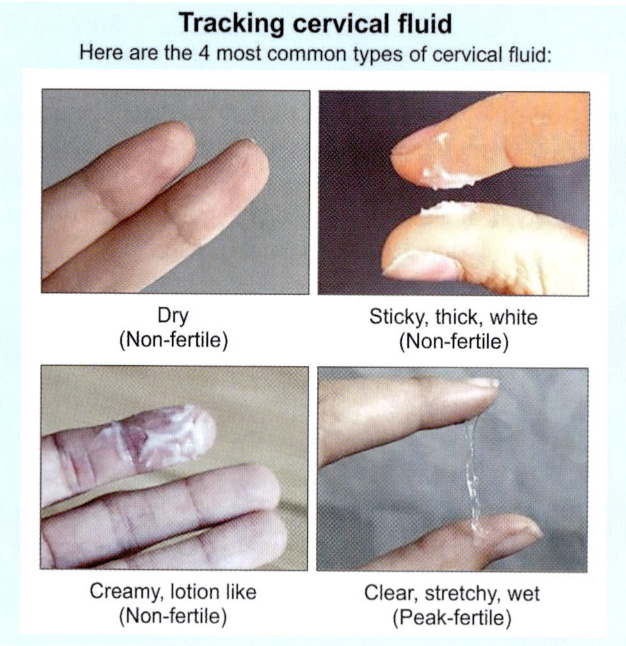

- **Biochemical Tests:**
  - **LH Surge Monitoring:** Urinary LH kits detect ovulation within 48 hours (92% positive, 95% negative predictive value). Twice-daily testing improves accuracy but is less effective for irregular cycles.
  - **Midluteal Progesterone:** Levels >3 ng/mL on days 21–23 (28-day cycle) confirm ovulation; <2 ng/mL may indicate anovulation.

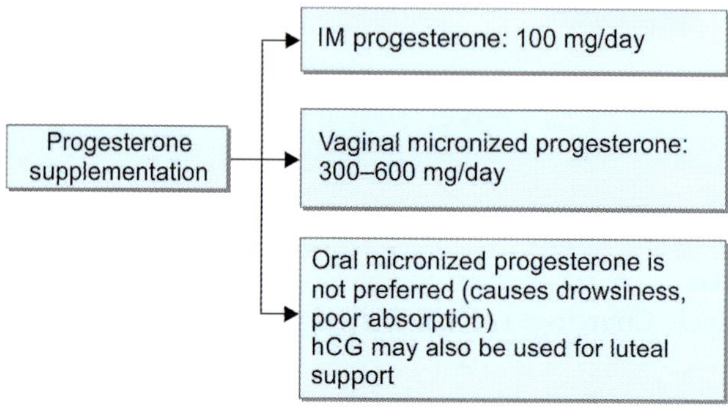

- **Pelvic Ultrasound:** Tracks follicular growth (17–19 mm in spontaneous cycles, 20–25 mm in induced cycles) and confirms ovulation via follicle collapse and cul-de-sac fluid. Reserve for complex cases.
- **Additional Methods:**
  - **Salivary Ferning:** Low-accuracy (42–53%) microscope-based fern pattern detection.
  - **Temperature Sensors:** Vaginal/underarm sensors predict ovulation with high sensitivity (89–100%).
  - **Smartphone Apps:** Combine temperature, urine, or saliva data for ovulation prediction.

Ovarian Reserve

Ovarian reserve reflects the primordial follicle pool and oocyte quality/quantity. No single test is ideal, so multiple tests are used:

- **Day 3 FSH:** <10 mIU/mL indicates good reserve; 10–15 mIU/mL is borderline.
- **Day 3 Estradiol:** <80 pg/mL suggests good reserve; >80 pg/mL correlates with poor outcomes.
- **Anti-Müllerian Hormone (AMH):** Declines with age; <0.5 ng/mL indicates poor reserve, >3.5 ng/mL risks overstimulation.
- **Antral Follicle Count (AFC):** <4 follicles (2–10 mm) predicts poor IVF response.
- **Clomiphene Citrate Challenge Test (CCT):** FSH >10 mIU/mL on day 3 or 10 suggests poor reserve.

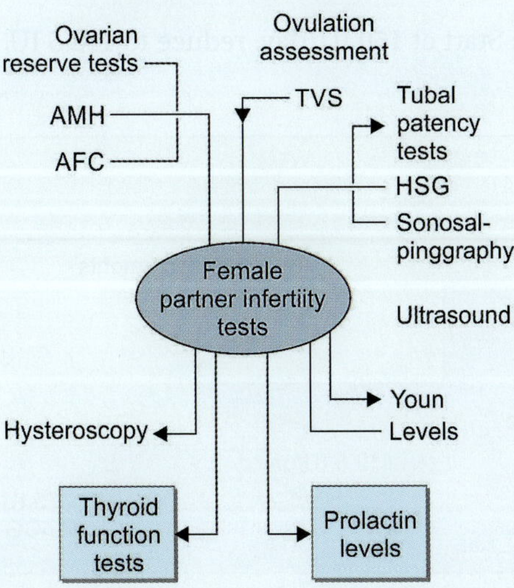

Gonadotropins for Ovulation Induction

Used for anovulatory PCOS or hypogonadotropic women resistant to oral agents, gonadotropins achieve 43–83% ovulation and 21–29% pregnancy rates. Preparations include hMG (75 IU FSH + 75 IU LH) and recombinant FSH/LH, administered subcutaneously.

Contraindications

Primary ovarian failure, uncontrolled thyroid/adrenal issues, pituitary tumors, undiagnosed uterine bleeding, ovarian cysts (non-PCOS), hypersensitivity, sex hormone-dependent tumors, pregnancy.

Protocols

- **Low-Dose Step-Up:** Start at 37.5–75 IU/day, increase by 50% after 7 days if no follicle >10 mm, up to 225 IU/day.

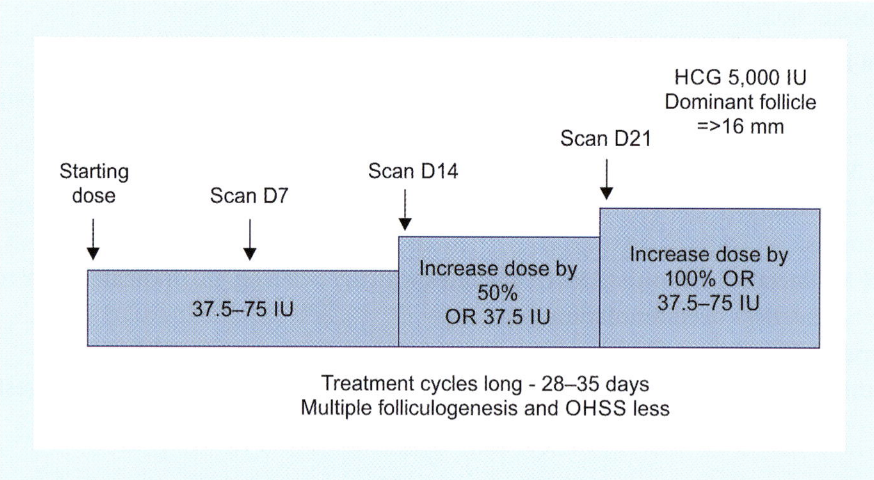

- **Low-Dose Step-Down:** Start at 150 IU/day, reduce to 112.5 IU, then 75 IU when a dominant follicle appears.

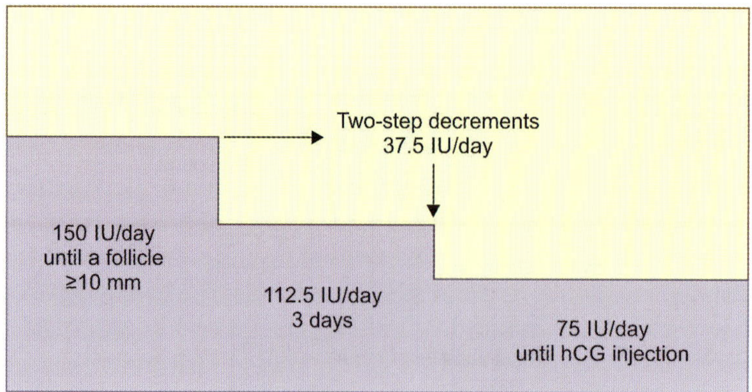

Monitoring: Use transvaginal ultrasound to track follicles. Administer hCG when a follicle reaches 11 mm or estradiol is 200 pg/mL. Stop if ≥3 follicles >15 mm to avoid multiple pregnancies or ovarian hyperstimulation syndrome (OHSS).

Outcomes: Similar live birth rates to clomiphene, but PCOS patients face higher risks of multiple gestation (36%), OHSS (4.6%), and cycle cancellation (10%).

Adjuvant Treatment: GnRH agonists suppress pituitary gonadotropins in IVF to prevent premature LH surges, optimizing follicular maturation.

Ovarian Hyperstimulation Syndrome (OHSS)

OHSS is a serious complication of ovulation induction in assisted reproductive technologies (ART), characterized by enlarged, hyperstimulated ovaries.

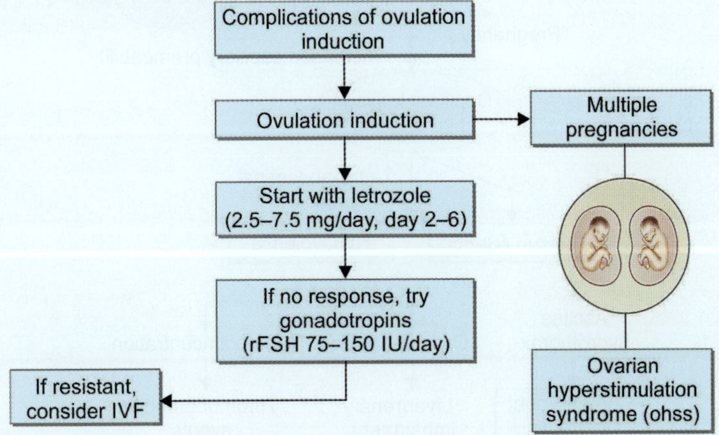

Risk Factors:

- Primary: Young age, low body weight, PCOS, high gonadotropin doses, prior OHSS.
- Secondary: >20 follicles (>10 mm), high/rapidly rising estradiol (>2,500 pg/mL), many oocytes retrieved, hCG use for luteal support, pregnancy, AMH >3.3 ng/mL, AFC >8.

Pathogenesis: High-dose gonadotropins disrupt normal menstrual cycle feedback, causing multiple follicle development. hCG administration for oocyte maturation triggers excessive VEGF and vasoactive substance production, increasing vascular permeability. This leads to:

- Massive luteinization of granulosa cells.
- Perifollicular neovascularization and fluid leakage into the peritoneal cavity.
- Fluid shift to the third space, causing hypovolemia, edema, ascites, hydrothorax, or pericardial effusion.
- Potential cardiac, renal, pulmonary, liver, or coagulation dysfunction.
- Pregnancy exacerbates OHSS via placental hCG.

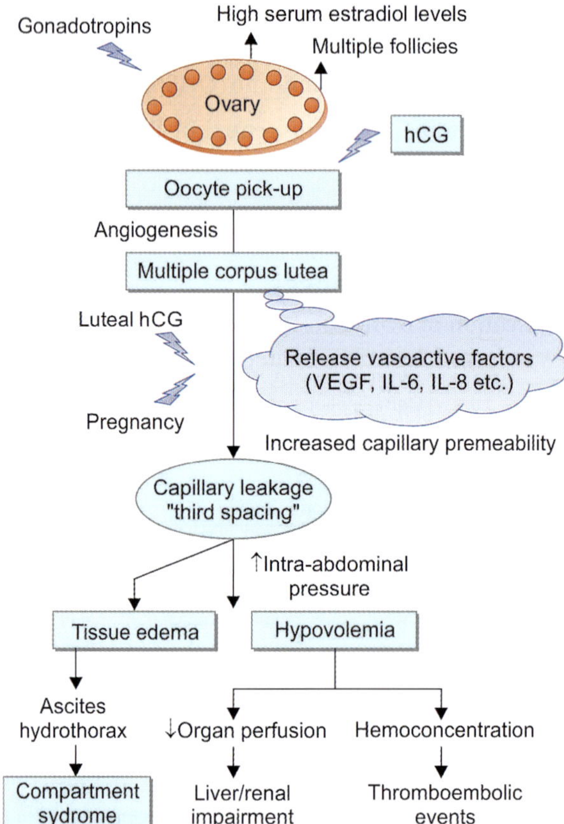

Clinical Features: Symptoms include abdominal pain/distension, rapid weight gain, ascites, dyspnea, oliguria, and hemodynamic instability due to enlarged ovaries and fluid shifts. Early OHSS (<7 days post-hCG) is milder; late OHSS (≥9 days) is often more severe due to pregnancy-related hCG.

Complications: Life-threatening issues include renal failure, ARDS, ovarian rupture, thromboembolism, and ovarian torsion.

Classification:

- **Mild:** Ovarian enlargement, mild abdominal discomfort, nausea; no biochemical abnormalities.
- **Moderate/Severe/Critical:** Escalating symptoms (e.g., severe pain, tense ascites, organ dysfunction).
- **Self-limiting:** No major complications.
- **With comorbidities:** Includes thromboembolism, ARDS, cerebral edema, or organ failure.

Differential Diagnosis: Ectopic pregnancy, ovarian cyst rupture, ovarian torsion.

Prevention:

- Identify at-risk patients.
- Use individualized stimulation protocols.
- Replace hCG with GnRH agonists for oocyte maturation.

Management:

- **Mild:** Outpatient, symptomatic relief (analgesics), activity restriction, monitor for worsening.
- **Moderate:** Hospitalization, 1–2 L/day oral fluids, no diuretics, monitor weight/abdominal circumference/urine output, lab tests (CBC, electrolytes, creatinine, albumin, liver/coagulation) every 48 hours, drain ascites (2–4 L) if needed, consider cabergoline (0.5 mg/day) for prevention.
- **Severe/Critical:** Hospitalize if hematocrit >55%, leukocytes >25,000/L, creatinine >1.6 mg/dL, or severe symptoms (e.g., oliguria, dyspnea, hypotension). Provide IV fluids, thromboprophylaxis, antibiotics for peritonitis, and ICU for critical cases. Monitor fluid balance, weight, labs, and imaging daily. Resolution signs: normalized hematocrit, reduced ascites, improved symptoms.

Unexplained Infertility

Unexplained infertility is diagnosed when no cause is found after 12 months (or 6 months if >35 years) of trying to conceive, despite normal ovulation, tubal patency, uterine cavity, ovarian reserve, and semen analysis.

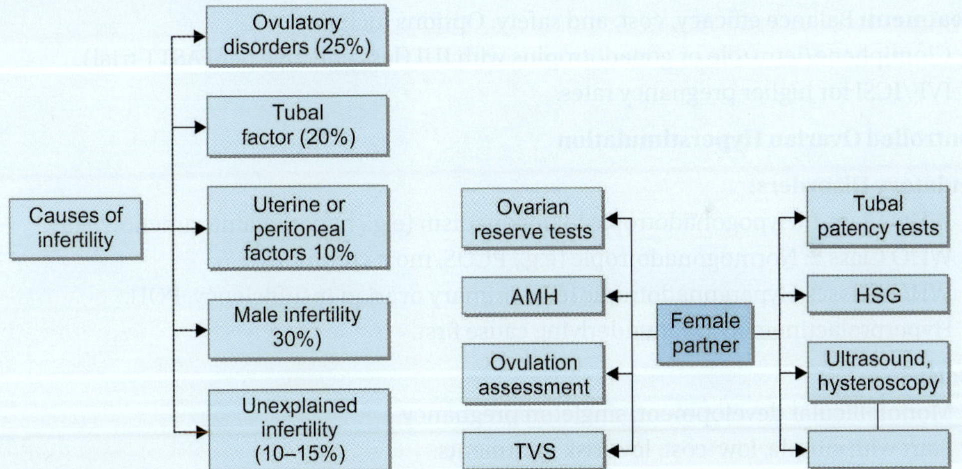

Proposed Causes:

- **Luteinized Unruptured Follicle Syndrome:** Follicle luteinizes without oocyte release, treatable with IVF.
- **Immunological Factors:** Th1:Th2 imbalance impairs endometrial receptivity; no validated biomarkers. Untreated celiac disease, antiphospholipid/antithyroid antibodies, or antisperm antibodies may contribute.
- **Infections:** Subclinical chlamydia, ureaplasma, or mycoplasma; consider doxycycline (100 mg BID, 4 weeks). Chronic endometritis may cause implantation failure.
- **Undiagnosed Pelvic Pathology:** Hysterolaparoscopy to check for adhesions or endometriosis.
- **Occult Factors:** Sperm DNA damage, zona hardening, mitochondrial dysfunction, or aberrant spindle formation.
- **Genetic Factors:** Requires further research.

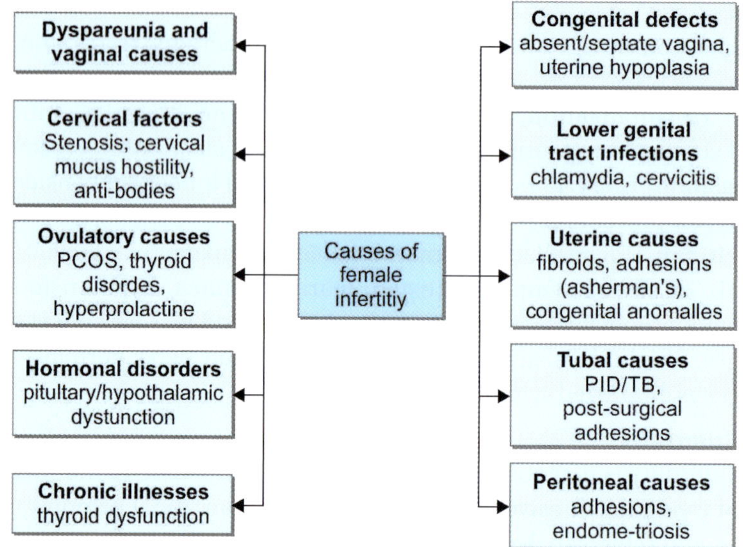

Treatment: Balance efficacy, cost, and safety. Options include:

- Clomiphene/letrozole or gonadotropins with IUI (less effective per FASTT trial).
- IVF/ICSI for higher pregnancy rates.

Controlled Ovarian Hyperstimulation

Ovulatory Disorders:

- WHO Class 1: Hypogonadotropic hypogonadism (e.g., hypothalamic amenorrhea).
- WHO Class 2: Normogonadotropic (e.g., PCOS, most common).
- WHO Class 3: Hypergonadotropic (e.g., primary ovarian insufficiency, POI).
- Hyperprolactinemia: Treat underlying cause first.

Goals:

- Monofollicular development, singleton pregnancy.
- Start with simple, low-cost, low-risk treatments.
- Minimize OHSS and multiple pregnancies.

Approach:

- **Hypothalamic Amenorrhea:** Pulsatile GnRH (first-line) or gonadotropins; clomiphene ineffective.
- **PCOS:** Lifestyle changes, weight loss, letrozole (first-line, higher live birth rates than clomiphene), or gonadotropins.
- **POI:** Ovulation induction ineffective; offer donor oocyte IVF.
- **Hyperprolactinemia:** Treat cause, then induce ovulation.

Ovulation Induction Agents:

- **Letrozole** (Aromatase Inhibitor):
  - Blocks estrogen synthesis, increasing FSH.
  - Dose: 2.5-7.5 mg/day, days 3–7 or 5–9.
  - Fewer endometrial side effects, higher live birth rates than clomiphene.

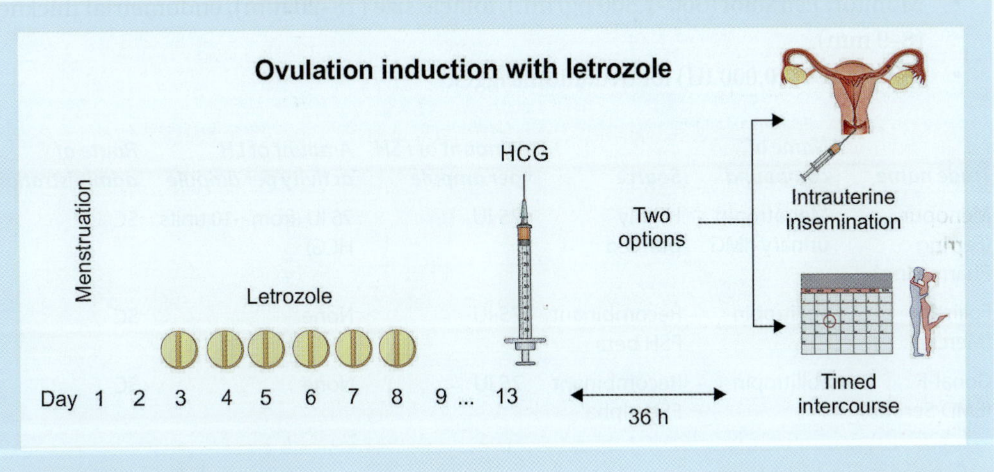

- **Clomiphene Citrate (SERM):**
  - Blocks estrogen receptors, increasing GnRH/FSH/LH.
  - Dose: 50–150 mg/day (up to 250 mg), days 1–5; stair-step dosing if no response.
  - Antiestrogenic effects on endometrium/cervix lower pregnancy rates.
- **Pulsatile GnRH:**
  - For hypothalamic amenorrhea; IV/SC via pump, 2.5–5 μg/pulse every 60–90 min.
  - 80% pregnancy rate after 6 cycles, 5% multiples, 30% miscarriage risk.
- **GnRH Agonists** (e.g., Buserelin, Nafarelin):
  - For gonadotropin-resistant cases or premature LH surge.
  - Downregulate pituitary; 75% ovulation, 25% pregnancy rate.
- Mechanism of action: GnRH analogs used in short or long protocol, mainly for down-regulation of pituitary by desensitization of pituitary GnRH receptors. Initial phase flare effect is seen which last for 2–3 weeks, where pituitary is stimulated to secrete gonadotropin. Adequate pituitary suppression is achieved when serum estradiol level is less than 10 pg/mL and FSH level is less than 10 mIU/mL. Then stimulation is done by administering gonadotropins.
- **GnRH Antagonists** (e.g., Cetrorelix):
  - Block pituitary GnRH receptors without flare; used in short protocols.

- **Gonadotropins:**
    - For WHO Class 1, clomiphene/letrozole failures, unexplained infertility, or older women.
    - Preparations: hMG, uFSH, rFSH, rLH (75 IU FSH/LH, subcutaneous).
    - Dose: 75 IU/day from days 2–5, adjust for 7–10 days.
    - Monitor: Estradiol (500–1,500 pg/mL), follicle size (18–20 mm), endometrial thickness (8–9 mm).
    - hCG (5,000–10,000 IU) for ovulation trigger.

Trade name	*Name of compound*	*Source*	*Amount of FSH per ampule*	*Amount of LH activity per ampule*	*Route of administration*
Menopur (Ferring Pharma Inc.)	Menotropin urinary hMG	Highly purified	75 IU	75 IU (from ~10 units HCG)	SC
Follistim (Merck)	Follitropin	Recombinant FSH beta	75 IU	None	SC
Gonal-F (EMD Serono)	Follitropin	Recombinant FSH alpha	75 IU	None	SC

Adjuvant Therapies:

- Metformin for hyperinsulinemia in PCOS.
- Dopamine agonists for hyperprolactinemia.

1. Most reliable method to document ovulation is

a. BBT
b. LH-KIT
c. Cervical mucus
d. USG

Ans: d. USG

Dose schedule:

- Stimulation is started any time from D2–D5 of the cycle and is continued for 7–10 days depending upon the response
- HMG stimulates follicular growth with a variable dose schedule starting with a low dose (75 IU IM/day)
- Follicular growth is monitored with serum estradiol estimation and follicular number and size are measured by TVS:
    - Serum estradiol 500–1,500 pg/mL
    - Follicular size 18–20 mm
    - Endometrial thickness 8–9 mm
- HCG 5,000–10,000 IU/IM administered for ovulation trigger

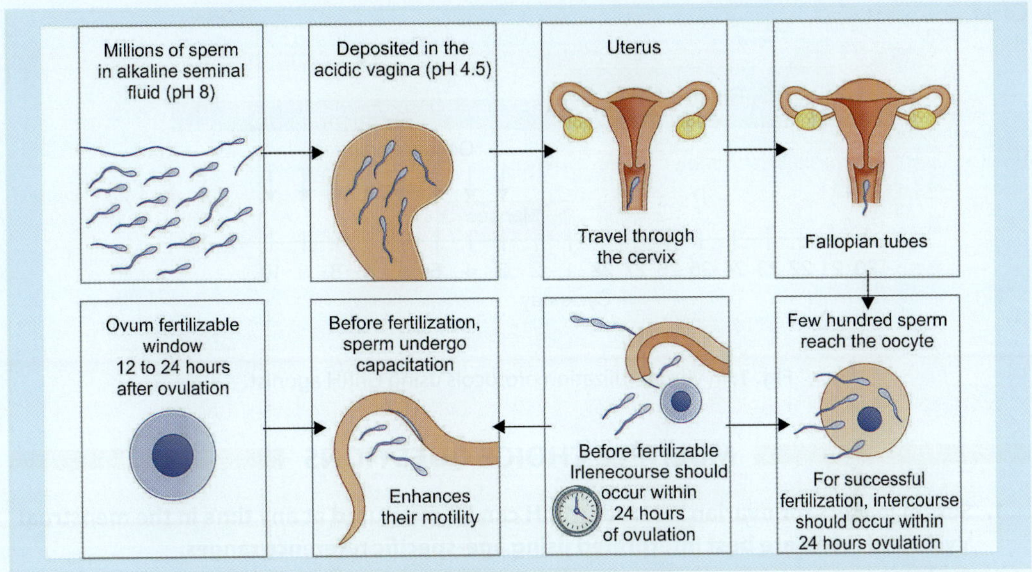
Millions of sperm in alkaline seminal fluid (pH 8)
Deposited in the acidic vagina (pH 4.5)
Uterus
Travel through the cervix
Fallopian tubes
Few hundred sperm reach the oocyte
For successful fertilization, intercourse should occur within 24 hours ovulation
Before fertilizable Irlenecourse should occur within 24 hours of ovulation
Before fertilization, sperm undergo capacitation
Enhances their motility
Ovum fertilizable window 12 to 24 hours after ovulation

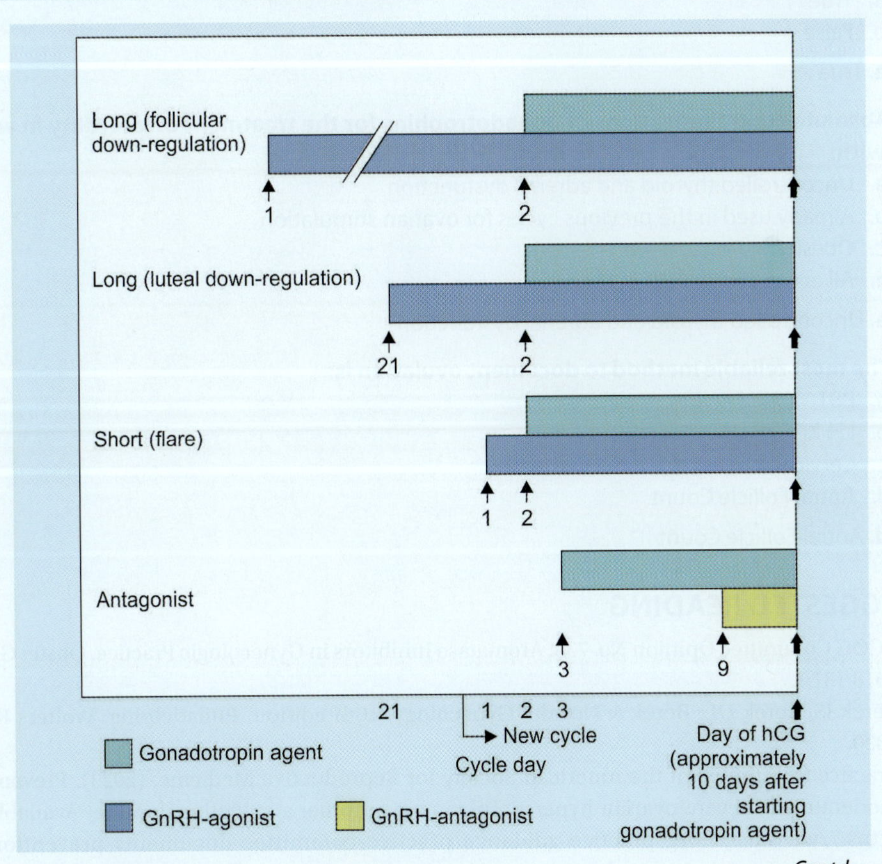
Long (follicular down-regulation)
1
2
Long (luteal down-regulation)
21
2
Short (flare)
1
2
Antagonist
3
9
21
1
2
3
New cycle
Cycle day
Day of hCG (approximately 10 days after starting gonadotropin agent)
Gonadotropin agent
GnRH-agonist
GnRH-antagonist

Contd...

Contd...

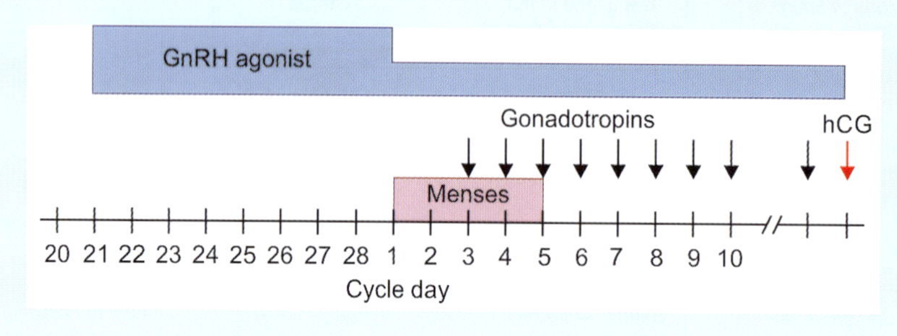

Fig. 1: In vitro fertilization protocols using GnRH agonist.

MULTIPLE CHOICE QUESTIONS

1. **Serum makers for ovarian reserve—AMH can be measured at any time in the menstrual cycle and levels are best interpreted using age-specific reference ranges.**
   a. True
   b. False

Ans. a. True

2. **Absolute contraindications of gonadotrophins for the treatment of infertility in women with:**
   a. Uncontrolled thyroid and adrenal dysfunction
   b. Already used in the previous cycles for ovarian stimulation
   c. Obesity
   d. All of the above

Ans. a. Uncontrolled thyroid and adrenal dysfunction

3. **The most reliable method to document ovulation is:**
   a. BBT
   b. LH-KIT
   c. Cervical mucus
   d. Antral Follicle Count

Ans. d. Antral Follicle Count

SUGGESTED READING

1. ACOG Committee Opinion No. 738: Aromatase Inhibitors in Gynecologic Practice. Obstet Gynecol. 2018;131:1.
2. Berek JS, Berek DL. Berek & Novak's Gynecology, 16th edition. Philadelphia: Wolters Kluwer; 2020.
3. Practice Committee of the American Society for Reproductive Medicine. (2023). Prevention of moderate and severe ovarian hyperstimulation syndrome: a guideline. [online] Available from https://www.asrm.org/practice-guidance/practice-committee-documents/prevention-and-treatment-of-moderate-and-severe-ovarian-hyperstimulation-syndrome-a-guideline/ [Last accessed December, 2025=

4. Royal College of Obstetricians and Gynaecologists. The management of ovarian hyperstimulation syndrome (Green-top Guidelines no 5). [online] Available from https://www.rcog.org.uk/guidance/browse-all-guidance/green-top-guidelines/the-management-of-ovarian-hyperstimulation-syndrome-green-top-guideline-no-5/ [Last accessed December, 2025]
5. Seshadri L. Essentials of Gynecology, 3rd edition. Gurgaon: Wolters Kluwer; 2021.
6. Taylor HS, Pal L, Seli E. South Asian edition of Speroff's Clinical Gynecologic Endocrinology and Infertility, 9th edition. Philadelphia: Wolters Kluwer; 2019.

Ovarian Hyperstimulation Syndrome

Shreedevi Tanksale, Tejal Poddar

LONG QUESTIONS AND ANSWERS

1. What is OHSS? Define OHSS. What is the pathophysiology of OHSS? What are the symptoms and signs of OHSS?

(DNB Oct 23, April 23)

What is OHSS?

Ovarian hyperstimulation syndrome (OHSS) is a common and severe iatrogenic complication of ovarian hyperstimulation. The syndrome consists of enlargement of the ovaries and a shift of fluid to the third space from intravascular compartment due to either increased capillary permeability or ovarian neoangiogenesis.

With the aim of increasing the number of oocytes available for fertilization, superovulation protocols were introduced. These protocols introduced a new iatrogenic and serious complication of ovarian hyperstimulation. With severe morbidity and mortality associated with OHSS, measures to reduce the incidence and management protocols were developed for OHSS.

What is the pathophysiology of OHSS?

The exact pathophysiology of OHSS is uncertain. But the single most important factor responsible for OHSS is the administration of human chorionic gonadotropin (hCG).

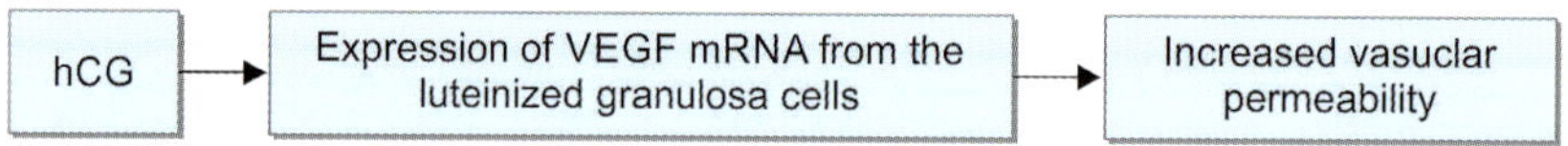

Various vasoactive substances such as interleukins, tumor necrosis factor-α, endothelin-1, and **vascular endothelial growth factor (VEGF)** secreted by the ovaries have been implicated in **increased vascular permeability**.

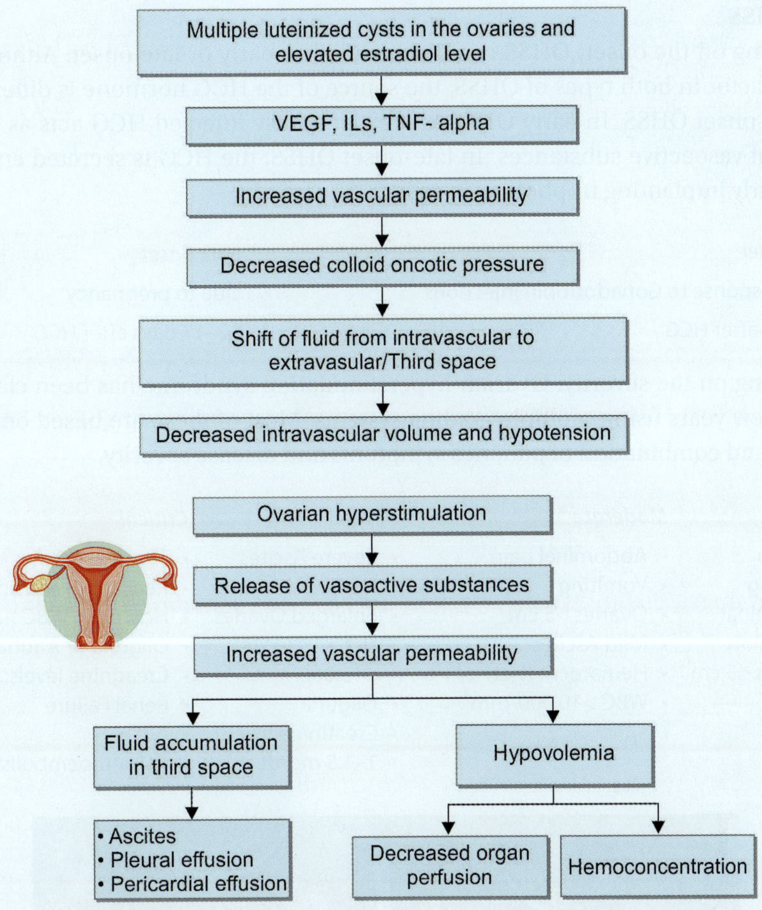

The movement of fluid into the third space causes pericardiac effusion, pleural effusion, ascites and dependent edema.

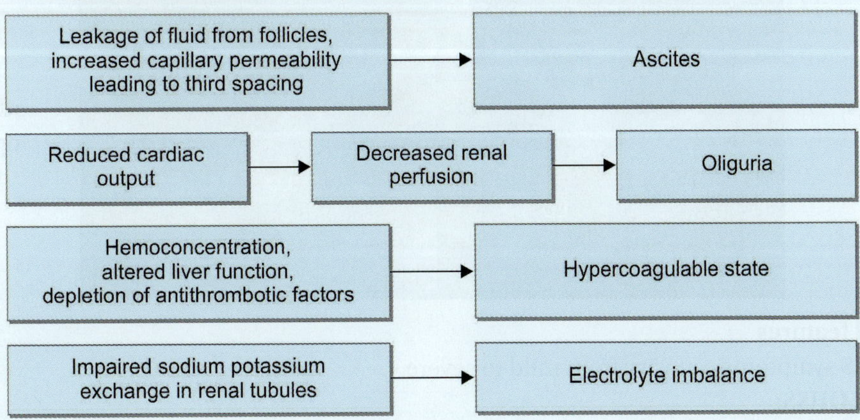

Types of OHSS

A. Depending on the onset: OHSS can be classified as early or late onset. Although HCG is the key factor in both types of OHSS, the source of the HCG hormone is different in early and late-onset OHSS. In early OHSS, the exogenously injected HCG acts as a trigger for release of vasoactive substances. In late-onset OHSS, the HCG is secreted endogenously by the early implanting trophoblastic cells.

Early onset	*Late onset*
Excess response to Gonadotropin injections	Due to pregnancy
3–7 days after HCG	12–17 days after HCG

B. Depending on the severity: Ovarian hyperstimulation syndrome has been classified over the last few years using multiple grading systems. Most of these are based on the disease severity and combination of patient's symptoms and disease severity.

Mild	*Moderate*	*Severe*	*Critical*
• Nausea • Bloating • Abdominal distension • Ovaries ≤5 cm	• Abdominal pain • Vomiting • Ovaries >5 cm • Mild Ascites • Hematocrit (Hct) <41% • WBC >10,000/mm³	• Severe Ascites • Hydrothorax • Enlarged Ovaries • Hct >45% WBC >15,000/mm³ • Oliguria • Creatinine levels: 1–1.5 mg/dL	• Tense Ascites • Pericardial effusion • Hct >55% WBC >25,000/mm³ • Oliguria or Anuria • Creatinine levels: >1.5 mg/dL • Renal Failure • ARDS • Thromboembolism

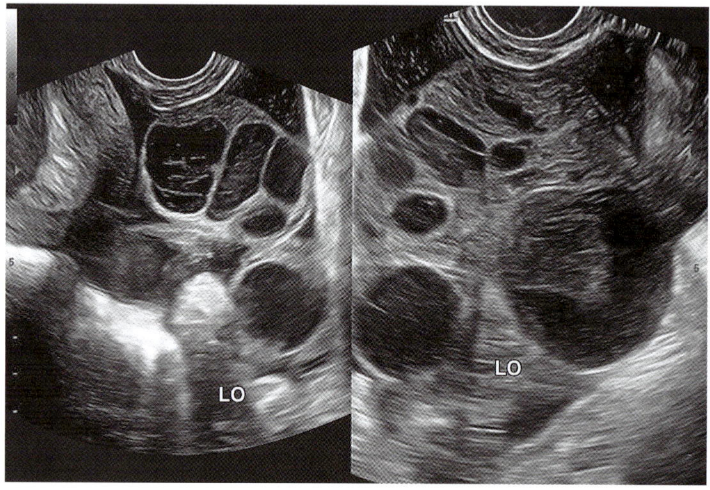

Clinical features

- OHSS symptoms can vary from mild to severe.
- **Mild OHSS:**
  - Nausea
  - Bloating
  - Minimal abdominal distension

- **Moderate OHSS:**
  - Abdominal pain (ranging from mild to moderate)
  - Abdominal bloating or increased waist size
  - Vomiting
  - Diarrhea
  - Tenderness around the ovaries
- **Severe OHSS:**
  - Rapid weight gain (more than 2.2 pounds or 1 kilogram in 24 hours)
  - Severe abdominal pain: May be due to ovarian torsion, intraperitoneal hemorrhage, or rupture of cysts
  - Persistent nausea and vomiting
  - Oliguria
  - Dyspnea
  - Ascites

2. Discuss the management of OHSS and newer agents in the management of OHSS.

OHSS patients should be managed by an IVF specialist. Counsel the patients and emphasize the importance of regular monitoring.

Management:

Initial Assessment:

- Daily weight, Abdominal girth at the level of umbilicus
- Auscultate chest to rule out pulmonary edema, pleural effusion
- Palpate Abdomen for tense ascites
- Urine output charting

Baseline Investigations:

- Compete Blood count—Check Hematocrit
- Liver function tests—Elevated enzymes and low albumin
- Serum electrolytes—Hyponatremia and hyperkalemia
- Ultrasound—Ovarian Size, presence of free fluid.
- Other tests in case of moderate to severe OHSS—Coagulation profile: elevated fibrinogen and reduced antithrombin, D dimer, Serum Osmolality, ABG, Chest X-ray

Treatment:

1. Mild OHSS

   Supportive management. Send all investigations. If mild OHSS is not monitored and treated, then it may progress to moderate or severe OHSS.

   Especially if the patient gets pregnant, then OHSS will be complicated to manage.

   Monitor changes in the hemodynamic pattern.

   Baseline ultrasound to check the ovarian size and presence of free fluid and ascites.

   Watch out for:

   - Enlarging abdominal girth
   - Acute weight gain
   - Abdominal discomfort
   - Increased abdominal pain

2. Moderate OHSS

   Bed rest and observe any changes in the lab investigations

   Adequate fluids: Fluid input <1,000 mL/day and output <1,000 mL/day or deficit >1,000 mL/day needs admission and further evaluation.

   Investigations: Altered hemodynamic parameters that need attention are:
   - Increasing hematocrit levels: >45–55%
   - Elevated creatinine levels: >1-1-2 ng/dL

   Continued weight gain: >2 lb/day

   Paracetamol 1,000–1,500 mg/day for pain relief

   Repeat ultrasound to check for ovarian size and check for ascites and other third space fluid accumulation.

   Patients can be managed on an outpatient basis with daily follow-up.

   Patients who need admission:
   - Continued abdominal pain and discomfort
   - Inadequate oral intake due to nausea and resultant fluid deficit
   - Patient unable to follow up on outpatient basis
   - Worsening of laboratory parameters and progress to severe or critical OHSS
3. Severe OHSS

   Admission and continued monitoring of all laboratory parameters. Patient should be managed in a hospital with all facilities available.

   Ascites: Paracentesis is done vaginally. Multiple paracentesis may be needed.

   Hydrothorax: Pleural tapping

   Hemoconcentration: Anticoagulant therapy: unfractionated heparin 5,000 IU twice daily or low molecular weight Heparin (LMWH) 40–60 IU/day

   Gonadotropin-releasing hormone antagonist 0.25 sc daily for 5–7 days
4. Critical OHSS: Multidisciplinary approach

   Critical OHSS requires admission in critical care unit and multidisciplinary approach.

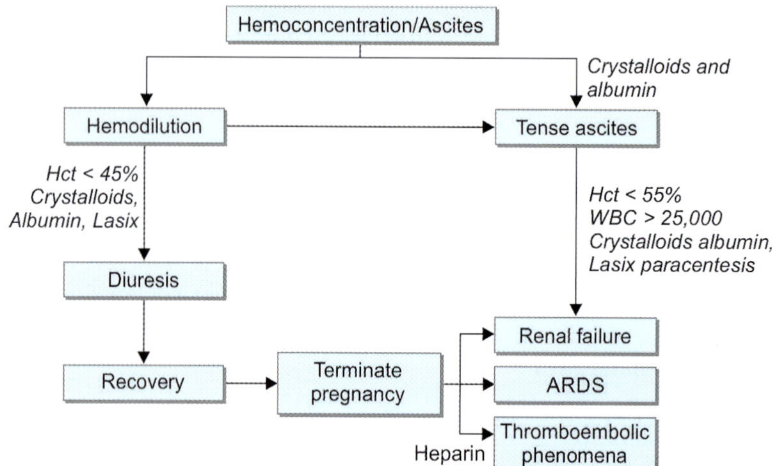

Refer to Short question no 2.

SHORT QUESTIONS AND ANSWERS

1. Describe the Modified Golan Classification of OHSS.

The **modified Golan classification of ovarian hyperstimulation syndrome**, employing clinical findings and imaging appearances, is used to categorize ovarian hyperstimulation syndrome (OHSS) into the following three categories of severity with five grades:

- **Mild OHSS:** Characterized by bilateral multicystic ovarian enlargement
  - **Grade 1:** Abdominal distention and discomfort
  - **Grade 2:** Grade 1 with nausea, vomiting and/or diarrhea, and ovarian enlargement from 5 to 12 cm
- **Moderate OHSS:** Characterized by ascites and abdominal distension
  - **Grade 3:** Features of mild OHSS with ultrasonographic evidence of ascites
- **Severe OHSS:** Characterized by hypovolemia, hemoconcentration, thrombosis, oliguria, pleural and pericardial effusion
  - **Grade 4:** Moderate OHSS with clinical evidence of ascites and/or hydrothorax and dyspnea
  - **Grade 5:** Grade 4 with change in blood volume, hemoconcentration, coagulation abnormalities, and diminished renal perfusion and function.

2. What is critical OHSS? How to manage critical OHSS?

Ovarian Hyperstimulation syndrome is the most serious complication of ovulation induction which results in a spectrum of symptoms ranging from mild to severe. It is most commonly seen due to hyper-response to ovulation in patients undergoing assisted reproductive techniques.

Overall Incidence: 2–3%

Pathogenesis: The principal mediator in development of OHSS is Vascular Endothelial Growth Factor (VEGF). hCG increases the VEGF levels.

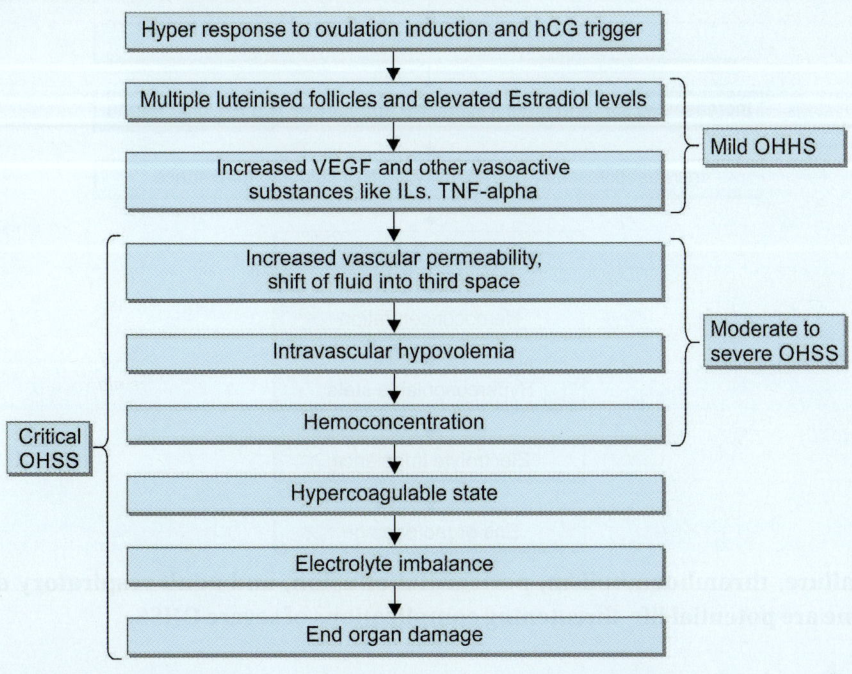

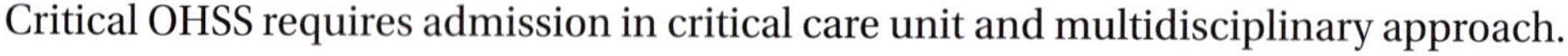

Critical OHSS requires admission in critical care unit and multidisciplinary approach.

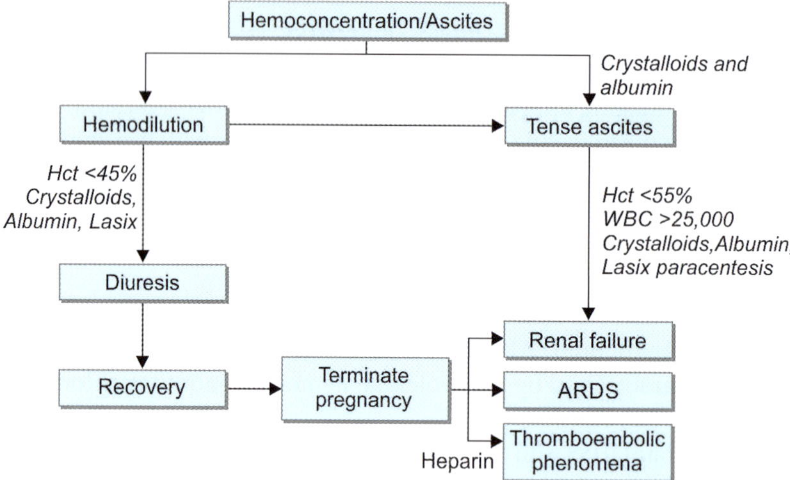

3. Ovarian Hyperstimulation Syndrome.

Definition: Ovarian hyperstimulation syndrome (OHSS) is an iatrogenic complication of assisted reproduction technology.

The syndrome is characterized by cystic enlargement of the ovaries and a shift of fluid from the intravascular to the third space due to increased capillary permeability and ovarian neoangiogenesis.

Pathogenesis

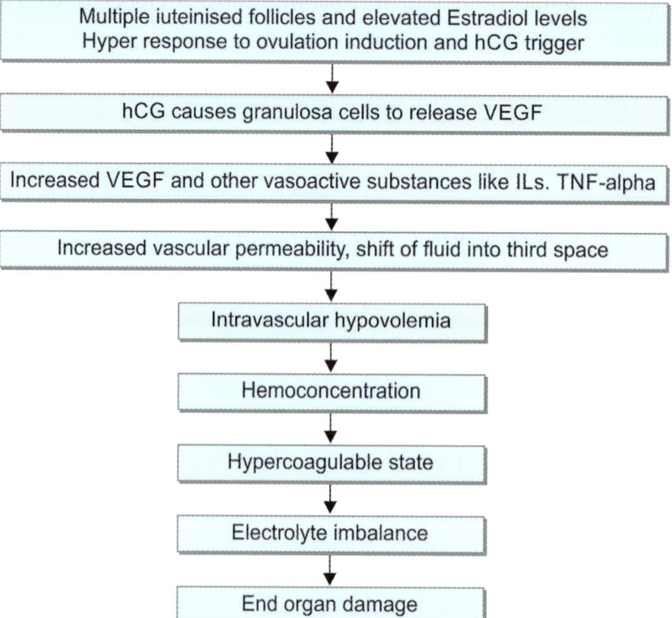

Renal failure, thromboembolism, pericardial effusion, and adult respiratory distress syndrome are potential life-threatening complications of severe OHSS.

Clinical Features and Classification

OHSS can be classified as:

- Mild (abdominal distension and discomfort),
- Moderate (ascites revealed only by ultrasound),
- Severe (ascites revealed by physical examination, or the presence of pleural or pericardial effusion associated with hemoconcentration), and
- Critical (the symptoms described above are accompanied by hypotension, acute renal failure, and thromboembolic disorders)

Management

Due to the wide spectrum of clinical features, management of OHSS can be done on Outpatient or Indoor basis as per the severity of the condition.

Treatment

Mild	*Moderate*	*Severe/critical*
• Supportive • Baseline investigations • Consider admission if there is tachycardia, hypotension, reduced urine output, dyspnea and worsening of abdominal pain	• Bedrest • Check electrolytes and creatinine • Maintain fluid balance • Paracetamol for pain	• Admission • Complete workup • Paracentesis • Prophylactic anticoagulation if Hct >55% • Multidisciplinary approach and ICU admission in critical OHSS

4. What are the methods to prevent OHSS?

Preventive measures to decrease the risk of OHSS are:

- **Choice of protocol:** Numerous studies have shown that there is a significant decrease in the incidence of OHSS in gonadotropin-releasing hormone (GnRH) antagonist protocol. As GnRH agonist ca be used as a trigger in this protocol, the chances of developing OHSS reduce significantly.
- **Coasting:** Coasting consists of withholding gonadotropin stimulation at the end of the stimulation for around 4 days but continuing suppression with antagonist or agonist as per the protocol used. This causes atresia of smaller follicles without affecting the large follicles.
- **Choice of Trigger:** The use of GnRH agonist as a trigger can prevent the development of OHSS.
- **Dopamine agonist:** Cabergoline started on the day of hCG injection has also been shown to reduce the risk of severe OHSS. Cabergoline reduces VEGF activity which is a crucial part of development of OHSS.
- **Cryopreservation:** Pregnancy worsens OHSS. Therefore, it is extremely important to postpone the embryo transfer. Cryopreserved embryos can be used later and Frozen embryo transfers are also giving very good clinical pregnancy and live birth rates.
- **Intravenous fluids:** IV albumin infusion on the day of pickup. A meta-analysis of five trials demonstrated a significant reduction in severe OHSS on administration of albumin at the time of oocyte retrieval in high-risk patients. Crystalloids help in stabilizing

hemodynamic changes. IV Calcium infusion—10 mL of 10% calcium gluconate in 200 mL NS on the day of oocyte pickup and up to 3 days after has shown to be of use.

5. **What are the newer agents in management of OHSS?**

- **Cabergoline:** The pathophysiology of OHSS is largely attributed to an increased vascular permeability of the ovarian and peritoneal capillaries caused by elevated levels of VEGF. Treatment with a dopamine-receptor agonist such as cabergoline may result in a reduction of VEGF production and subsequently reduce OHSS. In patients at risk for moderate-to-severe OHSS, it is recommended to start a dopamine agonist such as cabergoline on the day of the hCG trigger and continue for 7–10 days. Several studies reported a reduction in OHSS incidence when a dopamine agonist is administered alone or in combination with other risk-reducing strategies.
- **GnRH antagonist:** After the hCG trigger injection, administration of a GnRH antagonist during the luteal phase has been proposed as a potential intervention to accelerate luteolysis, reduce ovarian VEGF secretion, and promote regression of symptoms associated with OHSS. There is insufficient evidence that the administration of a GnRH antagonist after the hCG trigger leads to a statistically significant reduction in rates of moderate to severe OHSS. It is not recommended to administer a luteal GnRH antagonist alone to reduce rates of moderate-to-severe OHSS. It can be used along with Cabergoline.

SUGGESTED READING

1. Patel NH, Esteves SC> Advances in Assisted Reproductive Technology, 1st edition. New Delhi: Jaypee Brothers Medical Publishers; 2020.
2. Practice Committee of the American Society for Reproductive Medicine. Prevention of moderate and severe ovarian hyperstimulation syndrome: a guideline. [online] Available from https://www.asrm.org/practice-guidance/practice-committee-documents/prevention-and-treatment-of-moderate-and-severe-ovarian-hyperstimulation-syndrome-a-guideline/ [Last accessed December, 2025]
3. Royal College of Obstetricians and Gynaecologists. (2016). The Management of Ovarian Hyperstimulation Syndrome (Green-top Guideline No. 5). [online] Available from https://www.rcog.org.uk/media/or1jqxbf/gtg_5_ohss.pdf [Last accessed December, 2025]

Tubal Factor Infertility

Ruchika Garg, Neelansha Varshney

- **Fertilization Site:** Occurs in the ampullary part of the fallopian tubes.
- **Tubal Role:** Transports gametes (egg and sperm) via tubal endothelium; any damage or blockage impairs fertilization, a critical step in conception.
- **Infertility Impact:** Tubal disease accounts for 25–35% of female infertility and 10–30% of overall infertility.
- **Primary Cause:** Salpingitis (inflammation of the fallopian tubes).
- **Noninfectious Causes:**
  - Tubal endometriosis
  - Salpingitis isthmica nodosa (SIN)
  - Tubal polyps
  - Tubal spasm
  - Intratubal mucous debris

Fallopian Tube Structure

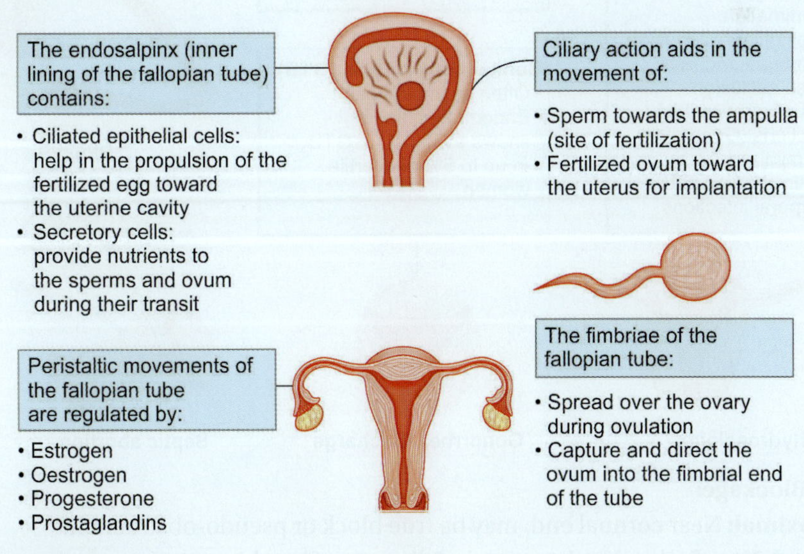

- **Mucous Membrane:**
  - Secretes fluids to support fertilization and embryo development.
  - Contains cilia (hair-like structures) that move eggs, sperm, and embryos.

- **Muscular Layer:**
  - Outer layer: Smooth, long muscle fibers.
  - Inner layer: Circular fibers.
  - Contracts to aid gamete/embryo movement, assisted by cilia.

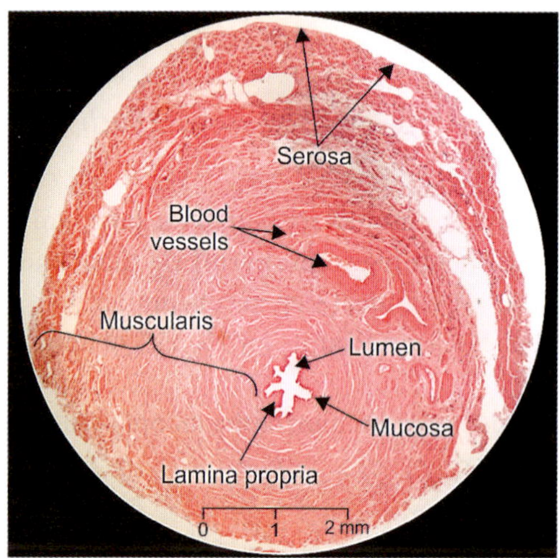

Fig. 1: Cross section of fallopian tube.

Common Tubal Causes of Infertility

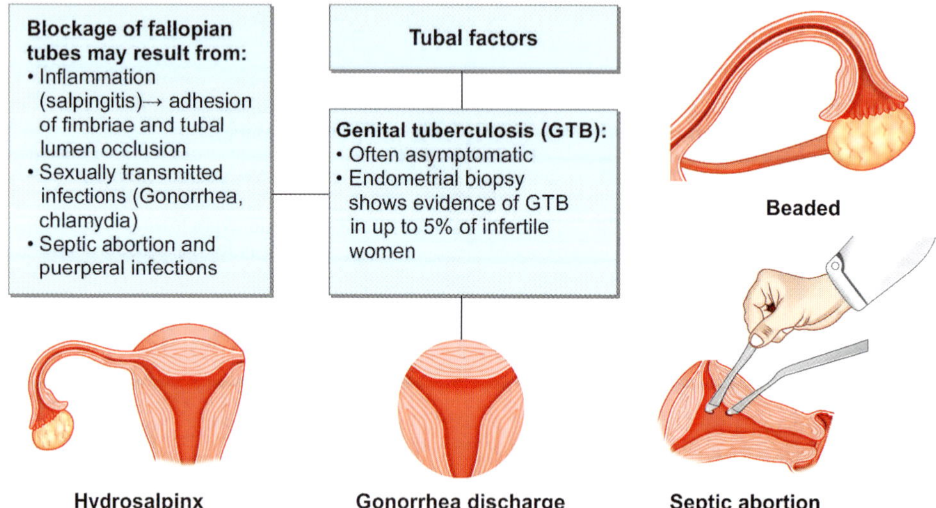

- **Tubal Blockage:**
  - **Proximal:** Near cornual end; may be true block or pseudo-obstruction.
  - **Distal:** Near fimbrial end; most tubal diseases affect this region.
- **Pelvic Inflammatory Disease (PID):**
  - Often caused by STIs (*Chlamydia trachomatis, Neisseria gonorrheae*).
  - Other pathogens: *Mycoplasma hominis, Ureaplasma urealyticum* (less clear role).

- Chronic inflammation causes scarring/blockages.
- Tubal infertility risk: 8% after 1 PID episode, 19.5% after 2, 40% after 3.

- **Endometriosis:** Endometrial tissue outside the uterus causes tubal involvement or adhesions, altering tubo-ovarian anatomy.
- **Tubal Surgery:**
  - Prior surgeries (e.g., for ectopic pregnancy, tubal ligation) may cause blocks or adhesions.
  - Recurrent blocks may occur postrecanalization.
- **Hydrosalpinx:**
  - Fluid-filled tube due to end-stage disease, causing distal blockage and fimbrial phimosis.
  - Fluid is toxic to embryos, impairing development and implantation.
  - Diagnosed via ultrasound or laparoscopy; may be asymptomatic.
- **Tubal Ectopic Pregnancy:**
  - Implantation in a damaged tube worsens tubal damage.
  - May require partial/complete salpingectomy.
- **Congenital Abnormalities:**
  - Rare structural issues (e.g., absent tubes, accessory tubes, rudimentary tubes).
  - Often associated with uterine malformations; most require no treatment.
- **Adhesions (Scar Tissue):** Caused by surgeries, infections, or endometriosis; distorts or blocks tubes.
- **Salpingitis Isthmica Nodosa (SIN):** Inflammation and nodular thickening, mainly in proximal tubes, causing fibrosis and blockage.

Genital Tuberculosis (TB)

- **Cause:** Chronic PID, often spread via lymphatic/hematogenous routes from lungs.
- **Impact:** Infertility, menstrual irregularities, dyspareunia.
- **Prevalence:** Rare in developed countries; common in developing countries (e.g., India).
- **Diagnosis Challenges:**
  - Often asymptomatic; low sensitivity/specificity of tests.
  - May mimic PID (elevated erythrocyte sedimentation rate).
  - Nonresponse to broad-spectrum antibiotics may suggest TB.
- **Treatment:**
  - Four drugs (rifampicin, isoniazid, ethambutol, pyrazinamide) for 2 months.
  - Three drugs (rifampicin, isoniazid, ethambutol) for 4 months.
  - Shorter regimens for multidrug-resistant TB (MDR-TB) or rifampicin resistance.

Evaluation of Tubal Factor

- **When to Evaluate:** Suspect tubal issues if no conception after 3 cycles of timed intercourse with confirmed ovulation and normal semen analysis.
  - **Methods:**
    - **Ultrasound:**
      - Healthy tubes not visible; inflamed or fluid-filled tubes appear as adnexal masses (e.g., hydrosalpinx with cogwheel appearance).
      - May be misdiagnosed as ovarian/paraovarian cysts.

- **Tubal Patency Tests** (ideal in follicular phase, days 7–11):
  - **Hysterosalpingography (HSG):**
    - Uses radiocontrast and X-rays to visualize tube patency.
    - Detects proximal blocks and severe hydrosalpinx (70–80% sensitive).
    - Less accurate for distal pathology or adhesions; cornual spasm reduces accuracy.
    - Contraindicated in PID, known hydrosalpinx, or pregnancy.

Flowchart 1: Bilateral patent fallopian tubes in HSG.

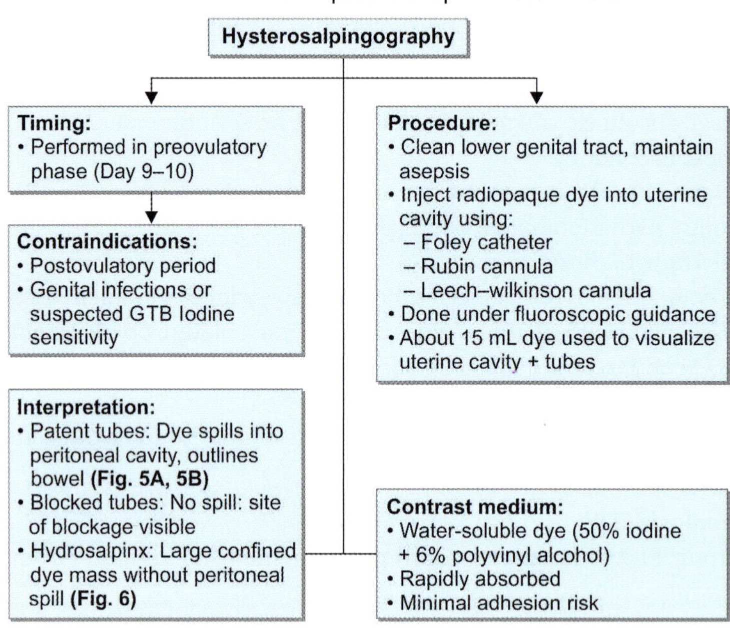

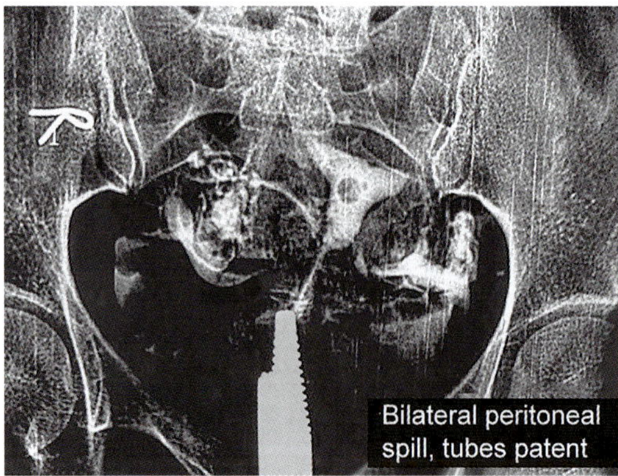

- **Sonosalpingography (SSG):**
  - Uses saline and Doppler/3D ultrasound to detect fluid flow.
  - 85–90% sensitive.

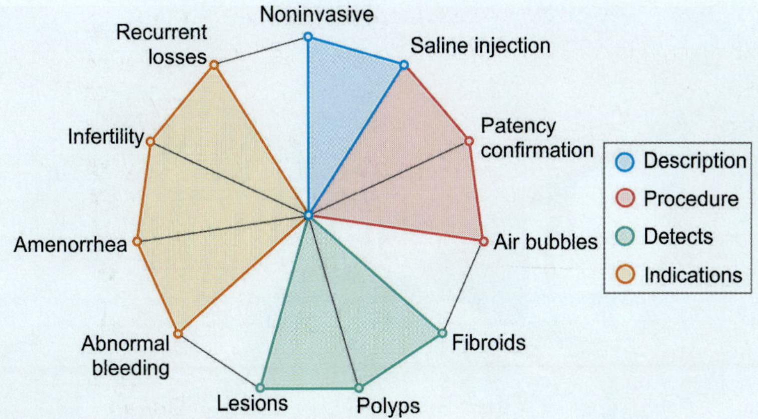

- **Laparoscopy:**
  - Gold standard for tubal/pelvic evaluation.
  - Allows diagnostic and operative procedures (e.g., tubal cannulation, adhesiolysis, endometriotic spot fulguration).
  - Can be combined with hysteroscopy for uterine cavity assessment.
  - Grading of salpingitis: Minimal, mild, moderate, severe (Jacobson & Westrom criteria).

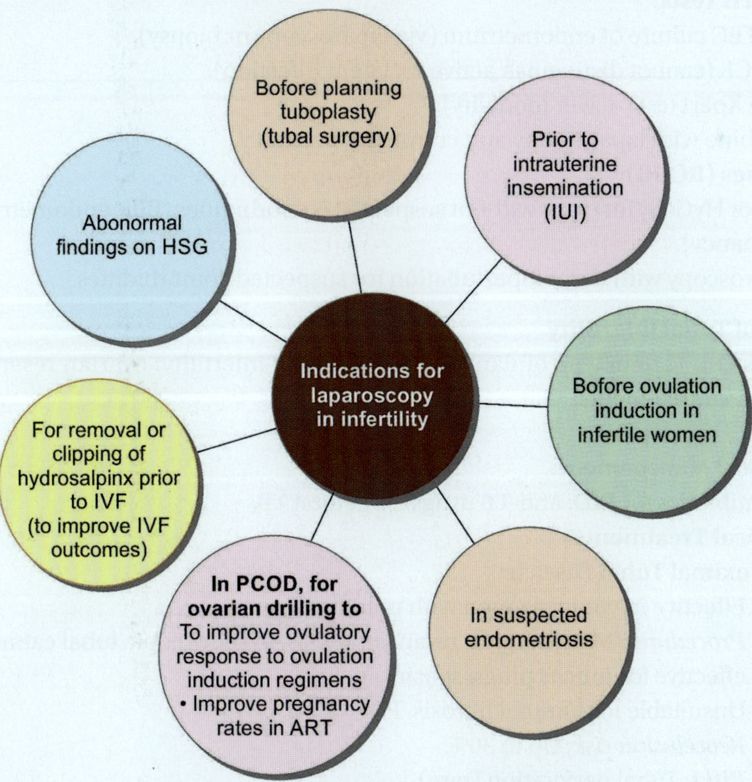

Fig. 2: Indications of laparoscopy in infertility.

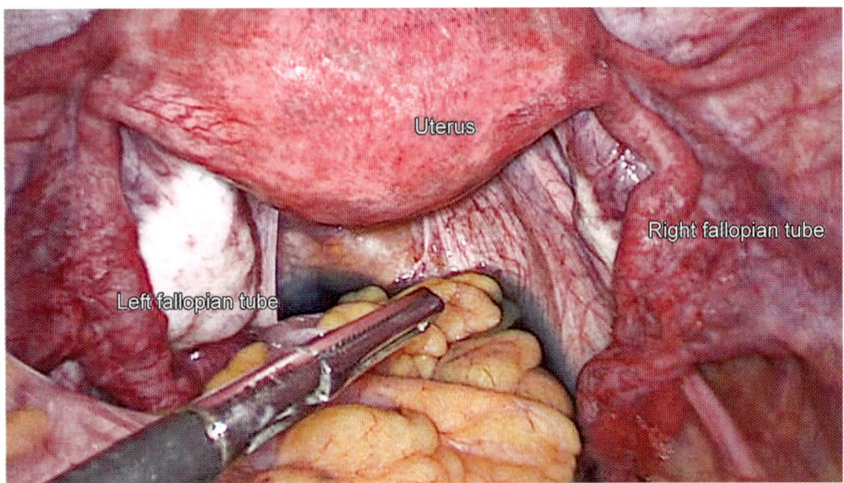

Laparoscopic chromopertubation.

- **Pelvic Infection Tests:** Chlamydia (common cause): Detected via antibodies (micro-immunofluorescence preferred; low sensitivity, high negative predictive value).
- **Genital TB Tests:**
  - BACTEC culture of endometrium (via laparoscopy or biopsy).
  - TB-PCR (cannot distinguish active vs. latent infection).
  - Gene Xpert test (newer modality).
  - Combine with laparoscopy and culture for accuracy.
- **Guidelines (RCOG):**
  - HSG or HyCoSy for cases without suspected comorbidities (PID, endometriosis, ectopic pregnancy).
  - Laparoscopy with chromopertubation for suspected comorbidities.

Treatment of Tubal Infertility

- **Depends On:** Extent/type of damage, age, years of infertility, ovarian reserve, obstetric history, prior treatments.
- **Options:**
  - **Medical Management:**
    - Antibiotics for PID; anti-TB drugs for genital TB.
  - **Surgical Treatments:**
    - **Proximal Tubal Disease:**
      - Effective in young women with mild damage.
      - *Procedures:* Microsurgical re-anastomosis, hysteroscopic tubal cannulation (85% effective for mucus plugs, spasms, debris).
      - Unsuitable for luminal fibrosis, PID, or TB.
      - *Reocclusion risk:* Up to 30%.
      - *Risks:* Tubal perforation (rare).

Persistent/recurrent blocks may require IVF. A guidewire is passed through both ostia under hysteroscopic guidance in tubal cannulation; tubal perforation can occur rarely. Catheterization involves passing a soft catheter through tubal ostia. If block persists or recurs, then IVF is advisable.

- **Distal Tubal Disease:**
  - Caused by endometriosis, infections, or prior surgeries.
  - Requires ≥50% healthy tubal endosalpinx/wall for reconstruction.
  - **Procedures:**
    - **Fimbrioplasty:** Lysis of fimbrial adhesions or dilation of phimosis.
    - **Salpingostomy:** Creates new tubal opening in occluded tubes.
    - **Tubocornual Anastomosis:** Excision of tubal isthmus and reimplantation (up to 68% pregnancy rate).
  - Increased ectopic pregnancy risk post procedure.
  - *Best candidates:* Age <35 years, mild disease, intact mucosa, minimal adhesions.
  - IVF recommended for older patients, severe damage, or additional infertility factors.
- **Hydrosalpinx:**
  - Salpingectomy before IVF improves pregnancy/live birth rates.
  - Laparoscopic tubal occlusion is a viable alternative.
- **Assisted Reproductive Technologies:** IVF for severe tubal damage, recurrent blocks, or other infertility factors.

Key Notes

- Early evaluation and tailored treatment are critical for tubal infertility.
- Surgical outcomes depend on patient selection and tubal health.
- IVF is often the best option for complex cases or poor surgical candidates.

LONG QUESTIONS

Q1. Evaluate tubal factors in infertility and outline the management of tubal block in a 25-year-old nulliparous woman. *RGUHS, 2004 (20 marks)*

Q2. Genital tuberculosis and its correlation with Infertility.
(MS Summer ph 2-2023, DNB ph 3-Aug 2021, DNB ph 2-Dec 2021)

Male Infertility

Ruchika Garg, Neelansha Varshney

INTRODUCTION

Male infertility affects 15% of couples globally, with oxidative stress (OS) from reactive oxygen species (ROS) implicated in 30–80% of cases.[1] ROS impair sperm function, while antioxidants in seminal fluid counterbalance OS to maintain redox equilibrium.[2] Hormonal therapies, including gonadotropins and selective estrogen receptor modulators (SERMs), address specific etiologies like hypogonadotropic hypogonadism (HH).

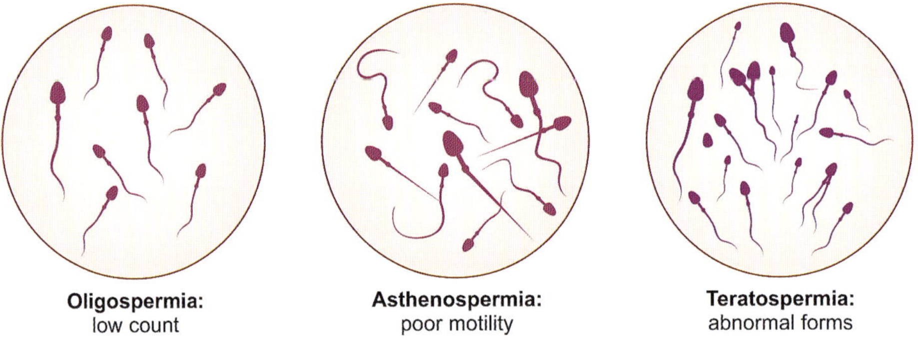

Common sperm abnormalities and their effects on fertility.

EPIDEMIOLOGY

- **Global:** Male factor contributes to 50% of infertility cases; OS affects 25–50% of infertile men.[3]
- **India:**
    - *Male infertility prevalence:* 10–15% of couples.[4]
    - *OS-related sperm dysfunction:* ~40% of cases in tertiary centers.[5]
    - Limited antioxidant use due to cost and awareness; hormonal therapies underutilized.[6]
- **Trends:** Increasing focus on OS and sperm DNA fragmentation (SDF) in infertility workup.[7]

Reactive Oxygen Species (ROS) and Antioxidants

- **ROS Role:** Excess ROS from leukocytes, immature sperm, or environmental factors (smoking, radiation) causes lipid peroxidation, DNA damage, and reduced motility.[8]
- **Antioxidant Systems:**[9]

- **Enzymatic:** Glutathione peroxidase (GPx), superoxide dismutase (SOD), catalase; prostate-derived.[10]
- **Nonenzymatic:** Vitamin C, vitamin E, zinc, selenium, carnitines, CoQ10, lycopene; diet/supplement-derived.[11]

TABLE 1: Mechanisms of common antioxidants.[12,13]

Antioxidant	*Mechanism*
Vitamin C	Neutralizes hydroxyl, superoxide, hydrogen peroxide radicals
Vitamin E	Quenches free radicals, reduces lipid peroxidation in membranes
Folate	Scavenges free radicals, supports nucleic acid synthesis
Selenium	Enhances GPx activity, protects sperm DNA
Zinc	Inhibits NADPH oxidase, antagonizes redox-active metals
Carnitines	Scavenges superoxide/hydrogen peroxide, enhances sperm motility
CoQ10	Inhibits superoxide in mitochondria, supports energy production
NAC	Boosts glutathione, directly scavenges hypochlorous acid/hydroxyl radicals
Lycopene	Quenches ROS, protects testicular tissue

CLINICAL APPLICATIONS OF ANTIOXIDANTS

TABLE 2: Antioxidants by clinical scenario.[14,15]

Condition	*Antioxidants (Doses)*
Oligozoospermia	Vitamin E (300 mg), NAC (600 mg), CoQ10 (300 mg), LC (2 g), folic acid (5 mg) + zinc (66 mg)
Asthenozoospermia	Vitamin E (400 mg) + selenium (200 μg), LC (2 g) + LAC (1 g), NAC (600 mg), lycopene (2 mg)
Teratozoospermia	Vitamin E (400 mg) + selenium (200 μg), NAC (600 mg), zinc (400 mg), lycopene (8 mg)
High SDF	Vitamin E (1 g) + vitamin C (1 g), zinc (10 mg), selenium (50 μg), LC (1,500 mg)
Oxidative Stress	Vitamin E (300 mg), NAC (600 mg), vitamin C (10 mg) + zinc (400 mg), selenium (225 μg)
ART Success	Vitamin E (200 mg), lycopene (6 mg), CoQ10 (20 mg), folate (0.5 mg), zinc (25 mg)
Live Birth Rate	CoQ10 (300 mg), vitamin E (1 g) + vitamin C (1 g), LC (2 g) + LAC (1 g), zinc (5,000 mg)

- **Evidence:**
  - *Vitamin E/C:* Improve motility, reduce ROS; limited impact on live birth.[16]
  - *Carnitines:* Enhance motility/viability in vitro; lower levels in infertile men.[17]
  - *CoQ10:* Correlates with sperm count/motility; reduces hydrogen peroxide.[18]
  - *NAC/Selenium:* Reduce SDF, improve motility via glutathione enhancement.[19]
  - *Zinc:* Protects sperm structure; deficiency linked to flagellar abnormalities.[20]
  - *Lycopene:* High in testes; lower in infertile men.[21]

- **Limitations:**
  - Heterogeneous studies, small sample sizes, variable doses.[22]
  - No strong evidence for routine use; counsel on questionable clinical utility.[23]

HORMONAL THERAPIES IN MALE INFERTILITY

- **Hypogonadotropic Hypogonadism (HH):**
  - **Congenital (IHH):** GnRH deficiency; treat with hCG (1,500–2,500 IU twice weekly) ± FSH to restore testosterone/spermatogenesis.[24]
  - **Secondary Causes:** Pituitary tumors, hyperprolactinemia, trauma; treat underlying disorder.[25]
- **Non-HH Idiopathic Infertility:**
  - **SERMs (e.g., Clomiphene):** Increase LH/FSH via hypothalamic–pituitary stimulation; off-label for adult-onset IHH.[26]
  - **Aromatase Inhibitors (AIs, e.g., Letrozole):** Reduce estradiol, increase testosterone; used in low testosterone with high estradiol.[27]
  - **hCG:** Stimulates Leydig cells; used in low/normal LH.[28]
  - **FSH Analogs:** Improve sperm concentration in idiopathic infertility; 150 IU daily for 12 weeks.[29]
- **Nonobstructive Azoospermia (NOA):**
  - SERMs/AIs/hCG/FSH used off-label to optimize spermatogenesis presurgical retrieval; limited data.[30]
  - *Clomiphene:* 11% sperm recovery in ejaculate; 57.7% surgical retrieval rate.[31]
  - *Letrozole:* Sperm recovery in NOA but no unassisted pregnancies.[32]
  - *FSH:* 64% surgical retrieval rate versus 33% control.[33]

TABLE 3: Hormonal therapies.[34,35]

Therapy	*Mechanism*	*Indication*	*Evidence*
hCG	LH analog, stimulates testosterone	HH, low/normal LH	Restores spermatogenesis in HH
SERMs	Blocks estrogen feedback, increases LH/FSH	IHH, idiopathic infertility	Limited pregnancy data
AIs	Inhibits aromatase, increases testosterone	Low testosterone, high estradiol	Improves testosterone, no strong pregnancy data
FSH	Stimulates spermatogenesis	HH, idiopathic infertility, NOA	Improves sperm concentration

GUIDELINES

- **AUA/ASRM (2020)**[36]
  - *Antioxidants:* Questionable clinical utility; counsel on limited evidence.
  - *HH:* hCG ± FSH first-line; SERMs/AIs off-label for IHH.
  - *Idiopathic Infertility:* Consider FSH analogs for sperm concentration improvement.

- *NOA:* Limited data for SERMs/AIs/hCG/FSH presurgery; inform patients of uncertainty.
- *Sperm Banking:* Encourage before gonadotoxic therapy (e.g., chemotherapy).[37]
- **EAU (2023):**[38]
  - *Antioxidants:* Not routinely recommended; consider in high OS/SDF.
  - *Hormonal Therapy:* Reserve for HH or specific indications; avoid empiric use.[39]

Indian Context

- **Burden:** Male infertility affects 12–18 million couples; OS in 30–50%.[40]
- **Challenges:**
  - Over-the-counter antioxidant use without prescription; variable formulations.[41]
  - Limited access to hormonal therapies (hCG/FSH) due to cost.[42]
  - Low sperm banking awareness before cancer treatment.[43]
- **2022 Study:** Antioxidant use in 60% of infertile men in urban India; only 10% prescribed evidence-based doses.[44]

CLINICAL CASE SCENARIO

Case: A 32-year-old man presents with oligoasthenozoospermia (count: 10 million/mL, motility: 30%). No HH; normal testosterone, high ROS on semen analysis.

Management:

- **Counseling:** Explain OS role, limited antioxidant evidence, and lifestyle (quit smoking, reduce alcohol).
- **Antioxidants:** Prescribe vitamin E (400 mg) + selenium (200 μg) daily for 3 months; discuss questionable efficacy.
- **Lifestyle:** Recommend weight loss (BMI 28 kg/m^2), exercise, and antioxidant-rich diet (fruits, vegetables).
- **Follow-Up:** Repeat semen analysis in 3 months; consider ART if no improvement.
- **Outcome:** Motility improves to 45%; couple referred for IUI.

Exam Tip: Highlight OS as a common cause, limited antioxidant evidence, and AUA's conditional recommendations.

KEY POINTS

- **Prevalence in India:** Male infertility in 12–18 million couples; OS in 30–50%.
- **Antioxidants:** Counter ROS; vitamin E, C, carnitines, CoQ10 used but limited pregnancy data.
- **Hormonal Therapies:** hCG/FSH for HH; SERMs/AIs/FSH off-label for idiopathic infertility/NOA.[45]
- **Guidelines:** AUA/ASRM caution on antioxidants; hormonal therapies for specific indications.[46]
- **Challenges:** Overuse of antioxidants, limited access to hormonal therapies, low sperm banking.

BOX 1: Important exam points.

- *ROS:* Cause lipid peroxidation, SDF, and motility loss.
- *Antioxidants:* Vitamin E/C, CoQ10, NAC improve motility/SDF; no strong live birth evidence.
- *HH Treatment:* hCG ± FSH first-line; SERMs/AIs off-label.
- *Sperm Banking:* Mandatory before gonadotoxic therapy.[47]

REFERENCES

1. Agarwal A, Makker K, Sharma R. Oxidative stress in male infertility. Fertil Steril. 2019;112(4):618-27.
2. Tremellen K. Oxidative stress and male infertility. Hum Reprod Update. 2018;24(1):1-12.
3. World Health Organization. (2023). Infertility prevalence estimates, 1990–2021. Geneva: World Health Organization; 2023.
4. Kumar N, et al. Male infertility in India: epidemiology and challenges. Indian J Urol. 2020;36(4):243-9.
5. Majumdar G, et al. Oxidative stress in male infertility: Indian perspective. J Hum Reprod Sci. 2019;12(2):87-94.
6. Sharma R, et al. Antioxidant use in India: a survey. Andrology. 2021;9(3):789-95.
7. Esteves SC, et al. Sperm DNA fragmentation: clinical implications. Andrology. 2021;9(1):30-44.
8. Suleiman SA, et al. Vitamin E and sperm motility. Hum Reprod. 2018;13(5):991-5.
9. Kessopoulou E, et al. Vitamin E in infertile men. Fertil Steril. 2017;67(3):553-8.
10. Jacob RA, et al. Vitamin C in seminal plasma. J Androl. 2016;13(4):344-9.
11. Fraga CG, et al. Vitamin C protects sperm DNA. Proc Natl Acad Sci. 2019;89(22):11069-73.
12. Abdollahzadeh M, et al. Vitamin C and asthenozoospermia. Andrologia. 2018;50(6):e13024.
13. Balercia G, et al. Carnitines and sperm motility. Fertil Steril. 2016;85(6):1756-9.
14. Lenzi A, et al. Carnitine supplementation in infertility. Hum Reprod. 2017;18(3):638-43.
15. De Rosa M, et al. Carnitines in oligoasthenoteratozoospermia. Andrology. 2018;36(2):221-6.
16. Mancini A, et al. CoQ10 in seminal plasma. Biofactors. 2019;37(3):178-83.
17. Lafuente R, et al. CoQ10 and sperm motility. Andrologia. 2017;45(6):371-8.
18. Aruoma OI, et al. NAC as an antioxidant. Free Radic Biol Med. 2016;24(8):1395-404.
19. Erkkilä K, et al. NAC and germ cell survival. Biol Reprod. 2018;61(4):1016-22.
20. Oeda T, et al. NAC improves sperm motility. Andrologia. 2017;29(3):127-32.
21. Foresta C, et al. Selenium and selenoproteins in sperm. Hum Reprod Update. 2019;15(6):762–75.
22. Ursini F, et al. Selenoprotein glutathione peroxidase. J Biol Chem. 2017;274(36):25959-68.
23. Behne D, et al. Selenium in sperm structure. J Reprod Fertil. 2016;106(2):291-7.
24. Moslemi MK, et al. Selenium and sperm motility. Urol J. 2018;8(1):28-32.
25. Fallah A, Mohammad-Hasani A, Colagar AH. Zinc is an Essential Element for Male Fertility: A Review of Zn Roles in Men's Health, Germination, Sperm Quality, and Fertilization. J Reprod Infertil. 2018;19(2):69-81.
26. J Hum Reprod Sci. 2019;11(4):308-14.
27. Powell SR, et al. Zinc as an antioxidant. Free Radic Biol Med. 2016;33(6):746-52.
28. Chia SE, et al. Zinc in fertile vs. subfertile men. Hum Reprod. 2017;15(3):677-82.
29. Colagar AH, et al. Folic acid and glutathione ratio. J Androl. 2018;29(5):557-63.
30. Di Mascio P, et al. Lycopene as an antioxidant. Arch Biochem Biophys. 2019;274(2):532-8.
31. Palan P, et al. Lycopene in seminal plasma. Fertil Steril. 2016;65(4):826-9.
32. Fraietta R, et al. HH treatment with hCG. Asian J Androl. 2017;15(1):88-93.
33. Burris AS, et al. hCG in IHH. Fertil Steril. 2018;49(5):881-7.
34. Finkel DM, et al. hCG and spermatogenesis. J Clin Endocrinol Metab. 2016;65(6):1141-7.
35. Shiraishi S, et al. SERMs in adult-onset IHH. Fertil Steril. 2019;92(5):1693-9.
36. Raman JD, et al. Clomiphene in IHH. J Urol. 2017;167(2):637-40.

37. Sabanegh ES, et al. Secondary HH: causes and management. Urol Clin North Am. 2018;35(2):165-76.
38. Tapanainen JS, et al. AIs in male infertility. J Clin Endocrinol Metab. 2016;83(5):1477-82.
39. EAU. Male infertility guidelines. Arnhem: EAU; 2023.
40. Schlegel PN, et al. SERMs and AIs in men. Fertil Steril. 2019;94(7):2417-25.
41. Attia AM, et al. FSH in idiopathic male infertility. Cochrane Database Syst Rev. 2017;5:CD005071.
42. Hussein A, et al. Clomiphene in NOA. J Urol. 2016;185(4):1307-11.
43. Saylam B, et al. Letrozole in NOA. Andrologia. 2017;43(4):273-7.
44. Reifsnyder JE, et al. hCG in NOA. J Urol. 2018;187(4):1364-8.
45. Aydos K, et al. FSH in NOA. Fertil Steril. 2016;75(6):1178-83.
46. AUA/ASRM. Male infertility guidelines. Linthicum: AUA; 2020.
47. Kumar R, et al. Sperm banking in India. Indian J Cancer. 2019;56(4):307-12.

Intrauterine Insemination

Ruchika Garg

INTRODUCTION

Intrauterine insemination (IUI) is a relatively simple, minimally invasive, and cost-effective assisted reproductive technique used to treat various types of infertility. It involves the placement of washed, motile sperm directly into the uterine cavity through the cervix, thereby bypassing cervical barriers and increasing the concentration of healthy sperm near the site of fertilization. The procedure is mostly combined with mild ovarian stimulation to improve the chances of pregnancy.[1]

IUI is widely indicated for infertility cases such as mild-to-moderate male factor infertility, unexplained infertility, cervical factor infertility, ovulatory disorders with patent tubes, and in specific situations using donor sperm.

PREREQUISITES FOR IUI

To undertake IUI successfully, several conditions should be met:

- A natural or stimulated ovulatory cycle.
- At least one patent and functional fallopian tube.
- Adequate total motile sperm count (usually >5 million post-wash).[2]
- Absence of active cervical, uterine, or pelvic infections.

INDICATIONS

Partner's Sperm

- Mild-to-moderate male factor infertility (e.g., with sufficient motile sperm)
- Retrograde ejaculation, erectile dysfunction, vaginismus
- Unexplained infertility
- Cervical factor infertility
- Minimal-to-mild endometriosis
- Unilateral tubal disease
- HIV serodiscordant couples

Donor Sperm

- Azoospermia
- Sex-linked genetic diseases in males
- Single women and LGBTQ+ couples (per ASRM donor guidelines).

CONTRAINDICATIONS

- Bilateral tubal blockage
- Severe oligoasthenoteratozoospermia (OAT) with very low total motile sperm count (<5 million).
- Stage III/IV endometriosis
- Active pelvic infections or severe uterine disorders
- Poor ovarian reserve or severe ovulatory dysfunction not responding to stimulation.

EFFECTIVENESS AND SUCCESS RATES

IUI success rates per cycle have improved over the years with better ovulation stimulation, timing, and sperm processing. Current data suggest:

- Clinical pregnancy rates (CPR) per cycle of 15–25% in well-selected patients undergoing optimized protocols.
- Cumulative live birth rates of around 40–60% after 3–6 IUI cycles.
- Success depends heavily on maternal age (<35 years having better outcomes), semen quality, ovarian stimulation response, and infertility etiology.
- After 3-4 unsuccessful cycles, IVF or ICSI are generally recommended.

SEMEN COLLECTION AND PREPARATION

- Semen should be collected after minimum 1 day of abstinence, which optimizes sperm motility and DNA integrity.
- Processing should occur within 30 minutes of ejaculation to minimize sperm damage.
- IUI should ideally be performed within 4 hours of semen processing to reduce DNA fragmentation and oxidative stress.
- Common preparation methods include simple wash and centrifugation, double density gradient, or swim-up techniques, with no clear evidence favoring one over another. The choice depends on raw sample characteristics.
- Post-wash inseminating motile count (TPMSC) >5 million correlates with higher success rates.

PROTOCOL OF IUI PROCEDURE

- **Ovarian Stimulation (OS)**
  - Mild stimulation using clomiphene citrate or letrozole, sometimes combined with low-dose gonadotropins, is preferred.
  - Stimulation aims to produce 1–3 mature follicles while minimizing risks of multiple pregnancy and OHSS.
  - Monitoring includes serial ultrasound and serum estradiol measurements.
- **Triggering Ovulation**
  - hCG injection (5,000–10,000 IU) administered when dominant follicle(s) reach 18–20 mm.
  - IUI is timed 24–40 hours after hCG trigger to coincide with ovulation.

- **Insemination**[3]
  - Using a soft catheter under sterile conditions, 0.3–0.5 mL of processed sperm is deposited transcervically into the uterine cavity near the fundus.
  - Bed rest of 10–15 minutes post procedure is common, though evidence suggests minimal effect on pregnancy rates.

TIMING AND NUMBER OF INSEMINATIONS

- Single insemination is generally preferred. Evidence shows no clear benefit with double insemination in terms of pregnancy rates, increasing cost and stress instead.
- Performing 3–6 consecutive IUI cycles is standard practice before considering alternative treatments.[4,5]

LUTEAL PHASE SUPPORT (LPS)

- Not usually required in natural or mildly stimulated cycles due to adequate corpus luteum function.
- In gonadotropin-stimulated cycles, vaginal progesterone supplementation may improve pregnancy and live birth rates and is recommended.

PROGNOSTIC FACTORS INFLUENCING SUCCESS

- **Female age:** Best results in women <35 years, with success declining sharply after 40 years.
- Male age may negatively influence sperm quality but has less impact if female partner is young.
- **Body mass index (BMI):** Obesity requires adjustment in stimulation dosage but does not substantially affect success once adjusted.
- **Duration and cause of infertility:** Longer infertility duration reduces chances; mild endometriosis responds better than severe forms.
- **Semen quality:** Higher motile sperm counts, better morphology, and total motile sperm counts >5 million increase success.

COMPLICATIONS

- IUI is low-risk but can rarely lead to infection, uterine cramping, or spotting.
- Multiple pregnancies and ovarian hyperstimulation syndrome risks exist with stimulation but are reduced with mild protocols and monitoring.

SUMMARY

Double IUI has no benefits over single IUI. IUI is a fundamental, patient-friendly assisted reproduction method suited to carefully selected patients, particularly those with mild male factor, unexplained infertility, or cervical infertility. Success depends on optimizing semen quality, stimulation, timing, and patient factors. Given its low complexity and cost, it serves as first-line therapy before advancing to IVF.

REFERENCES

1. ESHRE Capri Workshop Group. Intrauterine insemination. Hum Reprod Update. 2009;15(3):265-77.
2. Inceoglu C, Ozkaya E, Yilmaz MB. Intrauterine Insemination (IUI) Outcomes with Total Progressive Motile Sperm Count (TPMSC) Above and Below 5 Million. Cureus. 2025;17(4):e82580.
3. Ombelet W, Van Robays J. Artificial insemination history: hurdles and milestones. Facts Views Vis Obgyn. 2015;7(2):137-43.
4. Huniadi A, Bimbo-Szuhai E, Botea M, et al., Fertility Predictors in Intrauterine Insemination (IUI). J Pers Med. 2023;13(3):395.
5. Practice Committee ASRM. Evidence-based treatments for couples with unexplained infertility. Fertil Steril. 2020;113(2):305-22.

Semen Analysis and Sperm Function Test Overview

Ruchika Garg

Semen analysis (SA) is the first and most basic test used to assess male fertility. It measures sperm count, motility, shape, and other parameters to help identify potential causes of male infertility. All evaluations are performed according to guidelines in the World Health Organization (WHO) Laboratory Manual for the Examination and Processing of Human Semen, now in its 6th Edition (2021).

EVOLUTION OF WHO SEMEN ANALYSIS MANUAL

Since the first edition in 1980, WHO manuals have evolved to include improved techniques for semen testing, sperm preparation, cryopreservation, and quality control. The latest (6th) edition introduces new parameters like sperm DNA fragmentation (SDF) and oxidative stress (OS) testing, which provide better insights into sperm quality and fertility potential.

TABLE 1: WHO 6th edition semen parameter reference values (Lower 5th percentile).

Parameter	*WHO 2010 (5th Ed.)*	*WHO 2021 (6th Ed.)*
Semen volume (mL)	1.5 (1.4–1.7)	1.4 (1.3–1.5)
Total sperm number (million/ejaculate)	39 (33–46)	39 (35–40)
Total motility (%)	40 (38–42)	42 (40–43)
Progressive motility (%)	32 (31–34)	30 (29–31)
Immotile sperm (%)	22	20 (19–20)
Vitality (%)	58 (55–63)	54 (50–56)
Normal forms (%)	4 (3–4)	4 (3.9–4)

TABLE 2: Summary of key changes from WHO 5th to 6th edition.

Category	*Key updates*
Terminology	"Standard test" renamed Basic examination, "Optional test" → Extended examination "Research test" → Advanced examination
Basic examination	Addition of semen odor; subdivision of progressive motility into rapid/slow; morphology standardized with better imaging; vitality recommended when motility <40%; discontinuation of older terms like *oligozoospermia*, *asthenozoospermia*, etc.
Extended examination	Includes leukocyte counts, antisperm antibody testing, and sperm DNA damage tests (TUNEL, SCD, Acridine orange)
Advanced examination	Adds oxidative stress testing and refined CASA description; removes obsolete oocyte binding and penetration assays

SEMEN COLLECTION AND HANDLING

- Ideally, two samples are collected at least 2–3 weeks apart.
- Abstinence period should be consistent—recent data suggest that 1 day is optimal.
- Collection is via masturbation into a sterile cup; for cultural or religious restrictions, a special nontoxic condom may be used.
- After ejaculation, semen forms a coagulum that must liquefy within 30 minutes for assessment.
- **Color:** Normal is white/gray; yellow/green may indicate infection or medications; red or brown suggests blood.

Macroscopic Examination

Parameter	*Description*
Volume	Normal ≥1.4 mL. Low volume/aspermia requires evaluation for ejaculatory duct obstruction or retrograde ejaculation (via TRUS and postejaculatory urinalysis)
pH	Normal 7.2–8.2. Alkaline pH reflects seminal vesicle contribution; acidic may suggest obstruction or infection
Viscosity	Normally liquefies within 15–20 min. Delayed liquefaction (>2 h) suggests poor prostatic enzyme secretion; excessive thickness indicates hyperviscosity

MICROSCOPIC EXAMINATION

- **Sperm concentration:** Measured via hemocytometer; normal lower limit = 15 million/mL. If azoospermia suspected, centrifuge and re-examine the pellet.
- **Motility:** Evaluated at 37°C on fresh samples. The 6th edition reintroduces grading:
  - Grade a: Rapid progressive
  - Grade b: Slow progressive
  - Grade c: Nonprogressive
  - Grade d: Immotile
  - Normal lower reference for progressive motility = 30%.
- **Morphology:** Assessed using strict (Kruger) criteria. Only 4% or more normal forms are considered within fertile range. The 6th edition provides improved micrographs and systematic steps.
- **Leukocytospermia:** 1×10^6 leukocytes/mL indicates inflammation. Confirmed using peroxidase stain, as leukocytes generate reactive oxygen species detrimental to sperm function.

BIOCHEMICAL AND FUNCTIONAL EVALUATION

Accessory gland markers:

- Prostate: Zinc, citric acid
- Seminal vesicles: Fructose
- Epididymis: Alpha-glucosidase:
  - Low levels suggest duct obstruction or glandular dysfunction.

- **Sperm DNA Fragmentation (SDF):** Integrity of sperm DNA is essential for fertilization and embryo development. Tests include TUNEL, SCD, and Acridine Orange assays (recommended for clinical use).
- **Genetic Studies:** FISH detects chromosomal abnormalities (13, 18, 21, X, Y) in cases of recurrent pregnancy loss, failed ART, or known translocations.
- **Oxidative Stress (OS) Testing:** Assesses the balance between ROS and antioxidants in seminal plasma, useful in idiopathic infertility.

COMPUTER-ASSISTED SEMEN ANALYSIS (CASA)

A computer-based system analyzing sperm motility and kinematics. Measures include:

- *VCL:* Curvilinear velocity
- *VAP:* Average path velocity
- *VSL:* Straight-line velocity
- *LIN:* Linearity (VSL/VCL × 100)
- *ALH:* Amplitude of lateral head displacement

Though CASA provides precise measurements, manual counting remains superior for identifying cell debris and dead sperm, provided strict quality control is maintained.

SPERM VIABILITY TESTING

Performed when motility is <10%.

- Dye exclusion tests (Eosin Y, Trypan blue): Nonviable sperm uptake dye.
- Hypo-osmotic swelling (HOS) test: Live sperm develop a swollen tail; useful for selecting viable sperm for ICSI.

  In normal semen, ≥60% of sperm should swell in HOS testing.

SEMEN ANALYSIS FLOWCHART (STEP-BY-STEP)

1. **Patient History and Counseling:** Understand clinical background, infertility duration, previous treatments.
2. **Sample Collection:**
   - Collect 2 samples at least 2–3 weeks apart.
   - Abstinence period should be consistent (1–3 days).
   - Use a sterile wide-mouthed container or nontoxic condom if culturally required.
3. **Macroscopic Examination:** Assess volume, pH, viscosity, color, and odor.
   - Liquefaction expected within 15–30 min.
4. **Microscopic Examination:** Assess sperm concentration, motility (rapid/slow progressive), morphology, and leukocytes.
5. **Sperm Functional Tests:** Evaluate DNA fragmentation, oxidative stress, viability tests (e.g., HOS test).
6. **Interpretation and Reporting:** Compare with WHO reference levels, correlate with clinical context, recommend management.

KEY TAKEAWAYS

- WHO 6th edition simplifies terminology and focuses on clinical relevance.
- Emphasis on sperm function (DNA integrity, oxidative balance) over mere morphology.
- Two properly collected samples remain the cornerstone of reliable interpretation.

Individual results must always be correlated with clinical history, female partner's evaluation, and reproductive outcomes.

Gynecologic Oncology

Benign Lesions of Cervix

Ruchika Garg

INTRODUCTION AND BURDEN OF DISEASE

Cervical cancer is the only gynecological malignancy that is almost 100% preventable through vaccination and screening.

- India: ~1,25,000 new cases and ~75,000 deaths annually (4th most common cancer in women)
- 99.7% cases are caused by persistent high-risk HPV infection
- Natural history gives a 10–20-year window between HPV infection → CIN → invasive cancer → ideal for intervention
- WHO launched the Global Strategy to Eliminate Cervical Cancer as a public health problem by 2030 (incidence <4/100,000)

WHO 2030 Elimination Targets—"90-70-90"

Target	*Description*	*2030 Goal*
90	Girls fully vaccinated with HPV vaccine by age 15 years	90%
70	Women screened with high-performance test by 35 and 45 years	70%
90	Women with precancer treated + invasive cancer managed	90%

Human Papillomavirus (HPV)—The Causative Agent

Feature	*Details*
Virus type	Double-stranded DNA virus, >220 genotypes
Oncogenic classification	15 high-risk (Group 1 carcinogens), HPV-16 and -18 cause ~70 % of cancers
HPV-16	55–60% of squamous cell carcinomas
HPV-18	10–15%, more adenocarcinomas and aggressive behavior
Transmission	Almost exclusively sexual (skin-to-skin genital contact)
Peak acquisition	Immediately after sexual debut
Natural course	70–90% clear within 12–24 months; 10% persist → risk of CIN3+
Co-factors for persistence	Smoking, immunosuppression (HIV), multiparity, long-term OCP, multiple HPV types

Transformation Zone—The Origin of 99% Cervical Neoplasia

Term	*Definition*
Original SCJ	Junction between native ectocervical squamous epithelium and metaplastic squamous epithelium
New SCJ	Junction between metaplastic squamous and columnar epithelium
Transformation zone (TZ)	Area between original and new SCJ—site of active metaplasia and maximum HPV susceptibility

Types of Transformation Zone (IFCPC 2024 nomenclature)

Type	*Description*	*Fully visible?*	*Suitable for ablation?*
1	Entirely ectocervical	Yes	Yes
2	Has endocervical component but fully visible	Yes	Yes (if lesion seen)
3	Partially or completely endocervical, not visible	No	No → excision mandatory

Natural History of CIN

Lesion	*Regression*	*Persistence*	*Progression to CIN3*	*Progression to Invasion*
CIN 1	60–90%	10–30%	<15%	<1%
CIN 2	40–50%	35–40%	20%	5%
CIN 3	30–40%	50–60%	–	10–30% (10–20 yrs)

Progression 5–10 times faster in HIV-positive women.

Normal Cervix:

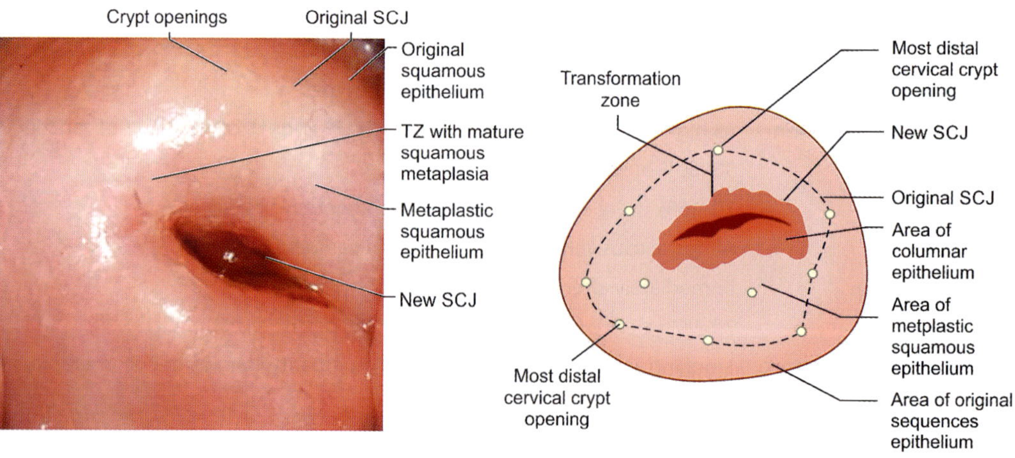

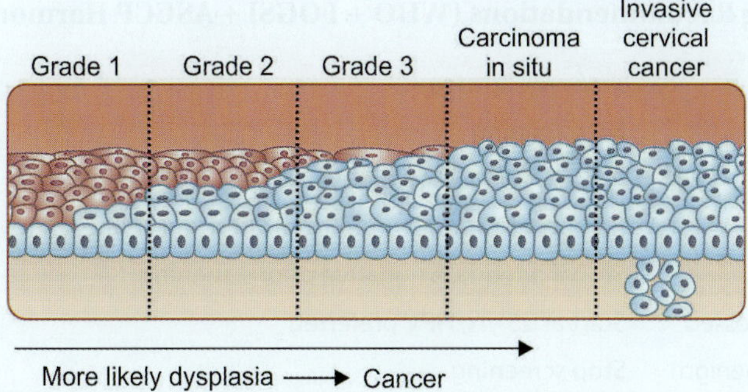

Bethesda 2014 Cytology Reporting (Still standard in India 2025)

Cytology result	*Interpretation*	*Next step (age ≥30 years)*
NILM	Normal	Routine screening
ASC-US	Atypical squamous cells	HPV triage preferred
ASC-H	Cannot exclude HSIL	Immediate colposcopy
LSIL	Low-grade SIL (HPV/CIN1)	Colposcopy
HSIL	High-grade SIL (CIN2/3)	Colposcopy + biopsy
AGC	Atypical glandular cells	Colposcopy + ECC ± endometrial sampling
AIS	Adenocarcinoma in situ	Excision (cold-knife preferred)

Current Screening Recommendations (WHO + FOGSI + ASCCP Harmonized)

Age group	*Preferred strategy*	*Interval*
<25 yrs	No screening	–
25–29 yrs	Primary HPV OR cytology	5 yrs/3 yrs
30–65 yrs	Primary HPV alone (preferred) OR co-test OR cytology	5 yrs/5 yrs/3 yrs
>65 yrs	Stop if adequate negative prior screening	–
HIV+/Immunosuppressed	Start at 25 yrs, HPV preferred	Every 3 yrs
Posthysterectomy (benign)	Stop screening	–

HPV Genotypes (Top 8 in India 2025)

16 (58–62 %) > 18 (10–12 %) > 45 > 31 > 33 > 52 > 58 > 35

Primary Screening Modality

GOLD STANDARD – Primary hrHPV testing (clinician or self-collected) every 5 years (age 25/30–65)

Self-Collected HPV Testing

WHO 2025: Equivalent to clinician-collected for all validated PCR assays → Gamechanger for India

Limitations of Conventional and Liquid-Based Pap Smear (Very High-Yield)

Limitation	*Conventional Pap*	*LBC*	*Clinical Impact (Exam points)*
Low sensitivity for HSIL/CIN2+	50–70%	70–85%	30–50% false negative → missed precancers
High inadequate/unsatisfactory rate	5–15%	<2%	Repeat visit → loss to follow-up
Sampling error (missed TZ)	Very common	Less	Especially postmenopause (receded SCJ)
Screening and interpretation error	15–20%	5–10%	Subjective, interobserver variation
Cannot detect endocervical/glandular lesions well	Very poor	Moderate	AGC/AIS often missed
Cannot be used for HPV co-testing from same sample (conventional)	No	Yes	Major advantage of LBC
Poor performance in postmenopausal women	Worst	Better	Dry vagina, atrophic cells, recessed SCJ
Requires immediate fixation and transport	Critical	Not needed	Logistical issue in rural areas
No residual material for ancillary testing (conventional)	No	Yes	LBC allows HPV, genotyping, biomarkers

Pap smear is no longer recommended as primary screening in any resource setting where HPV testing is available (WHO, FOGSI, ASCCP, ICMR).

Why Lugol's Iodine (VILI) is no longer routinely recommended/taught in many high-resource settings?

Reason	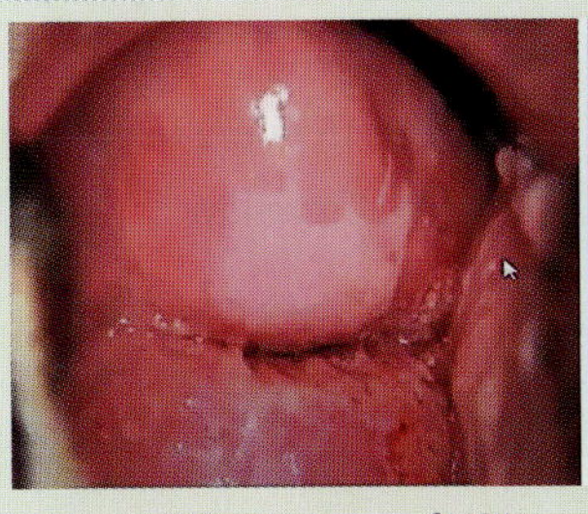 VIA positivity in a case of HSIL 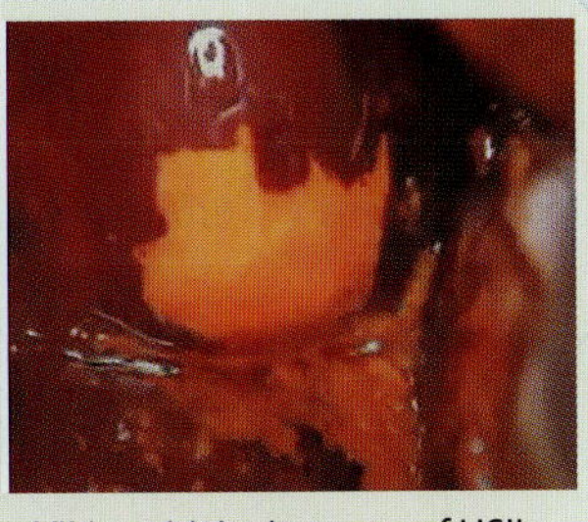 VILI positivity in a case of HSIL
Lower specificity than VIA	More false positives (nonglycogen areas mistaken)
Messy, stains patient and clinician	Poor acceptability
Allergic reactions (rare but reported)	Iodine sensitivity/anaphylaxis
Shelf-life and stability issues in hot climates	Turns ineffective fast in India
Not required when primary HPV or VIA available	Adds no extra yield
WHO 2021 and 2025 guidelines	Recommend VIA or HPV only; VILI optional and being phased out in most programs
India (NHSRC/NVCCP 2025)	VILI removed from training curriculum of ASHAs and staff nurses; only VIA taught

Current status:

- **LMICs with single-visit approach → still use VIA (acetic acid)**
- **VILI → largely abandoned except a few old state programs**

Updated Screening Modalities Comparison

Modality	*Sensitivity CIN2+*	*Specificity*	*Limitations/Disadvantages*	*Current Role*
Primary hrHPV	95–98 %	85–90%	Cost, lab infrastructure	Primary (global)
Self-collected HPV	94–97%	86–9%	Needs validated device and lab	Primary (India focus)
LBC	75–85%	95%	Low sensitivity, subjective	Only if HPV unavailable
Conventional Pap	55–75%	95%	All limitations listed above	Obsolete as primary
VIA	70–80 %	80–85%	Operator dependent, lighting	Single-visit LMICs only
VILI	80–90%	70–80%	Low specificity, allergy, stability	Phased out

Colposcopy—Swede Score (unchanged)

Parameter	*0*	*1*	*2*
Aceto-white	None/transparent	Thin	Thick, dense
Margins/surface	Diffuse	Sharp but irregular	Sharp + level difference (ridge)
Vessels	Fine	Absent	Coarse, bizarre
Lesion size	<5 mm	5–15 mm/2 quadrants	>15 mm/3–4 quadrants/endocervical
Iodine uptake	Brown	Faint yellow	Bright yellow

Score ≥7 → treat as CIN2+

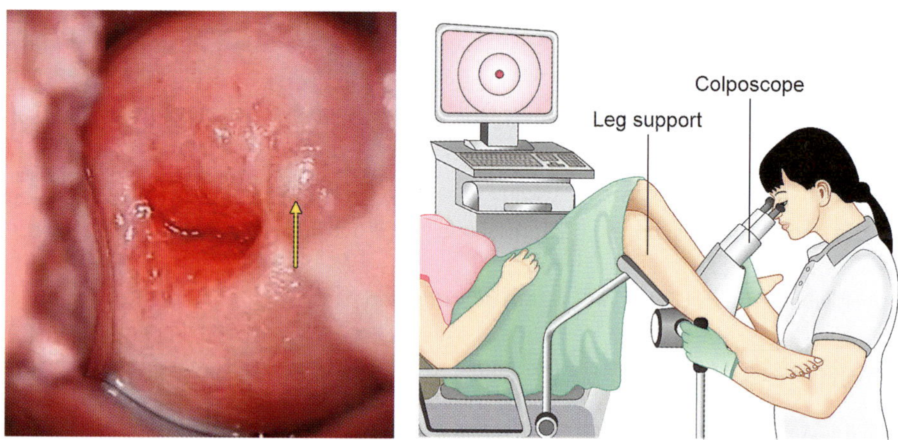

Screening Modalities—Quick Comparison

Method	*Sensitivity (CIN2+)*	*Specificity*	*Cost*	*Best setting*
Primary hrHPV testing	95–98%	85–90%	Moderate	Gold standard 2025
LBC/Conventional Pap	70–80%	95%	Moderate/Low	Where HPV not available
VIA/VILI	65–80%	80–85%	Very low	Single-visit LMICs

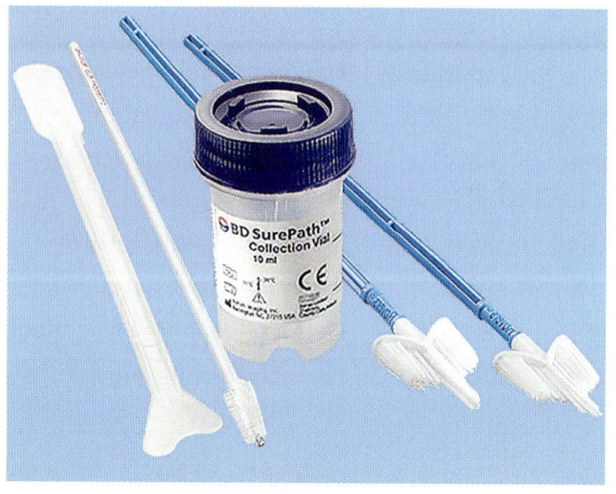

LBC

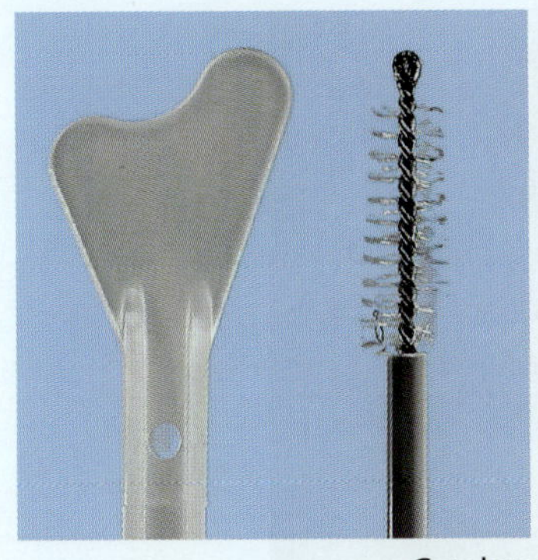
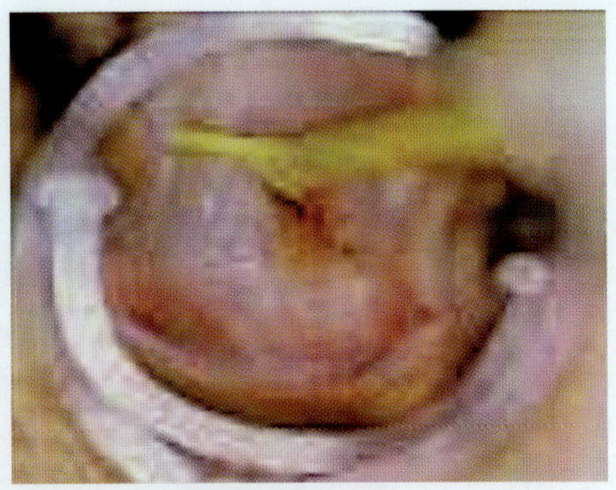

Cytobrush and ayres Spatula

Treatment Options for CIN2+

Method	*Depth*	*Fertility impact*	*Cure rate*	*Indication/Setting*
Thermal ablation	7 mm	Minimal	93–96%	New WHO favorite, single visit
Cryotherapy	7 mm	Minimal	90–95%	LMIC standard
LEEP/LLETZ	8–12 mm	1–5% stenosis	95–98%	OPD, histopathology needed
Cold-knife conization	15–20 mm	Highest risk preterm birth	>98%	Type 3 TZ, AIS, discrepancy
Hysterectomy	–	Loss of uterus	100%	Recurrent/postmenopausal + comorbidity

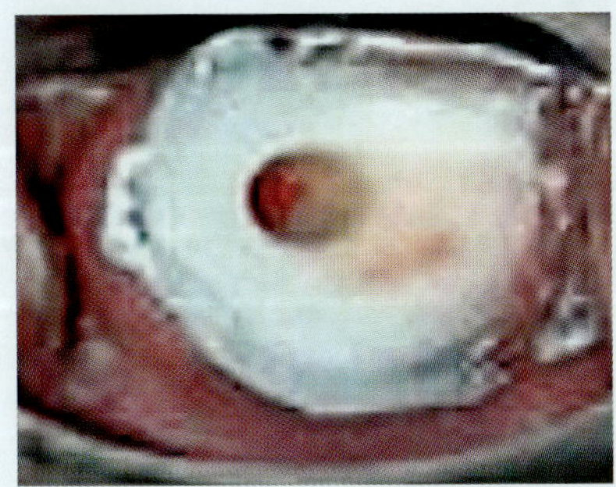

Postcryotherapy

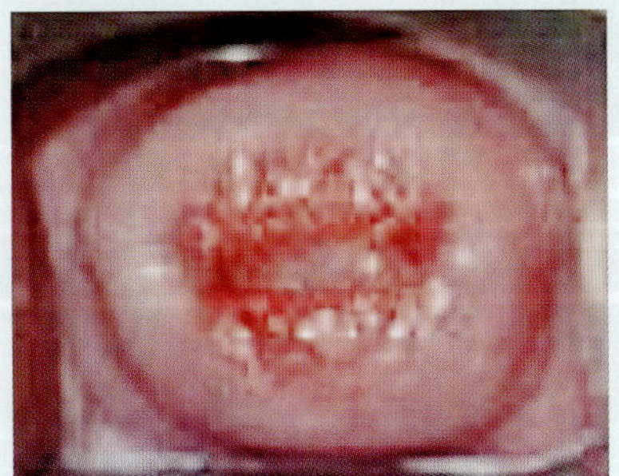

Precryotherapy

HPV Vaccines Available in India (2025)

Vaccine	*Valency*	*Types Covered*	*Age Group*	*Schedule (<15 yrs/ ≥15 yrs)*	*Remarks*
Cervarix	2	16, 18	9–45	2/3	—
Gardasil	4	6,11,16,18	9–45	2/3	—
Gardasil-9	9	6,11,16,18,31,33,45,52,58	9–45	2/3	Covers 90% cancers
Cervavac (SII)	4	6,11,16,18	9–26	2/3	Indigenous, free in NIP 2024 onward

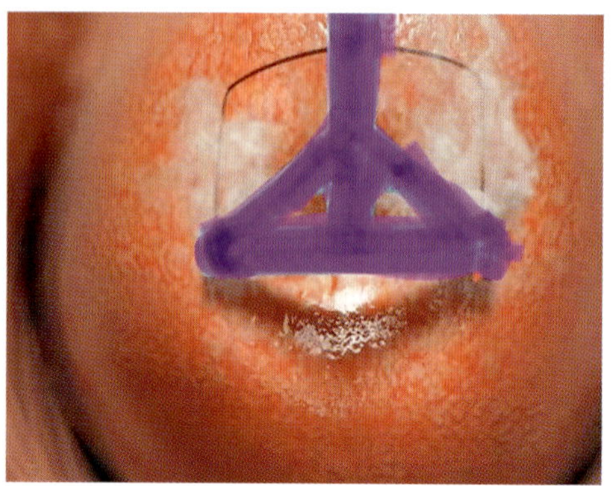

LEEP

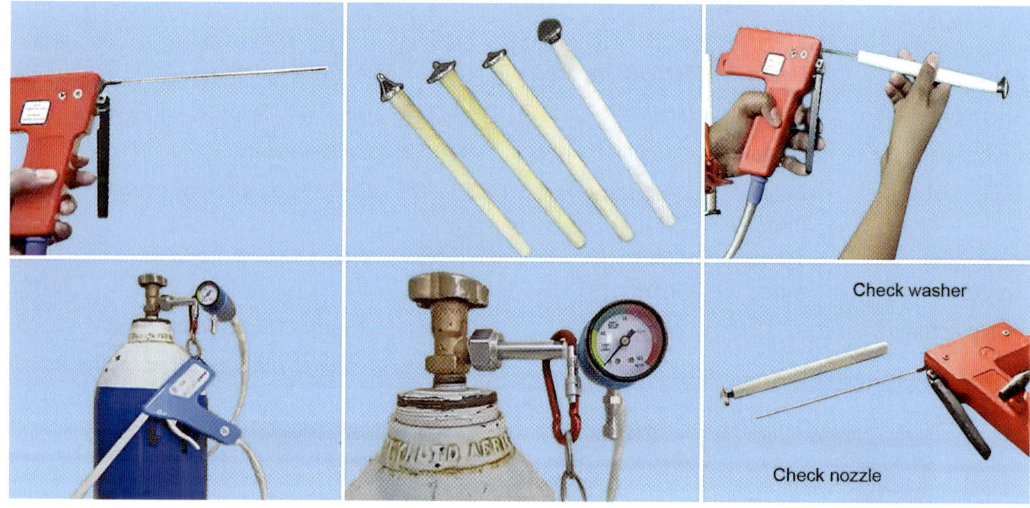

Cryotherapy

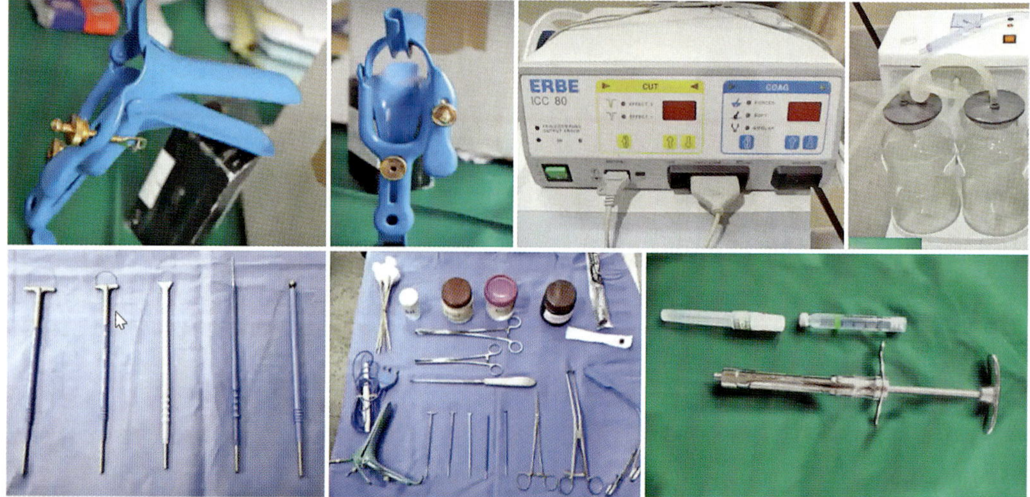

LEEP

Post-Treatment Follow-Up (Test of Cure)

- Preferred: hrHPV test at 12 months
- If negative → return to routine screening
- If positive → colposcopy ± repeat excision
- High-risk cases (CIN3, HIV+): Continue screening minimum 25 years

SUGGESTED READING

1. Bhatla N, Berek JS, Fredes MC, et al. Revised FIGO staging for carcinoma of the cervix uteri. Int J Gynecol Obstet 2025;168:213-9.
2. FOGSI GCPR. Cervical Cancer Screening and Treatment Guidelines 2024–2025.
3. ICMR. Consensus Document for Management of Cervical Cancer - 2024.
4. Perkins RB, Guido RS, Castle PE, et al. 2024 ASCCP Risk-Based Management Consensus Guidelines. J Low Genit Tract Dis. 2025;29:1-48.
5. World Health Organization. Guideline for screening and treatment of cervical pre-cancer lesions for cervical cancer prevention, 2nd edition. Geneva: WHO; 2025.

Preinvasive Lesions of Cervix and CIN

Ruchika Garg, Neelansha Varshney

Why Screening is Critical?

Cervical cancer has a long preinvasive phase (≥10 years), allowing detection and treatment of precancerous lesions before progression to invasive disease. Screening aims to identify asymptomatic individuals with precancer or early cancer.

Benefits of Screening

- Early detection and treatment
- Reduced morbidity and mortality

Cost-effective care with less radical treatment

WHO 2030 Elimination Strategy: 90–70–90 Targets

- 90% of girls fully vaccinated with HPV vaccine by age 15 years
- 70% of women screened by age 35 years and again by 45 years
- 90% of women with cervical disease treated

ETIOLOGY AND RISK FACTORS

- **Primary Cause:** High-risk HPV infection (HPV-16, -18 account for ~70% of cases).
- **Other Risk Factors:** Early sexual activity, multiple partners, multiparity, smoking, immunosuppression (e.g., HIV), low socioeconomic status.
- **HPV Pathogenesis:**
    - **Low-risk HPV** (6, 11): Cause genital warts; rarely progress to cancer.
    - **High-risk HPV** (16, 18, 31, 33, etc.): Integrate into host DNA, leading to oncogenic transformation.
- **Koilocytes:** HPV-infected squamous cells with perinuclear halos; seen in low-grade lesions (CIN1/LSIL).

TERMINOLOGY AND CLASSIFICATION

Old terminology	*CIN system*	*Bethesda system (2014)*
Mild dysplasia	CIN I	LSIL (Low-grade SIL)
Moderate dysplasia	CIN II	HSIL (High-grade SIL)
Severe dysplasia/CIS	CIN III	HSIL (High-grade SIL)

Key Definitions:

- **CIN:** Precancerous changes confined to epithelium; basement membrane intact.
- **LSIL (CIN I):** Lower 1/3 epithelial involvement; often regresses spontaneously.
- **HSIL (CIN II/III):** Involves ≥ lower 2/3 (CIN II) or full thickness (CIN III); higher risk of progression.
- **Natural History:**
  - **LSIL:** 60–80% regress; ~1% progress to cancer over years.
  - **HSIL:** 30% regress, 40% persist, 30% progress to invasion over 5–10 years.

SCREENING MODALITIES

- **Pap Smear (Cytology)**
  Procedure: Exfoliated cervical cells collected via Ayre's spatula/endocervical brush.
  Timing: Mid-cycle; avoid intercourse, douching, tampons 48 hours prior.
  Liquid-Based Cytology (LBC): Reduces inadequate samples; allows reflex HPV testing.
  Sensitivity: ~70–80% for HSIL; specificity 95–98%.
- **HPV Testing**
  Primary Screening: Preferred for women ≥30 years (higher sensitivity).
  Methods: DNA detection of 14 high-risk types; genotyping for 16/18.
  Advantages: High negative predictive value; allows longer screening intervals (5 years).
  Self-collection: Comparable sensitivity; improves access.
- **Visual Inspection with Acetic Acid (VIA)/Lugol's Iodine (VILI)**
  Use: Low-resource settings where cytology unavailable.
  Procedure: Apply 3–5% acetic acid (VIA) or Lugol's iodine (VILI); abnormal areas appear acetowhite or nonstaining.
  Limitations: Lower specificity; operator-dependent.
- **Colposcopy**
  Indication: Triage for abnormal screening (ASC-US, LSIL, HSIL, HPV 16/18+).
  Procedure: Magnified visualization after applying acetic acid (5%) and Lugol's iodine.
  Key Findings: Acetowhite epithelium, punctation, mosaicism, atypical vessels.
  Biopsy: Directed punch biopsy of abnormal areas for histologic confirmation.

SCREENING GUIDELINES

Organization	*Age to start*	*Recommended screening*	*Frequency*
ACOG (2020)	21 years	Pap alone	Every 3 years
30–65 years		Co-test (Pap + HPV) OR HPV primary	Every 5 years
WHO (2021)	30 years	HPV primary	Every 5–10 years

High-Risk Groups: More frequent screening if immunosuppressed, HIV+, prior CIN II/III, or DES exposure.

DIAGNOSTIC WORK-UP

Algorithm for Abnormal Screening:

Abnormal Screen → Colposcopy + Biopsy → Histology Report
↓
LSIL (CIN I) → Observation (repeat in 1 year)
HSIL (CIN II/III) → Excision (LEEP/Conization) or Ablation
Suspected Invasion → Cone Biopsy (Cold Knife/LEEP)

Cone Biopsy Indications:

- Nonvisible transformation zone
- Discrepancy between cytology, colposcopy, and biopsy
- Suspected microinvasion or glandular lesion

MANAGEMENT OF CIN

LSIL (CIN I)

- **Observation:** Repeat co-testing at 12 months (most regress).
- **Treatment:** Only if persistent ≥2 years or patient preference.

HSIL (CIN II/III)

- **Ablative Therapies (if criteria met):**
    - **Cryotherapy:** Freezes tissue; outpatient, low cost.
    - **Thermoablation:** Heated probe; minimal bleeding.
    - **Laser Ablation:** Less common due to cost.
- **Excisional Therapies (preferred):**
    - **LEEP/LLETZ:** Wire loop electrosurgical excision; outpatient, diagnostic and therapeutic.
    - **Cold Knife Conization (CKC):** Scalpel excision; used if microinvasion suspected.

Selection Criteria for Conservative Treatment

- Lesion fully visible on colposcopy
- No endocervical involvement
- No suspicion of invasion

Follow-Up Post-Treatment

- **HSIL:** Co-testing at 6 and 12 months, then annually for 20 years.
- **Persistent/Recurrent:** Repeat excision or hysterectomy (if no fertility desire).

PREVENTION

Primary Prevention

- **HPV Vaccination**
    - **Target age:** 9–14 years (2 doses) or 15–45 years (3 doses).
    - **Vaccines:**
        - **Bivalent (Cervarix):** HPV 16, 18
        - **Quadrivalent (Gardasil/Cervavac):** HPV 6, 11, 16, 18
        - **Nonavalent (Gardasil 9):** HPV 6, 11, 16, 18, 31, 33, 45, 52, 58
- **Efficacy:** Near 100% protection against targeted HPV types if given before exposure.

Secondary Prevention

- Population-based screening per guidelines.
- Treatment of precancerous lesions.

Tertiary Prevention

Management of invasive cancer (beyond this chapter).

NEET PG/EXAM HIGHLIGHTS

- **Koilocytes:** Perinuclear halo → HPV effect; seen in LSIL.
- **CIN III/CIS:** Full-thickness dysplasia; basement membrane intact.
- **LEEP vs. CKC:** LEEP is outpatient, lower morbidity; CKC used if microinvasion suspected.
- **Primary HPV screening:** Recommended ≥30 years; more sensitive than cytology.
- **WHO 90–70–90:** Vaccination, screening, treatment targets for 2030 elimination.

KEY POINTS

- **HPV is necessary** for cervical carcinogenesis; vaccination prevents infection.
- **Screening saves lives:** Pap, HPV testing, or VIA detect precancer.
- **LSIL often regresses;** HSIL requires treatment to prevent invasion.
- **Colposcopy directs biopsy** for abnormal screens.
- **Excision (LEEP) preferred** for HSIL; ablation options exist if criteria met.
- **Lifelong follow-up** after HSIL treatment due to persistent risk
- Quadrivalent **Gardasil** protect against HPV types 6/11 (90% of genital warts) and 16/18 (cervical cancer).
- Cervavac launched by Serum Institute of India is a Quadrivalent vaccine covering HPV-6, 11, 16, and 18 and has achieved license from 9-26 years of age and has much less cost compared to Gardasil.

Vaccines Available:

- **Gardasil (Quadrivalent):** Ages 9–45 years.
- **Gardasil 9:** Covers HPV 6/11/16/18/31/33/45/52/58. Broader cancer protection, ages 9–45 years.
- **Cervavac (Quadrivalent):** Serum Institute of India, targets HPV 6/11/16/18. Licensed for ages 9–26 years, cost-effective.

Side Effects (Gardasil 9)

- **Common:** Injection site pain/redness/swelling, headache, fever, fatigue, nausea.
- **Rare:** Allergic reactions, syncope, mild myalgia/dizziness.
- No link to serious long-term effects (e.g., infertility).

Recommendations

- **Dosing:** 2 doses (6–12 months apart) for ages 9–14 years; 3 doses (0, 1–2, 6 months) for ages 15–45 years.
- Use in both genders to prevent HPV-related cancers/warts.

Cancer Cervix

Ruchika Garg, Neelansha Varshney

EPIDEMIOLOGY

In India, cervical cancer accounts for ~21% of global cases.

- Annual new diagnoses (2022): ~127,500; age-standardized incidence rate: 17.7 per 100,000 women.
- Annual deaths: ~79,900 (government estimate: 35,691).
- Prevalence (2023): >340,000 women living with cervical cancer.
- Cumulative lifetime risk: Development 2.5%; death 1.4%.
- Global comparison: India's incidence (14–18 per 100,000) exceeds global average (13.1 per 100,000) and WHO elimination threshold (≤4 per 100,000). Invasive disease is often preceded by preinvasive lesions (e.g., CIN) lasting years.

RISK FACTORS

High-risk groups include women with:

1. **HPV Infection:** Primary risk; high-risk strains (HPV-16, 18); sexually transmitted; persistent infection causes dysplasia.
2. **Multiple Sexual Partners/Early Sexual Debut:** Increases HPV exposure.
3. **Smoking:** Damages cervical DNA; impairs HPV clearance.
4. **Immunosuppression:** HIV or medications hinder HPV resolution.
5. **Long-Term Oral Contraceptives:** ≥5 years slightly elevates risk; reversible post-discontinuation.
6. **High Parity:** Hormonal/immunological changes increase HPV susceptibility.
7. **Low Socioeconomic Status:** Limited screening/vaccination access.
8. **Family History:** Minor genetic role.
9. **Irregular Screening:** Misses CIN.
10. **Early Marriage/Childbearing:** Linked to early HPV exposure.
11. **Co-infections:** Chlamydia, HSV potentiate HPV persistence.

PATHOLOGY

- **Histological Types:** Squamous cell carcinoma (SCC) 80–90%; adenocarcinoma 10–20% (increasing due to OCP/progestogen use).
- **FIGO 2021 Classification:**
  - **Squamous:** HPV-associated, HPV-independent, NOS.

- **Glandular:** Adenocarcinoma (HPV-associated/independent: gastric, clear cell, mesonephric), endometrioid, carcinosarcoma, adenosquamous, mucoepidermoid, adenoid basal, undifferentiated.
- **Gross Features:** SCC: Cauliflower-like (exophytic, friable, bleeding), ulcerative, or flat/indurated. Endocervical: Barrel-shaped, protrudes through os.
- **Histology:** SCC graded as well (G1: pearls), moderately (G2), or poorly differentiated (G3). Nonkeratinizing common; keratinizing with pearls.
- **Precursor:** CIN 1–3 progresses to microinvasive then invasive SCC.
- **Microinvasive (FIGO IA):** Microscopy-only; IA1: ≤3 mm depth, ≤7 mm width; IA2: >3–≤5 mm depth, ≤7 mm width. No gross lesion; no LVSI in IA1.

MODE OF SPREAD

- **Direct:** Adjacent (vagina, parametrium, uterus); advanced: bladder/rectum.
- **Lymphatic:**
  - *Primary:* Parametrial, obturator, internal/external iliac.
  - *Secondary:* Common iliac.
  - *Tertiary:* Para-aortic, presacral.
- **Hematogenous:** Lung/liver (rare early); ovarian metastasis: 1% SCC, 10% adenocarcinoma.
- **Stage Patterns:** I: Minimal nodes; II: Obturator/internal iliac; III: External/common iliac/para-aortic; IV: Distant (supraclavicular/mediastinal rare).
- **Prognostic Impact:** Nodal involvement key; influences RT/surgery.

EVALUATION AND INVESTIGATIONS

Clinical

- **History:** Postcoital/intermenstrual/postmenopausal bleeding; foul discharge; pelvic pain; dyspareunia; advanced: leg edema, hematuria, flank pain, weight loss.
- **Exam:** Speculum: Growth/ulcer/bleeding. Bimanual: Cervix size/mobility, parametrial/vaginal involvement. Rectovaginal: Pelvic wall extension.

Diagnostic

- **Pap Smear:** Screening; shows tadpole cells, fibers, malignant cells, hemorrhage/necrosis.
- **Colposcopy/Biopsy:** Directed punch/wedge; gold standard for invasion.
- **ECC/Cone Biopsy:** For occult lesions/microinvasive.

Staging (FIGO 2018)

- Incorporates clinical, imaging (r), pathologic (p) findings.
- **Imaging:**

Modality	*Purpose*
MRI (gold standard)	*Local:* Tumor size, parametrium/vagina invasion, nodes
CT	Nodes, distant metastasis
PET-CT	Nodes/distant; RT planning
USG (TVS/renal)	Size, hydronephrosis
Chest X-ray/CT	Lung metastasis
IVU	Ureteric obstruction (IIIB)

- **Labs:** CBC (anemia), RFT/LFT (organ function), HIV, SCC antigen (monitoring).
- **Endoscopy**: Cystoscopy/proctoscopy for IVA suspicion.

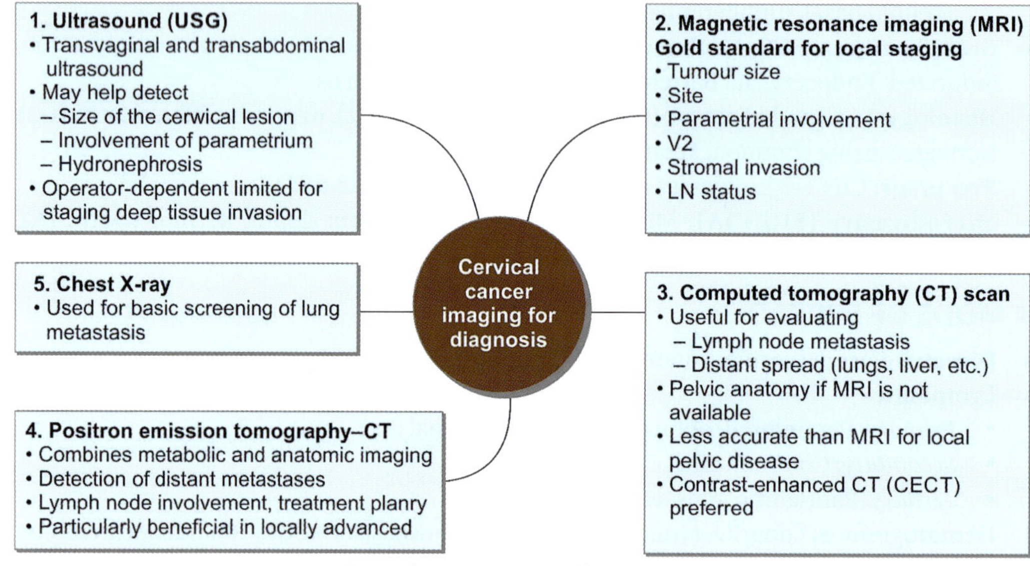

Cervical cancer imaging for diagnosis

Staging (FIGO 2018)

- **I:** Confined to cervix.
  - IA: Microscopic; IA1 ≤3 mm depth; IA2 >3–≤5 mm.
  - IB: Visible/>5 mm; IB1 ≤2 cm; IB2 >2–≤4 cm; IB3 >4 cm.
- **II:** Beyond cervix, not pelvic wall/lower 1/3 vagina.
  - IIA: No parametrium; IIA1 ≤4 cm; IIA2 >4 cm.
  - IIB: Parametrium (not wall).
- **III:** Pelvic wall/lower 1/3 vagina/hydronephrosis/nodes.
  - IIIA: Lower vagina.
  - IIIB: Wall/hydronephrosis.
  - IIIC: Nodes; IIIC1 pelvic; IIIC2 para-aortic (add r/p).
- **IV**: Adjacent organs/distant.
  - IVA: Bladder/rectum.
  - IVB: Distant.

Lymph Node Metastasis Incidence

Stage	*Pelvic LN (%)*	*Para-aortic LN (%)*
IA1	<1–2	Rare
IA2	5–10	Rare
IB1	10–15	Rare
IB2	15–25	~5
IB3	20–35	10–15
II	25–40	20
III	50–70	30
IV	>65	>40

Risks: LVSI, size >2 cm, deep invasion, parametrium, poor differentiation.

Clinical Features

- **Early:** Asymptomatic; screening essential.
- **Invasive:** Postcoital bleeding (most common), intermenstrual/menorrhagia, foul discharge, pelvic pain.
- **Advanced:** Urinary (dysuria/hematuria), bowel (constipation/bleeding), back pain, leg edema, cachexia.
- **Signs:** Friable growth, barrel cervix, parametrial nodularity, anemia.

Microscopic Features

- **SCC:** Invasive nests/sheets; pleomorphic/hyperchromatic nuclei; high N:C ratio; mitoses; keratin pearls (well-differentiated); desmoplasia.
- **Subtypes:** Keratinizing (pearls), nonkeratinizing (sheets), basaloid (aggressive), papillary, verrucous.
- **IHC:** p16+ (HPV surrogate), Ki-67 high, CK5/6/p63/p40+ (squamous).
- **Mutations:** PIK3CA (worse prognosis).
- **Precursor:** CIN III (no invasion); stromal invasion/LVSI prognostic.

Differential Diagnosis

Condition	*Features*
Cervicitis	Erythema, discharge; responds to antibiotics
Polyp	Pedunculated, benign histology
Ectropion	Velvety red; no ulcer
Nabothian cysts	Mucus-filled, asymptomatic
TB cervix	Granulomas/caseation on biopsy
CIN III	Dysplasia, no invasion
Endometrial Ca extension	CK7+/ER+, p16 focal
Metastatic (e.g., Colon)	CK20+/CDX2+
Melanoma	S100/HMB-45+
Lymphoma	CD20/CD3+

Management

- **Principles:** Stage-based; avoid dual modalities to minimize morbidity.
- **Stage-Wise:**
    - **IA1:** Conization/trachelectomy (fertility); simple hysterectomy; SLN/PLND if LVSI+.
    - **IA2:** Modified radical hysterectomy (Type II) + PLND; trachelectomy (fertility); BT if inoperable.
    - **IB1:** Radical hysterectomy (Type III) + PLND; trachelectomy (select).
    - **IB2/IIA1:** Radical hysterectomy (Type III) + PLND; RT if unfit.
    - **IB3/IIA2–IVA:** Chemoradiation (platinum-based) + BT; exenteration (select IVA).
    - **IVB:** Palliative chemo/immunotherapy/targeted; RT for bleeding.
- **Surgery Types (Piver-Rutledge/Querleu-Morrow):**

Type	Features	Use
I/A	Simple	IA1 no LVSI
II/B	Modified radical	IA1 LVSI+/IA2
III/C1–C2	Radical/nerve-sparing	IB1–IIA
IV/D	Extended	Limited invasion
V	Exenteration	Recurrence

- **MIS Caution:** LACC trial showed higher recurrence versus open; avoid routine.
- **NSRH:** Preserves nerves; reduces bladder/bowel/sexual dysfunction.
- **Complications:** Intraoperative (hemorrhage, ureter/bladder injury); early (UTI, fistula, lymphocele); late (dysfunction, lymphedema).
- **Radiotherapy:** EBRT (45–50 Gy) + BT (80–90 Gy total); concurrent cisplatin.
  - Adjuvant (PORT): High-risk (Peters: LN+/margins+/parametrium); intermediate (Sedlis: Size ≥4 cm/LVSI/deep invasion).
- **Neoadjuvant Chemo:** Not standard; trials ongoing (e.g., paclitaxel/ifosfamide).
- **Fertility-Sparing:** Trachelectomy + PLND (IA2–IB1 ≤2 cm, no LVSI/nodes); cerclage; risks: miscarriage/preterm.
- **Pregnancy:** Biopsy confirm; <24 wk: Hysterectomy/RT post-termination; >24 wk: CS at 34 wk + radical surgery/RT.
- **Endocervical AdenoCa:** Younger; barrel cervix; early spread; chemoradiation + hysterectomy; no ovarian preservation.
- **Stump Ca:** Post-subtotal hysterectomy; difficult management; trachelectomy + RT.

Recurrence

- **Risk:** 20–25% early stages; peaks 2 years post-treatment.
- **Types:** Central (vault), regional (wall/nodes), distant (lung/liver/bone).
- **Symptoms:** Bleeding, pain, edema, cough/hemoptysis.
- **Investigations:** Exam, smear, MRI/PET-CT, SCC antigen.
- **Management:** Central: Exenteration (anterior/posterior/total); lateral: RT (if prior surgery); distant: Chemo (paclitaxel + platinum).
- **Contraindications to Exenteration:** Wall fixation, distant mets, poor status.

Follow-Up

- Years 1–2: Every 3–4 months (history, exam, Pap, labs).
- Years 3–5: Every 6 months.
- 5 years: Annual.
- Imaging/labs as indicated.

Palliative Care

- **Symptoms:** Pain (WHO ladder/opioids), bleeding (RT/packing), discharge (hygiene/antibiotics), obstruction (stents/colostomy).

- **Therapy:** Palliative RT/chemo (cisplatin/paclitaxel ± bevacizumab); immunotherapy (pembrolizumab PD-L1+).
- **Support:** Psychosocial, family involvement, hospice/DNR.

Future Developments

- **Targeted:** Bevacizumab (anti-VEGF; approved); PD-1 inhibitors (pembrolizumab/cemiplimab); EGFR/PI3K/mTOR/PARP inhibitors in trials.
- **HPV Vaccines:** Therapeutic (E6/E7 targeted).
- **Precision:** NGS/liquid biopsy for mutations (PIK3CA/PTEN); biomarkers (PD-L1/TMB/MSI).
- **Challenges:** Access, resistance; focus on combinations/neoadjuvant.

CHAPTER 16

Benign Ovarian Tumors

Ruchika Garg

INTRODUCTION

Benign ovarian tumors are common, presenting across all age groups from infancy to postmenopause **(Fig. 1)**. They may be asymptomatic (incidental findings) or cause symptoms like abdominal pain, distension, palpable mass, or abnormal uterine bleeding.[1] These tumors range from physiologic cysts to benign neoplasms, with up to 10% of women undergoing surgery for ovarian masses in their lifetime.[2] Most premenopausal ovarian masses are benign, with malignancy risk low (1:1,000, rising to 3:1,000 at age 50 years).[3] Timely diagnosis and management are critical to minimize complications and future risks. This chapter covers the anatomy, histopathology, classification, diagnosis, and management of benign ovarian tumors, emphasizing evidence-based guidelines.

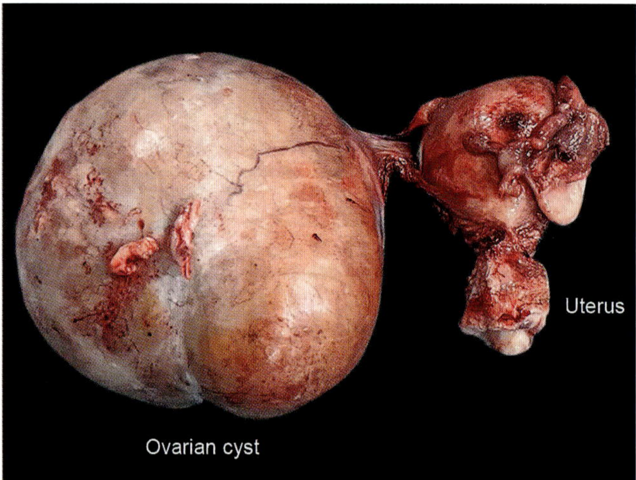

Fig. 1: A benign ovarian cyst.

ANATOMY

The ovaries are located posterolaterally to the uterus, attached to the pelvic wall by the infundibulopelvic ligament (containing ovarian artery, vein, lymphatics, and nerves) and to the uterus medially by the utero-ovarian ligament. The mesovarium connects the ovary to the broad ligament. During reproductive years, ovaries measure 2.5–5 cm long, 1.5–3 cm thick, and 0.7–1.5 cm wide, varying with hormonal activity.[4]

HISTOPATHOLOGY

The ovary comprises a cortex (stroma with follicles, corpora lutea, and corpora albicantia) and medulla (fibromuscular tissue with blood vessels), lined by cuboidal/columnar epithelium.[5] Benign ovarian tumors are classified by histological origin:

- **Surface Epithelial-Stromal Tumors:** 65–70% of ovarian tumors.[6]
- **Sex Cord-Stromal Tumors:** 15–20%.[7]
- **Germ Cell Tumors:** 5–10%.[8]
- **Metastatic Tumors:** ~5%.[6]

CLASSIFICATION

Benign ovarian tumors are categorized by age group and histological type, with rare outliers **(Table 1)**.

TABLE 1: Age-based classification of benign ovarian tumors.[1,6]

Age group	*Common benign tumors*
Children/Adolescents	Simple cysts (60%), mature cystic teratoma, gonadoblastoma, endometrioma **(Fig. 3)**
Reproductive Age	Functional cysts, serous/mucinous cystadenoma, mature cystic teratoma, endometrioma, Brenner tumor, granulosa cell tumor
Postmenopausal	Functional cysts, serous/mucinous cystadenoma, Brenner tumor

Citation in text: **Table 1** outlines age-specific benign ovarian tumors, guiding differential diagnosis.[1,6]

DIFFERENTIAL DIAGNOSIS

- **Gynecologic:** Fibroids, uterine tumors, hydrosalpinx, hematosalpinx.
- **Nongynecologic:** Urinary tract (e.g., bladder cysts), bowel (e.g., appendiceal mucocele), retroperitoneal masses.[9]

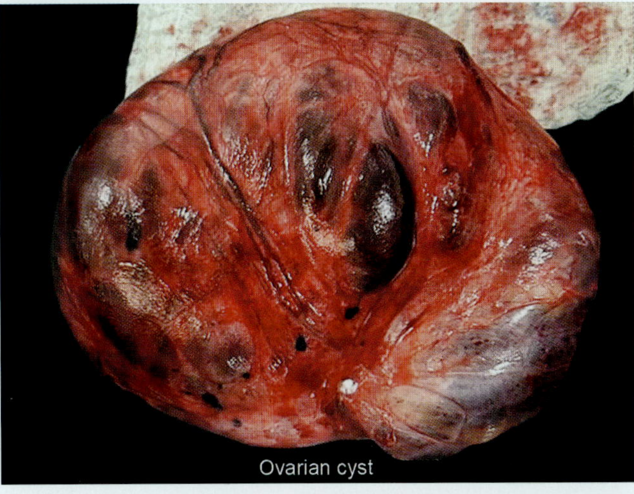

Fig. 2: Twisted ovarian cyst.

DIAGNOSIS

Clinical Evaluation

- **History:** Assess symptoms (pain, distension, bleeding), risk factors (family history of breast/ovarian/colorectal cancer), and reproductive status.[3]
- **Examination:** General physical, breast, and gynecologic (bimanual/rectovaginal) to detect masses or ascites.[9]

Imaging

- **Transvaginal Ultrasound (TVUS):** First-line for presumed benign ovarian tumors; assesses size, morphology, and vascularity.[10]
- **MRI:** Second-line for indeterminate masses or those >7 cm; superior for complex cysts.[11]
- **CT:** Used for suspected nongynecologic origins or staging malignancy (e.g., omental/peritoneal implants).[12]

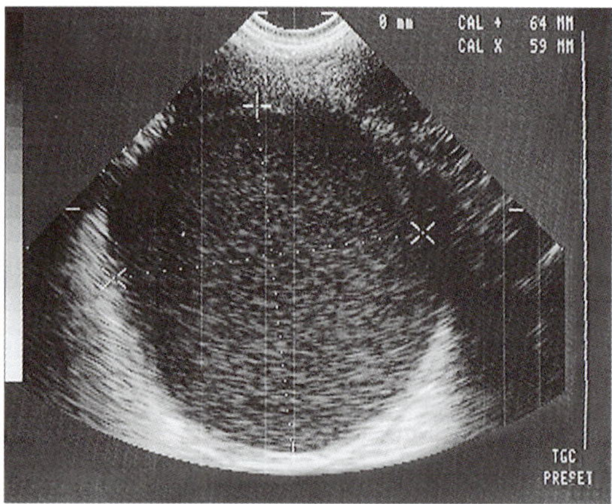

Fig. 3: An ultrasound image of an endometrioma.

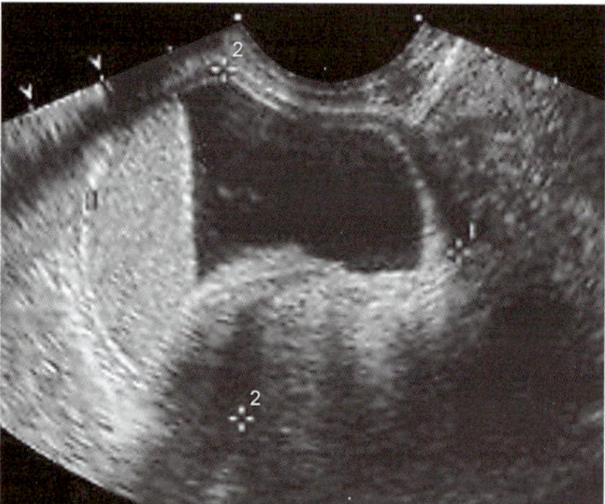

Fig. 4: An ultrasound image of a dermoid cyst.

Tumor Markers

- **CA-125:** Nonspecific; not routine in premenopausal women with simple cysts due to elevation in benign conditions (e.g., endometriosis, fibroids).[13] >35 IU/mL
- **LDH, AFP, β-hCG:** Indicated in women <40 years with complex masses to rule out germ cell tumors.[14]
- **HE4:** More specific than CA-125; fewer false positives in benign disease (e.g., endometriosis).[15]

IOTA ULTRASOUND RULES

The International Ovarian Tumor Analysis (IOTA) group provides criteria to differentiate benign from malignant masses **(Table 2; Fig. 5)**.[16]

TABLE 2: IOTA ultrasound rules for benign versus malignant ovarian tumors.[16]

Benign (B-rules)	*Malignant (M-rules)*
Unilocular cyst	Irregular solid tumor
Solid components <7 mm	Ascites
Acoustic shadowing	≥4 papillary structures
Smooth multilocular tumor <100 mm	Irregular multilocular tumor ≥100 mm
No blood flow	Very strong blood flow

Citation in text: IOTA ultrasound rules **(Table 2)** enhance diagnostic accuracy for ovarian masses.[16]

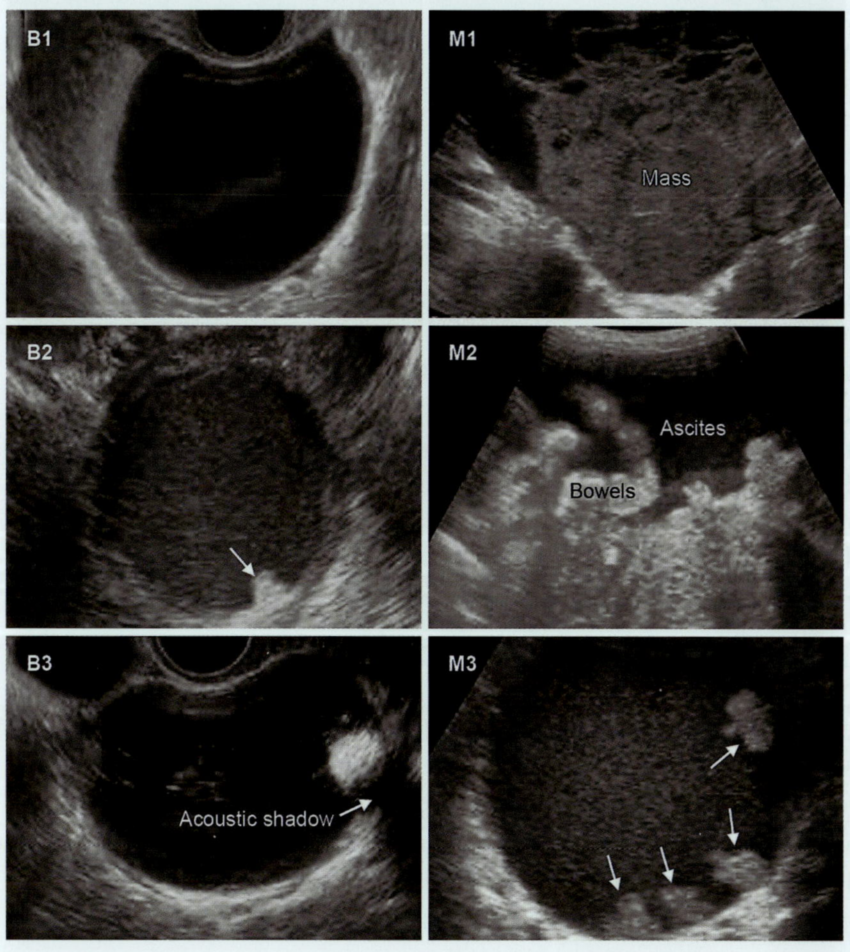

Contd...

Contd...

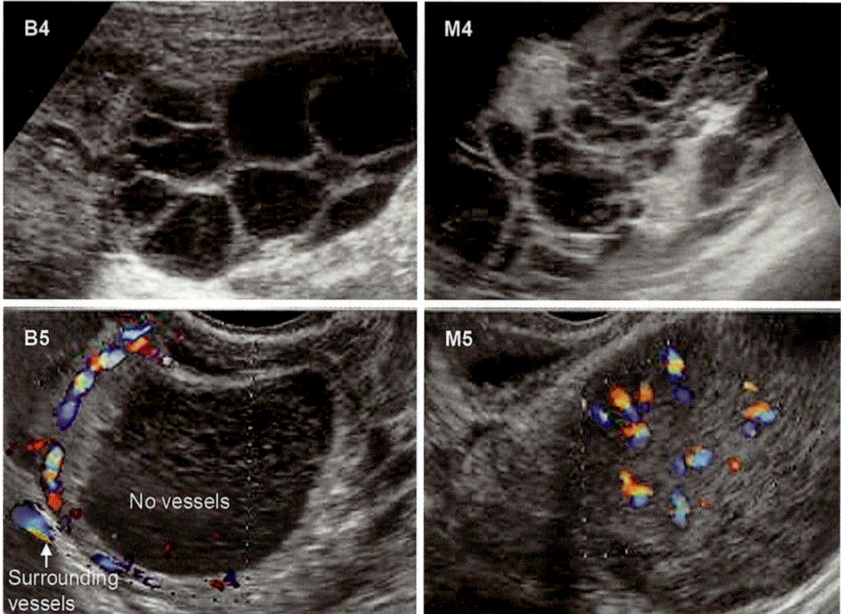

Fig. 5: IOTA ultrasound rules for benign versus malignant ovarian tumors.

RISK OF MALIGNANCY INDEX (RMI)

RMI I = U × M × CA-125:[17]

- **U (Ultrasound Score):** 0 (score 0), 1 (score 1), 3 (score 2–5); scored for multilocular cysts, solid areas, metastases, ascites, bilateral lesions.
- **M (Menopausal Status):** 1 (premenopausal), 3 (postmenopausal).
- **CA-125:** >35 Serum level (IU/mL).
- **Threshold:** RMI >200 indicates referral to gynecologic oncology.[3]

TYPES OF BENIGN OVARIAN TUMORS

TABLE 3: Classification of benign ovarian tumors.[6-8]

Category	*Tumors*
Functional cysts	Simple follicular cyst, corpus luteal cyst
Epithelial tumors	Serous cystadenoma, mucinous cystadenoma, cystadenofibroma, Brenner tumor
Sex cord-stromal tumors	Fibroma, thecoma, fibrothecoma, Leydig cell tumor, stromal luteoma
Germ cell tumors	Mature cystic teratoma (dermoid cyst)
Others	Endometrioma

Citation in text: **Table 3** categorizes benign ovarian tumors by histological origin.[6-8]

Functional Cysts

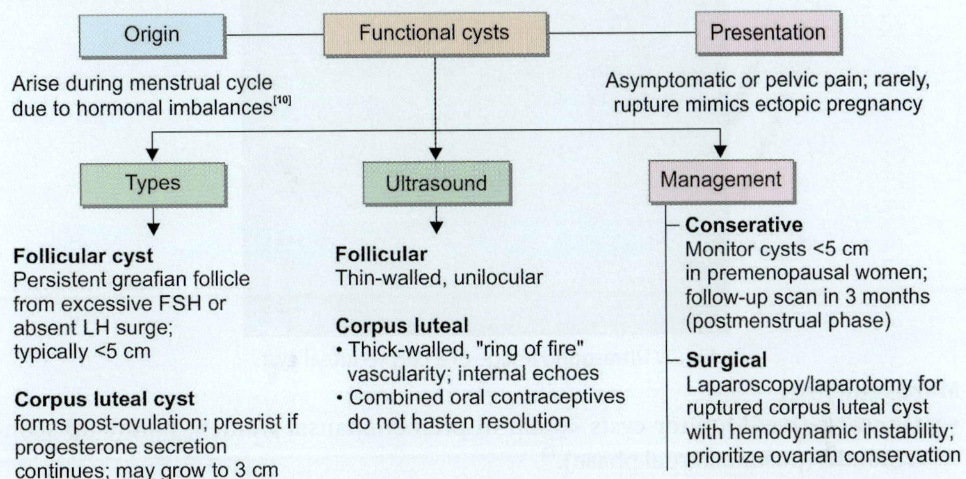

- **Origin:** Arise during menstrual cycle due to hormonal imbalances.[18]
- **Types:**
  - **Follicular Cyst:** Persistent Graafian follicle from excessive FSH or absent LH surge; typically <5 cm **(Fig. 6)**.
  - **Corpus Luteal Cyst:** Forms postovulation; persists if progesterone secretion continues; may grow to 3 cm **(Fig. 7)**.
- **Presentation:** Asymptomatic or pelvic pain; rarely, rupture mimics ectopic pregnancy.
- **Ultrasound:** Follicular: Thin-walled, unilocular; Corpus luteal: Thick-walled, "ring of fire" vascularity, internal echoes.[10]

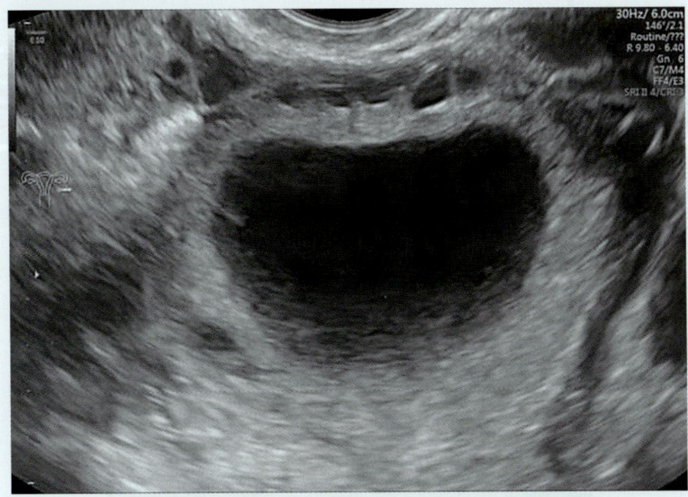

Fig. 6: Ultrasound image of a follicular cyst.

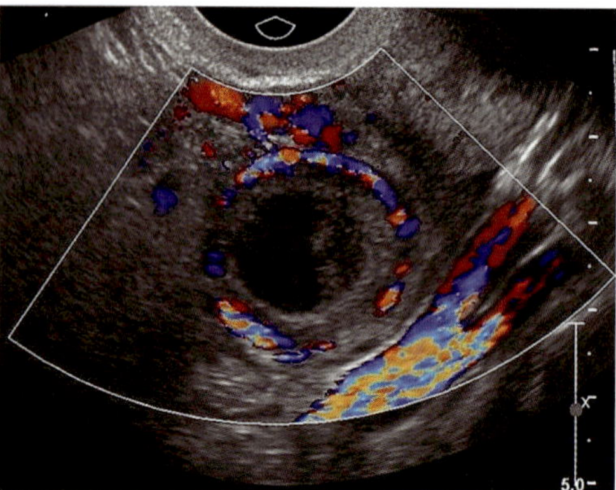

Fig. 7: Ultrasound image of a corpus luteal cyst.

- **Management:**
  - **Conservative:** Monitor cysts <5 cm in premenopausal women; follow-up scan in 3 months (postmenstrual phase).[18]
  - **Surgical:** Laparoscopy/laparotomy for ruptured corpus luteal cyst with hemodynamic instability; prioritize ovarian conservation.[19]
  - **Note:** Combined oral contraceptives do not hasten resolution.[20]

Epithelial Ovarian Tumors

- **Prevalence:** 65–75% of ovarian tumors; 15% in pediatric populations.[6]
- **Types:**
  - **Serous Cystadenoma (Fig. 8):**
    - **Incidence:** 40% of ovarian tumors; 10% bilateral; common in reproductive age.[6]
    - **Presentation:** Pelvic heaviness/pain or incidental; unilocular/multilocular cysts with thin walls.[10]
    - **Risk:** 7–13% malignancy risk (premenopausal), 8–45% (postmenopausal).[21]
    - **Management:** Observe cysts <5 cm in premenopausal women; laparoscopy for fertility preservation, laparotomy for large/suspicious masses (RMI <200).[22]

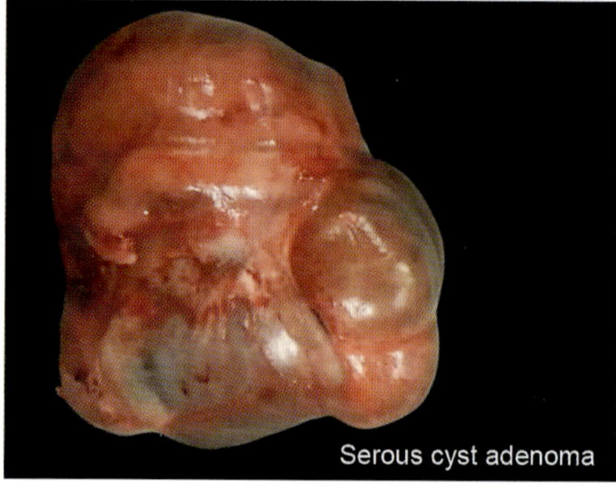

Fig. 8: Benign serous cyst adenoma.

- **Mucinous Cystadenoma (Fig. 9):**
  - **Incidence:** 15–20% of epithelial tumors; 10% bilateral; middle-aged women.[6]
  - **Presentation:** Pelvic pressure/pain; large multilocular cysts without surface invasion.[10]
  - **Complications:** Torsion, rupture (risk of pseudomyxoma peritonei).[23]
  - **Management:** Cystectomy or salpingo-oophorectomy; laparotomy for suspected malignancy.[22]

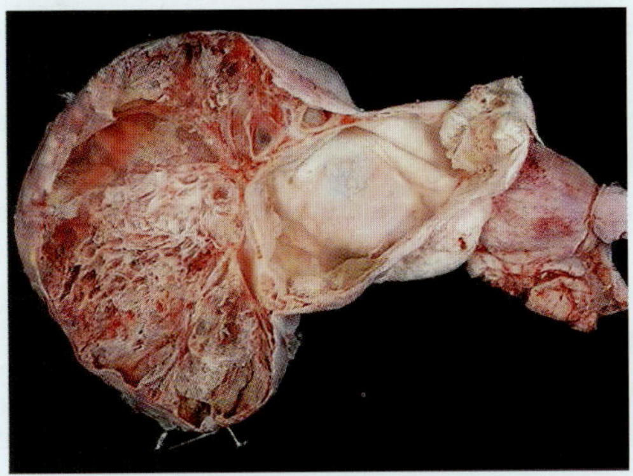

Fig. 9: Image of mucinous cyst adenoma.

- **Cystadenofibroma:**
  - **Incidence:** 1.7% of benign tumors; 15% bilateral; age 15–65 years.[6]
  - **Ultrasound:** Cystic with septations (30%), papillary projections (50%), peripheral vascularity.[11]
  - **Management:** Oophorectomy with frozen section to rule out malignancy.[24]
- **Brenner Tumor (Fig. 10):**
  - **Incidence:** 2–3% of ovarian tumors; fifth–sixth decades.[6]
  - **Presentation:** Incidental, abdominal mass, or postmenopausal bleeding; 20% coexist with other tumors.[10]
  - **Imaging:** Solid/cystic with low T2 signal on MRI due to fibrous content.[11]
  - **Management:** Surgical resection; histopathological diagnosis.[25]

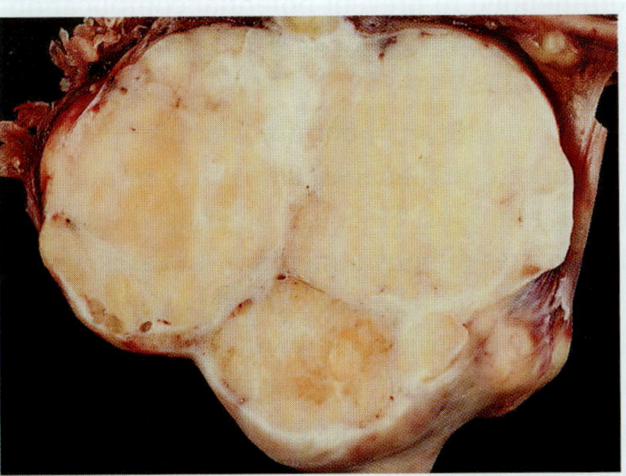

Fig. 10: An image of Brenner tumor.

Sex Cord-Stromal Tumors

- **Prevalence:** <4% of benign ovarian neoplasms; perimenopausal presentation.[7]
- **Types:**
  - **Fibroma:**
    - **Incidence:** 4% of ovarian neoplasms; unilateral.[7]
    - **Presentation:** Ascites (10–15%), Meigs syndrome (ascites + hydrothorax).[26]
    - **Management:** Oophorectomy; cystectomy if fertility desired.[27]
  - **Thecoma:**
    - **Presentation:** Postmenopausal; estrogen excess (abnormal bleeding, endometrial neoplasia).[7]
    - **Management:** Hysterectomy + bilateral salpingo-oophorectomy (due to endometrial cancer risk); unilateral oophorectomy in young patients.[27]
- **Fibrothecoma, Leydig Cell Tumor, Stromal Luteoma:** Rare; managed similarly.[7]
- **Sertoli-Leydig Cell Tumor:**
  - **Presentation:** Young women (<40 years); virilization (33%) or estrogen excess.[7]
  - **Management:** Oophorectomy; cystectomy if fertility-preserving.[27]

Germ Cell Tumors

- **Mature Cystic Teratoma (Dermoid Cyst):**
  - **Incidence:** 20% of benign ovarian tumors; 10–15% bilateral; common in pregnancy.[8]
  - **Presentation:** Pain or asymptomatic; ultrasound shows dermoid plug, mesh, or fat-fluid levels.[10]
  - **Risk:** 1–2% malignancy.[8]
  - **Management:** Conservative for asymptomatic cysts < 4–6 cm; laparoscopic cystectomy for larger/symptomatic cysts.[28] Small, asymptomatic dermoid cysts may not require immediate surgical intervention, as they can remain stable for extended periods or even regress spontaneously. Nevertheless, because these cysts typically enlarge over time, complete excision by an experienced surgeon—ensuring the cyst wall remains intact—is generally recommended to prevent potential complications. Performing surgery at an early stage can also minimize the extent of dissection, allowing for a smaller incision and better cosmetic results.
- Surgical removal further provides an opportunity for histopathological confirmation, which is important since some rare malignant lesions may mimic a dermoid cyst in the head and neck region of children. Most cysts can be excised through a direct approach, with meticulous dissection at sites of bony adherence. In cases where rupture of the cyst wall occurs intraoperatively, the residual tissue should be thoroughly curetted and irrigated to prevent recurrence. When vital structures are involved, partial excision may be necessary.
- Incomplete removal of a dermoid cyst is associated with a higher risk of recurrence; therefore, early surgical management offers the advantage of achieving complete excision with intact capsule integrity. For small cysts, endoscopic excision is emerging as a minimally invasive alternative technique.

Endometrioma

- **Origin:** Endometriotic tissue in ovaries; reproductive age.[2]
- **Presentation:** Subfertility, dysmenorrhea, dyspareunia; "kissing ovaries" on laparoscopy.[10]
- **Ultrasound:** Diffuse low-level echoes, hyperechoic wall foci ("chocolate cyst").[10]
- **Management**:
  - **Conservative:** Monitor small/asymptomatic cysts; continuous/cyclic COCs reduce recurrence post-cystectomy.[29]
  - **Surgical:** Laparoscopic cystectomy by advanced surgeons; avoid GnRH agonists presurgery.[30]

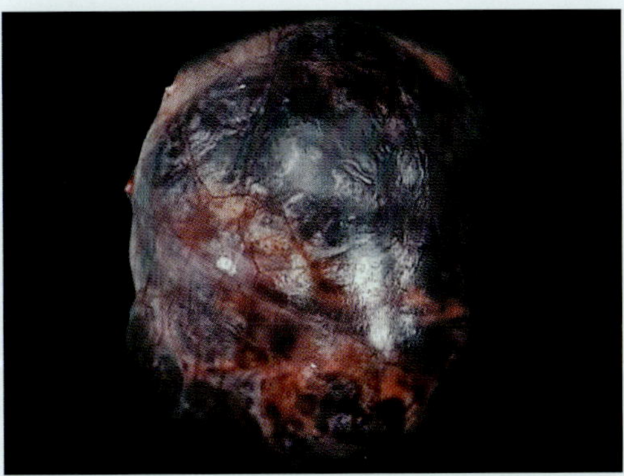

Fig. 11: Hemorrhagic ovarian cyst.

Complications

- **Torsion:** Common in dermoids/mucinous cysts; presents with acute pain.[23]
- **Rupture:** Risk of pseudomyxoma peritonei (mucinous) or hemoperitoneum (corpus luteal cyst).[19]
- **Malignancy:** Increased risk with benign epithelial tumors (RR 1.39, 95% CI 1.01–1.90).[21]

EMERGING TRENDS AND GUIDELINES

- **IOTA ADNEX Model:** Predicts malignancy risk with higher accuracy than RMI.[31]
- **Minimally Invasive Surgery:** Laparoscopy preferred for PBOT; reduces morbidity.[22]
- **Fertility Preservation:** Cystectomy prioritized in reproductive-age women.[28]
- **ACOG/NICE Guidelines (2023):** Recommend TVUS, RMI, and conservative management for low-risk cysts.[3,10]
- **ESHRE (2022):** Nonsurgical diagnosis for endometriomas. Laparoscopy is no longer the gold standard for diagnosis. COCs for recurrence prevention.[29]

CONCLUSION

Benign ovarian tumors are diverse, ranging from functional cysts to complex neoplasms. Most are manageable conservatively or with minimally invasive surgery, guided by TVUS, IOTA rules, and RMI. Multidisciplinary care, incorporating patient preferences and fertility goals, optimizes outcomes. Advances in imaging and surgical techniques continue to improve diagnosis and management.

KEY POINTS

- Benign ovarian tumors are common; malignancy risk is low (1:1,000 premenopausal).[3]
- TVUS and IOTA rules are first-line for diagnosis; MRI for indeterminate masses.[10,16]
- Functional cysts often resolve spontaneously; surgical intervention for complications.[18]
- Laparoscopy is preferred for PBOT; laparotomy for suspected malignancy.[22]
- Endometriomas require tailored management to preserve fertility.[29]

REFERENCES

1. Timmerman D, Testa AC, Bourne T, et al. Simple ultrasound-based rules for the diagnosis of ovarian cancer. Ultrasound Obstet Gynecol. 2016;47(6):751-9.
2. Muto MG. Management of the adnexal mass. Gynecol Oncol. 2017;144(3):615-22.
3. National Institute for Health and Care Excellence. Ovarian cancer: Recognition and initial management. NICE guideline [NG122]. 2023.
4. Clement PB, Young RH. Ovarian anatomy and histology. In: Kurman RJ, Ellenson LH, Ronnett BM. (Eds). Blaustein's Pathology of the Female Genital Tract. New York: Springer; 2019.
5. Kurman RJ, Shih IM. The dualistic model of ovarian carcinogenesis. Am J Pathol. 2016;186(4):733-47.
6. Prat J. Pathology of benign and malignant ovarian epithelial tumors. Int J Gynecol Pathol. 2018;37(1):1-10.
7. Young RH. Sex cord-stromal tumors of the ovary: An update. Adv Anat Pathol. 2018;25(3):178-91.
8. Horta M, Cunha TM. Germ cell tumors of the ovary: A review. Diagn Interv Imaging. 2017;98(4):291-302.
9. Spencer JA, Gore RM. Non-ovarian causes of adnexal masses. Radiology. 2016;280(2):345-57.
10. American College of Obstetricians and Gynecologists. Management of adnexal masses. ACOG Practice Bulletin No. 174. Obstet Gynecol. 2016;128(5):e210-26.
11. Thomassin-Naggara I, Aubert E, Rockall A, et al. MRI characterization of adnexal masses. Eur Radiol. 2019;29(5):2338-47.
12. Forstner R, Meissnitzer M, Cunha TM. Update on imaging of ovarian cancer. Curr Radiol Rep. 2016;4(6):31.
13. Buys SS, Partridge E, Black A, et al. Effect of CA-125 screening on ovarian cancer mortality. JAMA. 2017;317(18):1901-12.
14. Shaaban AM, Rezvani M, Elsayes KM, et al. Ovarian germ cell tumors: Imaging features. AJR Am J Roentgenol. 2016;207(5):1033-44.
15. Moore RG, Miller MC, Steinhoff MM, et al. HE4 in the differential diagnosis of ovarian masses. Clin Chem Lab Med. 2017;55(9):1307-14.
16. Van Calster B, Van Hoorde K, Valentin L, et al. Evaluating the risk of ovarian cancer before surgery using the ADNEX model. BMJ. 2019;367:l5720.
17. Jacobs I, Oram D, Fairbanks J, et al. Risk of malignancy index in ovarian cancer. Br J Obstet Gynaecol. 2016;123(Suppl 1):25-30.
18. Grimes DA, Jones LB, Lopez LM, et al. Oral contraceptives for functional ovarian cysts. Cochrane Database Syst Rev. 2016;4:CD006134.
19. Bottomley C, Bourne T. Diagnosis and management of ovarian cyst accidents. Best Pract Res Clin Obstet Gynaecol. 2017;41:66-76.

20. Levine D, Brown DL, Andreotti RF, et al. Management of asymptomatic ovarian cysts. Radiology. 2019;293(2):251-62.
21. Wentzensen N, Poole EM, Trabert B, et al. Ovarian cancer risk associated with benign ovarian tumors. J Natl Cancer Inst. 2016;108(9):djw109.
22. Canis M, Rabischong B, Houlle C, et al. Laparoscopic management of adnexal masses. J Gynecol Surg. 2018;34(3):109-16.
23. Nezhat CR, Kalan A, Nezhat CH. Mucinous cystadenoma complications: A review. J Minim Invasive Gynecol. 2017;24(7):1035-41.
24. Cho SM, Byun JY, Rha SE, et al. CT and MRI findings of cystadenofibromas. AJR Am J Roentgenol. 2016;207(3):597-604.
25. Green GE, Mortele KJ, Glickman JN, et al. Brenner tumors of the ovary: Imaging features. Abdom Imaging. 2016;41(8):1547-56.
26. Meigs JV. Fibroma of the ovary with ascites and hydrothorax. Am J Obstet Gynecol. 2017;216(3):S1-S5.
27. Schultz KAP, Harris AK, Schneider DT, et al. Management of ovarian sex cord-stromal tumors. Gynecol Oncol. 2016;142(1):178-87.
28. Telischak NA, Yeh BM, Joe BN, et al. Mature cystic teratoma: Imaging and management. Radiographics. 2017;37(4):1247-63.
29. Dunselman GAJ, Vermeulen N, Becker C, et al. ESHRE guideline: Management of women with endometriosis. Hum Reprod. 2022;37(2):233-55.
30. Becker CM, Bokor A, Heikinheimo O, et al. ESHRE guideline: Endometriosis. Hum Reprod Open. 2022;2022(2):hoac009.
31. Timmerman D, Van Calster B, Testa A, et al. Predicting the risk of malignancy in adnexal masses based on the ADNEX model. Am J Obstet Gynecol. 2016;214(4):424.e1-424.e14.

Ovarian Malignancy

Richa Bansal, Sumedha Sharad Pathade

INTRODUCTION

Ovarian cancer is a significant gynecological malignancy characterized by high mortality due to late diagnosis.

EPIDEMIOLOGY

Ovarian cancer ranks as the eighth most common malignancy and the eighth leading cause of cancer-related mortality among women worldwide, accounting for approximately 3.7% of all female cancers and 4.7% of cancer deaths as of 2020. Globally, 324,603 new cases were reported in 2022, with incidence projected to rise to nearly half a million annually by 2050, particularly in Asia and Africa. In the United States, the age-adjusted incidence rate stands at 10.3 per 100,000 women per year, with the highest frequency of diagnosis among women aged 55–64 years. High-grade serous carcinoma is the predominant histological subtype.

ETIOPATHOGENESIS

Ovarian cancer is now understood as a heterogeneous disease with divergent molecular pathways and origins. The dualistic model classifies tumors as Type I (low-grade serous, endometrioid, mucinous, and clear cell carcinomas) and Type II (high-grade serous carcinoma, carcinosarcoma, undifferentiated carcinoma). Type I tumors arise via stepwise malignant transformation of benign or borderline precursors and frequently harbor mutations in KRAS, BRAF, PTEN, or ARID1A. Conversely, Type II tumors—often high-grade serous carcinomas—are typified by TP53 mutations and are thought to originate from the distal fallopian tube epithelium; nearly half show germline or somatic BRCA1/2 mutations. Chronic inflammation—termed "inflammaging", altered immune surveillance, and dysbiosis (oncobiosis)—contribute to pathogenesis through continuous exposure to reactive oxygen species, cytokines, and growth factors, promoting genomic instability and neoplastic transformation. The gonadotropin hypothesis implicates sustained ovarian epithelial proliferation under high gonadotropin levels, especially postmenopause.

RISK FACTORS

Several risk factors modulate ovarian cancer susceptibility:

- Advancing age, with majority of cases occurring postmenopause.
- Genetic predisposition: Germline mutations in BRCA1/2, genes associated with Lynch syndrome, RAD51C, RAD51D increase lifetime risk. Family history of ovarian, breast, or colorectal cancers heightens risk.

- Personal history of breast cancer.
- Reproductive factors: Nulliparity, delayed childbearing (first full-term pregnancy after 35 years), and infertility increase risk, whereas multiparity and oral contraceptive use confer protection.
- Hormone replacement therapy in postmenopausal women.
- Obesity and high BMI.
- Endometriosis, particularly linked to clear cell and endometrioid subtypes.
- Fertility treatments have a debated but possible association.

CLINICAL FEATURES

Ovarian cancer is often dubbed the "silent killer" because early-stage disease is frequently asymptomatic or manifests vague, nonspecific symptoms. Classic presenting features include:

- Abdominal bloating or distention.
- Pelvic pain or discomfort.
- Early satiety and anorexia.
- Urinary urgency or frequency.
- Altered bowel habits (constipation, indigestion).
- Unintentional weight loss and fatigue.
- Abnormal vaginal bleeding, especially postmenopausal, though less common. At advanced stages, signs may include palpable abdominal or pelvic mass, ascites, cachexia, and paraneoplastic syndromes (e.g., subacute cerebellar degeneration). CA-125 serum levels are elevated in the majority of advanced-stage cases, though only half of early-stage cancers exhibit this marker

Diagnostic Work-up

- **Imaging:**

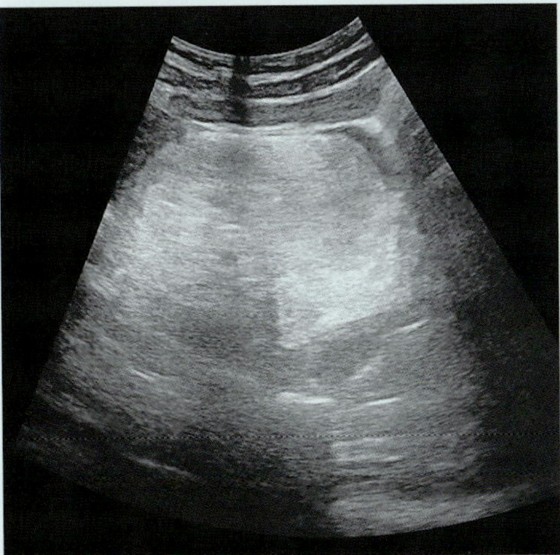

Ultrasound showing a large solid ovarian mass in a 16-year-old presenting with acute urinary retention; 1.5 L urine drained on catheterization. Tumor size: approximately 10 × 8 cm.

- **Transvaginal Ultrasound:** First-line imaging modality
    - Assesses mass characteristics (size, solid/cystic components, septations, papillary projections)

 - ♦ **O-RADS (Ovarian-Adnexal Reporting and Data System):** Standardized risk stratification system
- **CT Scan:** For staging (assesses peritoneal deposits, lymph nodes, distant metastases)
- **MRI:** Problem-solving tool for characterizing indeterminate masses **(Fig. 1)**

- **Biomarkers:**
  - **CA-125:** Primary tumor marker (elevated in ~80% of epithelial ovarian cancers)
    - ♦ Limitations: Can be elevated in benign conditions (endometriosis, PID, fibroids)
  - **HE4:** Often used with CA-125 in ROMA (Risk of Ovarian Malignancy Algorithm)
  - **ROMA Score:** Combines CA-125, HE4, and menopausal status to predict malignancy risk
- **Risk Assessment Tools:**
  - **ROMA Algorithm:** Stratifies patients into high-/low-risk categories
  - **RMI (Risk of Malignancy Index):** Combines CA-125, ultrasound findings, and menopausal status
- **Definitive Diagnosis**
- **Histopathological confirmation** via:
  - Surgical biopsy (laparoscopic or open)
  - Analysis of ascitic fluid (if present)
  - **Note:** FNAC is generally avoided due to risk of rupture and spillage
- **Multimodal Approach:**
  - No single test is diagnostic
  - Combination of clinical assessment, imaging, and biomarkers guides management
  - High index of suspicion required for at-risk women (BRCA mutations, family history)

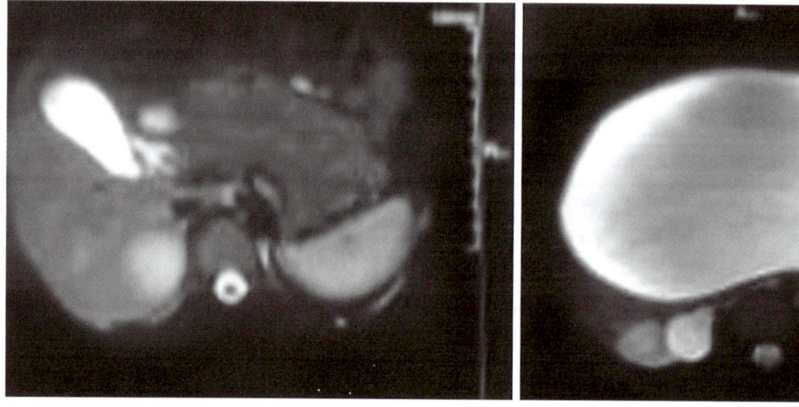
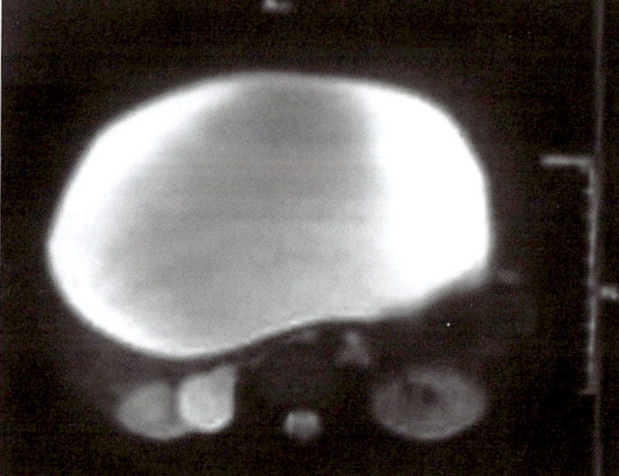

Fig. 1: MRI showing a huge ovarian cyst.

LONG QUESTIONS

1. a. **Latest FIGO staging of ovarian cancer**
   b. **How will you manage a case of a 56-year-old woman with Stage IIIC epithelial ovariancancer?**
2. **Molecular classification of ovarian cancer and its clinical implications.**

SHORT QUESTIONS

1. **Tumor markers for ovarian cancer**
2. **HIPEC**
3. a. **Classification of ovarian germ cell tumors.**
   b. **Dermoid cyst.**
4. a. **Classification of Sex cord tumors.**
   b. **Granulosa cell tumor.**

LONG ANSWERS

***Ans.* 1a.** The FIGO (International Federation of Gynecology and Obstetrics) staging for ovarian cancer. It helps in guiding treatment decisions and predicting prognosis. It is as follows:

Stage I: Tumor confined to the ovary.

- **IA:** Tumor confined to one ovary; no tumor on the surface of the other ovary; capsule intact; no malignant cells in ascites or peritoneal washings.
- **IB:** Tumor confined to both ovaries; capsule intact; no malignant cells in ascites or peritoneal washings.
- **IC:** Tumor either on one or both ovaries with at least one of the following: Tumor on one or both surfaces of one or both ovaries, capsule ruptured, malignant cells in ascites or peritoneal washings, or tumor involves the liver surface.

Stage II: Tumor involves one or both ovaries with pelvic extension.

- **IIA:** Tumor involves one or both ovaries with extension to the uterus and/or fallopian tubes.
- **IIB:** Tumor involves one or both ovaries with extension to other pelvic tissues (e.g., bladder or rectum).
- **IIC:** Tumor involves one or both ovaries with at least one of the following: Tumor on one or both surfaces of one or both ovaries, capsule ruptured, malignant cells in ascites or peritoneal washings.

Stage III: Tumor involves one or both ovaries with peritoneal implants outside the pelvis and/ or regional lymph node metastasis.

- **IIIA:** Tumor involves one or both ovaries with microscopically confirmed spread to the peritoneum outside the pelvis.
- **IIIB:** Tumor involves one or both ovaries with macroscopic peritoneal implants beyond the pelvis but no larger than 2 cm in greatest dimension.
- **IIIC:** Tumor involves one or both ovaries with peritoneal implants larger than 2 cm and/or regional lymph node metastasis.

Stage IV: Tumor involves one or both ovaries with distant metastasis.

- **IVA:** Tumor involves one or both ovaries with malignant pleural effusion (fluid in the pleural cavity).
- **IVB:** Tumor involves one or both ovaries with distant metastases to organs such as liver parenchyma or distant lymph nodes.

***Ans.* 1b.** This classification system is crucial for treatment planning and provides an important prognostic indicator for patients.

Management of Stage IIIC ovarian cancer, which involves peritoneal implants larger than 2 cm and/or regional lymph node metastasis, typically involves a combination of surgery and chemotherapy. The goal is to achieve optimal debulking of the tumor and to address any residual cancer cells with systemic treatment. Here is a general overview of the management approach.

- **Surgical Management**
  - **Primary Debulking Surgery:** The primary treatment for Stage IIIC ovarian cancer is often surgical. The aim is to remove as much of the tumor as possible (debulking). Ovarian cancer has surgical staging. This includes:
    - Total abdominal hysterectomy (TAH) with bilateral salpingo-oophorectomy (BSO).
    - Omentectomy (removal of the omentum).
    - Peritoneal washings for cytology.
    - Possible resection of any involved bowel, bladder, or other affected organs.
    - Removal of any large peritoneal implants.
  - **Cytoreductive Surgery:** Surgeons aim to leave no visible tumor. Complete cytoreduction is associated with improved outcomes.
- **Adjuvant Chemotherapy**
  - **Combination Chemotherapy:** After surgery, patients typically receive a combination of chemotherapy drugs. The standard regimen includes:
    - **Carboplatin:** AUC 5
    - **Paclitaxel:** Commonly used in combination with carboplatin. Dose 175 mg/m^2

    Chemotherapy is usually administered every 3 weeks for 6–8 cycles.
  - **Neoadjuvant Chemotherapy:** In some cases, particularly if the tumor is initially deemed unresectable, patients may receive chemotherapy before surgery to shrink the tumor. Afterward, they undergo debulking surgery followed by additional chemotherapy.
- **Targeted Therapy and Maintenance Therapy**
  - **Bevacizumab (Avastin):** This antiangiogenic agent is sometimes used in combination with chemotherapy or as a maintenance therapy to inhibit blood vessel growth in tumors.
  - **PARP Inhibitors:** For patients with BRCA1/2 mutations or other homologous recombination repair deficiencies, PARP inhibitors like olaparib or niraparib may be used as maintenance therapy after chemotherapy to prolong remission.
- **Supportive Care**
  - **Pain Management:** Addressing pain and discomfort through medications and supportive therapies.
  - **Nutritional Support:** Ensuring adequate nutrition, which may involve dietary adjustments or supplements.
- **Follow-Up Care**
  - **Regular Monitoring:** Include physical examination, imaging studies (e.g., CT scans), and blood tests (such as CA-125 levels) to monitor for recurrence and assess response to treatment.

- **Patient Education:** Educating patients on signs of recurrence and when to seek medical help.

Ans. **2. Molecular classification of ovarian cancer and its clinical implications.**

The molecular classification of ovarian cancer has advanced significantly, providing insights into the distinct biological behavior, prognosis, and therapeutic responses of different subtypes. Here is an overview of the major molecular subtypes and their clinical implications:

Molecular Subtypes

- High-Grade Serous Carcinoma (HGSC)
  - Genetic Alterations: TP53 mutations (nearly universal), BRCA1/2 mutations (both germline and somatic), and homologous recombination deficiency (HRD).
  - Pathway Involvement: PIK3CA, RAS, and NOTCH signaling pathways.
  - Clinical Implications:
  - Often diagnosed at an advanced stage.
  - Responsive to platinum-based chemotherapy.
  - BRCA-mutated tumors may respond well to PARP inhibitors (e.g., olaparib).
  - HRD testing can guide the use of targeted therapies.
- Endometrioid Carcinoma
  - Genetic Alterations: PTEN mutations, CTNNB1 (beta-catenin), ARID1A, and PIK3CA mutations.
  - Pathway Involvement: PI3K/AKT/mTOR pathway.
  - Clinical Implications:
  - Often associated with endometriosis.
  - Generally presents at an earlier stage with a better prognosis.
  - Potential response to PI3K/AKT/mTOR inhibitors.
- Clear Cell Carcinoma
  - Genetic Alterations: ARID1A and PIK3CA mutations.
  - Pathway Involvement: PI3K/AKT/mTOR and MET signaling pathways.
  - Clinical Implications:
  - Often resistant to standard platinum-based chemotherapy.
  - Poor prognosis compared to other subtypes.
  - Potential for targeted therapies focusing on the PI3K/AKT/mTOR pathway.
- Mucinous Carcinoma
  - Genetic Alterations: KRAS mutations.
  - Pathway Involvement: MAPK/ERK pathway.
  - Clinical Implications:
  - Less common subtype.
  - Often diagnosed at an earlier stage.
  - Limited response to standard ovarian cancer chemotherapy regimens.
  - Targeted therapies against KRAS and MAPK/ERK pathway are under investigation.
- Low-Grade Serous Carcinoma (LGSC)
  - Genetic Alterations: BRAF and KRAS mutations.
  - Pathway Involvement: MAPK/ERK pathway.
  - Clinical Implications:

- Slower progression compared to high-grade serous carcinoma.
- Often less responsive to conventional chemotherapy.
- MEK inhibitors (e.g., trametinib) have shown some efficacy in treatment.

Implications for Treatment and Prognosis

- Targeted Therapy: Understanding specific genetic alterations allows for the use of targeted therapies (e.g., PARP inhibitors for BRCA-mutated tumors, PI3K/AKT/mTOR inhibitors for endometrioid and clear cell carcinomas, MEK inhibitors for low-grade serous carcinomas).
- Personalized Medicine: Molecular profiling enables personalized treatment plans, potentially improving outcomes and reducing unnecessary toxicity from ineffective treatments.
- Prognostic Information: Molecular subtyping provides prognostic information, helping to identify patients at higher risk for aggressive disease who may benefit from more intensive monitoring and treatment.
- Clinical Trials: Molecular classification allows for more precise inclusion criteria in clinical trials, leading to the development of novel therapies tailored to specific genetic alterations.

In summary, the molecular classification of ovarian cancer has significant implications for diagnosis, prognosis, and treatment, enabling a more personalized and effective approach to managing this complex disease.

Classification of Epithelial Ovarian Cancer

Epithelial ovarian cancers, comprising over 90% of ovarian malignancies, are classified histologically into major subtypes:

- High-grade serous carcinoma (most common, aggressive, often diagnosed late)
- Low-grade serous carcinoma
- Endometrioid carcinoma
- Clear cell carcinoma
- Mucinous carcinoma

These subtypes vary in molecular profile, clinical behavior, and prognosis, guiding tailored management.

Meigs Syndrome and Pseudo-Meigs Syndrome

- Meigs Syndrome is characterized by the triad of a benign ovarian fibroma (or similar solid tumor), ascites, and pleural effusion, with resolution of effusions after tumor removal.
- Pseudo-Meigs Syndrome resembles Meigs syndrome clinically but involves other ovarian or pelvic tumors (benign or malignant) causing ascites and pleural effusion[knowledge].

Surgical Staging of Ovarian Cancer

Surgical staging follows FIGO (International Federation of Gynecology and Obstetrics) guidelines and involves:

- Total abdominal hysterectomy with bilateral salpingo-oophorectomy,
- Omentectomy,
- Peritoneal biopsies,
- Pelvic and para-aortic lymphadenectomy,
- Inspection and biopsy of diaphragmatic peritoneum and other suspicious areas,
- Evaluation of ascitic fluid or peritoneal washings.

Accurate staging determines prognosis and guides adjuvant therapy [knowledge].

Solid Ovarian Tumors

Solid ovarian tumors, generally of stromal or germ cell origin or benign solid epithelial variants, include:

- Fibroma,
- Thecoma,
- Granulosa cell tumor,
- Sertoli-Leydig cell tumor,
- Brenner tumor,
- Dysgerminoma,
- Teratoma (solid variants),
- Small cell carcinoma of the ovary

SHORT ANSWERS

1. Tumor markers for ovarian cancer

Tumor markers are substances often found in higher levels in the blood or other body fluids of people with certain types of cancer. For ovarian cancer, several tumor markers are used in diagnosis, monitoring treatment, and assessing prognosis. Here are the main tumor markers for ovarian cancer and their significance:

1. **CA-125 (Cancer Antigen 125)**
   - **Significance:**
     - **Diagnosis:** Elevated levels of CA-125 are often associated with ovarian cancer, particularly in advanced stages. It is not specific to ovarian cancer alone and can be elevated in other cancers or benign conditions.
     - **Monitoring:** Used to monitor the response to treatment and check for recurrence. A significant decrease in CA-125 levels after treatment can indicate a positive response, while rising levels may suggest disease progression or recurrence.
     - **Screening:** CA-125 is not generally used for routine screening in the general population due to its lack of specificity and the potential for false positives and negatives. However, it may be used in conjunction with other tests for women at high risk (e.g., those with a family history or BRCA mutations).
2. **HE4 (Human Epididymis Protein 4)**
   - **Significance:**
     - **Diagnosis:** HE4 levels can be elevated in ovarian cancer, and it may be used alongside CA-125 to improve diagnostic accuracy. HE4 is particularly useful in distinguishing between ovarian cancer and benign pelvic conditions.
     - **Monitoring:** Like CA-125, HE4 levels can help monitor treatment response and disease recurrence. HE4 is often used in combination with CA-125 and other factors in a risk assessment model known as the ROMA (Risk of Ovarian Malignancy Algorithm).
3. **AFP (Alpha-Fetoprotein)**
   - **Significance:**
     - **Diagnosis:** AFP is more commonly associated with germ cell tumors of the ovary, such as endodermal sinus tumors (yolk sac tumors) rather than epithelial ovarian cancer.

- **Monitoring:** AFP levels can be used to monitor treatment response and disease progression in germ cell tumors.

4. **hCG (Human Chorionic Gonadotropin)**
   - **Significance:**
     - **Diagnosis:** Elevated levels of hCG are associated with germ cell tumors, particularly choriocarcinoma and certain other germ cell tumors of the ovary.
     - **Monitoring:** hCG levels are monitored to evaluate response to treatment and check for recurrence in patients with germ cell tumors.
5. **LDH (Lactate Dehydrogenase)**
   - **Significance:**
     - **Diagnosis:** LDH is not specific to ovarian cancer but can be elevated in a variety of cancers, including ovarian cancer, particularly in cases with high tumor burden.
     - **Monitoring:** Used to monitor disease progression and response to treatment, especially in cases where the tumor is known to be aggressive.

CLINICAL USE AND LIMITATIONS

- **Complementary Role:** Tumor markers are used in conjunction with imaging studies and clinical evaluation rather than as standalone diagnostic tools. They are more effective for monitoring disease rather than initial diagnosis.
- **False Positives/Negatives:** Tumor markers can be elevated in conditions other than cancer or remain normal in some patients with cancer. Hence, results are interpreted in the context of other clinical findings.
- **Individual Variability:** Not all ovarian cancer patients will have elevated levels of these markers, and marker levels can vary depending on the type and stage of the cancer.
- Risk of Malignancy Index (RMI), Risk of Ovarian Malignancy Index (ROMI), and CA 125 are important clinical tools and biomarkers utilized in the assessment of ovarian masses, particularly for preoperative differentiation of benign from malignant tumors in gynecological practice.
- Risk of Malignancy Index (RMI): RMI is a widely used scoring system that combines three parameters: Serum CA 125 level, menopausal status, and ultrasound findings of the ovarian mass. It was developed to estimate the probability of malignancy in adnexal masses before surgery. The classical formula is:

$$RMI = U \times M \times CA125\text{RMI} = U \times M \times CA125$$

Where:

- *UU* is the ultrasound score (assigned 1 for 0–1 abnormal ultrasound features such as multilocular cysts, solid areas, bilateral lesions, ascites, metastases; and 3 or 4 for 2 or more features depending on the RMI type),
- *MM* is menopausal status (1 for premenopausal, 3 or 4 for postmenopausal), CA 125 level in IU/mL.
- Various versions of RMI exist (RMI 1, 2, 3, 4), differing slightly in scoring weights and inclusion of tumor size for RMI 4. A commonly accepted cutoff is an RMI score ≥200 indicating high risk of malignancy. RMI has demonstrated sensitivities around 75-90%, specificities 77–90%, and diagnostic accuracy over 80% in multiple studies.

1. Risk of Ovarian Malignancy Index

- ROMI is a similar predictive model incorporating serum CA 125 and human epididymis protein 4 (HE4) levels along with menopausal status. ROMI improves diagnostic accuracy compared to CA 125 alone by integrating these biomarkers and menopausal status, with different formulas applied for premenopausal and postmenopausal women. ROMI is less commonly used than RMI but offers enhanced specificity.
- CA 125: CA 125 is a high-molecular-weight glycoprotein antigen elevated in the majority of epithelial ovarian cancers, particularly advanced stages. It is the most widely used tumor marker for ovarian cancer. However, it lacks specificity since elevated CA 125 can occur in benign gynecological conditions (endometriosis, pelvic inflammatory disease, menstruation) and other malignancies. Its sensitivity for detecting early-stage ovarian cancer is limited, making it less useful as a standalone screening tool. CA 125 levels are most valuable when used in conjunction with clinical findings and imaging for monitoring disease progression or response to therapy.

In summary, tumor markers like CA-125, HE4, AFP, hCG, and LDH play important roles in managing ovarian cancer, particularly in monitoring treatment response and detecting recurrence. However, they are used alongside other diagnostic and clinical information to provide a comprehensive approach to patient care.

2. HIPEC

Hyperthermic Intraperitoneal Chemotherapy (HIPEC) is a treatment approach used for ovarian cancer, especially in cases of advanced disease where the cancer has spread within the peritoneal cavity. HIPEC involves delivering heated chemotherapy directly into the abdominal cavity after the surgical removal of visible tumors. Here is an overview of HIPEC and its role in managing ovarian cancer **(Fig. 2)**:

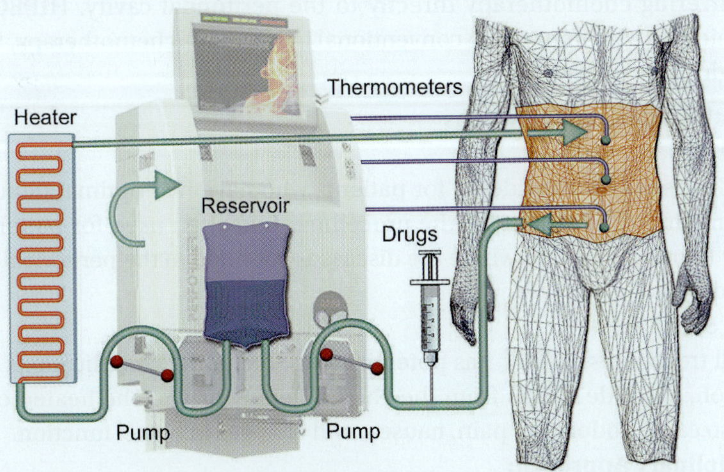

Fig. 2: Hyperthermic Intraperitoneal Chemotherapy (HIPEC)

- **Procedure:**
  - **Surgical Debulking:** First, a surgeon performs cytoreductive surgery (debulking surgery) to remove as much of the tumor as possible from the abdominal cavity.

- **HIPEC Administration:** After debulking, a heated chemotherapy solution is circulated within the peritoneal cavity. This solution is usually heated to around 41–43°C (105.8–109.4°F) to enhance the effectiveness of the chemotherapy drugs.
- **Duration:** The heated chemotherapy is typically circulated for about 60–90 minutes.
- **Drainage and Closure:** The solution is then drained and the abdominal cavity is closed.

- **Chemotherapy Agents:**
  - Common agents used in HIPEC include cisplatin, carboplatin, and docetaxel. The choice of agent may depend on the specific type of ovarian cancer and the patient's overall treatment plan.

Significance of HIPEC in Ovarian Cancer

- **Local Treatment:**
  - HIPEC targets cancer cells that may be present in the peritoneal cavity but are not visible or detectable through imaging. It aims to destroy microscopic cancer cells remaining after debulking surgery.
- **Enhanced Drug Delivery:**
  - The heat helps to enhance the absorption and effectiveness of chemotherapy drugs. It also improves drug penetration into cancerous tissues and potentially increases their cytotoxicity.
- **Improved Survival Outcomes:**
  - Studies have shown that HIPEC can improve progression-free survival and overall survival in patients with optimally debulked ovarian cancer. The benefit is often observed in patients with peritoneal carcinomatosis, where cancer has spread throughout the abdominal cavity.
- **Reduced Systemic Toxicity:**
  - By delivering chemotherapy directly to the peritoneal cavity, HIPEC may reduce systemic toxicity compared to conventional intravenous chemotherapy, as lower doses of the drug are needed.

Patient Selection and Considerations

- **Patient Criteria:**
  - HIPEC is generally considered for patients who have had optimal debulking surgery and who are otherwise fit for the procedure. It is often used for patients with Stage IIIC or IV ovarian cancer where the disease is confined to the peritoneal cavity but not beyond.
- **Risks and Side Effects:**
  - Like all treatments, HIPEC has potential risks, including complications from surgery, infection, and side effects from the chemotherapy drugs. The heated chemotherapy can also cause abdominal pain, nausea, and changes in bowel function.
- **Multidisciplinary Approach:**
  - HIPEC is typically part of a broader treatment plan that includes initial chemotherapy, surgery, and sometimes additional systemic therapy. A multidisciplinary team including gynecologic oncologists, surgical oncologists, and medical oncologists usually manages the treatment.

- **Clinical Trials:**
  - Ongoing research and clinical trials continue to evaluate the effectiveness of HIPEC, refine techniques, and explore combinations with other therapies.

SUMMARY

HIPEC is an advanced treatment modality used in the management of ovarian cancer, particularly for cases with extensive peritoneal involvement. It aims to improve survival outcomes by directly targeting cancer cells in the abdominal cavity with heated chemotherapy. The procedure is typically performed after debulking surgery and is part of a comprehensive treatment plan tailored to the individual patient's needs. As with all cancer treatments, it is essential for patients to discuss the potential benefits and risks with their healthcare team to determine the most appropriate approach for their specific condition.

3. a. Classification of ovarian germ cell tumors.
b. Dermoid cyst (Fig. 3)

Germ Cell Tumor Classification

I. Gonadal Germ Cell Tumors

A. Ovarian Germ Cell Tumors

1. Benign Tumors
   - Mature Cystic Teratoma (Dermoid Cyst): Contains differentiated tissues such as hair, skin, and teeth.
2. Malignant Tumors
   - Immature Teratoma: Contains immature or embryonal-type tissues.
   - Dysgerminoma: The ovarian counterpart to testicular seminoma, often seen in younger women.
   - Endodermal Sinus (Yolk Sac) Tumor: Aggressive tumor with elevated alpha-fetoprotein (AFP).
   - Embryonal Carcinoma: Rare and highly malignant, with elements of early embryonic cells.
   - Choriocarcinoma: Highly malignant tumor producing human chorionic gonadotropin (hCG).
   - Mixed Germ Cell Tumor: Contains two or more types of germ cell tumor components.

B. Testicular Germ Cell Tumors

1. Seminoma: The most common type, often slow-growing and responsive to treatment.
2. Non-Seminomatous Germ Cell Tumors (NSGCTs)
   - Embryonal Carcinoma: Aggressive and poorly differentiated.
   - Yolk Sac Tumor: Common in young children, with elevated AFP.
   - Choriocarcinoma: Rare but highly malignant, with elevated hCG.
   - Teratoma: Can be mature (benign) or immature (malignant).
   - Mixed Germ Cell Tumors: Combination of different germ cell tumor types.

II. Extragonadal Germ Cell Tumors

1. Mediastinal Germ Cell Tumors
   - Located in the anterior mediastinum, more common in males.
   - Can be seminomatous or nonseminomatous.

2. Retroperitoneal Germ Cell Tumors
   - Located in the retroperitoneum, often associated with metastasis from gonadal tumors.
3. Central Nervous System (CNS) Germ Cell Tumors
   - Located in areas like the pineal or suprasellar regions.
   - Includes germinomas and nongerminomatous germ cell tumors (NGGCTs).

III. Classification Based on Histological Types
1. Teratoma
   - Mature Teratoma: Benign, containing well-differentiated tissues.
   - Immature Teratoma: Malignant, containing immature embryonic-like tissues.
2. Dysgerminoma/Seminoma
   - Resembling primordial germ cells, highly responsive to radiation therapy.
3. Yolk Sac Tumor (Endodermal Sinus Tumor)
   - Produces AFP, aggressive, common in children.
4. Choriocarcinoma
   - Highly malignant, characterized by trophoblastic cells, producing hCG.
5. Embryonal Carcinoma
   - Poorly differentiated, aggressive, and can differentiate into other germ cell tumor types.6. Mixed Germ Cell Tumors
   - Contains a mixture of different germ cell tumor components, each with its own characteristics and markers.

Dermoid Cysts

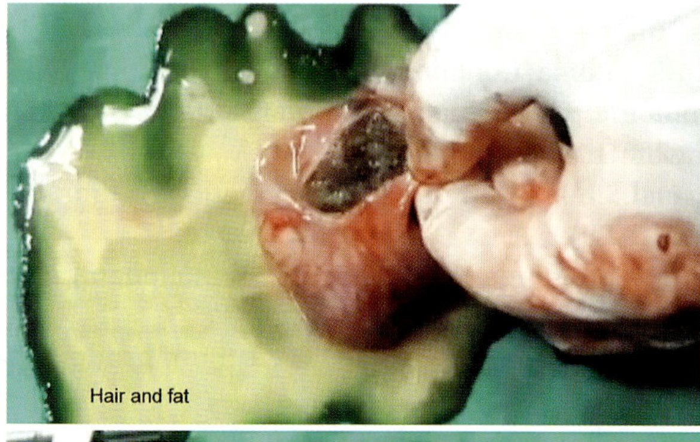

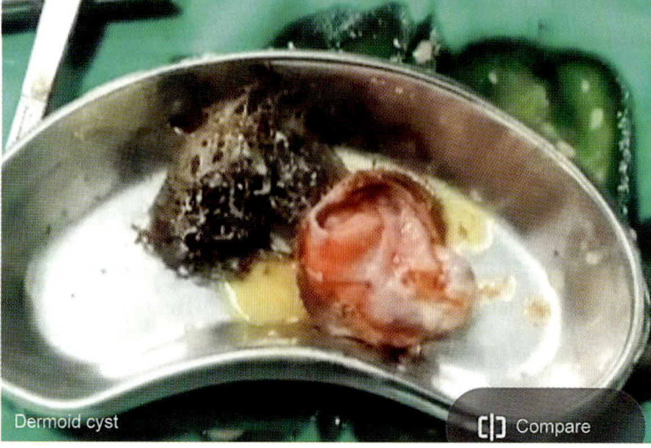

Fig. 3: A specimen of dermoid cyst.

Definition

A dermoid cyst, also known as a mature cystic teratoma, is a benign tumor most commonly found in the ovaries. These cysts can contain a variety of tissues such as hair, skin, teeth, and sometimes even bone or neural tissue.

Causes

Dermoid cysts develop from totipotent germ cells, which are capable of developing into any type of tissue. These cells become misplaced during fetal development, leading to the formation of a cyst that can contain different tissue types.

Symptoms

Dermoid cysts are often asymptomatic and found incidentally during imaging studies or surgeries. When symptoms do occur, they might include:

- Abdominal or pelvic pain, often from the pressure of the cyst on surrounding organs.
- A palpable mass in the lower abdomen.
- Nausea or vomiting, especially if the cyst causes ovarian torsion.
- Irregular menstrual cycles.
- Pain during intercourse or during menstrual periods.

Diagnosis

- Pelvic Examination: A physical examination to check for masses.
- Ultrasound: The primary imaging tool used to visualize the cyst and its contents.
- CT Scan or MRI: These imaging techniques can provide more detailed information about the cyst, especially if there are concerns about its nature.
- Laparoscopy: A minimally invasive procedure that allows direct visualization and often the treatment of the cyst.

Treatment

- Observation: Small, asymptomatic dermoid cysts can be monitored with regular follow-up appointments and imaging studies.
- Surgical Removal: Indicated for larger cysts, symptomatic cysts, or those causing complications like torsion or rupture. Surgical options include:
- Laparoscopy: Preferred for its minimally invasive nature and quicker recovery times.
- Laparotomy: Used for larger or more complicated cysts.

Complications

- Ovarian Torsion: The cyst can cause the ovary to twist, cutting off its blood supply and causing severe pain and potential loss of the ovary if not treated promptly.
- Rupture: Though rare, a dermoid cyst can rupture, leading to peritonitis and requiring emergency surgery.
- Infection: Rarely, a dermoid cyst can become infected, leading to pain and fever.

Prognosis

The prognosis for individuals with dermoid cysts is generally very good. These cysts are benign, and once removed, the risk of recurrence is low. However, regular follow-up is recommended to monitor for any new cyst development, especially in younger women of reproductive age.

Fertility

Most dermoid cysts do not affect fertility. However, if the cyst requires surgical removal, care is taken to preserve as much ovarian tissue as possible.

Preventive Measures

There are no specific preventive measures for dermoid cysts since they are congenital and develop from germ cells. Regular gynecological exams and imaging studies can help in early detection and management.

4. a. Classification of Sex cord tumors.
b. Granulosa cell tumor

1. Granulosa-stromal cell tumors
   A. Granulosa cell tumor
   B. Tumors in thecoma-fibroma group
      a. Thecoma
      b. Fibroma
      c. Unclassified
2. Androblastoma; Sertoli-Leydig cell tumors
   A. Well differentiated
      a. Sertoli cell tumor
      b. Sertoli-Leydig cell tumor
      c. Leydig cell tumor; hilus cell tumor
   B. Moderately differentiated
   C. Poorly differentiated (Sarcomatoid)
   D. With heterologous elements
3. Gynandroblatoma
4. Sex cord tumor with annular tubules

Granulosa cell tumors (GCTs) are a type of sex cord-stromal tumor of the ovary. They arise from the granulosa cells of the ovarian follicle, which are involved in the maturation of the egg and hormone production. Granulosa cell tumors are known for their distinctive histological features, potential for hormonal activity, and variable clinical behavior. Here is a detailed overview.

Characteristics of Granulosa Cell Tumors

Histology

- **Cell Type:** Granulosa cell tumors consist of cells that resemble the granulosa cells of the ovarian follicle. These cells often have small, round nuclei with scant cytoplasm.
- **Patterns:** The tumors commonly show trabecular or insular patterns. The trabecular pattern resembles trabeculae or cords of cells, while the insular pattern consists of nests or follicles filled with eosinophilic material.
- **Call-Exner Bodies:** These are small structures resembling immature Graafian follicles and can be seen in many granulosa cell tumors. They are filled with eosinophilic material and are a characteristic feature.
- **Fibrosis:** The stroma of the tumor can be fibrous or myxoid.

Hormonal changes

- **Estrogen Production:** Granulosa cell tumors often produce estrogen, which can lead to symptoms such as:
  - **Abnormal Uterine Bleeding:** This may include heavy menstrual bleeding or bleeding between periods.
  - **Precocious Puberty:** In prepubescent girls, high estrogen levels can lead to early onset of menstruation and breast development.
  - **Postmenopausal Bleeding:** In postmenopausal women, these tumors can cause vaginal bleeding.

Clinical presentation

- **Benign to Malignant:** Granulosa cell tumors are usually low-grade and indolent. However, they can exhibit malignant behavior, particularly if there is evidence of invasive growth or metastasis.
- **Recurrence:** These tumors have a tendency to recur many years after the initial diagnosis, making long-term follow-up essential.

Diagnosis

- **Imaging:** Ultrasound, CT scans, or MRI can be used to evaluate the extent of the tumor and to assess for possible metastases.
- **Histological Examination:** The definitive diagnosis is made through histopathological examination of the tumor tissue. Immunohistochemical staining can support the diagnosis by highlighting the characteristic cellular features of granulosa cells.
- **Endometrial sampling**

Treatment

- **Surgical Management:** The primary treatment is surgical removal of the tumor. This typically involves:
  - **Total Abdominal Hysterectomy (TAH) and Bilateral Salpingo-Oophorectomy (BSO):** In most cases, the uterus and ovaries are removed.
  - **Tumor Debulking:** Removal of as much of the tumor as possible, which might involve resection of adjacent tissues if the tumor has spread.
- **Follow-Up**: Regular follow-up is crucial due to the potential for late recurrence. Monitoring typically includes physical exams, imaging studies, and serum tumor markers (like CA-125) if indicated.
- **Chemotherapy—Low risk**—No need

High Risk- Stage 1 (High mitotic index, capsular rupture, surface involvement, large tumor size, incomplete stage), Stage II, Stages III and IV if not completely resected

BEP for 3 cycles

Bleomycin—3,000 IU IV days 1, 8, 15

- Etoposide—100 mg/m^2 for 5 days
- Cisplatin—20 mg/m^2 for 5 days

Prognosis

- **Survival Rates:** The prognosis for granulosa cell tumors is generally good, especially for early-stage disease. Long-term survival rates are favorable, but the risk of late recurrence means that ongoing surveillance is necessary.

- **Factors Influencing Prognosis:**
  - **Tumor Size and Stage:** Larger tumors or those with advanced stage may have a worse prognosis.
  - **Histological Features:** Certain features, such as high mitotic activity or extensive invasion, can influence the outcome.

Granulosa cell tumors are ovarian sex cord-stromal tumors with unique histological features and potential hormonal effects. They often present with estrogen-related symptoms and can have a variable clinical course. Effective management usually involves surgical resection and long-term follow-up to monitor for recurrence. Understanding the characteristics and behavior of granulosa cell tumors helps in providing appropriate treatment and surveillance for affected patients.

Prognosis in ovarian cancer is closely linked to stage at diagnosis, residual disease after primary cytoreduction, tumor biology, and response to platinum-based chemotherapy. Second-look laparotomy (SLL) historically aimed to refine prognostication and guide further therapy, but its role has markedly declined in the era of modern imaging, CA-125 monitoring, and maintenance therapies.

Prognosis of ovarian cancer

- Overall 5-year survival for epithelial ovarian cancer is approximately 90% in stage I, 70–80% in stage II, 30–50% in stage III, and <20% in stage IV, reflecting the heavy impact of advanced stage at presentation.
- The single-most powerful prognostic factor is volume of residual disease after primary debulking; optimal cytoreduction to no macroscopic residual tumor confers the best progression-free and overall survival.
- Additional adverse prognostic factors include high-grade serous histology, platinum resistance, suboptimal response to first-line chemotherapy, BRCA-wild type status, poor performance status, and presence of ascites or extensive peritoneal carcinomatosis.

Second-look laparotomy: concept and indications

- Second-look laparotomy is a planned re-exploration of the abdomen after completion of first-line surgery and chemotherapy in women who are in clinical and radiologic remission, intended to detect residual or recurrent disease, obtain histologic confirmation of response, and allow secondary cytoreduction where feasible.
- It typically includes systematic inspection of peritoneal surfaces, biopsies from suspicious areas, peritoneal washings, and lymph node sampling ± debulking of macroscopic deposits.

Prognostic information from second-look laparotomy

- SLL is the most accurate method to determine pathologic response: Series report complete pathologic response in roughly 20–30%, microscopic residual disease in about one-third, and macroscopic residual disease in the remaining patients.
- Even with a negative SLL (no macroscopic or microscopic disease), recurrence occurs in approximately 40–50% of patients, but disease-free and overall survival are significantly longer than in those with positive SLL (residual microscopic or macroscopic disease).

Impact on survival and current role

- Although SLL provides powerful prognostic stratification, multiple studies have failed to demonstrate a clear overall survival advantage for routine SLL compared with careful clinical, biochemical (CA-125), and imaging follow-up, largely because salvage and consolidation regimens have limited curative potential.
- Consequently, contemporary guidelines regard routine SLL as obsolete in standard practice; its use is now largely confined to research settings, for evaluation of novel regimens or when results would directly alter management (e.g., consideration of further cytoreductive surgery in selected patients with suspected residual disease)

MULTIPLE CHOICE QUESTIONS

1. Which of the following indicates Stage IC ovarian cancer?

a. Cancer limited to one ovary, capsule intact, no tumor on the surface
b. Cancer limited to both ovaries, capsule intact, no tumor on the surface
c. Cancer limited to one or both ovaries with surgical spill, capsule rupture, or malignant cells in ascites
d. Cancer spread to pelvic organs

Ans. c. Cancer limited to one or both ovaries with surgical spill, capsule rupture, or malignant cells in ascites

Reference: International Federation of Gynecology and Obstetrics. (2014). FIGO staging for ovarian cancer. https://www.figo.org/resources/figo-staging

2. Which RMI score indicates a high risk of malignancy in an ovarian mass?

a. >50 b. >100
c. >150 d. >200

Ans. d. >200

RMI-1 (Risk of Malignancy Index 1)

RMI-1 combines three factors:

1. ***Menopausal Status:***
   - ***Premenopausal: 1 point***
   - ***Postmenopausal: 4 points***
2. ***Ultrasound Findings:***
   - ***Unilocular Cyst: 1 point***
   - ***Multilocular Cyst: 2 points***
   - ***Solid Tumor: 4 points***
   - ***Evidence of Extra-Ovarian Tumor Spread: 4 points***
3. ***Serum CA-125 Level:***
   - ***<35 U/mL: 1 point***
   - ***≥35 U/mL: 4 points***

RMI-1 Formula:

RMI-1 = Menopausal Status × Ultrasound Findings × Serum CA-125 Level\text {RMI-1} = \text{Menopausal Status} \times \text{Ultrasound Findings} \times \text{Serum CA-125 Level}RMI-1 = Menopausal Status×Ultrasound Findings×Serum CA-125 Level

RMI-2 (Risk of Malignancy Index 2)

RMI-2 is an updated version that incorporates additional factors for potentially greater accuracy:

1. ***Menopausal Status:***
   - ***Premenopausal: 1 point***
   - ***Postmenopausal: 3 points***
2. ***Ultrasound Findings:***
   - ***Unilocular Cyst: 1 point***
   - ***Multilocular Cyst: 2 points***
   - ***Solid Tumor: 4 points***
   - ***Evidence of Extra-Ovarian Tumor Spread: 4 points***
3. ***Serum CA-125 Level:***
   - ***<35 U/mL:*** *1 point*
   - ***35–200 U/mL:*** *2 points*
   - ***>200 U/mL:*** *4 points*
4. ***Ascites:***
   - ***Absent:*** *1 point*
   - ***Present:*** *2 points*
5. ***Tumor Type*** *(based on ultrasound):*
   - ***Cystic:*** *1 point*
   - ***Solid: 2*** *points*

RMI-2 Formula:

RMI-2 = Menopausal Status × Ultrasound Findings × Serum CA-125

Interpreting RMI Scores

- ***Thresholds:*** *The interpretation of RMI scores is typically based on thresholds that predict the likelihood of malignancy. For example:*
  - ***RMI-1:*** *A score greater than 200 is generally considered indicative of a high risk of malignancy.*
  - ***RMI-2:*** *Scores are categorized to assess risk levels, with higher scores suggesting a greater likelihood of ovarian cancer.*

Reference: Jacobs I, Oram D. RMI 1: Risk of malignancy index for the pre-operative assessment of ovarian masses. British J Obstet Gynaecol. 1993;100(6):697-701.

3. What is the most common genetic mutation associated with hereditary ovarian cancer?

a. TP53
b. BRCA1
c. BRCA2
d. HER2

Ans. b. BRCA1

Explanation in question 6

Reference: King MC, Marks JH, Mandel J. Breast and ovarian cancer risks due to inherited mutations in BRCA1 and BRCA2. Science. 2003;302(5645):643-6.

4. What is the ROMA (Risk of Ovarian Malignancy Algorithm) score based on?

a. Age and menopausal status
b. CA-125 and HE4 levels
c. Ultrasound findings and CA-125
d. Genetic markers and family history

Ans. b. CA-125 and HE4 levels

Components of the ROMA Score

The ROMA score is based on the following factors:

1. Serum Biomarkers:
- **CA-125 (Cancer Antigen 125):** A protein often elevated in ovarian cancer and other conditions.
- **HE4 (Human Epididymis Protein 4):** A protein that can be elevated in ovarian cancer and has been found to be useful in differentiating between malignant and benign pelvic masses.

2. Menopausal Status:
- **Premenopausal:** Women who have not yet reached menopause.
- **Postmenopausal:** Women who have gone through menopause.

Reference: Moore RG, Goebel EA, Wright AA. The Risk of Ovarian Malignancy Algorithm (ROMA) for evaluating risk of ovarian cancer in patients with pelvic masses. Gynecol Oncol. 2012;127(2):257-64.

5. Which scoring system is used to assess the surgical outcome in ovarian cancer?

a. RMI score
b. ROMA Score
c. FIGO staging
d. Fagotti score (Peritoneal Cancer Index)

Ans. d. Fagotti score (Peritoneal Cancer Index)

The Fagotti Index is designed to predict whether a patient with ovarian cancer is likely to achieve optimal debulking surgery. It evaluates various factors to help guide surgical planning, rather than staging the cancer, evaluating chemotherapy response, or determining the need for radiation therapy.

Reference: Fagotti A, Ferrandina G, Gubbini G. A scoring system for the evaluation of ovarian cancer patients: The Fagotti score. Gynecol Oncol. 2008;109(1):87-92.

6. Which of the following is a risk factor for ovarian cancer?

a. Early menopause
b. Nulliparity
c. Use of oral contraceptives
d. Multiparity

Ans. b. Nulliparity

Genetic Factors

1. *Family History:*
- ***Hereditary Breast and Ovarian Cancer Syndrome (BRCA1 and BRCA2 mutations):*** *Mutations in these genes significantly increase the risk of ovarian cancer, as well as breast cancer. BRCA 1 > BRCA 2*
- ***Lynch Syndrome:*** *Also known as hereditary nonpolyposis colorectal cancer (HNPCC), this syndrome increases the risk of ovarian cancer and other cancers such as colorectal cancer.*
- ***Other Genetic Syndromes:*** *Mutations in genes such as RAD51C, RAD51D, and BRIP1 may also be associated with increased ovarian cancer risk.*

2. *Family History of Ovarian Cancer:*
- *Having a close relative (mother, sister, daughter) with ovarian cancer increases an individual's risk. The risk is higher if multiple family members or multiple generations are affected.*

Reproductive Factors

1. *Age:*
- *The risk of ovarian cancer increases with age, particularly after the age of 50 years. Most cases are diagnosed in women who are postmenopausal.*

2. *Menstrual History:*
- ***Early Menarche.***
- ***Late Menopause***

3. *Pregnancy and Childbirth:*
- ***Nulliparity***

Hormonal Factors

1. ***Hormone Replacement Therapy (HRT):***
   - *Long-term use of estrogen-only hormone replacement therapy (HRT) has been linked to a higher risk of ovarian cancer.*
2. ***Oral Contraceptives:***
   - *Use of oral contraceptives (birth control pills) has been associated with a decreased risk of ovarian cancer, especially with long-term use.*

Lifestyle and Environmental Factors

1. ***Obesity***
2. ***Smoking:***
3. ***Diet:***

Medical History

1. ***Endometriosis:***
2. ***Previous Cancer Diagnosis:***
   - *Women who have been previously diagnosed with breast, colon, or other cancers may have an increased risk of ovarian cancer, particularly if they have certain genetic mutations.*

Reference: Risch HA. Hormonal factors and risk of ovarian cancer. J Natl Cancer Inst. 2003;95(23): 1715-6.

7. Which of the following is a protective factor against ovarian cancer?

a. Late menopause
b. Early menarche
c. Use of oral contraceptives
d. Family history of breast cancer

Ans. c. Use of oral contraceptives

Explanation as Question 6

Reference: Aune D, Chan DSM, Vieira AR, et al. Oral contraceptive use and ovarian cancer risk: A systematic review and meta-analysis. Cancer Causes Control. 2012;23(4):539-50.

8. What is the first-line chemotherapy regimen for advanced epithelial ovarian cancer?

a. Methotrexate and leucovorin
b. Doxorubicin and cyclophosphamide
c. Carboplatin and paclitaxel
d. Cisplatin and etoposide

Ans. c. Carboplatin and paclitaxel

Carboplatin and Paclitaxel are the most commonly used first-line chemotherapy regimen for treating advanced ovarian cancer. This combination is effective at targeting ovarian cancer cells and has become the standard treatment. Doxorubicin and Cyclophosphamide are used for other cancers, while Cisplatin and Etoposide, and Methotrexate and 5-Fluorouracil, are not standard regimens for ovarian cancer.

Reference: Berek JS, Hacker NF. Chemotherapy for ovarian cancer. In: Berek JS, Hacker NF (Eds). Gynecologic Oncology, 6th edition. Philadelphia: Wolters Kluwer; 2021. pp. 425-54

9. Which of the following symptoms is most commonly associated with ovarian cancer?

a. Weight gain
b Persistent bloating
c. Persistent cough
d. Hematuria

Ans. b. Persistent bloating

Abdominal bloating is one of the most common presenting symptoms of ovarian cancer. Women with ovarian cancer often experience a sensation of fullness or bloating in the abdomen. Other common symptoms include pelvic pain, difficulty eating, and frequent urination. Hematuria, persistent cough, and joint pain are not typical symptoms of ovarian cancer.

Reference: Berek JS, Novak E. Berek & Novak's Gynecology, 16th edition. Philadelphia: Wolters Kluwer; 2020

10. Which of the following procedures is typically used to confirm the diagnosis of ovarian cancer?

a. Fine needle aspiration
b. Excisional biopsy
c. Laparotomy
d. Laparoscopy with biopsy

Ans. d. Laparoscopy with biopsy

Diagnosis of ovarian cancer can be confirmed by performing laparoscopy with biopsy

Reference: Berek JS, Novak E. Berek & Novak's Gynecology, 16th edition. Philadelphia: Wolters Kluwer; 2020.

11. Which ovarian tumor is characterized by the presence of Call-Exner bodies?

a. Serous carcinoma
b. Granulosa cell tumor
c. Mucinous carcinoma
d. Dysgerminoma

Ans. b. Granulosa cell tumor

Granulosa cell tumors are known for containing Call-Exner bodies, which resemble immature Graafian follicles and are a distinctive histological feature of this tumor type. Endometrioid, clear cell, and Sertoli-Leydig cell tumors have different histological features and do not typically present with Call-Exner bodies.

Reference: Berek JS, Novak E. Berek & Novak's Gynecology, 16th edition. Philadelphia: Wolters Kluwer; 2020.

12. Which type of ovarian cancer is associated with the presence of Schiller-Duval bodies?

a. Serous carcinoma
b. Mucinous carcinoma
c. Endometrioid carcinoma
d. Yolk sac tumor

Ans. d. Yolk sac tumor

The presence of Schiller-Duval bodies is highly indicative of yolk sac tumors, which are a type of germ cell tumor.

Reference: Berek JS, Novak E. Berek & Novak's Gynecology, 16th edition. Philadelphia: Wolters Kluwer; 2020

13. Which type of ovarian cancer is most commonly associated with psammoma bodies on histopathological examination?

a. Serous carcinoma
b. Mucinous carcinoma
c. Endometrioid carcinoma
d. Clear cell carcinoma

Ans. a. Serous carcinoma

Serous papillary ovarian carcinoma is characterized by the presence of psammoma bodies, which are calcified structures that appear as concentric layers. Call-Exner bodies are more typical of granulosa cell tumors, mucinous pools are seen in mucinous ovarian carcinoma, and solid sheets of cells with scant cytoplasm are indicative of small cell ovarian carcinoma.

Reference: Berek JS, Novak E. Berek & Novak's Gynecology, 16th edition. Philadelphia: Wolters Kluwer; 2020.

14. Which of the following statements is true about the FIGO staging system for ovarian cancer?

a. It includes biochemical markers
b. It assesses surgical resectability
c. It is based on the extent of disease spread
d. It incorporates genetic mutations

Ans. c. It is based on the extent of disease spread

Explanation as question 1

Reference: International Federation of Gynecology and Obstetrics. (2014). FIGO staging for ovarian cancer. https://www.figo.org/resources/figo-staging

15. What parameters are included in the Risk of Malignancy Index (RMI) for ovarian cancer?

a. Age, CA-125, ultrasound findings
b. Tumor size, lymph node involvement, metastasis
c. CA-125, ultrasound findings, menopausal status
d. Serum AFP, HCG levels, tumor size

Ans. c. CA-125, ultrasound findings, menopausal status

Explanation as question 2

Reference: Jacobs I, Oram D. RMI 1: Risk of malignancy index for the pre-operative assessment of ovarian masses. British J Obstet Gynaecol. 1993;100(6):697-701.

16. What is the role of bevacizumab in the management of ovarian cancer?

a. Hormonal therapy
b. Anti-angiogenesis therapy
c. Immunotherapy
d. Chemotherapy

Ans. b. Anti-angiogenesis therapy

Bevacizumab is a monoclonal antibody that acts as an angiogenesis inhibitor by blocking vascular endothelial growth factor (VEGF), which is involved in the formation of blood vessels that tumors need to grow. It is used in combination with chemotherapy for advanced ovarian cancer. It is not a platinum-based or taxane chemotherapy drug, nor is it a hormone therapy.

Reference: Berek JS, Hacker NF. Chemotherapy for ovarian cancer. In: Berek JS, Hacker NF (Eds). Gynecologic Oncology, 6th edition. Philadelphia: Wolters Kluwer; 2021. pp. 425-54.

17. In ovarian cancer, the presence of BRCA1 or BRCA2 mutations may make a patient eligible for which type of targeted therapy?

a. PARP inhibitors
b. Tyrosine kinase inhibitors
c. Immunotherapy
d. Hormonal therapy

Ans. a. PARP inhibitors

PARP inhibitors are particularly effective in ovarian cancer patients with BRCA1 or BRCA2 mutations because these mutations impair the homologous recombination repair pathway. The inhibition of PARP further compromises DNA repair, leading to increased cancer cell death. HER2 overexpression, p53 mutations, and KRAS mutations are not directly related to the effectiveness of PARP inhibitors.

Reference: Berek JS, Hacker NF. Chemotherapy for ovarian cancer. In: Berek JS, Hacker NF (Eds). Gynecologic Oncology, 6th edition. Philadelphia: Wolters Kluwer; 2021. pp. 425-54.

18. Which of the following is a common side effect of chemotherapy with carboplatin and paclitaxel in ovarian cancer patients?

a. Nephrotoxicity
b. Neuropathy
c. Cardiotoxicity
d. Hypercalcemia

Ans. b. Neuropathy

Paclitaxel can cause neuropathic pain due to its impact on peripheral nerves, leading to symptoms such as tingling, burning, and pain in the extremities.

Reference: Berek JS, Hacker NF. Chemotherapy for ovarian cancer. In: Berek JS, Hacker NF (Eds). Gynecologic Oncology, 6th edition. Philadelphia: Wolters Kluwer; 2021. pp. 425-54.

19. Which of the following factors is considered when deciding to perform neoadjuvant chemotherapy (NACT) before surgery in ovarian cancer?

a. Tumor size and spread
b. Patient's age
c. CA-125 level
d. Menopausal status

Ans. a. Tumor size and spread

A key consideration when planning NACT is to assess how the treatment will impact tumor resectability. This includes evaluating whether the chemotherapy will sufficiently shrink the tumors to allow for optimal debulking surgery. Genetic testing for BRCA mutations may guide treatment but is not the primary consideration for planning NACT. Radiation therapy and hormone therapy are not typically involved in the NACT process for ovarian cancer.

Reference: Berek JS, Hacker NF. Chemotherapy for ovarian cancer. In: Berek JS, Hacker NF (Eds). Gynecologic Oncology, 6th edition. Philadelphia: Wolters Kluwer; 2021. pp. 425-54.

20. What is the typical role of secondary cytoreductive surgery in ovarian cancer management?

a. Initial treatment for early-stage disease
b. Treatment for recurrent ovarian cancer
c. Routine follow-up procedure
d. Pretreatment staging

Ans. b. Treatment for recurrent ovarian cancer

Secondary cytoreductive surgery in ovarian cancer management is used for the treatment for recurrent ovarian cancer.

Reference: Berek JS, Hacker NF. Chemotherapy for ovarian cancer. In: Berek JS, Hacker NF (Eds). Gynecologic Oncology, 6th edition. Philadelphia: Wolters Kluwer; 2021. pp. 425-54.

SUGGESTED READING

1. Aghajanian C, Blank SV, Goff BA, et al. Olaratumab plus doxorubicin in advanced soft-tissue sarcoma. N Engl J Med. 2017;377(5):453-60.
2. American Cancer Society. Ovarian cancer. [online] Available from: https://www.cancer.org/cancer/ovarian-cancer.html. [Last accessed December, 2025].
3. Berek JS, Novak E. Berek & Novak's Gynecology, 16th edition. Philadelphia: Wolters Kluwer; 2020.
4. Chan J, Singh G, Oza AM. Intraperitoneal chemotherapy for ovarian cancer: a systematic review. Gynecol Oncol. 2021;161(3):842-51.
5. ClinicalTrials.gov. Study of the efficacy of pazopanib versus standard chemotherapy in ovarian cancer. [online] Available from https://clinicaltrials.gov/ct2/show/NCT03317111. [Last accessed December, 2025]

6. Colombo N, Morrow CP, Scarfone G, et al. A phase III trial of pegylated liposomal doxorubicin versus carboplatin-paclitaxel as first-line treatment for ovarian cancer. J Clin Oncol. 2018;36(9):928-34.
7. EudraCT. A study evaluating the safety and efficacy of new ovarian cancer therapies. [online] Available from https://www.clinicaltrialsregister.eu/ctr-search/search?query=eudract_number:2020-002508-40. [Last accessed December, 2025]
8. European Society for Medical Oncology (ESMO). ESMO Clinical Practice Guidelines for the management of ovarian cancer. [online] Available from https://www.esmo.org/guidelines/gynaecological-cancers/ovarian-cancer. [Last accessed December, 2025]
9. Hoskins WJ, Perez CA, Young RC (Eds). Principles and Practice of Gynecologic Oncology, 6th edition. Philadelphia: Lippincott Williams & Wilkins; 2018.
10. Kauff ND, Satagopan JM, Robson ME, et al. The incidence of ovarian cancer in BRCA1 and BRCA2 mutation carriers. Cancer. 2020;116.
11. Lheureux S, Gourley C, Vergote I, et al. Epithelial ovarian cancer. Lancet. 2019;393(10186):1240-53.
12. Liu JF, Miao Q, Hughes T, et al. Long-term survival outcomes and safety of niraparib in ovarian cancer patients. J Clin Oncol. 2020;38(13):1515-22.
13. Mallen AR, Gordon AN, Ovarian Cancer: Current Management and Emerging Therapies. Expert Rev Anticancer Ther. 2021;21(5):589-600.
14. Moore K, Colombo N, Scambia G, et al. Maintenance olaparib in patients with newly diagnosed ovarian cancer. N Engl J Med. 2018;379(26):2495-505.
15. Morrow CP, Berek JS (Eds). Ovarian Cancer: Principles and Practice, 3rd edition. New York: Springer; 2021.
16. National Cancer Institute. Ovarian cancer treatment (PDQ®)–health professional version. [online] Available from: https://www.cancer.gov/types/ovarian/hp/ovarian-treatment-pdq. [Last accessed December, 2025].
17. National Comprehensive Cancer Network (NCCN). NCCN Clinical Practice Guidelines in Oncology: Ovarian Cancer. [online] Available from https://www.nccn.org/professionals/physician_gls/pdf/ovarian.pdf. [Last accessed December, 2025]
18. Poveda A, Reimer D, Harter P, et al. Efficacy and safety of bevacizumab in the treatment of recurrent ovarian cancer. Ann Oncol. 2017;28(5):1014-21.
19. Society of Gynecologic Oncology. Ovarian cancer. [online] Available from: https://www.sgo.org/for-patients/about-ovarian-cancer/. [Last accessed December, 2025].
20. Tinker AV, Gourley C, McNeish IA, et al. PARP inhibitors for the treatment of ovarian cancer: a review. J Clin Oncol. 2020;38(20):2260-9.

Endometrial Hyperplasia

Ruchika Garg

INTRODUCTION

Endometrial hyperplasia (EH) is a precancerous condition characterized by excessive, noninvasive proliferation of the endometrium, driven by unopposed estrogen exposure. It disrupts the delicate balance between endometrial growth and apoptosis, regulated by estrogen and progesterone, leading to abnormal uterine bleeding (AUB) and increased risk of endometrial cancer.[1]

EPIDEMIOLOGY

- **Global:**
  - Prevalence: 1–5% in premenopausal women; 10–20% in postmenopausal women.[2]
  - Risk of progression to endometrial cancer: 1–5% (simple EH without atypia), 20–30% (atypical EH).[3]
- **India:**
  - Prevalence: 5–15% in women with AUB; higher in obese, diabetic populations.[4]
  - **2023 Study:** 12% prevalence in Indian women with postmenopausal bleeding; 25% had atypical EH.[5]
  - **Risk Factors:** Obesity, PCOS, unopposed estrogen therapy, tamoxifen, nulliparity.[6]

PATHOPHYSIOLOGY

- **Mechanism:**
  - Estrogen drives endometrial epithelial proliferation; progesterone promotes differentiation and apoptosis.[7]
  - Unopposed estrogen (e.g., anovulation, hormone therapy) causes excessive proliferation, altering glandular architecture and increasing gland-to-stroma ratio (>1:1).[8]
- **Classification (WHO, 2014):**[9]
  - **Hyperplasia without atypia:** Simple or complex; low cancer risk.
  - **Atypical hyperplasia/Endometrial intraepithelial neoplasia (EIN):** High cancer risk.
- **Molecular Pathways:** PTEN mutations, PI3K/AKT pathway activation in atypical EH.[10]

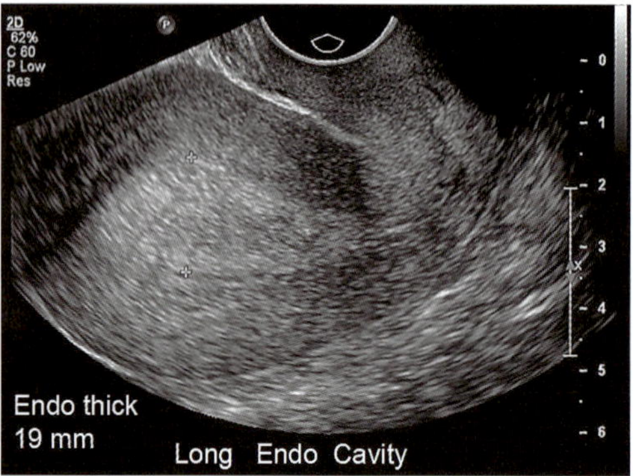

Fig. 1: Ultrasound showing endometrial hyperplasia.

TABLE 1: WHO 2014 classification of EH.[9,11]

Type	*Features*	*Cancer risk*
Simple without atypia	Crowded glands, minimal architectural change	1–3%
Complex without atypia	Complex glandular crowding, no atypia	3–5%
Atypical hyperplasia/EIN	Cytological atypia, architectural complexity	20–30%

CLINICAL FEATURES

- **Symptoms:**
  - **Abnormal Uterine Bleeding (AUB):** Menorrhagia, intermenstrual bleeding, postmenopausal bleeding, irregular bleeding on hormone replacement therapy (HRT) or tamoxifen.[12]
  - Asymptomatic: Rare, detected incidentally on imaging/biopsy.[13]
- **Risk Groups:**
  - Premenopausal: PCOS, obesity-related anovulation.
  - Postmenopausal: Unopposed estrogen, tamoxifen use.[14]

DIAGNOSIS

- **Investigations:**
  - **Transvaginal Ultrasound (TVUS):** Endometrial thickness (ET) >4 mm in postmenopausal women prompts biopsy.[15]
  - **Endometrial Biopsy:** Gold standard; outpatient Pipelle or dilatation and curettage (D&C).[16]
  - **Hysteroscopy:** Visualizes endometrial cavity; useful for focal lesions..[17]
- **Indications for Biopsy:**
  - Postmenopausal bleeding.
  - AUB in women >40 years or <40 with risk factors (obesity, PCOS).
  - ET >10 mm in premenopausal women with AUB.[18]

Flowchart 1: Investigation of EH.[19]

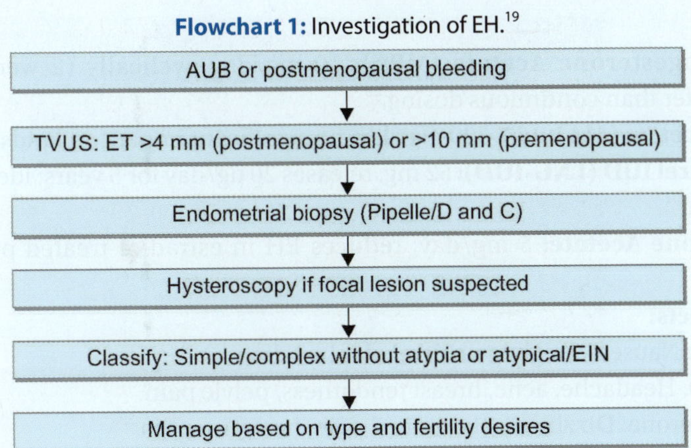

MANAGEMENT

Progestin Therapy

- **Indications:**
  - EH without atypia (first-line).
  - Atypical EH in women desiring fertility preservation or unfit for surgery.[20]
- **Mechanism:**
  - Induces apoptosis, reduces glandular cellularity, inhibits angiogenesis.[21]
  - Prevents EH progression in unopposed estrogen states.[22]
- **Delivery:** Oral, intramuscular, vaginal cream, levonorgestrel-intrauterine device (LNG-IUD).[23]
- **Response:**
  - 61% regression in atypical EH; 80–90% in non-atypical EH.[24]
  - Median resolution time: 6 months; response seen after 10–12 weeks.[25]
- **Monitoring:**
  - Repeat biopsy every 3–6 months during treatment.
  - Annual biopsy if positive response.[26]

TABLE 2: Progestin dosing for EH.[27,28]

Progestin	*Common name*	*Dose (Simple EH)*	*Dose (Atypical EH)*
Progesterone	Crinone, Endometrin	300 mg/day × 14 days/month	300 mg/day
Medroxyprogesterone acetate	Provera, Depo-Provera	10 mg/day × 14 days/month	100 mg/day or 1,000 mg/week IM
Megestrol acetate	Megace	80 mg/day × 14 days/month	160 mg/day
Levonorgestrel IUD	Mirena	20 µg/day × 6 months–2 years	20 µg/day × 6 months–2 years

Specific Agents

- **Medroxyprogesterone Acetate (MPA):** 10 mg/day cyclically (2 weeks/month) for 3 months; safer than continuous dosing.[29]
- **Megestrol Acetate (MA):** 160–320 mg/day; no significant impact on lipids/glucose.[30]
- **Levonorgestrel IUD (LNG-IUD):** 52 mg, releases 20 μg/day for 5 years; ideal for long-term management.[31]
- **Norethisterone Acetate:** 5 mg/day; reduces EH in estradiol-treated postmenopausal women[32]
- **Adverse Effects:**
  - MPA/MA: Nausea, weight gain, irregular bleeding.
  - LNG-IUD: Headache, acne, breast tenderness, pelvic pain.
  - Norethisterone: Dizziness, abdominal pain, heavy menses.[33]

Nonprogestin Therapies

- **Danazol:**
  - Synthetic androgen; induces endometrial atrophy via hypoestrogenic/hypoandrogenic state.
  - Dose: 200–400 mg/day for 3–6 months.
  - Side Effects: Weight gain, acne, hirsutism, voice deepening; possible ovarian cancer risk.[34]
- **Genistein:**
  - Soy-derived isoflavonoid; inhibits estrogen-induced genes (c-fos, c-jun).
  - Dose: 54 mg/day for 6 months; 42% response in non-atypical EH.
  - Side Effects: Minimal; GI upset rare.[35]
- **Metformin:**
  - Biguanide; reduces IR, enhances progestin response in atypical EH.
  - Dose: 500–1,500 mg/day.
  - Side Effects: GI upset, lactic acidosis (rare).[36]
- **Gonadotropin-Releasing Hormone (GnRH) Agonists:**
  - Suppress estrogen via hypothalamic-pituitary-ovarian axis inhibition.
  - Dose: 3.75 mg IM every 28 days for 6 months.
  - Side Effects: Menopausal symptoms, bone loss; high cost limits use.[37]
- **Aromatase Inhibitors:**
  - Letrozole, anastrozole reduce estrogen production; effective in obese postmenopausal women.
  - Dose: Letrozole 2.5 mg/day; anastrozole 1 mg/day.
  - Side Effects: Joint pain, hot flashes, osteoporosis risk.[38]

SURGICAL MANAGEMENT

- **Indications:**
  - Atypical EH in women not desiring fertility or nonresponsive to progestins.
  - Postmenopausal women with atypical EH.[39]

- **Options:**
  - **Hysterectomy:** First-line for atypical EH; include bilateral salpingo-oophorectomy in postmenopausal women.[40]
  - **Endometrial Ablation:** For nonatypical EH in high-risk surgical candidates.[41]
  - **Resectoscopic Surgery:** Effective for nonatypical EH; removes focal lesions.[42]
  - **Follow-Up:** Annual TVUS/biopsy postablation to monitor recurrence.[43]

TABLE 3: Management options for EH.[44,45]

Therapy	Indication	Advantages	Disadvantages
Progestins	Nonatypical EH, fertility preservation	High regression rate, noninvasive	Side effects, need for monitoring
LNG-IUD	Nonatypical/atypical EH	Long-term, effective	Irregular bleeding, cost
Metformin	Atypical EH with IR	Enhances progestin response	GI upset, limited efficacy alone
GnRH Agonists	Atypical EH (experimental)	Anti-proliferative	High cost, menopausal symptoms
Hysterectomy	Atypical EH, postmenopausal	Definitive	Invasive, fertility loss

Complications

- **Progression to Cancer:** 20–30% in atypical EH; 1–5% in nonatypical EH.[46]
- **Recurrence:** 10–20% postprogestin therapy; higher in obese patients.[47]
- **Infertility:** Chronic anovulation in premenopausal EH.[48]

Guidelines

- **RCOG (2016):**[49]
  - **Diagnosis:** TVUS for AUB; biopsy if ET >4 mm (postmenopausal) or >10 mm (premenopausal).
  - **Management:**
    - Nonatypical EH: Progestins (LNG-IUD preferred); monitor with biopsy every 6 months.
    - Atypical EH: Hysterectomy; progestins if fertility desired, with close follow-up.
  - **Prevention:** Avoid unopposed estrogen; use combined HRT in postmenopausal women.
- **NICE (2018):**[50]
  - **Investigation:** Hysteroscopy for focal lesions; biopsy for all postmenopausal bleeding.
  - **Treatment:** LNG-IUD for non-atypical EH; hysterectomy for atypical EH unless fertility preservation needed.
  - **Follow-Up:** Annual biopsy post-progestin therapy; TVUS if symptoms recur.

Indian Context

- **Burden:** 5–15% prevalence in AUB; obesity, diabetes increase risk.
- **Challenges:**
  - Delayed diagnosis due to stigma, limited TVUS access in rural areas.
  - High hysterectomy rates for atypical EH; fertility preservation less prioritized.

- **Strategies:**
  - ASHA workers for AUB awareness; subsidized LNG-IUDs in public hospitals.
  - **2024 Study:** 30% of Indian women with EH untreated due to cost; 40% had recurrence post-progestins.

CLINICAL CASE SCENARIO

Case: A 48-year-old postmenopausal woman presents with bleeding for 3 months. BMI 34 kg/m^2, no HRT.
TVUS: ET 8 mm.
Biopsy: Complex EH without atypia.

Management:

- **Diagnosis:** Nonatypical EH (biopsy-confirmed).
- **Counseling:** Explain EH, cancer risk, and treatment options.
- **Treatment:** LNG-IUD (Mirena) insertion; lifestyle modification (weight loss).
- **Follow-Up:** Biopsy at 6 months; annual TVUS/biopsy thereafter.
- **Outcome:** Bleeding resolves in 4 months; biopsy at 6 months shows normal endometrium.

Exam Tip: Highlight LNG-IUD as first-line for nonatypical EH, hysterectomy for atypical EH, and biopsy follow-up.

KEY POINTS

- **Prevalence in India:** 5–15% in AUB; obesity-driven.
- **Diagnosis:** TVUS (ET >4 mm postmenopausal); biopsy confirms EH type.
- **Management:**
  - Nonatypical EH: LNG-IUD or oral progestins.
  - Atypical EH: Hysterectomy; progestins for fertility preservation.
- **Complications:** 20–30% cancer risk in atypical EH; recurrence post-progestins.
- **Guidelines:** RCOG/NICE advocate LNG-IUD, biopsy monitoring, and hysterectomy for atypical EH.

BOX 1: Important points to remember.

- **EH Classification:** Simple/complex without atypia (low risk); atypical/EIN (high risk)
- **LNG-IUD:** Preferred for nonatypical EH; 20 µg/day for 5 years
- **Hysterectomy:** First-line for atypical EH in postmenopausal women
- **Follow-Up:** Biopsy every 6 months during progestin therapy; annual thereafter

REFERENCES

1. Kurman RJ, et al. Endometrial hyperplasia. WHO Classification of Tumours. 2014;6:126-31.
2. Sanderson PA, et al. EH prevalence. BJOG. 2017;124(7):1043-51.
3. Lacey JV, et al. EH cancer risk. J Clin Oncol. 2019;37(12):1012-20.
4. Mishra S, et al. EH in Indian women. J Obstet Gynaecol India. 2018;68(4):276-82.
5. Gupta A, et al. EH in postmenopausal bleeding. Indian J Med Res. 2023;158(3):234-41.
6. Reed SD, et al. EH risk factors. Obstet Gynecol. 2018;132(4):949-57.

7. Horn LC, et al. EH pathophysiology. Int J Gynecol Pathol. 2017;36(5):411-20.
8. Chandra V, et al. Estrogen-progesterone balance in EH. Endocr Rev. 2019;40(3):776-89.
9. World Health Organization. Classification of endometrial hyperplasia. Geneva: WHO; 2014.
10. Mutter GL, et al. Molecular pathways in EH. Gynecol Oncol. 2020;158(2):467-75.
11. Sobczuk K, et al. EH classification update. Arch Gynecol Obstet. 2018;298(3):455-62.
12. Auclair MH, et al. AUB in EH. Am J Obstet Gynecol. 2017;217(6):642-50.
13. Trimble CL, et al. Asymptomatic EH. Obstet Gynecol. 2019;134(5):1031-9.
14. Lethaby A, et al. EH in postmenopausal women. Cochrane Database Syst Rev. 2017;8:CD000402.
15. Timmermans A, et al. TVUS in EH. Ultrasound Obstet Gynecol. 2018;52(1):12-20.
16. Clark TJ, et al. Endometrial biopsy techniques. BJOG. 2019;126(5):611-8.
17. Di Spiezio Sardo A, et al. Hysteroscopy in EH. Fertil Steril. 2020;113(3):492-501.
18. ACOG. AUB evaluation. Obstet Gynecol. 2021;137(4):e78-e87.
19. RCOG. AUB investigation. Green-top Guideline No. 67. London: RCOG; 2016.
20. Gallos ID, et al. Progestins in EH. Cochrane Database Syst Rev. 2019;5:CD012458.
21. Kim MK, et al. Progestin mechanisms in EH. Gynecol Endocrinol. 2017;33(8):573-9.
22. Orbo A, et al. Progestin regression in EH. Int J Gynecol Cancer. 2018;28(4):789-96.
23. Dominick S, et al. LNG-IUD in EH. Contraception. 2020;101(5):297-304.
24. Reed SD, et al. Progestin efficacy in atypical EH. Obstet Gynecol. 2019;113(3):655-62.
25. Emarh M, et al. Cyclic MPA in EH. Arch Gynecol Obstet. 2017;292(6):1339-43.
26. Gunderson CC, et al. EH monitoring. Gynecol Oncol. 2018;151(2):321-8.
27. Kim JJ, et al. Progestin dosing in EH. Fertil Steril. 2020;114(3):456-64.
28. Abu Hashim H, et al. Progestin regimens in EH. Eur J Obstet Gynecol Reprod Biol. 2019;236:103-10.
29. Randall TC, et al. MPA in EH. Obstet Gynecol. 2018;132(2):377-84.
30. Gallos ID, et al. MA in EH. BJOG. 2021;128(6):987-94.
31. Wildemeersch D, et al. LNG-IUD efficacy. Gynecol Endocrinol. 2019;35(7):567-73.
32. Depypere H, et al. Norethisterone in EH. Maturitas. 2017;102:1-7.
33. Wheeler DT, et al. Progestin side effects. Clin Obstet Gynecol. 2020;63(2):258-66.
34. Beaumont H, et al. Danazol in EH. Eur J Obstet Gynecol Reprod Biol. 2018;224:156-62.
35. Bitzer J, et al. Genistein in EH. Climacteric. 2019;22(3):287-93.
36. Clement NS, et al. Metformin in EH. Gynecol Oncol. 2021;162(3):749-55.
37. Scarpello B, et al. GnRH in EH. Fertil Steril. 2018;110(4):678-84.
38. Barker LC, et al. Aromatase inhibitors in EH. Menopause. 2020;27(5):576-83.
39. Armstrong AJ, et al. Surgery in atypical EH. Am J Obstet Gynecol. 2019;220(1):86-93.
40. Giampaolino P, et al. Hysterectomy in EH. Int J Gynecol Obstet. 2021;154(2):189-97.
41. Wortman M, et al. Endometrial ablation in EH. J Minim Invasive Gynecol. 2018;25(6):974-81.
42. Vilos GA, et al. Resectoscopic surgery in EH. J Obstet Gynaecol Can. 2020;42(5):611-8.
43. Lethaby A, et al. EH recurrence post-treatment. Cochrane Database Syst Rev. 2021;3:CD012064.
44. Management of endometrial hyperplasia. Am J Obstet Gynecol. 2022;226(3):S789-S796.
45. Doherty MT, et al. EH treatment options. Clin Obstet Gynecol. 2019;62(4):684-93.
46. Baquedano L, et al. EH cancer progression. Eur J Cancer. 2020;130:140-8.
47. Wise MR, et al. EH recurrence rates. BJOG. 2019;126(8):1023-30.
48. Palmer JE, et al. EH and infertility. Hum Reprod Update. 2017;23(4):412-25.
49. RCOG. EH management. Green-top Guideline No. 67. London: RCOG; 2016.
50. NICE. Heavy menstrual bleeding (NG88). London: NICE; 2018.

Endometrial and Uterine Corpus Cancers

Ruchika Garg

INTRODUCTION

Endometrial cancer is a malignancy of the uterine lining, primarily affecting postmenopausal women (50–65 years). In India, it is the third most common gynecological cancer after cervical and ovarian cancers. Uterine sarcomas, such as leiomyosarcoma, are rare but aggressive.

EPIDEMIOLOGY

- **Prevalence:** Higher in high-income countries.
- **Age:** Predominantly postmenopausal women (50–65 years).
- **Survival:** 5-year survival ~95% for localized disease (Stage I).

Risk and Protective Factors

- **Risk Factors:**
  - Unopposed estrogen exposure (e.g., HRT without progesterone, tamoxifen).
  - Obesity, diabetes, hypertension (metabolic syndrome).
  - Nulliparity, early menarche, late menopause, PCOS.
  - Lynch syndrome (hereditary nonpolyposis colorectal cancer), Cowden syndrome.
- **Protective Factors**:
  - Multiparity, combined oral contraceptives, LNG-IUD, breastfeeding, early menopause (<49 years).

Pathophysiology

- **Type I (Endometrioid, 75–80%):**
  - Associated with unopposed estrogen, endometrial hyperplasia, and EIN.
  - Common mutations: PTEN, KRAS, microsatellite instability (MMRd).
  - Better prognosis, hormone receptor-positive.
- **Type II (Serous, Clear Cell, 10–15%):**
  - Linked to p53 mutations, atrophic endometrium.
  - Poor prognosis, aggressive behavior.
- **Endometrial Hyperplasia:**
  - Caused by unopposed estrogen, leading to glandular proliferation.
  - WHO 2014 Classification: Hyperplasia without atypia (1–3% progression risk) vs. Atypical hyperplasia/EIN (19–29% progression risk).

Classification

- **Histologic:**
  - *Type I:* Endometrioid adenocarcinoma (most common, low-grade).
  - *Type II:* Serous, clear cell, carcinosarcoma (high-grade, aggressive).

- **Molecular (WHO 2020):**
  - *POLEmut:* Best prognosis (>96% 5-year survival), high-grade endometrioid.
  - *MMRd/MSI-H:* Intermediate prognosis, responsive to immunotherapy.
  - *NSMP:* Intermediate prognosis, hormone-responsive.
  - *p53abn:* Poor prognosis (50% 5-year survival), often serous.
- **Molecular Classification:**
  - **POLEmut:** Ultramutated tumors with high mutation rates, excellent prognosis due to immune activation. Often high-grade but rarely recur.
  - **MMRd/MSI-H:** Associated with Lynch syndrome (MLH1, MSH2, MSH6, PMS2 mutations). Responds to immune checkpoint inhibitors (e.g., pembrolizumab).
  - **NSMP:** Estrogen-driven, hormone receptor-positive, responsive to progestins in low-grade cases.
  - **p53abn:** Aggressive, often serous, with TP53 mutations. Poor response to standard therapies, higher recurrence rates.
  - **Clinical Utility:** Molecular profiling guides adjuvant therapy (e.g., immunotherapy for MMRd, hormonal therapy for NSMP) and identifies hereditary syndromes (Lynch).

FIGO STAGING (2023)

- Stage I: Confined to uterus/ovary (IA: <50% myometrial invasion; IB: >50%; IC: aggressive histology)
- Stage II: Cervical stroma invasion or substantial LVSI.
- Stage III: Local/regional spread (e.g., lymph nodes, adnexa).
- Differentiating between adnexal versus uterine serosa infiltration; (IIIB) infiltration of vagina/parametria and pelvic peritoneal metastasis; and
- (IIIC) refinements for lymph node metastasis to pelvic and para-aortic lymph nodes, including micrometastasis and macrometastasis.
- Stage IV: (IVA): Locally advanced disease infiltrating the bladder or rectal mucosa; (IVB) extrapelvic peritoneal metastasis; and (IVC) Distant metastases (e.g., bladder, lungs).
- Molecular staging: Stage IAmPOLEmut (POLEmut tumors), IICmp53abn (p53abn tumors).

Clinical Features

- **Primary Symptom:** Abnormal uterine bleeding (AUB), especially postmenopausal bleeding (90% of cases).
- **Advanced Disease:** Pelvic/abdominal pain, ascites, metastases (lungs, liver, bones).

DIAGNOSIS

- **History and Examination:**
  - Focused history for AUB, risk factors (e.g., obesity, nulliparity, Lynch syndrome).
  - Pelvic examination to assess uterine size, mobility, and cervical/vaginal involvement.
- **Investigations:**
  - **Transvaginal Ultrasound (TVUS):** First-line, endometrial thickness ≥4 mm in postmenopausal women warrants biopsy.

- **Endometrial Biopsy:** Via Pipelle aspiration or D&C with hysteroscopy (ACOG recommends hysteroscopy for accuracy).
- **Imaging:** MRI/CT/PET-CT for staging, assessing myometrial invasion, or metastases.
- **Molecular Testing:** Universal MMR testing, POLEmut/p53 IHC for high-grade tumors.

Management

- **Surgical:**
  - **Standard:** Total hysterectomy with bilateral salpingo-oophorectomy (THBSO).
  - **Staging:** Includes pelvic cytology, sentinel lymph node biopsy (SLNB) for low- to intermediate-risk cases, or full lymphadenectomy for high-risk cases. The cornerstone of treatment for endometrial cancer is total hysterectomy combined with bilateral salpingo-oophorectomy (THBSO). Surgical staging typically involves pelvic cytology analysis and assessment of lymph nodes. For low- to intermediate-risk patients, sentinel lymph node biopsy (SLNB) offers a less invasive staging option, while patients categorized as high risk usually require comprehensive pelvic and para-aortic lymph node dissection.
- **Adjuvant Therapy:**
  - **Low Risk (Stage IA, POLEmut/NSMP):** No adjuvant therapy.
  - **Intermediate Risk:** Vaginal brachytherapy if LVSI present.
  - **High Risk (Stage III–IV, serous/clear cell):** External beam radiotherapy (EBRT) + chemotherapy (carboplatin + paclitaxel).
  - **Advanced/Recurrent:** Immunotherapy (pembrolizumab/dostarlimab for MMRd/MSI-H) or hormonal therapy (megestrol acetate, everolimus + letrozole).
  - Postoperative management is tailored according to the risk profile of the tumor:
- Patients with early-stage disease (Stage IA) exhibiting POLEmut or NSMP molecular subtypes generally do not require additional therapy.
- Those in the intermediate-risk category, especially if lymphovascular space invasion (LVSI) is present, benefit from vaginal brachytherapy to reduce local recurrence.
- High-risk groups, including advanced-stage disease (Stages III–IV) or histologies such as serous and clear cell carcinoma, are treated with a combination of external beam radiotherapy (EBRT) and chemotherapy, commonly carboplatin with paclitaxel.
- In cases of advanced or recurrent cancer, immunotherapy agents such as pembrolizumab or dostarlimab are indicated, particularly in tumors with mismatch repair deficiency (MMRd) or microsatellite instability-high (MSI-H). Hormonal regimens like megestrol acetate or combinations of everolimus and letrozole also represent viable therapeutic options.
  - Fertility-Sparing Approach
  - For younger patients desiring fertility preservation, treatment is limited to specific criteria: A well-differentiated (Grade 1) endometrioid carcinoma confined to the endometrium without evidence of spread. Management involves progestin-based therapy delivered either via levonorgestrel-releasing intrauterine devices (LNG-IUDs) or orally administered progestins. Close surveillance with endometrial sampling every 3–6 months is essential, and definitive surgery is recommended once childbearing is complete.
    - Criteria: Grade 1 endometrioid carcinoma, confined to endometrium, no metastases.

- Treatment: Progestin therapy (LNG-IUD, oral progestins), surveillance every 3–6 months, hysterectomy post-childbearing.
- **Fertility-Sparing Management**

- **Criteria:** Strict selection (grade 1 endometrioid, confined to endometrium, no metastases) ensures safety.
- **Monitoring:** Endometrial sampling every 3–6 months; MRI preferred for assessing confinement.
- **Outcomes:** 70–80% response rate to progestins; recurrence risk remains, necessitating hysterectomy post-childbearing.
- **Emerging Therapies**

- **Immunotherapy:** Pembrolizumab and dostarlimab improve progression-free survival in MMRd/MSI-H advanced/recurrent endometrial cancer (NEJM, 2023).
- **Targeted Therapies:** DNA repair inhibitors (e.g., PARP inhibitors) and pathway-specific agents (e.g., mTOR inhibitors like everolimus) are under investigation for p53abn and recurrent cases.
- **Hormonal Therapy:** Alternating megestrol acetate and tamoxifen or everolimus + letrozole for low-grade, hormone receptor-positive tumors.

Uterine Sarcomas

- **Types:**
  - **Leiomyosarcoma (LMS):** Most common, aggressive, presents with AUB, pelvic mass, or pain.
  - **Endometrial Stromal Sarcoma (ESS):** Low-grade (slow-growing) or high-grade (aggressive) **(Fig. 1)**.
  - **Undifferentiated Uterine Sarcoma (UUS):** Highly aggressive, no specific differentiation.
- **Management:** Total hysterectomy with BSO; adjuvant therapy (chemotherapy/radiotherapy) is controversial.
- **Staging:** FIGO system (I: confined to uterus; II–IV: pelvic/abdominal/distant spread).

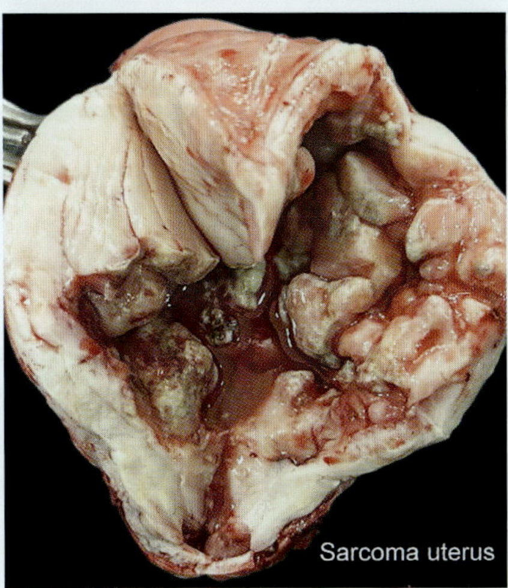

Fig. 1: Endometrial Stromal Sarcoma.
Courtesy: Shivani Singh, Bundela, Lucknow.

Prognosis

- **Stage I:** 93–95% 5-year survival.
- **Stage IC:** 77% 5-year survival.
- **Recurrence:** 7–15% in early-stage disease; locoregional (vagina, pelvis), abdominal, or distant (lungs, liver).

Key points

- Postmenopausal bleeding is the hallmark symptom, requiring urgent evaluation.
- Endometrial thickness ≥4 mm on TVUS in postmenopausal women indicates biopsy.
- Type I (endometrioid) has better prognosis than Type II (serous/clear cell).
- Molecular classification (POLEmut, MMRd, NSMP, p53abn) guides prognosis and therapy.
- THBSO is the cornerstone of treatment; SLNB is standard for staging low-risk cases.
- Lynch syndrome screening via MMR testing is critical for hereditary risk assessment.

Lynch Syndrome Screening

- Universal MMR immunohistochemistry (IHC) is recommended for all endometrial cancers to identify Lynch syndrome, which increases the risk of colorectal, ovarian, and other cancers.
- Germline testing for MLH1, MSH2, MSH6, PMS2 mutations is indicated if MMRd is detected, especially in women <50 years or with a family history of related cancers.

UTERINE SARCOMAS: DIAGNOSTIC CHALLENGES

- **Preoperative Diagnosis:** LMS mimics benign leiomyomas; rapid growth in postmenopausal women raises suspicion.
- **Molecular Markers:** Emerging markers (e.g., BCOR, YWHAE in HG-ESS) aid in distinguishing sarcoma subtypes but are not routine in undergraduate curricula.

International Ovarian Tumour Analysis (IOTA) Criteria

Kavita Chaudhary, Anusha Singh

SHORT QUESTIONS AND ANSWERS

1. Discuss the advances in imaging modalities for gynecological malignancy.
(April 2023 DNB) (5 marks)

Role of Ultrasound in Diagnosing Ovarian Tumors.

Postmenopausal patients

After menopause, even ovarian cyst 1 cm or more has to be investigated to rule out malignancy. The recommended tests for triage of patients for the risk of ovarian cancer are CA125 and TVS.[1]

Transvaginal pelvic ultrasound is the single-most important imaging investigation in assessing postmenopausal ovarian cysts. Transabdominal ultrasound should not be used in isolation. It should be used as a supplement to transvaginal ultrasound, particularly when ovarian cysts are large or beyond field of vision of TVS. On TVS, the morphology description and subjective assessment of the ultrasound features should be clearly documented to allow calculation of the risk of malignancy index.

CA125 levels are done to investigate patients with the following symptoms if present persistently or frequently (more than 12 times per month): Bloating, early satiety, pelvic pain, urinary frequency or urgency.[2] It is particularly important for women over the age of 50 years, if there is new onset of irritable bowel syndrome symptoms and all postmenopausal ovarian cysts are 1 cm or more in size.

CA125 is the only tumor marker for postmenopausal cysts. However, it cannot be used in isolation.[1] A very high value may assist in diagnosis, but a normal value does not rule out the diagnosis. It is raised in 80% of epithelial ovarian cancer, but only in 50% early ovarian cancer.[3]

The RMI score takes into account the menopausal status, CA125 levels, and morphological features of the ovarian cyst on TVS. The scoring system is:

Menopausal status: Premenopausal status—the score is 1; poatmenopausal status—the score is 3.

CA125 measured in IU/L is used.

Ultrasound features: A score of 1 point is given for each of the following solid areas, ascites, bilateral lesions, metastasis, and multilocular cysts.

- U = 0 for an ultrasound score of 0.
- U = 1 for an ultrasound score of 1.
- U +3 for an ultrasound score of 2–5.

The RMI Score was first introduced in 1990. Since then, RMI I, RMI II, RMI III, and RMI IV evolved. But RMI I is being used now and has been found to be most effective.[2] It is not useful in premenopausal women, as CA125 may be nonspecifically raised by other pathologies like PID, TB, endometriosis, and many others. Also, CA125 does not rise in nonepithelial ovarian cancers.

Color flow doppler studies are not essential for routine initial assessment of ovarian cysts in postmenopausal women.

MRI should be used as a second-line imaging modality for characterization of indeterminate ovarian cysts when ultrasound is inconclusive.

The SIGN guideline recommends that for epithelial ovarian cancer, a cutoff value of 200 should guide further management. The sensitivity and specificity for prediction of ovarian cancer were 78% and 87%, respectively.

If a malignancy is suspected, then CT scan may be arranged and the patient referral to a gynecological oncologist.

Premenopausal patients

In premenopausal patients, the international ovarian tumor analysis B-rules and M-rules criteria are used to distinguish between benign and malignant tumors. The IOTA (International Ovarian Tumor Analysis) classification system provides a *structured approach to assessing ovarian masses.*

It uses specific morphological features to distinguish between benign and malignant tumors without CA125. Using these rules, the sensitivity was 95%, specificity 91%, positive likelihood ratio 10.37, and negative likelihood ratio 0.06.

Subjective assessment by experts may be needed if not clearly classifiable.

Some tumors have a typical appearance like a "honey comb" appearance in a mucinous cyst and the "dot-dash appearance" in a teratoma to hint at the diagnosis.

The system is based on several approaches:

- *Simple Rules:* A series of ultrasound characteristics classified as B-rules (benign) and M-rules (malignant).
- *Adnex model* (Assessment of Different Neoplasias in the Adnexa): A multivariate model to predict the risk of malignancy. It is a statistical tool that predicts the probability of malignancy in an ovarian mass. It considers factors such as age, CA125 levels, and ultrasound features to classify masses into benign, borderline, stage I cancer, stages II–IV cancer, and metastatic cancer.

Various models are proposed for assessment of tumors:

- *Simple models* use CA125, Pulsatility index, and resistance index.
- *Intermediate models* use morphological scoring and RMI.
- *Advanced models* use multiple logistic regression model where each variable has an independent relation with the dependent variable.

IOTA group ultrasound rules are as follows (Fig. 1):

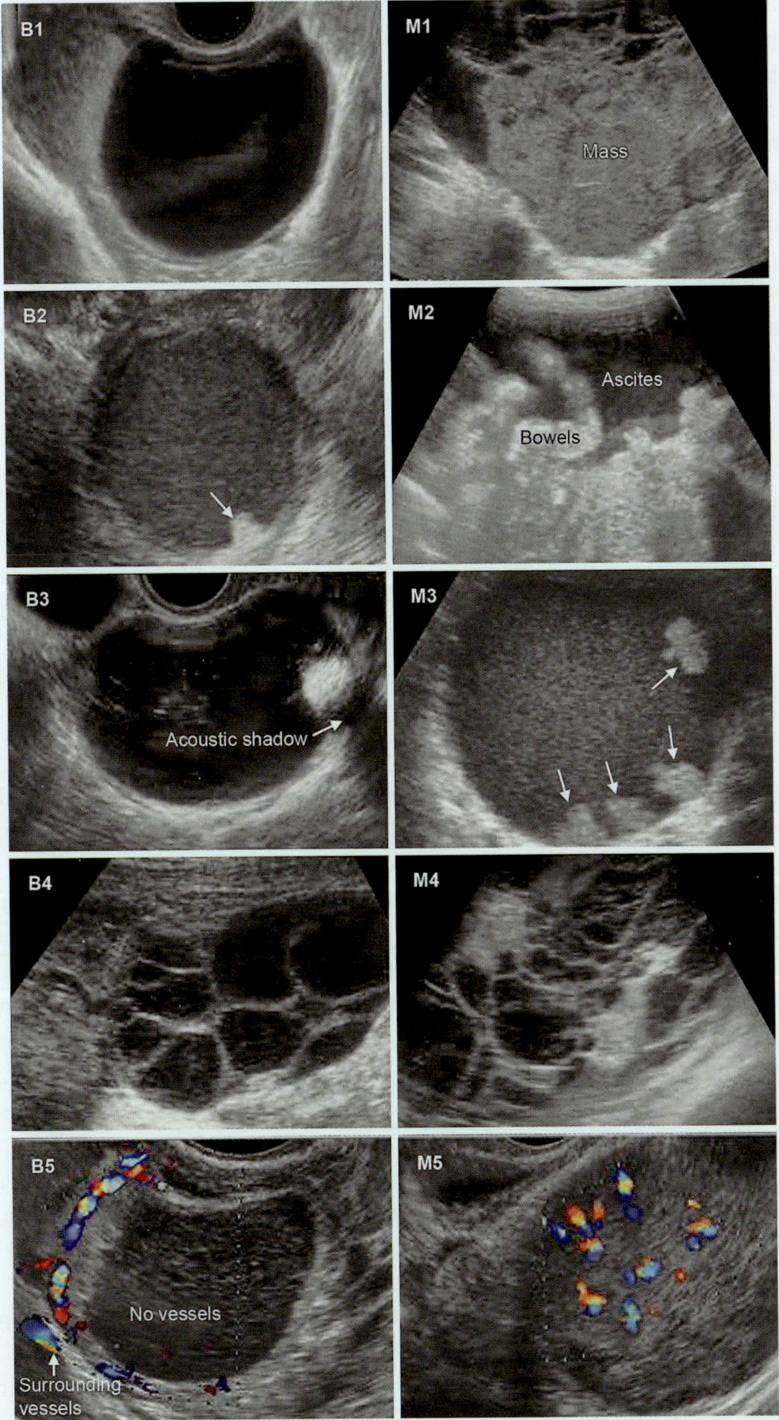

Fig.1: IOTA classification.

B-rules (Benign):

- Unilocular cyst.
- Solid components are absent or very small (largest less than 7 mm)
- Presence of posterior acoustic shadows.
- Smooth multilocular tumor with largest diameter less than 10 cm.
- No blood flow or very minimal blood flow on Doppler examination.

M-rules (Malignant):

- Irregular solid tumor.
- Ascites present.
- At least four papillary structures.
- Irregular multilocular solid tumor largest diameter more than or equal to 10 cm.
- Very strong blood flow.

Doppler ultrasound assesses blood flow within the ovarian mass. It is useful is differentiating benign and malignant tumors using parameters like Resistive index, Pulsatility index, and flow velocity.

Strong blood flow (high vascularization) is often a sign of malignancy and is one of the key features in the IOTA M-rules. Minimal or no blood flow suggests a benign mass (B-rule).

- If at least one B-rule applies without any M-rule, the mass is likely benign.
- If at least one M-rule applies without any B-rule, the mass is likely malignant. They are referred to gynecological oncologist.
- If both B- and M-rules are present or none apply, the results are inconclusive, and further evaluation is needed.

Accuracy

The IOTA system is highly accurate, with studies showing over 90% sensitivity and specificity for distinguishing benign from malignant ovarian tumors. The simple rules have proven to be reliable when interpreted by both expert and nonexpert clinicians.

The IOTA system is generally not validated for use in pregnant women, and specific adaptations may be necessary to assess ovarian masses in pregnancy.

The IOTA system was primarily developed for adult women, and its application in children or adolescents is not well validated. Ovarian masses in younger patients tend to have different characteristics, so pediatric-specific diagnostic criteria may be needed.

The IOTA simple rules are designed to be user-friendly and can be used by clinicians with basic ultrasound training. However, when inconclusive results arise, expert consultation is recommended.

When the IOTA rules are inconclusive, further evaluation is needed. This can include **subjective assessment by an expert sonographer, additional imaging (such as MRI),** or **referral to a gynecological oncologist** for further investigation.

The main advantages of the IOTA classification are its high diagnostic accuracy, structured approach, and ability to standardize the evaluation of ovarian masses across various clinical settings.

This system is an important tool for clinicians to make informed decisions about managing ovarian masses, **reducing unnecessary surgeries, and ensuring timely intervention for malignancies**.

IOTA versus RMI

The IOTA system has been shown to be more accurate and reliable than other commonly used methods, such as RMI (Risk of Malignancy Index) and simple ultrasound evaluation. While RMI combines CA125, menopausal status, and ultrasound findings, IOTA incorporates more detailed and specific ultrasound features that improve diagnostic accuracy.

- The IOTA system helps differentiate:
- Benign ovarian cysts (e.g., functional cysts, dermoid cysts).
- Borderline tumors (low-malignant potential tumors).
- Primary malignant ovarian tumors (such as epithelial ovarian cancer).
- Metastatic ovarian tumors (cancer that has spread to the ovaries from other organs).

Limitations of the IOTA classification system

- Inconclusive Results: If both benign and malignant features are present, the classification may be inconclusive.
- Dependence on Operator Expertise: While simple rules can be used by nonexperts, the accuracy is higher when performed by experienced sonographers.
- Limited Use in Certain Populations: The system is less validated for use in pregnant women or for diagnosing rare ovarian tumors.

Additional subjective assessment

Subjective assessment involves the experience of the clinician interpreting the ultrasound findings. Even when the IOTA rules are inconclusive, an expert clinician can often accurately diagnose the nature of the mass based on their experience and the overall appearance of the mass. Expert subjective assessment has been shown to have a diagnostic accuracy comparable to IOTA rules.

Follow-up

IOTA criteria can be applied during follow-up ultrasound examinations to monitor changes in an ovarian mass over time. For example, a benign-appearing cyst can be monitored for any suspicious changes in size, structure, or vascularization that could suggest malignancy.

Significance of CA125 levels in the IOTA system

The IOTA ADNEX model integrates CA125 (a tumor marker often elevated in ovarian cancer) to improve the predictive accuracy for malignancy. However, CA125 is not specific to ovarian cancer and can be elevated in benign conditions such as endometriosis or inflammation, so it is used in conjunction with ultrasound features.

IOTA system contributes to surgical decision-making

The IOTA system helps clinicians decide whether an ovarian mass requires surgical intervention. For benign-appearing masses, conservative management or monitoring may be appropriate. For masses suspected of being malignant, referral to a gynecological oncologist for surgical management (often including staging or debulking surgery) is essential.

IOTA Simple Rules for borderline ovarian tumors

Borderline ovarian tumors (BOTs) are challenging to diagnose with ultrasound alone, but the IOTA system has shown moderate success. 20% of borderline ovarian tumors appear like simple cyst.[2] The ADNEX model helps differentiate BOTs from benign and malignant masses by including specific risk categories, although definitive diagnosis typically requires histopathology after surgical removal.

IOTA improve patient outcomes by providing a structured and accurate assessment of ovarian masses. It reduces the number of unnecessary surgeries for benign masses. It ensures that malignant masses are identified earlier, leading to prompt treatment. It improves presurgical planning by identifying high-risk patients who need referral to specialized oncological care. It lowers the risks associated with misdiagnosis and delayed treatment of ovarian cancer.

Research to improve the IOTA classification

Researchers continue to refine the IOTA models by incorporating advanced imaging techniques (such as MRI and 3D ultrasound) and integrating new biomarkers. Efforts are also underway to improve IOTA's predictive power for rare ovarian tumors and to adapt it for use in diverse populations, including pregnant women and adolescents.

- Other diagnostic tools that may complement IOTA include:
  - Lactate dehydrogenase, Alpha fetoproteins and human chorionic gonadotrophin should be measured in patient under 40 years of age with complex ovarian masses because the possibility of germ cell tumor has to be ruled out.[3]
  - MRI (Magnetic Resonance Imaging): Useful for detailed characterization of complex masses, especially when ultrasound findings are inconclusive.
  - Tumor markers: Besides CA-125, markers like HE4 (human epididymis protein 4) are also being explored to improve diagnostic accuracy.
  - CT scans or PET scans: Typically used for staging cancer once malignancy is confirmed.
- Many clinical guidelines, including those from the European Society of Gynaecological Oncology (ESGO) and the Royal College of Obstetricians and Gynaecologists (RCOG), recommend the use of the IOTA Simple Rules in the diagnostic evaluation of ovarian masses, recognizing their high accuracy and ease of use.

The IOTA classification continues to evolve as more data is collected, and it remains an important part of modern gynecological practice, especially in differentiating between benign and malignant ovarian tumors.

Please see chapter on imaging in gynecology for role of CT scan, MRI, and PET scan.

MULTIPLE CHOICE QUESTIONS

Q1. Which scoring system is recommended to assess ovarian cyst in a postmenopausal patient to diagnose a malignancy?

a. IOTA Group
b. RMI I
c. RMI II
d. RMI III

Ans. b. RMI I

Q2. Which scoring system is recommended to assess ovarian cyst in a premenopausal patient to diagnose a malignancy?

a. IOTA Group
b. RMI I
c. RMI II
d. RMI III

Ans. a. IOTA Group

Q3. Which investigation is recommended for patient with RMI Score of 300 to assess ovarian cancer?

a. CT scan
b. MRI scan
c. PET scan
d. Doppler studies

Ans. a. CT scan

REFERENCES

1. Royal College of Obstetricians and Gynaecologists. Ovarian cysts in postmenopausal women (Green-Top Guideline, No 34) July 2016. [online] Available from https://www.rcog.org.uk/guidance/browse-all-guidance/green-top-guidelines/ovarian-cysts-in-postmenopausal-women-green-top-guideline-no-34/ [Last accessed December, 2025].
2. Royal College of Obstetricians and Gynaecologists. (2012). The Initial Management of Chronic Pelvic Pain (Green-top Guideline No. 41). [online] Available from https://www.rcog.org.uk/guidance/browse-all-guidance/green-top-guidelines/the-initial-management-of-chronic-pelvic-pain-green-top-guideline-no-41/ [Last accessed December, 2025].
3. Royal College of Obstetricians and Gynaecologists. (2011). Management of suspected ovarian masses in premenopausal women (Green-Top Guideline No 62). online] Available from https://www.rcog.org.uk/media/yhujmdvr/gtg_62-1.pdf [Last accessed December, 2025].

Vulvar and Vaginal Cancer

Ruchika Garg

INTRODUCTION

Vulvar squamous intraepithelial lesions (VSIL), previously termed vulvar intraepithelial neoplasia (VIN), are noninvasive, precancerous squamous lesions of the vulva with potential to progress to invasive vulvar squamous cell carcinoma (SCC). The abnormal cells are confined to the epithelium, excluding the keratinized layer, and are restricted by the basement membrane, preventing dermal invasion. Notably, invasive vulvar cancer may arise de novo without a preceding preinvasive lesion. VSIL is typically seen in women around 40 years but is increasingly reported in younger women due to rising HPV infections.

CLASSIFICATION (ISSVD 2015)

The International Society for the Study of Vulvovaginal Diseases (ISSVD) updated the terminology in 2015, categorizing VSIL into:

- **Low-grade squamous intraepithelial lesion (LSIL):** Associated with low-risk HPV types.[6,11] Minimal risk of malignant transformation.
- **High-grade squamous intraepithelial lesion (HSIL):** Linked to high-risk HPV types (e.g., HPV 16 in >70% cases). Higher risk of progression to invasive SCC.
- **Differentiated VIN (dVIN):** HPV-independent, often associated with chronic dermatoses like lichen sclerosus. Higher malignant potential despite lower prevalence.
    - Includes differentiated exophytic vulvar intraepithelial lesion (DEVIL) and vulvar acanthosis with altered differentiation (VAAD).

WHO 2020 Terminology

Aligns with ISSVD 2015, emphasizing LSIL, HSIL, and dVIN for standardized histopathological reporting.

EPIDEMIOLOGY AND ETIOLOGY

- **Incidence:** Vulvar cancer accounts for 2–5% of female genital tract malignancies, with lower incidence in developing countries. VSIL incidence is rising due to increased awareness, improved diagnostics, and higher life expectancy.
- **Risk Factors:**
    - *HPV-related (HSIL):* High-risk HPV serotypes (16, 18, 31, 33; HPV 16 in >70% cases). Associated with smoking, immunosuppression (e.g., HIV, pregnancy), and concurrent cervical neoplasia (50% of cases).

- *HPV-independent (dVIN):* Chronic vulvar dermatoses (lichen sclerosus, lichen planus), oxidative stress, and immune dysregulation.
- *Other factors:* Obesity, diabetes, chronic vulvar irritation, and herpes simplex virus (HSV) infection.

HISTOPATHOLOGY

- **LSIL:** Atypia in the lower third of the epithelium, with acanthosis and minimal malignant potential.
- **HSIL:** Atypia extending beyond the lower third, with increased mitotic activity and nuclear pleomorphism.
- **dVIN:** Subtle basal layer atypia, often misdiagnosed as chronic dermatoses. Immunohistochemistry (e.g., p16, p53) aids diagnosis.
- **Key Features:** Basal layer atypia, enlarged nuclei, hyperchromasia, and increased mitoses in both HSIL and dVIN. Intraepithelial pearl formation and dermal inflammation may be present.

CLINICAL FEATURES

- **Symptoms:** Pruritus (most common), irritation, pain, bleeding, or visible lesions. Asymptomatic in early stages.
- **Lesion Characteristics:**
  - *LSIL:* Flat, warty, or condylomatous lesions, often multifocal.
  - *HSIL:* Multifocal, multicentric (vulva, cervix, vagina, perianal), warty or papular, well-defined edges, common in younger women.
  - *dVIN:* Unifocal, hyperkeratotic plaques with ill-defined edges, often in older women with chronic dermatoses.

INVESTIGATIONS

- **Biopsy:** Gold standard for diagnosis. Recommended: 4 mm wide, 5 mm deep (hair-bearing areas) or 3 mm deep (hairless areas). Multiple biopsies for multifocal lesions with acetic acid-guided mapping.
- **Colposcopy:** Limited utility due to keratinization but useful for persistent symptoms or to assess disease extent.
- **HPV DNA Testing:** Combined with cytology, improves detection rate to 95%.
- **Additional Tests:** Proctoscopy/anoscopy for perianal involvement; screening for cervical/vaginal neoplasia to rule out multicentric disease.

MANAGEMENT

The management of VSIL aims to relieve symptoms, prevent progression to invasive cancer, and avoid mutilating surgery (e.g., radical vulvectomy) to preserve sexual function, especially in younger women.

Type	Management strategy	Follow-up
LSIL	Observation unless symptomatic; topical treatments (e.g., imiquimod) if needed	Regular monitoring; no treatment required if asymptomatic
HSIL	Wide local excision (2 cm margin), laser ablation, or topical imiquimod	Long-term follow-up (6-monthly for 5 years, then annually) to detect recurrence
dVIN	Surgical excision preferred due to high malignant potential	Lifelong follow-up to monitor for recurrence and progression to invasive SCC

- **Conservative Approaches:**
  - *Young women with multifocal euploid HSIL:* Observation for up to 6 months, as 90% regress spontaneously (especially postpregnancy or immunosuppression).
  - *Unifocal HSIL/dVIN:* Wide local excision or laser ablation (CO_2 laser, photodynamic therapy).
  - Topical treatments (e.g., imiquimod 5%, 5-FU) are alternatives but require lifelong follow-up due to recurrence risk (20–30%).
  - *Elderly Patients:* Simple vulvectomy for dVIN or persistent HSIL to prevent progression.
  - *Prophylaxis:* HPV vaccination reduces VSIL incidence by targeting high-risk serotypes.

VULVAR CANCER

- **Epidemiology:** Accounts for 2–5% of genital tract cancers, primarily affecting women >60 years. Increasing incidence in younger women due to HPV-related risk factors.
- **Types:**
  - Squamous cell carcinoma (90%)
  - Melanoma (1–5%)
  - Basal cell carcinoma (1%)
  - Adenocarcinoma (Paget disease-related, 1%)
  - Sarcoma (2%)

Clinical Features of Invasive Vulvar Cancer

- **Symptoms:** Pruritus (80%), vulvar lump, ulcer, bleeding, discharge, or pain. Late symptoms: Dysuria, rectal bleeding, or lower limb edema.
- **Signs:**
  - Solitary lesions (98%) on labia majora (70%), less commonly labia minora, clitoris, or perineum.
  - Appearance: Papule, plaque, ulcer, or warty growth (white, red, or pigmented).
  - Surrounding skin may show dystrophy or leukoplakia.

Staging (FIGO)

Stage	*Description*	*Lymph node involvement*
IA	Single lesion ≤2 cm, invasion ≤1 mm (microinvasive)	None
IB	Lesion >2 cm or invasion >1 mm	None
II	Tumor of any size with extension to adjacent structures (e.g., urethra, vagina)	None
III	Tumor with regional lymph node metastasis	Ipsilateral or bilateral
IV	Distant metastasis or invasion of bladder/rectum	100%

Spread

- **Direct:** To adjacent structures (urethra, vagina, anal canal).
- **Lymphatic:**
  - *Lateral lesions:* Ipsilateral inguinal nodes.
  - *Midline lesions (<2 cm from midline):* Bilateral inguinal nodes.
  - *Clitoral lesions:* Direct pelvic node drainage.
  - *Involvement:* Stages I (10%), II (30%), III (70%), IV (100%).
  - *Hematogenous:* Rare, occurs in advanced stages.

Investigations for Vulvar Cancer

- **Biopsy:** Punch or excisional biopsy to confirm SCC, melanoma, or Paget disease.
- **Imaging:** CT/MRI for lymph node metastasis; PET scan for staging.
- **Lymphatic Mapping:** Sentinel lymph node biopsy with blue dye or radioactive tracer (100% detection rate).
- **Additional:** Cystoscopy (urethral involvement), anoscopy/proctoscopy (perianal involvement), chest X-ray, and bone imaging for metastasis.

Management of Vulvar Cancer

FIGO stage	*Primary surgery*	*Lymph node strategy*	*Adjuvant treatment*
IA	Wide local excision (2 cm margin)	No dissection required	None
IB–II	Radical wide local excision	Ipsilateral (lateral lesions) or bilateral (midline/large lesions) lymphadenectomy	Radiotherapy if nodes positive
III–IV	Evaluate resectability; chemoradiation if unresectable	Bilateral lymphadenectomy; omit full dissection if nodes enlarged	Radiotherapy to groin/pelvis for positive nodes

- **Microinvasive (Stage IA):** Wide local excision without lymphadenectomy.
- **Stage IB–II:** Radical vulvectomy with inguinofemoral lymphadenectomy; radiotherapy if nodes are positive.

- **Stage III–IV:** Chemoradiation (5-FU, mitomycin-C) or radiotherapy (4,000–5,000 rad) to shrink tumors, followed by local excision. Exenteration is rarely performed.
- **Chemotherapy:** Bleomycin, methotrexate, trastuzumab for advanced stages.
- **Melanoma:** Vulvectomy with lymphadenectomy; test for c-KIT/BRAF mutations for immunotherapy (e.g., nivolumab).

Paget Disease: Local excision or vulvectomy; **radiotherapy** for inoperable cases. Search for underlying adenocarcinoma (20–30%).

Bartholin's Gland Tumor: Radical vulvectomy with lymphadenectomy (poor prognosis).

Sarcoma: Local excision; high metastasis risk.

Follow-Up

- **VSIL:** 6-monthly visual inspection for 5 years, then annually. Pap smear, colposcopy, or biopsy as needed. Recurrence rate: 20–30%; progression to invasive cancer: 5–10% in 8 years.
- **Invasive Cancer:** Similar follow-up with additional imaging for nodal recurrence. Recurrence (30%) is common within 2 years, treated with **excision**, radiotherapy, or chemotherapy.

Prognosis

- **VSIL:** HSIL (10% progression), dVIN (higher risk). LSIL has negligible malignant potential.
- **Invasive Cancer:** 5-year survival is 90% without lymph node involvement, decreasing with nodal metastasis. Groin node status is the most critical prognostic factor.

VAGINAL CANCER

- **Epidemiology:** Rare (<0.2% of female cancers), primarily in women >70 years. Associated with HPV, prior cervical cancer, or in utero DES exposure (clear cell adenocarcinoma, now rare).
- **Histology:** Squamous cell carcinoma (90%), adenocarcinoma, or sarcoma (e.g., sarcoma botryoides in children).
- **Clinical Features:** Asymptomatic early; later presents with watery discharge, postcoital bleeding, or ulcers. Often multifocal in the upper third of the posterior vaginal wall.
- **Diagnosis:** Schiller's test, colposcopy, and biopsy. CT/MRI for staging.
- **Management:**
    - *VAIN:* Local excision, CO_2 laser, or 5-FU cream.
    - *Invasive:* Radiotherapy, Wertheim hysterectomy with colpectomy or exenteration for advanced cases. Chemotherapy (VAC regimen) for sarcoma.
    - *Prophylaxis:* Treat decubitus ulcers and monitor pessary use to prevent malignancy.
    - *Prognosis:* 30–40% overall survival due to late diagnosis.

KEY POINTS FOR POSTGRADUATE EXAM

- VSIL (ISSVD 2015) includes LSIL, HSIL, and dVIN; HSIL and dVIN are premalignant.
- HPV 16 drives HSIL (>70%); dVIN is linked to lichen sclerosus.
- Pruritus is the hallmark symptom; HSIL is multifocal, dVIN is unifocal.
- Biopsy is mandatory; HPV DNA testing enhances detection.
- Conservative management (excision, ablation) is preferred for young women; vulvectomy for elderly or dVIN.
- Vulvar cancer (2–5% of genital cancers) is treated with radical vulvectomy and lymphadenectomy if nodes are involved.
- Prognosis hinges on lymph node status; 90% 5-year survival without nodal involvement.
- Vaginal cancer is rare, often HPV-related, and requires radiotherapy or surgery.
- HPV vaccination reduces VSIL and vulvar cancer incidence.
- Lifelong follow-up is essential due to high recurrence rates (20–30%).

Urological Injuries in Obstetrics and Gynecology

Ruchika Garg

INTRODUCTION

Urological injuries, though rare, are serious complications in obstetric and gynecological procedures, significantly impacting quality of life. These injuries, affecting the bladder, ureters, or urethra, occur during childbirth, cesarean sections, hysterectomies, or other pelvic surgeries. Early recognition and prompt management are essential to reduce morbidity and long-term complications.

- **Incidence:** Urological injuries vary by procedure, surgeon experience, and patient factors. Bladder injuries occur in 0.05–0.66% of major gynecological surgeries and 0.27% (primary) to 0.43–0.81% (repeat) cesarean sections. Ureteral injuries are rarer, affecting 0.3% of gynecological surgeries and <0.1% of cesarean sections. Risk increases in complex cases like large fibroid hysterectomies, endometriosis, or malignancies.
- **Anatomy:** The bladder lies anterior to the uterus, with ureters running lateral to the uterine arteries before entering the bladder. The ureters' proximity to the uterine arteries ("water under the bridge") makes them vulnerable during hysterectomies, cesarean sections, or pelvic floor repairs.
- **Risk Factors and Prevention**
  - **Risk Factors:**
    - Prior pelvic surgeries: Adhesions distort anatomy.
    - Endometriosis/Pelvic inflammatory disease: Cause scarring/fibrosis.
    - Large fibroids/Malignancies: Alter bladder/ureter positions.
    - Emergency surgeries: Increase risk due to urgency.
    - Thermal injuries: More common with monopolar cautery.
  - **Prevention:**
    - Understand anatomical variations for precise dissection.
    - Use sharp dissection for adhesions; prefer harmonic cautery to minimize thermal injury.
    - Prevent ureteral injury by tracing the ureter from the pelvic brim, avoiding blind clamping, opening the vesicouterine pouch, and using preoperative ureteric stenting for complex cases (e.g., broad ligament/cervical fibroids).
- **Bladder Injuries**
  - **Etiology:** Most common urological injury, occurring during cesarean sections, hysterectomies, or pelvic surgeries due to sharp dissection, suturing, or electrosurgical thermal damage. Distended or adherent bladders (from prior surgeries) are particularly at risk.

- **Diagnosis:** Often detected intraoperatively via inspection or cystoscopy. Postoperative signs include hematuria, urinary leakage, or peritonitis.
  Imaging (cystogram/CT cystography) confirms delayed injuries.
- **Management:** Intraoperative repair involves two- or three-layer closure with absorbable polydioxanone 3-0 sutures, followed by Foley catheter drainage (7–14 days). Delayed injuries (e.g., vesicovaginal fistula) may require further surgery.

- **Ureteral Injuries**
  - **Etiology:** Less common but harder to manage, occurring during hysterectomies, lymph node dissections, or endometriosis surgeries. Injury sites include the pelvic brim, iliac artery bifurcation, uterosacral ligament, broad ligament, ureteric canal, bladder insertion, or upper vagina, caused by ligation, transection, or thermal damage.
  - **Diagnosis:** Intraoperative signs include absent urine output, visible transection, or ischemia. Postoperative symptoms include flank pain, fever, or urinary leakage **(Fig. 1)**. Diagnosis uses IVP, CT urogram, or retrograde pyelogram.

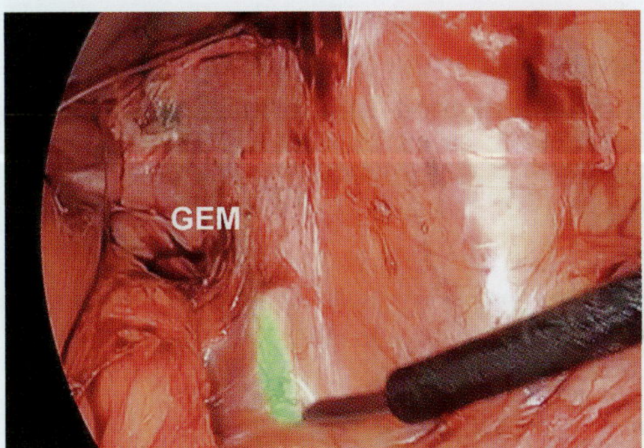

Fig. 1: ICG dye during Laparoscopy to visualize ureter. It is seen as green.

  - **Management:** Immediate intraoperative repair (reanastomosis or reimplantation with stenting) is ideal. Postoperative cases may need percutaneous nephrostomy and delayed repair.

Repair Principles

- Preserve ureteric sheath/blood supply.
- Use gentle handling, tension-free anastomosis, and fine absorbable sutures.
- Support with peritoneum/omentum, stent for 3–4 weeks and use a closed suction drain.
- Consider proximal diversion for severe injuries.

Techniques

- Partial transection/crushing: Cystoscopic stenting.
- Upper/middle ureter transection: Ureteroureterostomy with DJ stent.
- Extensive resection: Ureteroileal interposition.
- Middle third injury: Transureteroureterostomy.
- Lower third transection (<6 cm from bladder): Ureteroneocystostomy, psoas hitch, or Boari flap.

- **Urethral Injuries** Rare, typically from difficult forceps deliveries, prolonged obstructed labor, or bladder neck dissection. Symptoms include incontinence, hematuria, or retention. Repair involves careful suturing to maintain urethral patency.
- **Prevention Strategies**
  - **Preoperative:** Identify high-risk patients (prior surgeries, endometriosis, fibroids) for tailored planning.
  - **Intraoperative:** Minimize tissue handling, use delicate dissection, confirm bladder/ ureter integrity via cystoscopy.
  - **Imaging:** Use preoperative CT/MRI in complex cases to map anatomy.
- **Postoperative Care and Outcomes**

  Monitor urinary function and educate patients on signs of complications (leakage, infection, obstruction). Early detection and timely repair improve outcomes, but delayed management risks fistulas, strictures, or renal dysfunction.

Conclusion

Urological injuries, though uncommon, significantly affect quality of life. Prompt recognition, precise surgical techniques and preventive strategies are critical. With appropriate management, most patients achieve good functional recovery **(Fig. 2)**.

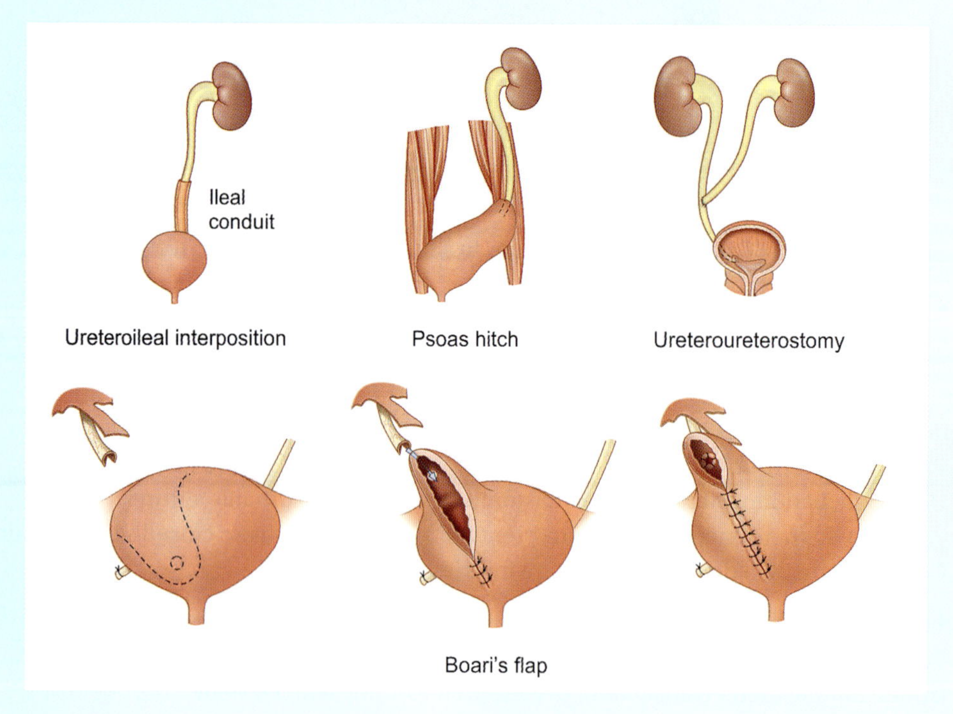

Fig. 2: Operations for ureteric injuries repair.

LONG QUESTIONS AND ANSWERS

Q1. Discuss the incidence, causes, and management of urological injuries in gynecological surgeries.

Ans:

Introduction

Urological injuries are not very common, but they can really impact a person's quality of life after gynecological surgeries. These injuries mostly happen to the bladder or ureters and sometimes to the urethra too. Most common urological problems occur during surgeries like hysterectomies or when treating endometriosis and pelvic cancers. It is very important to spot these issues early and manage them quickly to avoid long-term complication **(Fig. 2)**.

Incidence of Urological Injuries

The rate of urological injuries during gynecological surgeries changes based on the type of surgery and the patient. For major operations like hysterectomies or pelvic reconstruction, bladder injuries happen in about 1–2% of cases. Ureteral injuries are a bit rarer, showing up in roughly 0.5–1% of procedures. The likelihood increases when surgeries are more complex—like when dealing with large fibroids or severe endometriosis.

Causes and risk factors

A few different things can lead to urological injuries during surgeries:

- **Anatomical factors:** The bladder is in close relation with the uterus. So, this closeness means there is a higher chance of accidentally harming these organs during surgery.
- **Previous surgeries:** If the patient had previous pelvic surgery, it increases the risk of adhesions and distorting the anatomy and increases the risk of bladder and ureter injury during surgery.
- **Endometriosis:** This condition can cause thick adhesions in the pelvis that complicate surgery. Such situations raise the chance of injury to the bladder or ureters.
- **Pelvic malignancies:** Surgeries for cancer typically involve extensive tissue dissection. This increases the risk of accidentally injuring nearby urological parts.
- **Big Uterine Fibroids:** When fibroids grow large, they can push around the bladder and ureters, making it harder for surgeons for surgical access and increasing the risk of injury.

Bladder Injuries

Etiology

Bladder injuries are most common. They often happen during gynecological surgeries. These can be caused by accidental suture placement, sharp dissection, or thermal injury from electrocautery—especially during major surgeries like hysterectomies. If the bladder is stretched or adherent because of past surgeries, it can raise the chances of injuries too.

Diagnosis

Most of the time, a surgeon notices bladder injuries while performing surgery. It is clear if the bladder gets opened or damaged during the procedure. If the surgeon miss it then, then he might see the signs later on. This could be leaking urine, hematuria, or symptoms showing peritonitis. A surgeon can confirm the diagnosis using intraoperative cystoscopy or postoperative imaging like cystogram.

Management

When a bladder injury is recognized during surgery, it should be repaired right away. The usual way to do this is through a two- or three-layer closure using absorbable sutures. Then, a Foley catheter should be used for about 7–14 days after the surgery to help in healing. If the injury is not spotted immediately and leads to something like a vesicovaginal fistula, further surgical intervention might be needed later on.

Ureteral Injuries

Etiology

Ureteral injuries are not as common but can be trickier than bladder injuries. They usually happen during surgeries like hysterectomies, especially in spots where ureters are close to uterine arteries. These injuries might come from clamping, ligation of blood vessels transection, or thermal damage.

Diagnosis

Sometimes, ureteral injuries do not show up right away during the surgery. Intraoperative signs include lack of urine output from one kidney or visible damage to a ureter. Postoperative symptoms, including flank pain, fever, or leaking urine, could point to an issue. Diagnostic tests like an intravenous pyelogram (IVP) or retrograde pyelogram can help confirm the degree and location of the injury.

Management

If a ureteral injury is identified intraoperatively, immediate repair is preferred. Ureteral reanastomosis or reimplantation into the bladder may be necessary depending on the site and extent of the injury. Stenting of the ureter is often performed to promote healing. In cases where the injury is detected postoperatively, management options include percutaneous nephrostomy to divert urine, followed by delayed surgical repair.

Principles of Ureteric Injury Repair.

- Meticulous dissection preserving Ureteric sheath with its blood supply.
- Handle gently with noncrushing clamps/forceps.
- Tension free anastomosis by ureteric Mobilization.
- Minimum amount of fine absorbable interrupted sutures to attain a watertight closure.
- Use peritoneum/omentum to Support Anastomosis, especially if the periureteric tissue is rigid and fibrotic, for better healing.
- Stent the anastomotic site with a ureteric catheter (3–4weeks) and then remove by flexible cystoscopy and do IVP to confirm patency.
- Drain the anastomotic site with a closed suction drain to prevent urinoma (at least 2–3 days).
- Consider proximal urinary diversion (percutaneous nephrostomy) for large defect, severe inflammation, and complete transection.

Management depends on the type and site of ureter injury.

- When the ureter becomes inadvertently clamped or crushed and partially transected, placement of ureteric stents via cystoscopy is typically sufficient.
- The cut ends of the ureter are identified and mobilized to prevent tension in cases of ureteric transection in the upper and middle third of the ureter. Subsequently, a ureteric (DJ) stent is placed around them, and they are anastomosed using 3-0 vicryl suture (polyglactin) (ureteroureterostomy).
- Ileal segments can be used between the ureter's two ends or between the ureter and the bladder (ureteroileal interposition) in ureteric segment resection procedures.
- The ureter should be mobilized and anastomosed with the opposite ureter in the event of a middle third ureter damage (transureteroureterostomy).
  - The vascularity of the distal ureteral segment is severely damaged by transection of the bottom third of the ureter, particularly within 6 cm of the ureterovesical junction.
  - Ureteroneocystostomy is done directly, ideally over a ureteral stent, after the bladder is mobilized. A nonabsorbable suture ought to be used to bind the ureter's distal portion.
  - Psoas hitch operation: Bladder mobilization achieved by releasing the bladder's whole ventral surface from the retropubic region. To prevent strain, the bladder is secured to the psoas muscle using nonabsorbable suture. The bladder dome is used for a cystostomy procedure. Next, a cystostomy is created at the lower end of the upper ureter using a 3-0 vicryl (polyglactin) suture.
  - Bladder flap (Boari's flap) method: A tubular flap (Boari's) is extracted from the bladder and a ureter is placed in it to establish ureteroneocystostomy tension if, even after mobilization of the bladder, ureteroneocystostomy is not achievable without tension.

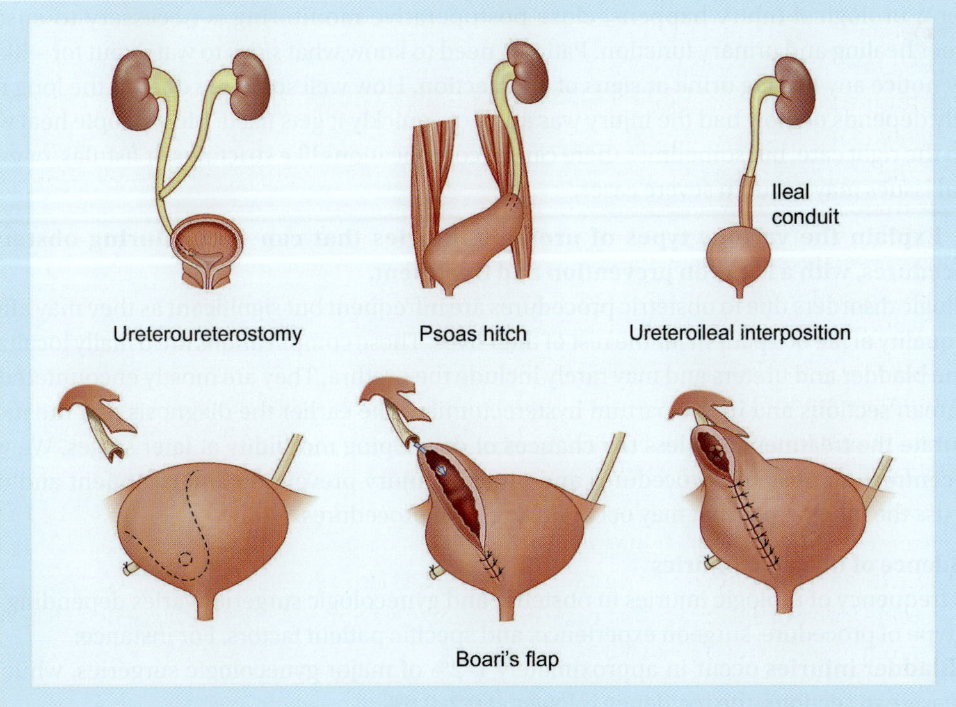

Ureteral injuries can have serious consequences, including ureteral strictures and loss of renal function if not treated promptly.

Urethral Injuries

Urethral injuries are not common. But they can happen, especially during big pelvic surgeries. People might notice symptoms like urinary incontinence, hematuria (i.e., blood in the urine), or urinary retention. Usually, management typically involves surgical repair of the urethra with careful suturing to preserve its integrity.

Preventing Urological Injuries

To avoid urological injuries during gynecological surgeries, prevention is key. Here are some important steps:

- **Preoperative Planning:** It is really helpful to identify patients who might be at risk. Those with previous pelvic surgeries, endometriosis, or big fibroids need special attention when planning for surgery.
- **Anatomical Awareness:** Understanding pelvic anatomy is essential. It is important to know the reproductive organs and urological structures' anatomical relationship.
- **Intraoperative Techniques:** During surgery, handling tissue gently helps! Careful cutting in areas with lots of adhesions (scar tissue) and using tools like cystoscopy for better visibility of the ureters can lower the chances of injuries.
- **Use of Ureteral Stents:** If a surgery is high risk, placing ureteral stents before surgery can help in identifying and protecting the ureters during the operation.

Postoperative Care and Long-Term Outcomes

After a urological injury happens, close postoperative monitoring is necessary to ensure proper healing and urinary function. Patients need to know what signs to watch out for—like if they notice any leaking urine or signs of an infection. How well someone does in the long run really depends on how bad the injury was and how quickly it gets fixed. Most people heal well with the right care, but sometimes there can be complications like strictures or fistulas, or even renal issues may occur in severe cases.

Q2. Explain the various types of urologic injuries that can occur during obstetric procedures, with a focus on prevention and treatment.

Urologic disorders due to obstetric procedures are infrequent but significant as they may affect the quality of life of a patient for the rest of their lives. These complications are usually localized in the bladder and ureters and may rarely include the urethra. They are mostly encountered in cesarean sections and in peripartum hysterectomies. The earlier the diagnosis and the more accurate the treatment, the less the chances of developing morbidity at later stages. We will concentrate on obstetric procedures and urologic injury prevention and treatment and will discuss the injury types that may occur during such procedures.

Incidence of Urologic Injuries

The frequency of urologic injuries in obstetric and gynecologic surgeries varies depending on the type of procedure, surgeon experience, and specific patient factors. For instance:

- **Bladder injuries** occur in approximately 1–2% of major gynecologic surgeries, while in cesarean sections, the incidence is lower at 0.2–0.6%.

- **Ureteral injuries** are less common, occurring in 0.5–1% of major gynecologic surgeries, and they are exceedingly rare (less than 0.1%) in cesarean sections.

  The likelihood of these injuries increases in more complex surgeries, such as hysterectomies performed for large fibroids, malignancies, or cases complicated by endometriosis.

Anatomical Considerations

The proximity of the urinary system to the reproductive organs makes the bladder, ureters, and occasionally the urethra vulnerable during obstetric procedures. Key anatomical relationships include the following:

- The bladder is located anterior to the uterus, making it susceptible to injury during lower-segment cesarean sections.
- The ureters pass near the uterine arteries, particularly in hysterectomies, creating potential risks during dissection and clamping.

  Understanding these relationships is essential for surgical planning and injury prevention.

Risk Factors and Prevention of Urologic Injuries

Risk Factors

Factors which increase the risk of urologic injuries during obstetric procedures are as follows:

- **Previous pelvic surgeries:** If a patient had previous pelvic surgery, which increases risk of adhesions and distorting the anatomy and increase risk of bladder and ureter injury during surgery.
- **Endometriosis:** This condition often causes dense adhesions and fibrosis, complicating pelvic dissection.
- **Pelvic inflammatory disease:** Scarring from chronic inflammation can distort the normal anatomy, increasing the risk of injury.
- **Large uterine fibroids or malignancies:** These can displace nearby organs, increasing the difficulty of surgical maneuvers.
- **Emergency surgeries:** Situations such as obstructed labor or uterine rupture require rapid surgical intervention, elevating the risk of unintended injuries.

Prevention

Preventive measures are critical to reducing the risk of urologic injuries:

- **Thorough anatomical knowledge** and identification of normal anatomical variations help the surgeon avoid injury.
- **Sharp dissection** is preferred in cases of adhesions, as blunt dissection increases the risk of accidental trauma to the urinary structures.
- **Use of advanced surgical technology:** Harmonic scalpel use can reduce thermal injuries compared to monopolar cautery.
- **Intraoperative techniques:** For ureteral protection, tracing the ureter from the pelvic brim and avoiding blind clamping are recommended. Preoperative ureteric stenting may be necessary in cases involving large fibroids or where ureter displacement is expected.

Bladder Injuries

- **Etiology:** Bladder injuries most frequently occur during cesarean sections, hysterectomies, or other pelvic surgeries, often due to sharp dissection, accidental suture placement, or thermal damage. The risk is particularly high when the bladder is distended or adherent to the uterus due to prior surgeries.
- **Diagnosis:** Bladder injuries are typically identified intraoperatively, but if missed, patients may present postoperatively with hematuria, urinary leakage, or peritonitis. Intraoperative cystoscopy can confirm bladder integrity, and postoperative imaging (e.g., cystograms) may be needed if an injury is suspected later.
- **Management:**
    - Intraoperatively detected injuries should be immediately repaired with a multilayer closure using absorbable sutures. Postoperative bladder drainage with a Foley catheter for 7–14 days is crucial to promote healing.
    - If the injury is diagnosed postoperatively (e.g., due to urinary leakage or fistula formation), further surgical intervention may be required.

Ureteral Injuries

- **Etiology:** Ureteral injuries are less common but more challenging to manage than bladder injuries. They typically occur during complex surgeries like hysterectomies. Common sites of injury include:
    - Near the pelvic brim during clamping of the infundibulopelvic ligament.
    - At the ureter's junction with the bladder or cervix.
- **Diagnosis:** Ureteral injuries are often not recognized immediately. Intraoperative signs include reduced urine output or visible ureteral trauma. Postoperatively, patients may present with flank pain, fever, or urinary leakage, and diagnostic tools such as CT urograms or intravenous pyelograms are used to confirm the injury.

Management

- If identified intraoperatively, ureteral repair should be performed immediately, with stenting often used to ensure patency.
- In cases where the injury is identified postoperatively, initial management may involve percutaneous nephrostomy for urinary diversion, followed by delayed surgical repair.

Urethral Injuries

Though rare, urethral injuries can occur during forceps-assisted vaginal deliveries or prolonged obstructed labor. These injuries are often associated with urinary incontinence or hematuria. Repair involves careful suturing of the urethral tissue, ensuring patency with postoperative monitoring.

Prevention of Urologic Injuries

Preventive strategies include:

- **Preoperative planning:** Identifying high-risk patients (e.g., those with previous surgeries or complex anatomy) and employing imaging such as MRI to define structures preoperatively.
- **Intraoperative techniques:** Gentle tissue handling and intraoperative cystoscopy to confirm the integrity of the bladder and ureters are recommended in high-risk surgeries.

- **Use of ureteral stents:** In complicated cases, preoperative stenting can help avoid accidental ureteral injuries.

Postoperative Management and Long-Term Outcomes

Postoperative care involves close monitoring for signs of urinary leakage, infection, or obstruction. While most patients recover fully with prompt management, delayed complications such as fistula formation, strictures, or even renal dysfunction can occur if injuries are not recognized and treated early.

SHORT QUESTIONS AND ANSWERS

Q1. What is the most commonly injured urologic structure during a gynecological surgery and its prevention?

Ans: Gynecological procedures association with ureteric injuries

Abdominal surgery

(1) Abdominal Hysterectomy, (2) Wertheim's hysterectomy, (3) Oophorectomy, (4) Uterine suspension, (5) Vesicovaginal fistula repair

Vaginal surgery

(1) Vaginal Hysterectomy, (2) Anterior colporrhaphy, (3) Vesicovaginal fistula repair, (4) Cervical biopsy

Laparoscopic surgery

(1) Laparoscopic Hysterectomy, (2) Colposuspension, (3) Treatment of endometriosis, (4) Sterilization (especially electrocoagulation)

Prevention

Abdominopelvic surgery

- Adequate exposure
- Most important axiom of surgery: Any important structure at risk of inadvertent injury must be carefully dissected and adequately exposed.
- To avoid blind clamping of blood vessels.
- To not damage the sheath of ureter; longitudinal vessels
- Recognized by pale glistening appearance, longitudinal vessels on surface, peristalsis.

Abdominal hysterectomy

- Divide the round ligament near the lateral pelvic sidewall; then open the lateral peritoneum in a cephalad direction.
- Place an index finger on the external iliac artery.
- By moving the finger upward (cephalad), the first structure to be exposed, crossing, and in contact with the iliac artery will be the ureter.
- As the index finger is placed on the ureter, the infundibulopelvic ligament should be behind the middle phalanx and can be safely clamped with the ureter clearly visible.
- Followed toward the cardinal ligament, where it passes under the uterine artery. Push laterally and downward moving it away from cervix.

Vaginal surgery
To develop an adequate vesicouterine space

To clamp, cut, and ligate only small bites of paracervical and parametrial tissue

In posterior culdoplasty ligation of uterosacral to support vaginal apex after the uterus is removed can kink or obstruct the ureters if not done carefully.

Anterior colporrhaphy: Not to start too laterally or to insert deep sutures; distance between needle and ureter in the upper third of vagina is only 0.9 cm (Hofmeister's fluoroscopic findings)

Laparoscopic Surgery
Retroperitoneal dissection to locate ureters

Electrocoagulation of bleeding points around the uterosacral ligaments is risky; might better be done with clips and sutures.

Sometimes, the width and length of the stapler make safe application difficult; uterine and cardinal ligaments are better ligated vaginally.

Q2. How can ureteral injuries be diagnosed postoperatively?
Ans: Many missed ureteric injury perioperatively but were diagnosed postoperatively.

Clinical features: (1) Anuria (bilateral ureteric injury), (2) Abdominal distention (urinoma), (3) Loin pain, (4) Infection, (5) Unexplained fever, (6) Hydronephrosis, and (7) Renal failure

Assessment: One must have a high degree of suspicion. If a unilateral ureteric injury is overlooked, the damaged kidney may eventually become nonfunctional. However, within 6 weeks after pelvic surgery, patients typically exhibit one or more of the previously listed symptoms and indicators. Abdominal distension along with urinoma (peritoneal cavity urine collection) and related fever or peritonitis may be seen in certain people.

- Renal function tests are performed; elevated blood urea and serum creatinine levels may indicate declining renal function.
- Leukocytosis may be evident in total leukocyte counts.
- A pelvic and abdominal ultrasonography is required and may reveal fluid in the peritoneal cavity (urinoma), hydronephrosis, and hydroureter.
- The gold standard for diagnosing ureteric obstruction and hydronephrosis is an intravenous Urogram.
- Hydronephrosis, hydroureter, and urinoma can also be found with magnetic resonance imaging or computerized axial tomography.
- Damage or obstruction of one or both ureters can be identified by cystoscopy and retrograde pyelography.

Management
Urine leaks should be stopped and obstructions relieved right away. By implanting stents either antegrade or retrograde, most small injuries can be treated. Nephrostomies are typically used to maintain renal function after ureteric damage surgery. Once the patient's overall health and renal function have stabilized, definitive surgery is performed as described in the intraoperative management section

Q3. What is the course of pelvic ureter and principle of management of ureteric repair?

Ans: Pelvis Course

- The ureter first travels along the anterior border of the larger sciatic notch in the pelvis, going laterally, backward, and downward.
- It curves forward and medially to reach the base of the bladder, in opposition to the ischial spine.
- The oblique entry point into the bladder wall.
- At the lateral angle of its trigone, it narrows, follows a serpentine path within the bladder wall and opens as the ureteric orifice into the bladder cavity.

Principle of Ureteric Injury Repair

- Meticulous dissection preserving Ureteric sheath with its blood supply.
- Handle gently with noncrushing clamps/forceps.

MULTIPLE CHOICE QUESTIONS

Q1. Which urological organ is most commonly injured during cesarean sections?

a. Ureter
b. Bladder
c. Urethra
d. Kidney

Ans. b. Bladder

Explanation: The bladder is the most commonly injured urological organ during cesarean sections due to its proximity to the lower uterine segment, with an incidence of 0.27% in primary CS and 0.43–0.81% in repeat CS.

Q2. What is the reported incidence of ureteral injuries in major gynecological surgeries?

a. 0.05–0.66%
b. 0.3%
c. 1–2%
d. Less than 0.1%

Ans. b. 0.3%

Explanation: Ureteral injuries occur in approximately 0.3% of major gynecological surgeries, making them less common than bladder injuries.

Q3. Which anatomical relationship is described as "water under the bridge"?

a. Ureter and ovarian artery
b. Ureter and uterine artery
c. Bladder and uterine artery
d. Bladder and ureter

Ans. b. Ureter and uterine artery

Explanation: The ureter passes beneath the uterine artery, a critical relationship during pelvic surgeries, referred to as "water under the bridge".

Q4. Which of the following increases the risk of urological injuries during pelvic surgery?

a. Use of harmonic cautery
b. Prior pelvic surgeries
c. Sharp dissection in adhesions
d. Preoperative ureteric stenting

Ans. b. Prior pelvic surgeries

Explanation: Prior pelvic surgeries cause adhesions that distort anatomy, increasing the risk of bladder and ureteral injuries.

Q5. What is the most common cause of bladder injuries during gynecological surgeries?

a. Thermal injury from monopolar cautery
b. Sharp dissection
c. Blunt dissection
d. Ureteric stenting

Ans. b. Sharp dissection

Explanation: Bladder injuries most commonly result from sharp dissection during procedures like hysterectomies or cesarean sections.

Q6. How is a bladder injury typically diagnosed intraoperatively?

a. CT cystography
b. Intravenous pyelogram
c. Careful inspection of the bladder
d. Retrograde pyelogram

Ans. c. Careful inspection of the bladder

Explanation: Intraoperative detection involves careful inspection of the bladder, especially near the dome or trigone, to identify injuries.

Q7. What is the recommended postoperative management for a repaired bladder injury?

a. Immediate removal of Foley catheter
b. Bladder drainage with a Foley catheter for 7–14 days
c. Percutaneous nephrostomy
d. Antibiotics without catheterization

Ans. b. Bladder drainage with a Foley catheter for 7–14 days

Explanation: Postoperative bladder drainage with a Foley catheter for 7–14 days promotes healing and prevents urinary leakage.

Q8. Which site is most vulnerable to ureteral injury during a hysterectomy?

a. Near the pelvic brim
b. At the ureterovesical junction
c. At the renal pelvis
d. In the mid-abdomen

Ans. b. At the ureterovesical junction

Explanation: The ureter is most vulnerable near the bladder where it inserts, especially during clamping or dissection close to the cervix.

Q9. What is a common postoperative symptom of an unrecognized ureteral injury?

a. Hematuria
b. Flank pain
c. Dysuria
d. Urinary retention

Ans. b. Flank pain

Explanation: Postoperatively, unrecognized ureteral injuries may present with flank pain due to obstruction or urinary leakage.

Q10. Which diagnostic tool is most commonly used to confirm a ureteral injury postoperatively?

a. Ultrasound
b. CT Urogram
c. X-ray KUB
d. Cystoscopy alone

Ans. b. CT Urogram

Explanation: A CT Urogram is highly sensitive for diagnosing ureteral injuries, identifying the site and extent of damage.

Q11. What is the primary principle of ureteric injury repair?

a. Use nonabsorbable sutures for anastomosis
b. Tension-free anastomosis with ureteric mobilization
c. Avoid stenting the ureter
d. Perform immediate nephrostomy

Ans. b. Tension-free anastomosis with ureteric mobilization

Explanation: A key principle is achieving a tension-free anastomosis by mobilizing the ureter, ensuring proper healing.

Q12. Which condition is most likely to cause urethral injuries during vaginal delivery?

a. Prolonged obstructed labor
b. Cesarean section
c. Endometriosis
d. Large fibroids

Ans. b. Prolonged obstructed labor

Explanation: Urethral injuries are rare but can occur during vaginal deliveries, particularly with prolonged obstructed labor or forceps-assisted delivery.

Q13. What is a key preventive strategy for avoiding ureteral injuries during pelvic surgery?

a. Routine use of monopolar cautery
b. Tracing the ureter from the pelvic brim
c. Blind clamping of blood vessels
d. Avoiding cystoscopy

Ans. b. Tracing the ureter from the pelvic brim

Explanation: Tracing the ureter from the pelvic brim helps identify its course and avoid injury during dissection.

Q14. Which guideline emphasizes routine intraoperative cystoscopy to detect urological injuries?

a. WHO Safe Surgery Guidelines
b. FIGO Global Surgery Initiative
c. ACOG Practice Bulletin No. 195
d. RCOG Green-top Guideline No. 53

Ans. c. ACOG Practice Bulletin No. 195

Explanation: ACOG recommends routine intraoperative cystoscopy after pelvic surgery to identify bladder and ureteral injuries early.

Q15. What is the most common long-term complication of untreated ureteral injuries?

a. Vesicovaginal fistula
b. Ureteral stricture
c. Bladder atony
d. Urethral prolapse

Ans. b. Ureteral stricture

Explanation: Untreated ureteral injuries can lead to ureteral strictures, causing obstruction and potential loss of renal function.

Q16. Which of the following is the most common site of ureteric injury during gynecological surgery?

a. Pelvic brim
b. Ureterovesical junction
c. Pelvic sidewall
d. Ureteropelvic junction

Ans. c. Pelvic Sidewall

Explanation: The ureter's ureteral vasculature is probably the most vulnerable part at the pelvic side wall since the uterine artery and other pelvic contents are closely situated during gynecological procedures like hysterectomy.

Q17. During a hysterectomy, which of the following structures is at the highest risk of injury to the ureter?

a. Infundibulopelvic ligament
b. Cardinal ligament
c. Round ligament
d. Uterosacral ligament

Ans. a. Infundibulopelvic Ligament

Explanation: When going in for hysterectomy, this is also due to the fact that they are more likely to have the ureter located because the ureter is next to the infundibulopelvic (suspensory) ligament, a frequent site of ureter injury in the process.

Q18. What is the initial step in managing a suspected ureteral injury during pelvic surgery?

a. Intraoperative cystoscopy
b. Ureteral stenting
c. Immediate nephrostomy
d. Observation

Ans. a. Intraoperative Cystoscopy

Explanation: If intraoperative cystoscopy is to diagnose ureteral injury or to rule out ureteral obstruction, it must be the first step undertaken before any other activities are extended.

Q19. The most common cause of vesicovaginal fistula in developing countries is:

a. Radiation therapy
b. Prolonged obstructed labor
c. Surgical injury
d. Malignancy

Ans. b. Prolonged obstructed labor

Explanation: In less developed nations, infection is associated with obstructed labor due to continuous compression of the bladder and the adjacent tissues resulting to falling off of the tissues.

Q20. Which of the following is the recommended diagnostic test for detecting a vesicovaginal fistula?

a. Intravenous pyelogram
b. CT scan
c. Retrograde cystography
d. MRI

Ans. c. Retrograde cystography

Explanation: For the diagnosis of vesicovaginal fistulas, retrograde cystography is regarded as the most definitive investigation since it depicts any bladder contrast that may escape into the vagina.

Q21. Which of the following types of urinary tract injury is most commonly associated with cesarean section?

a. Ureteral injury
b. Bladder injury
c. Urethral injury
d. Renal injury

Ans. b. Bladder injury

Explanation: Bladder injuries are also the most common injury to the urinary tract during CS since the bladder lies very close to the lower segment of the uterus.

Q22. What is the most common presentation of a ureteral injury after gynecological surgery?

a. Hematuria
b. Oliguria
c. Abdominal pain and fever
d. Clear vaginal discharge

Ans. d. Clear vaginal discharge

Explanation: One of the components of ureteral injury is the development of a ureterovaginal fistula; females who have undergone surgery experience continuous urinary incontinence via the vagina (clear vaginal discharge). Therefore, it is important to foresee this complication and provide help to the patients.

Q23. In which of the following conditions is a ureteric stent usually not indicated as the initial management?

a. Ureteric transection
b. Ureteric kinking
c. Ureteric obstruction due to edema

Ans. a. Ureteric transection

Explanation: In most cases where there is a complete transection of the ureter, surgical input is needed to repair the injury instead of stenting it because a stent will not resolve the situation since there is complete discontinuity.

Q24. When is the risk of urologic injury highest during a vaginal hysterectomy?

a. During clamping of the uterosacral ligament
b. During clamping of the uterine artery
c. During clamping of the infundibulopelvic ligament
d. During closure of the vaginal cuff

Ans. b. During clamping of the uterine artery.

Explanation: The urethra runs very close to the uterine artery, so it is more vulnerable when the fallopian tubes are being clamping in a vaginal cavity

Q25. Which imaging modality is most sensitive for diagnosing ureteral injury?

a. CT Urogram
b. IVP (Intravenous pyelogram)
c. Ultrasound
d. X-ray KUB (Kidneys, Ureters, Bladder)

Ans. a. CT Urogram

Explanation: The CT Urogram provides a more detailed image of the urethra and is much more sensitive to the diagnosis of ureteral injury.

Q26. In the context of gynecologic surgery, which of the following structures is closest to the ureter?

a. External iliac artery
b. Ovarian vessels
c. Internal iliac vein
d. Uterine artery

Ans. d. Uterine artery

Explanation: The ureter passes under the uterine artery, making this a critical anatomic relationship to keep in mind during gynecologic surgeries, often referred to as "water under the bridge".

Q27. What is the primary cause of stress urinary incontinence after obstetric trauma?

a. Urethral stricture
b. Pelvic floor muscle weakness
c. Urethral diverticulum
d. Bladder neck hypermobility

Ans. b. Pelvic floor muscle weakness

Explanation: Pelvic floor muscle weakness, usually after vaginal birth or birth trauma, is a major cause of stress urinary incontinence.

Q28. What is the most common symptom of a vesicovaginal fistula?

a. Hematuria
b. Continuous urinary leakage
c. Dysuria
d. Nocturia

Ans. b. Continuous urinary leakage

Explanation: The most prominent symptom of a vesicovaginal fistula is persistent, involuntary vaginal discharge.

Q29. Which of the following best describes the treatment for a small, simple vesicovaginal fistula?

a. Immediate surgery
b. Prolonged catheterization
c. Urethral dilation
d. Hormonal therapy

Ans. b. Prolonged catheterization.

Explanation: For small, uncomplicated vesicovaginal fistulas, prolonged bladder intubation is usually sufficient for spontaneous healing.

Q30. During which gynecologic procedure is bladder injury most likely to occur?

a. Oophorectomy
b. Abdominal myomectomy
c. Vaginal hysterectomy
d. Laparoscopic sterilization

Ans. c. Vaginal hysterectomy

Explanation: The bladder is likely to be injured during hysterectomy due to the proximity of the bladder to the surgical site.

Q31. What is the first step in the management of a recognized bladder injury during cesarean section?

a. Immediate catheterization
b. Bladder repair with sutures
c. Observation
d. Postoperative stenting

Ans. a. Immediate catheterization.

Explanation: This is done to drain the bladder and decompress it, allowing better visualization of the injury and reducing further damage.

- Catheterization helps prevent further leakage of urine and facilitates healing by keeping the bladder decompressed.
- Once the bladder is drained, the surgeon can assess the extent of the injury and determine the appropriate next steps, which often include repairing the bladder with sutures if necessary.

Q32. Ureteral stents are primarily used to manage which of the following complications?

a. Vesicovaginal fistula
b. Ureteric obstruction
c. Bladder atony
d. Urethral prolapse

Ans. b. Ureteric obstruction

Explanation: Ureteral stents are used to relieve ureteric obstruction, maintaining ureteral patency while allowing healing or resolving the cause of obstruction.

Q33. Which type of urologic injury is associated with a prolonged second stage of labor?

a. Vesicovaginal fistula
b. Ureteric injury
c. Stress incontinence
d. Urethral injury

Ans. a. Vesicovaginal fistula

Explanation: Prolonged pressure from obstructed labor, especially in the second stage, can lead to ischemic damage, resulting in vesicovaginal fistula formation.

Q34. The "water under the bridge" refers to the anatomic relationship between which two structures?

a. Ureter and uterine artery
b. Ureter and ovarian artery
c. Bladder and uterine artery
d. Bladder and ureter

Ans. b. Ureter and uterine artery

Explanation: This phrase refers to the ureter passing under the uterine artery, a crucial landmark in gynecological surgery.

Q35. What is the recommended timing for surgical repair of vesicovaginal fistula postdelivery?

a. Immediately
b. After 2–3 weeks
c. After 3–6 months
d. After 1 year

Ans. c. After 3–6 months

Explanation: Surgical repair of vesicovaginal fistulas is generally recommended after 3–6 months to allow tissue healing and resolution of inflammation.

SUGGESTED READING

1. American College of Obstetrics and Gynecology. (2018). Practice Bulletin No. 195: Prevention and Management of Obstetric Lacerations at Vaginal Delivery. [online] Available from https://www.acog.org/clinical/clinical-guidance/practice-bulletin/articles/2018/09/prevention-and-management-of-obstetric-lacerations-at-vaginal-delivery [Last accessed December, 2025].
2. Chan JD, Lefferts JA, Meeker MA, et al. Bladder injury during gynecologic surgery: incidence and risk factors. Am J Obstet Gynecol. 2010;203(6).
3. Harkki-Siren P, Sjoberg, J. Major complications in gynecological surgery: a nationwide analysis. Obstet Gynecol. 1995;85(4):543-7.
4. Neuman M, Lavy Y, Lavie O, et al. Ureteral injury in gynecologic surgery: the role of preoperative imaging. J Minim Invasive Gynecol. 2002;9(3):229-34.
5. Royal College of Obstetricians and Gynaecologists. (2009). Female Genital Mutilation and its Management (Green-top Guideline No. 53). [online] Available from https://www.rcog.org.uk/guidance/browse-all-guidance/green-top-guidelines/female-genital-mutilation-and-its-management-green-top-guideline-no-53/ [Last accessed December, 2025].
6. Sakellariou P, Protopapas A. Urologic injuries in laparoscopic gynecologic surgery. J Endourol. 2002;16(8):533-7.
7. Vakili B, Chesson RR, Kyle BL, et al. Ureteral injuries in gynecologic surgery: risk factors and management. J Urol. 2005;174(4):1480-4.
8. World Health Organization. (2016). Safe Childbirth Checklist and WHO Guidelines on Surgical Care.

Approach to Abdominopelvic Lump in Gynecology

Jyothi GS, Afreen Mahaboob

SECTION 1: HISTORY TAKING

Ovarian tumors exhibit varying characteristics and prevalence across various age groups. Understanding the presentation of these malignancies is crucial for the accurate diagnosis and management.

Patient's Particulars

TABLE 1: Age-wise distribution of ovarian tumors.

Type of ovarian malignancy	*Age*
Germ cell tumours	Less than 30 years of age
Borderline tumours	30–40 years of age
Epithelial ovarian tumours	Above the age of 50 years

Occupation: Exposure to asbestos and talc is proven to be a risk factor for ovarian malignancy.

Race: Highest incidence is seen in Northern Europe and North American women and least incidence is seen among Japanese women.

Chief complaints: Patient usually presents with complaints of lump in the abdomen.

History of nonspecific symptoms has been associated with ovarian cancer and given by:

Goff Symptom Index

TABLE 2: Goff symptom index.

- Frequency of symptoms reported >12 times per month for duration of <1 year
- Bloating/Abdominal distension
- Abdominal/pelvic pain
- Difficulty in eating
- Early satiety
- Urinary frequency/urgency

Associated symptoms due to pressure effect include urinary urgency, frequency, altered bowel habits.

Acute onset of abdominal pain is more likely to be due to torsion, rupture, or hemorrhage.

History of breathlessness, cough, yellowish discoloration of eyes, and seizures is significant in cases of metastasis to different organs.

History of Present Illness

A history of rapid progression of symptoms over a short interval, associated with loss of appetite and significant weight loss, is more commonly seen in cases of malignancies.

Obstetric History

Parity: Ovarian tumors are more common in nulliparous women. Multiparity is protective against ovarian cancer (30–60%).

Breastfeeding reduces the risk by 24–30%.

Menstrual History

Menstrual abnormalities are seen only in case of hormone-producing tumors like granulosa cell tumor, thecoma, and fibroma.

Early menarche and late menopause are risk factors for developing ovarian cancer.

7% of tumors in premenopausal and 30% in postmenopausal women have malignant potential.

Surgical History

Hysterectomy, tubal ligation, and salpingectomy are protective factors against ovarian malignancy.

Associated Conditions

Endometriosis and obesity are risk factors for ovarian cancer.

Family History

TABLE 3: Familial syndromes and risk of ovarian cancer.

BRCA1 gene mutation	39–46% Risk of ovarian cancer by 70 years	• Annual screening with CA125 and TVS in 1st-degree relatives. • TAH+BSO after completing family between 35 and 40 years due to increased risk
BRCA2 gene mutation	10–27% Risk of ovarian cancer by 70 years	
Lynch syndrome (MLH1, MSH2 mutation)	10–12% Risk of ovarian cancer	Associated with colorectal cancer and carries a 60–70% risk of endometrial cancer

Personal history: Cigarette smoking increases the risk of mucinous cystadenoma.

Contraceptive history: The use of Oral contraceptive pills reduces the risk of ovarian carcinoma.

SECTION 2: EXAMINATION

General Physical Examination

Signs of cachexia should be assessed.

BMI

- Pallor
- Icterus in cases of metastasis to the liver
- Lymphadenopathy: Enlargement of Virchow's node
- Edema due to mass effect and pressure on the inferior vena cava

- Breast examination: This is performed in all cases of ovarian cancer, as the BRCA1 gene mutation is associated with the risk of breast cancer. In cases of Krukenberg tumor, the primary site can be the breast
- Examination of thyroid and spine

Systemic Examination

The Cardiovascular system and the Respiratory system are examined.

In cases of Meigs syndrome, unilateral pleural effusion and ascites are associated with the ovarian mass.

In advanced ovarian malignancies, metastasis occurs in the lungs.

Abdominal Examination

Inspection:

There is fullness and localized distension of abdomen due to the lump, and in advanced cases, the presence of ascites may be noted.

Any dilated veins are looked for due to compression of the inferior vena cava by the mass.

Palpation:

Lower abdominal mass:

TABLE 4: Description of the abdominal lump.

- *Consistency:* Cystic/solid in consistency.
- *Surface:* Smooth or nodular.
- Size and shape of the mass.
- *Mobility:* Horizontal and vertical is tested.
- *Margins:* Lower margin is not palpated in pelvic masses.

The liver, spleen, and other abdominal organs are palpated for organomegaly.

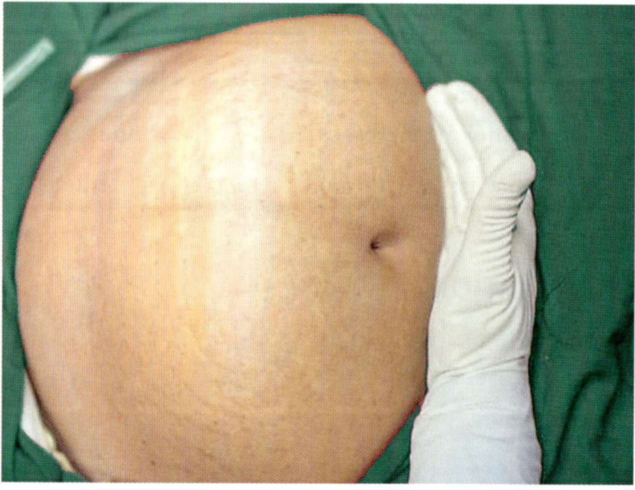

Fig. 1: Technique of palpation of abdominal mass.

Percussion

In the absence of ascites, a dull note is heard on percussion over the mass, and a resonant note is heard over the flank.

In the presence of ascites, dullness on percussion is heard over the flanks, and depending on the severity, shifting dullness or fluid thrill may be elicited.

Auscultation: The presence of any bruit is assessed.

Local Examination

The vulva and perineum are inspected.

Per Speculum Examination:

Cervix and vagina are inspected as a part of a routine examination.

Bimanual Examination

Uterine size, mobility, and consistency are noted.

The adnexal mass is felt as a fullness in the fornix and its consistency and mobility are tested.

The uterus is felt separately from the mass, and a groove is felt in between the mass and the uterus (groove sign).

Movements of the cervix are transmitted to the mass in the case of a fibroid uterus, which is not seen in cases of an ovarian mass.

The posterior fornix is palpated for presence of any nodularity/tenderness.

Per rectal examination: This is performed to look for any nodularity/metastatic deposits in the Pouch of Douglas (POD) and the involvement of rectal mucosa.

SECTION 3: DIFFERENTIAL DIAGNOSIS FOR ABDOMINOPELVIC LUMP

Differential Diagnosis for Abdominopelvic Lump

Benign ovarian	*Malignant ovarian*	*Benign non-ovarian*	*Malignant nonovarian*	*Nongynecological*
• Serous cystadenoma • Mucinous cystadenoma • Mature teratoma • Theca lutein cysts	• Borderline tumors • Epithelial carcinoma • Sex cord stromal tumor • Ovarian germ cell tumor	• Leiomyoma • Endometrioma • Tubo-ovarian mass • Hydrosalpinx • Ectopic pregnancy • Adenomyosis	• Fallopian tube carcinoma • Krukenberg tumor • Leiomyosarcoma • Retroperitoneal tumors • Endometrial cancer	• Primary peritoneal tumors • Desmoid tumor • Peritoneal cyst • Pelvic kidney • Appendicular mass • Full bladder • Encysted Ascites

SECTION 4: DIFFERENCE BETWEEN AN OVARIAN MASS AND A FIBROID

TABLE 5: Difference between fibroid and ovarian mass.

Factors	*Fibroid*	*Ovarian mass*
History	Complaints of heavy menstrual bleeding, pain abdomen, and dysmenorrhea	Complaints of lump in the abdomen, easy fullness, satiety, and weight loss in advanced malignancy
Progression	Slow progression over the years	Rapid progression over months
Age	Reproductive age	Extremes of age
Surface	Smooth	Irregular and nodular
Consistency	Firm	Solid to cystic in consistency
Mobility	Mobile, lower margin cannot be reached	Fixed, lower margin cannot be reached
Ascites	Absent	May be Present
Deposits in POD	Absent	Nodularity in POD in cases of metastasis
On bimanual examination	Movements of the cervix are transmitted to the mass and no grove is felt between uterus and mass	Movements of the cervix are not transmitted to the mass and a groove is felt between the mass and the uterus (groove sign)

Case Scenario 1

Mrs. XYZ, a 45-year-old P2L2 with complaints of mass per abdomen and pain abdomen since 2 years, radiating to the back

On Examination: Vitals stable

Per Abdomen: Localized distension is seen in the lower abdomen. A mass corresponding to 24 weeks' gravid uterus size occupying the hypogastric region felt, superior and lateral borders well defined and lower border not made out, firm in consistency with smooth surface, horizontally mobile.

Bimanual Examination: Uterus corresponding to 24 weeks' gravid uterus size, anteverted, mobile, firm, anterior fornix fullness present, lateral fornices free and nontender, movement of the cervix transmitted to the mass, no groove sign felt.

USG abdomen pelvis: Retroverted uterus, ET—6.7 mm, a heterogenous hyperechoic 15 × 14 × 11 cm mass seen arising from fundus with peripheral vascularity extending into the abdomen, bilateral ovaries normal.

Patient was evaluated and proceeded with bilateral DJ stenting and Total Abdominal Hysterectomy with bilateral salpingectomy.

Intraoperative findings: Uterus corresponding to 10 weeks' gravid uterus size. A subserosal fibroid measuring 14 × 10 × 7 cm seen arising from the fundus of the uterus. Bilateral tubes and ovaries were within normal limits.

- Sarcomatous change in a pre-existing fibroid is extremely rare, with an estimated incidence of less than 0.5%.

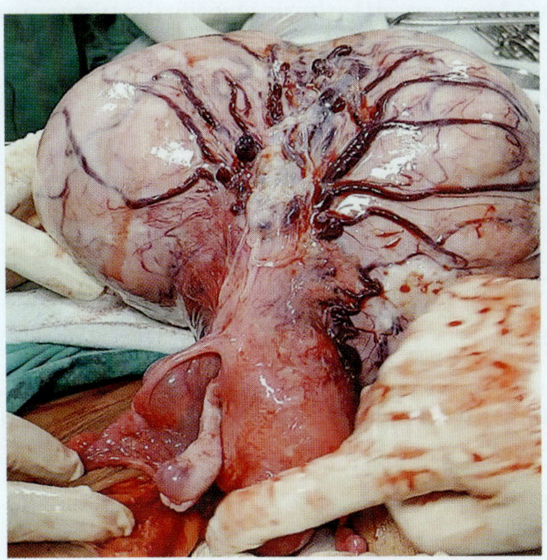

Fig. 2: Subserosal fibroid presenting as mass per abdomen.

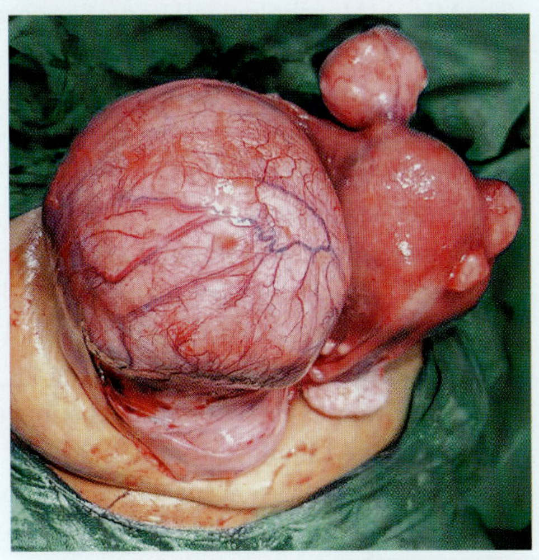

Fig. 3: Multiple uterine fibroids.

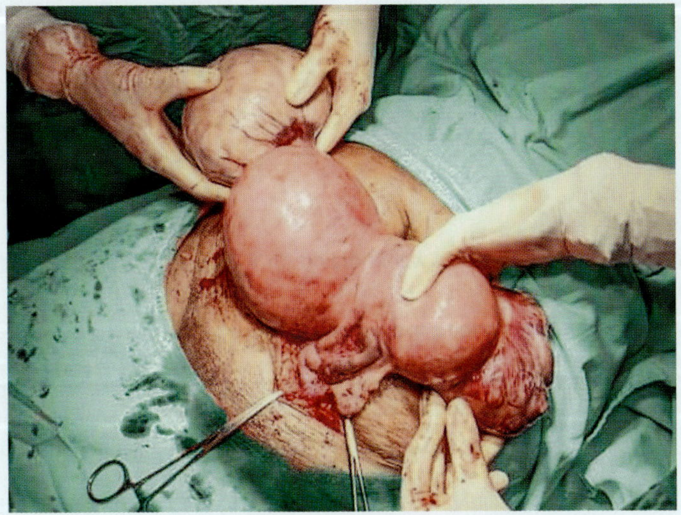

Fig. 4: Multiple subserosal fibroids.

SECTION 5: ADENOMYOSIS

It is a benign gynecological condition which is characterized by the presence of endometrial glands and stroma within the myometrium. It is commonly seen in multiparous women.

The classic triad of symptoms associated with adenomyosis includes:

- Dysmenorrhea
- Menorrhagia
- Uterine enlargement

The MUSA (Morphological Uterus Sonographic Assessment) criteria classify the ultrasound features of adenomyosis into two categories:

- **Direct features:** These features are due to presence of ectopic endometrial tissue within the myometrium
  - Myometrial cysts
  - Hyperechogenic islands
  - Echogenic subendometrial lines and buds
- **Indirect features:** These features are due to changes in the myometrium that occur secondary to the presence of endometrial tissue.
  - Globular enlargement of the uterus
  - Asymmetrical myometrial thickening usually involving the posterior wall of the uterus
  - Fan-shaped shadowing
  - Translesional vascularity on color doppler ultrasound.

  Irregular and interrupted junctional zone

TABLE 6: Difference between fibroid and adenomyosis.

Factors	*Fibroid*	*Adenomyosis*
Chief complaint	Heavy menstrual bleeding	Heavy menstrual bleeding with dysmenorrhea
Age	Reproductive age	>45 years of age
Surface	Irregularly enlarged uterus	Symmetrically enlarged uterus
Consistency	Firm	Soft and doughy in consistence
Tenderness on palpation	Absent	Present, called the Halban's sign
On examination size of the uterus	Grows beyond 12–14 weeks gravid uterus size	Does not grown beyond 12–14 weeks' gravid uterus size6.
On imaging	• Well circumscribed and hypoechoic • Peripheral vascularity • Calcification is common • Well-defined junctional zone • In T2-weighted MRI, adenomyosis often appears as hyperintense (bright) foci within the myometrium	• Poorly circumscribed and heterogenous • Translesional scattered vascularity • Calcification is uncommon • Poorly defined junctional zone with thickness >12 mm • In T2-weighted MRI, fibroids often appear as hypointense masses

Case Scenario 2

Mrs. XYZ, a 58-year-old postmenopausal P2L2 lady came with complaints of pain localized to the right side of lower abdomen since 2 months and mass per abdomen since 1 month.

On Examination: Vitals were stable

Per Abdomen Examination: On inspection localized distension seen in the hypogastric region.

On palpation: A mass corresponding to 20 weeks' gravid uterus size felt in the hypogastric lesion, cystic in consistency, smooth surface, horizontally mobile with restricted vertical mobility, lower border not felt.

No organomegaly.

On Bimanual Examination: Uterus was anteverted, normal size, firm and nontender.

A cystic mass of 16 × 20 cm felt through right fornix, mobile and nontender, a grove felt between the uterus and the movements of cervix not transmitted to the mass.

Ultrasonogram of abdomen pelvis: Uterus anteverted 6.2 × 3.6 × 1.8 cm with ET of 3 mm. A large well-defined cystic mass of 22 × 25 × 27 cm, 776 cc in volume, multiloculated, seen arising from the right ovary. Left ovary atrophic.

MRI abdomen pelvis: Large well-defined multiloculated cystic lesion in the midline pelvis likely right ovarian origin? Serous cystadenoma (ORADS-3), no evidence of ascites or lymphadenopathy.

CA125: 40.1 U/mL, CEA: 15.2 ng/mL.

Patient was taken up for Staging Laparotomy and Proceed along with frozen section.

Intraoperative findings: Left-sided multiloculated ovarian cyst of 20 × 18 cm, no evidence of any ascites or lymphadenopathy. Uterus: Postmenopausal. Left ovary: Atrophic. Omentum was healthy with no evidence of omental caking. Total Abdominal Hysterectomy with Bilateral salpingoophrectomy was done.

Frozen section: Benign tumor—Serous cystadenoma of the ovary.

SECTION 6: DIFFERENCE BETWEEN BENIGN AND MALIGNANT OVARIAN MASS

TABLE 7: Difference between benign and malignant ovarian mass.

Factors	*Benign*	*Malignant*
History	Long standing	Short history
Progression	Slow progression	Rapid progression of disease
Age	Reproductive age	Extremes of age
Site	Unilateral involvement	Bilateral involvement
Surface	Smooth	Irregular and nodular
Consistency	Cystic	Solid
Mobility	Mobile	Fixed
Ascites	Absent	May be Present
Deposits in pod	Absent	Nodularity in POD in cases of metastasis
Ultrasound features	Unilateral, simple, anechoic, unilocular with no solid components, calcification or mural nodules	Bilateral, multiloculated with thick septa, papillary excrescences, increased vascularity on doppler, mural nodules and calcification, ascites and lymphadenopathy are also present

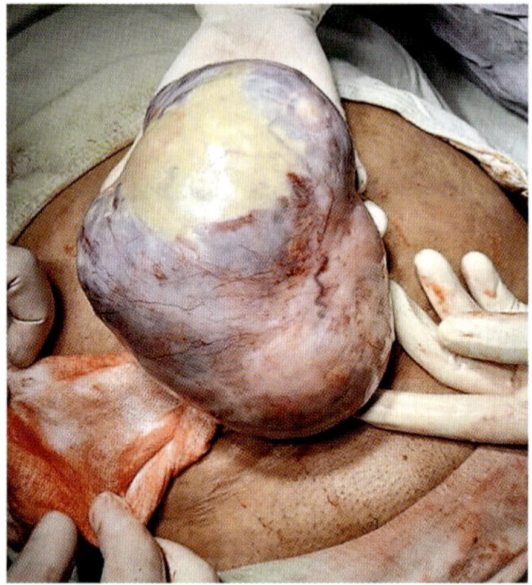

Fig. 5: Dermoid tumor of the ovary.

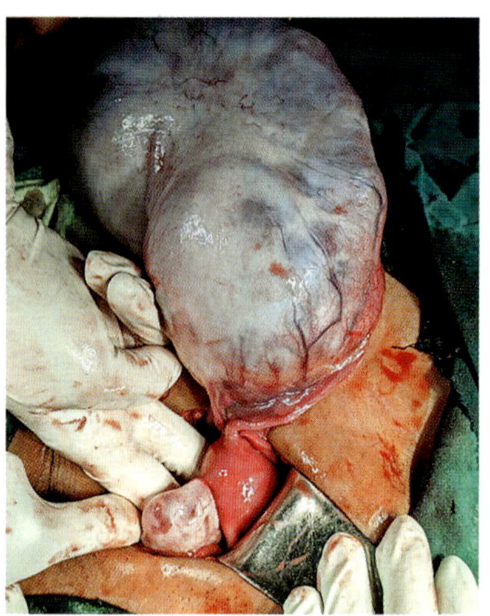

Fig. 6: Mucinous cystadenoma of ovary.

SECTION 7: INVESTIGATIONS IN A CASE OF OVARIAN MASS

Investigations:

- **Imaging**

TABLE 8: NCCN Guidelines for imaging in a case of ovarian mass.

- NCCN guidelines:
  - USG: first investigation
  - MRI: in case usg is inconclusive
  - CT: assessing the metastasis
  - Fluorodeoxyglucose pet: indeterminate lesions

USG: TVS with Doppler is the first modality of choice, and transabdominal sonography is preferred if the lesion extends beyond the pelvis.

Increased vascularity with strong blood flow (PI <1 and RI <0.4) indicates malignancy.

IOTA: Interational ovarian tumor analysis:

- IOTA simple rules
- IOTA logistic regression
- IOTA adnex model

This group has developed ultrasound-based models to help to classify ovarian mass as benign or malignant. It has a sensitivity of 95% and specificity of 91%.

IOTA Simple Rules

B rules	*M rules*
• B1: Unilocular cysts • B2: Presence of solid components with the largest being <7 mm • B3: Presence of acoustic shadowing • B4: Smooth multilocular tumor with largest diameter <10 cm • B5: No blood flow	• M1: Irregular solid tumor • M2 Ascites • M3: At least 4 papillary structures • M4: Irregular smooth multilocular tumor with largest diameter >10 cm • M5: No blood flow

Presence of only B rules, no M rules: Benign

Presence of M rules and no B rules: High risk of malignancy and referral to oncologist

IOTA logistic regression models l1 and L2 use clinical data along with ultrasound findings to assess the likelihood of malignancy.

IOTA adex model: This model uses

- 3 clinical variables- (Age, CA125 status, and whether the USG was from an oncology center)
- 6 ultrasound variables (maximum lesion diameter, maximum solid component diameter, number of papillary projections, acoustic shadowing, ascites and presence of >10 locules) it provides a risk score that differentiates between benign, borderline, stage 1, stages 2–4 and metastatic disease.

MRI: It is useful when USG is indeterminate.

Primary criteria:

- Wall thickness >3 cm
- Septal thickness >3 mm
- Necrosis

Ancillary criteria:

- Involvement of pelvic sidewall
- Involvement of the peritoneum, omentum, and mesentery
- Ascites
- Lymphadenopathy

CT: Most commonly used to optimize surgical planning and assess the resectability of ovarian cancer and provides information regarding metastasis. It is used to evaluate the following:

- Lymphadenopathy
- Peritoneal implants
- Omental caking
- Presence of ascites
- Liver/Spleen deposits

PET: Not used in the initial evaluation of patients. It is used for postoperative follow-up of patients.

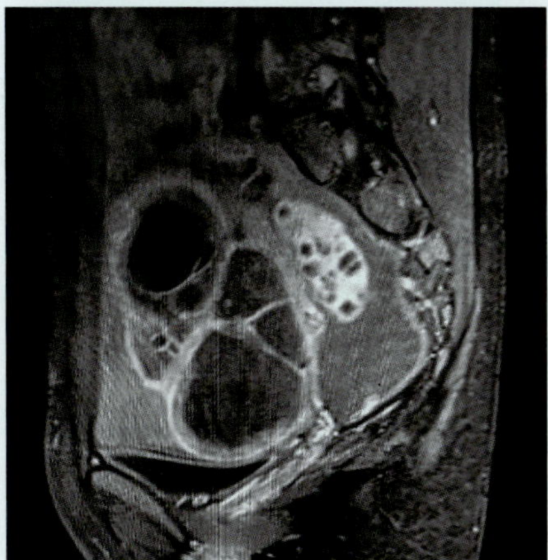

Fig. 7: MRI showing a large well-defined multiseptated, multiloculated solid cystic lesion arising from the pelvis.

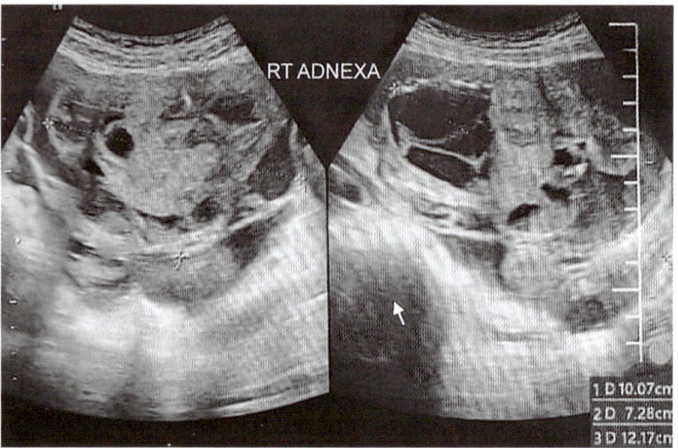

Fig. 8: USG showing a large solid cystic lesion arising from the adnexa.

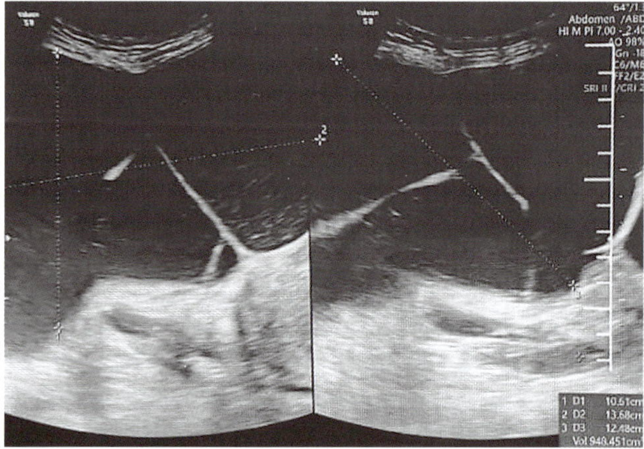

Fig. 9: USG showing a large cystic lesion in the pelvis with internal septations.

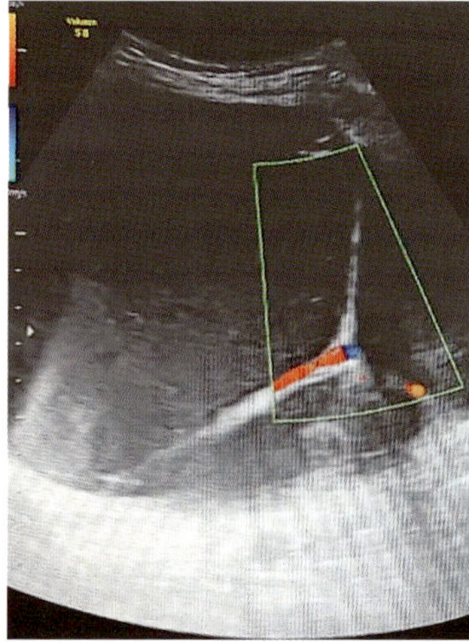

Fig. 10: USG showing increased septal vascularity within the ovarian cyst.

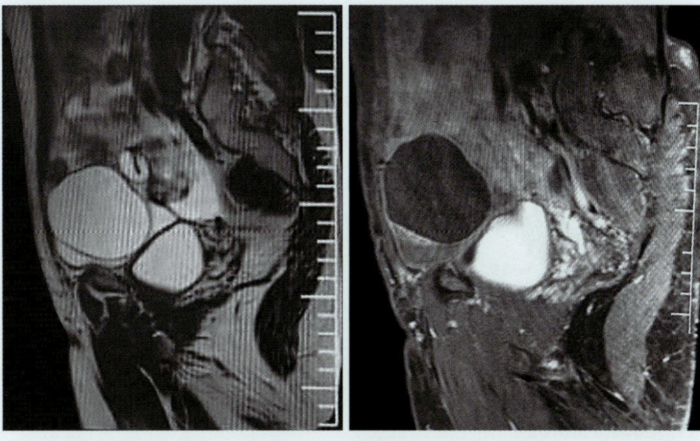

Fig. 11: MRI showing a large well-defined multiloculated cystic lesion in the pelvis, likely serous cystadenoma of right ovary.

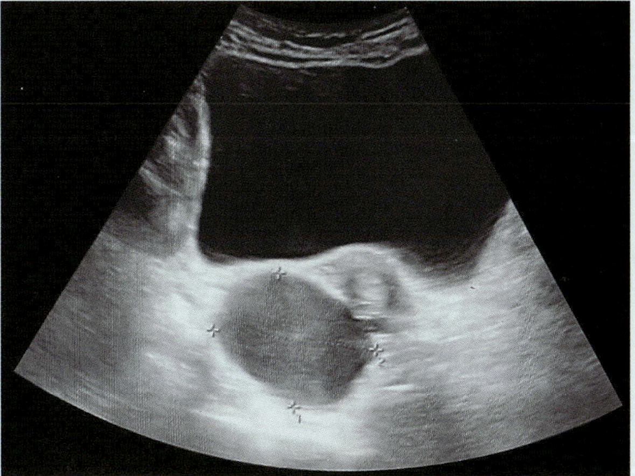

Fig. 12: USG showing an anechoic cystic lesion in the right adnexa.

SECTION 8: TUMOR MARKERS

Tumor markers in various ovarian tumors

TABLE 9: Tumor markers specific to ovarian tumors.

Type of ovarian tumor	*Specific tumor markers*
Epithelial ovarian tumors	CA125, CEA, HE4
Dysgerminoma	LDH, B-HCG, PLAP
Endodermal sinus tumor	AFP, LDH
Immature teratoma	AFP
Embryonal carcinoma	AFP, B-HCG, PLAP
Choriocarcinoma	B-HCG
Sex cord stromal tumors	Estradiol, testosterone
Granulosa cell tumor	Inhibin B

SECTION 9: RISK STRATIFICATION IN OVARIAN TUMORS

- **RMI score**: risk of malignancy index
  This score is determined by the multiplication of ultrasound score (U) × menopausal score (M) × CA125 level in U/Ml. A score of >200 is a high-risk score that requires referral to a gyne-oncologist.

> - Multilocular cyst
> - Presence of solid areas
> - Bilaterality of lesions
> - Presence of ascites
> - Presence of intra-abdominal metastasis
> - No abnormality = 0; One abnormality = 1; Two or more abnormalities = 3
>
> - Menopausal status
> - Premenopausal = 1
> - Postmenopausal = 3

- **ROMA**: Risk of malignancy algorithm
  It is used as a triage tool for adnexal mass.
  It includes CA125 and HE4.
  Sensitivity—92%, specificity-75%.
- **ROCA**: Risk of cancer algorithm
  It is a computerized algorithm based on serial monitoring of CA125 levels along with the age and menopausal status to calculate a risk score, and classify women into normal, intermediate, and elevated risk score.
  It is based upon the hypothesis that CA125 levels continue to rise in malignancy.
  It is used in screening of women with high risk factors for developing ovarian cancer.
- **OVA1 and Overa**

TABLE 10: Comparison between OVA1 and Overa.

OVA1	*Overa*
• CA125 • B2-MICROGLOBULIN • TRANSFERRIN • TRANSTHYRETIN • APOLIPOPROTEIN A1	• CA125 • FSH • TRANSFERRIN • HE4 • APOLIPOPROTEIN A1
• Premenopausal OVA1 >5 • Postmenopausal OVA1 >4.4 • Are suggestive of high risk of malignancy	It stratifies patients into high risk and low risk on a scale of 1–10
• Sensitivity—99% • Specificity—54%	• Sensitivity—94% • Specificity—69%

- **ORADS—OVARIAN ADNEXAL REPORTING AND DATA SYSTEM**
  The ORADS committee proposed guidelines for the management of ovarian masses in 2019.

TABLE 11: ORADS score and risk of malignancy.

ORADS Type	*Category*	*Risk of malignancy*	*Advise*
ORADS 0	Incomplete evaluation	–	Re-evaluation
ORADS 1	Normal ovary	0%	Reassessment in lesser frequency
ORADS 2	Almost certainly benign	<1%	
ORADS 3	Low risk	1-10%	Reassessment in 6 months
ORADS 4	Intermediate risk	10-50%	Refer to gyne-oncologist
ORADS 5	High risk	>50%	

SECTION 10: MANAGEMENT OF OVARIAN TUMORS

Management of ovarian cyst in an adolescent girl.

TABLE 12: Management guidelines for ovarian cyst in an adolescent girl.

Asymptomatic girl with a simple cyst	**Symptoms of acute abdomen and torsion is suspected:**	Asymptomatic girl with **a complex cyst**
• **3–5 cm:** Reassurance and repeat scan after 3 months • **5–7 cm:** If asymptomatic, rescan within 3 months. If persistent or when the size is between 5 and 7 cm and the patient is symptomatic, MRI and tumor markers are considered. • **Simple cyst of size >7 cm**—laparoscopic ovarian cystectomy due to chances of torsion	• Emergency USG abdomen and pelvis with doppler is done • In case of torsion—Emergency laparoscopy/laparotomy and ovarian sparing surgery are considered within 4 hours of admission to the hospital. • In case the vascularity is maintained, then detorsion with oophoropexy is done.	• **>5 cm:** Tumor markers with MRI is done • In case there is no suspicion of cancer, laparoscopic cystectomy and counseling for close follow-up are done. • In case of suspicion of cancer, the patient is referred to a multidisciplinary team/ gyne-oncologist

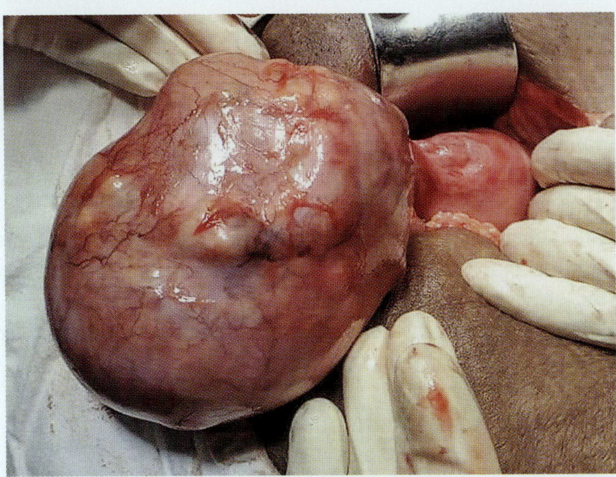

Fig. 13: Dermoid cyst of the ovary.

Management of an ovarian cyst in a postmenopausal lady.

TABLE 13: Management guidelines for ovarian cyst in a postmenopausal lady.

• RMI IS <200 LOW RISK OF MALIGNANCY • Asymptomatic cysts, unilateral, unilocular, simple anechoic cyst of <5 cm—plan for conservative management and repeat scan after every 4–6 months. • Symptomatic cysts >5 cm, multilocular, bilateral, complex features—consider bilateral salpingoophrectomy	• RMI IS >200 HIGH RISK OF MALIGNANCY • CT abdomen and pelvis is done to know the extent of disease and to look for any metastasis • The patient is then referred to a multidisciplinary team/gyne-oncologist and staging laparotomy with optimal debulking surgery done by a Gyne-Oncologist

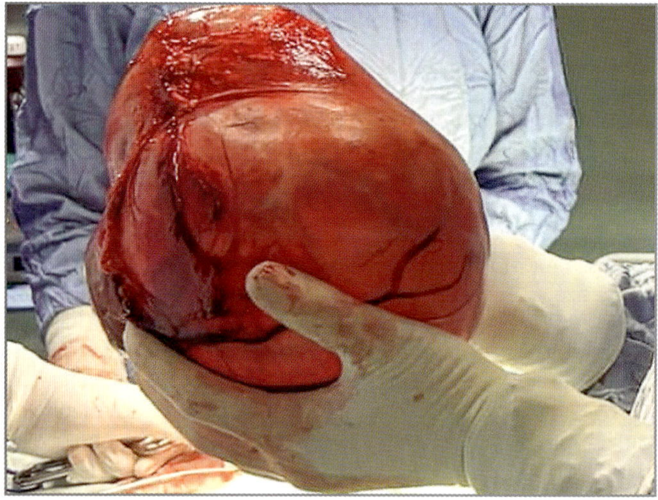

Fig. 14: Serous cystadenoma of the ovary.

SECTION 11: STEPS OF STAGING LAPAROTOMY

TABLE 14: Steps of staging laparotomy.

• Midline incision, abdomen is opened in layers • If ascites is present, ascitic fluid is sent for analysis. Otherwise, 100 mL of peritoneal wash is given and the washing is sent for cytology • Inspection and palpation of all organs in a clockwise manner in ceco-cephalad direction. • Multiple random peritoneal biopsies are taken from paracolic gutters, sub diaphragmatic surface, peritoneum, cul de sac, etc. • Extrafascial Type 1 Hysterectomy with bilateral salpingoophrectomy is done and specimen is sent for frozen section • Infracolic omentectomy is done • Pelvic and paraaortic lymph node dissection are done • After achieving hemostasis, abdomen is closed in layers

- In cases of advanced stage ovarian cancer, the mainstay of treatment is cytoreductive surgery/debulking surgery followed by 6 cycles of chemotherapy.

- If the patient is medically unfit for surgery and there is parenchymal involvement of liver and lung parenchyma, then neoadjuvant chemotherapy 3 cycles followed by Interval debulking followed by 3 cycles of completion chemotherapy is given.
  Goal must be to obtain complete cytoreduction—no visible residual disease.
  Optimal debulking—residual disease is less than 1 cm.
  Suboptimal debulking—Residual disease is more than 1 cm.

Second look surgery is performed after completion of chemotherapy with normal imaging and CA125 levels to look for any recurrence.

Fertility sparing surgery: Unilateral salpingoophrectomy with peritoneal washings and excision of enlarged lymph nodes is done in cases of germ cell tumors.

SECTION 12: CHEMOTHERAPY IN OVARIAN CANCER

Postoperative chemotherapy for ovarian cancer

- *Epithelial ovarian tumor:* Given in all stages except stages 1A and 1B
- 6 cycles of IV chemotherapy over 3 hours once in 3 weeks with carboplatin and paclitaxel
  - Carboplatin: AUC = 5–6
  - Paclitaxel: 175 mg/m sq.

TABLE 15: Calvert formula for calculation of carboplatin dose.

- **Calvert Formula: Carboplatin Dose = AUC × (GFR+25)**
- **Cockcroft Gault Formula: GFR = {[(140 – AGE) × Weight IN KG]/72 × Serum Creat} × 0.85**

- **HIPEC:** Hyperthermic Intraperitoneal Chemotherapy
  In this, the chemotherapeutic agents are heated to >41°C after optimal debulking surgery. It improves the penetration of the drugs through the peritoneal surface.
- **PIPAC:** Pressurized Intraperitoneal Aerosolized Chemotherapy
  In this technique, the chemotherapeutic agents are administered under high pressures in the form of aerosols directly into the abdominal cavity at normal temperature. It improves the penetration of the drugs through the peritoneal surface.
  - Germ cell tumors: Chemotherapy is given in all stages except in dysgerminoma stage 1 for 3–4 cycles.
  - Bleomycin: 30,000 IU weekly for 12 weeks
  - Etoposide: 100 mg/m sq./d for 5 days every 3 weeks
  - Cisplatin: 20 mg/m sq./d for 5 days every 3 weeks

TABLE 16: Difference between platinum-sensitive, platinum-refractory. and platinum-resistant diseases.

Platinum-sensitive disease	*Platinum-refractory disease*	*Platinum-resistant disease*
These tumors respond to platinum chemotherapy and have a relapse or reoccurrence after 6 months since the last dose	These tumors do not respond to platinum-based chemotherapy and show relapse during treatment/within 4 weeks from the last dose of chemotherapy	These tumors relapse/reoccur within 6 months since the last dose of chemotherapy
They are more likely to respond to second course of platinum-based chemotherapy	Alternative agents like liposomal doxorubicin and bevacizumab are considered	They have lower response rate to second course of platinum therapy

SECTION 13: SALIENT FEATURES OF OVARIAN TUMORS

TABLE 17: Salient features of various ovarian tumors.

Dysgerminoma	• Present at a young age and are highly chemosensitive • Bilateral in 15% of the cases • Most common malignancy in pregnancy	Elevated LDH HPE: Large polyhedral cells resembling primordial germ cells	Treatment includes unilateral salpingoophrectomy in the young and Total Abdominal Hysterectomy with bilateral salpingoophrectomy in the elderly along with lymphadenectomy (30% risk of metastasis) Postoperatively chemotherapy with BEP REGIMEN is given.
Krukenberg tumor	This is a bilateral metastatic tumor of the ovary with primaries in the stomach, intestine/breast	HPE: Signet ring appearance on microscopy	Treatment includes surgery—removal of the metastatic component and the primary site followed by chemotherapy
Yolk sac tumor	It is a unilateral solid tumor that is known for its rapid spread and recurrence	• Elevated alpha fetoprotein • HPE: Schiller–Duval body	Treatment includes surgery followed by chemotherapy in all stages
Sertoli leydig tumor	It is usually seen in young women and they present with symptoms of hoarse and deep voice, temporal baldness, acne, hirsutism, breast atrophy, and clitoromegaly	Elevated serum testosterone HPE: Sertoli cells and Leydig cells are seen in cords	Treatment includes unilateral salpingoophrectomy in young and TAH +BSO in the elderly
Thecoma and fibroma	They usually present as solid tumors in the postmenopausal age group	Associated with Meigs syndrome: triad of ovarian mass, unilateral pleural effusion, and ascites	Management includes excision of the mass and the pleural effusion and ascites resolve on their own as they are transudative in nature
Granulosa cell tumors	They are unilateral tumors of two types: Juvenile and Adult type. Symptoms of precocious puberty, menometrorrhagia, postmenopausal bleeding	• Associated with increased inhibin B levels • HPE: Coffee bean nuclei of cells arranged in rosettes—Call Exner's body	Management includes unilateral salpingoophrectomy and radical surgery followed by chemotherapy in advanced age group

SECTION 14: BORDERLINE OVARIAN TUMORS

- They have characteristics intermediate between benign and malignant tumors.
- They present a decade earlier than malignant tumors.
- There are nuclear atypia and stratification, but no features of stromal invasion.

- Management of borderline tumors includes conservative surgery in the form of unilateral salpingoophrectomy in the young and TAH + BSO in postmenopausal women.
- It has a good prognosis.

SECTION 15: COMPLICATIONS OF BENIGN OVARIAN TUMORS

TABLE 18: Complications of ovarian tumors.

- Torsion
- Intracystic hemorrhage
- Rupture
- Malignancy
- Pseudomyxoma peritonei
- Infection

SECTION 16: OVARIAN TORSION: DIAGNOSIS AND MANGEMENT

Ovarian Torsion

- Ovarian torsion is an acute gynecologic emergency that arises due to twisting of the ovary on its pedicle
- It is one of the differential diagnoses of acute abdomen
- If there is severe pain abdomen in the background of ovarian cyst of >5 cm, one should always suspect torsion. Patient also Complaints of low-grade fever with nausea and vomiting
- On examination, there is guarding and rigidity; forniceal fullness and tenderness are felt on bimanual examination
- Emergency USG is suggestive of a whirlpool sign/target sign due to the coiled appearance, and doppler is suggestive of absent vascularity
- Management includes detorsion and laparoscopic cystectomy followed by oophoropexy to the lateral pelvic wall/broad ligament/back of the uterus
- In case of a necrosed ovary, salpingoophrectomy is done

CASE SCENARIO 3

Mrs. ABC, a 42-year-old P2L2 with complaints of pain localized to the right side of lower abdomen radiating to the groin for 3 days, aggravated in the past 4 hours with 4 episodes of vomiting.

On Examination: pulse rate: 110/min BP, regular good volume of 110/60 mm Hg.

Per Abdomen: Cystic mass palpable in right iliac fossa, rebound tenderness present, guarding present, rigidity present.

No organomegaly.

On Bimanual Examination: Uterus anteverted, normal size, firm, nontender

Right forniceal fullness and tenderness present, A cystic mobile mass of 8 × 6 cm felt through the right fornix.

Emergency USG abdomen pelvis with doppler showed right adnexal cystic lesion: 7 × 6.1 × 5.8 cm with volume of 133 cc with absent vascularity raising suspicion of adnexal torsion.

Patient was taken up on emergency basis and proceeded with laparoscopy.

Intraoperative findings: Left-sided ovarian cyst of 7 × 6 × 6 cm, gangrenous, two and a half turns of the pedicle present, ovary could not be visualized separately and right salpingoophrectomy was done. Left ovary and uterus were within normal limits.

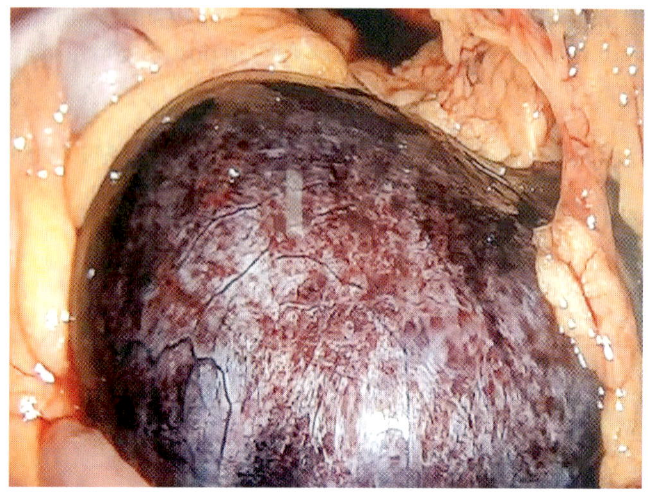

Fig. 15: Gangrenous ovary due to ovarian torsion visualized on laparoscopy.

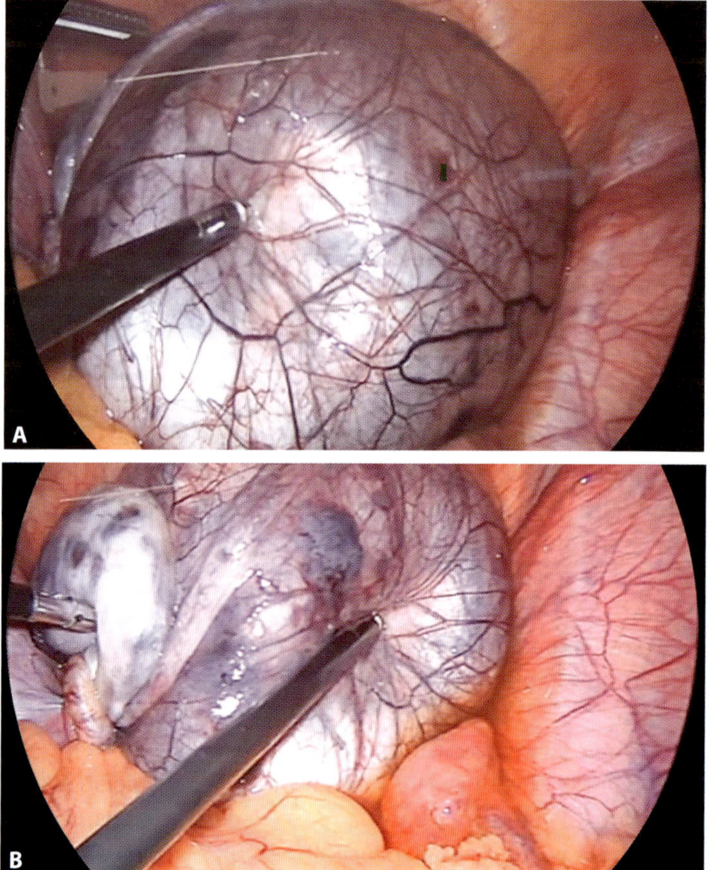

Figs. 16A and B: Torsion of a paraovarian cyst.

SECTION 17: KEYPOINTS

- History of nonspecific symptoms has been associated with ovarian cancer: **Goff symptom index**.
- Nulliparity, genetic syndromes like BRCA1 and 2 and Lynch syndrome are associated with ovarian cancer.
- Early menarche and late menopause and exposure to asbestos and talc are risk factors for development of ovarian cancer.
- Multiparity, OCPS, hysterectomy, and salpingectomy are protective factors against ovarian cancer.
- The MUSA classification system is specifically designed to provide a standardized approach to describing and assessing the morphological features of adenomyosis as seen on ultrasound.
- Sarcomatous change in a preexisting fibroid is extremely rare, with an estimated incidence of less than 0.5%.
- Adnexal masses maybe benign or malignant; therefore, risk stratification is of utmost importance.
- Most common benign tumor in pregnancy is dermoid cyst and malignant tumor is dysgerminoma.
- As per the NCCN guideline, USG is the first investigation of choice for evaluating ovarian masses.
- Goal of surgery in ovarian cancer is optimal debulking.
- All ovarian cancers are radioresistant except dysgerminoma.
- Sertoli Leydig cells present with features of virilization, whereas Granulosa cell tumor presents with precocious puberty/postmenopausal bleeding due to estrogen-secreting nature.
- Ovarian tumors are often diagnosed late due to their nonavailability of screening tests, nonspecific symptoms.
- Borderline tumors have characteristics midway between benign and malignant disease and present a decade earlier than their malignant counterparts and carry a better prognosis.
- Torsion is a gynecological emergency and is managed by emergency laparoscopy followed by cystectomy, detorsion, and oophoropexy.

10 MARKER QUESTIONS

1. **Describe the key clinical and imaging features that help differentiate a large uterine fibroid from a large ovarian cyst presenting as an abdominal lump.** ***(10 marks)***
2. **Discuss the emergency management of suspected ovarian torsion, including diagnostic clues and the principles of surgical intervention aimed at ovarian conservation.** ***(10 marks)***

3. **A 62-year-old postmenopausal woman presents with gradual abdominal distension, vague abdominal discomfort, and a feeling of early satiety. Physical examination reveals ascites and a fixed, irregular left adnexal mass. Her CA125 level is significantly elevated.**
   a. **Discuss the differential diagnoses for an adnexal mass in a postmenopausal woman with these presenting features.** ***(3 marks)***
   b. **Describe the role of imaging modalities (ultrasound, CT, MRI) and tumor markers (CA125, HE4, ROMA) in the risk stratification of adnexal masses in postmenopausal women.** ***(4 marks)***
   c. **Discuss the principles of surgical management for an adnexal mass highly suspicious for malignancy in this patient population, including the importance of referral to a Gyne-Oncologist.** ***(3 marks)***

5 MARKER QUESTIONS

1. **What are tumor markers? Enlist the ones that help in the diagnosis of ovarian malignancy.**
2. **What is RMI index? Write a short note on the newer risk stratification models.**
3. **Differentiate between benign and malignant ovarian masses.**
4. **Write a short note on dysgerminoma.**
5. **Add a brief note on role of chemotherapy in ovarian cancer.**
6. **What are the differences between Fibroid and Adenomyosis?**

MULTIPLE CHOICE QUESTIONS

Q1. Meigs' syndrome is characterized by which of the following?
a. Ovarian fibroma, ascites, and right-sided pleural effusion
b. Ovarian cystadenoma, ascites, and left-sided pleural effusion
c. Ovarian malignancy, ascites, and right-sided pleural effusion
d. Ovarian teratoma, ascites, and left-sided pleural effusion

Ans: a. Ovarian fibroma, ascites, and right-sided pleural effusion

Q2. A 60-year-old woman presents with a palpable abdominal mass and ascites. Her CA125 level is elevated, and imaging reveals a large, complex ovarian mass. Which of the following is the most likely diagnosis?
a. Ovarian fibroma
b. Ovarian endometrioma
c. Serous cystadenocarcinoma
d. Mature cystic teratoma

Ans: c. Serous cystadenocarcinoma

Q3. What is the most common source of a Krukenberg tumor?
a. Ovaries
b. Fallopian tubes
c. Gastrointestinal tract
d. Breast

Ans: c. Gastrointestinal tract

Q4. A 28-year-old nulliparous woman presents with acute, severe, unilateral lower abdominal pain, nausea, and vomiting. On ultrasound, a complex adnexal mass with a "whirlpool sign" is observed. Which of the following is the most appropriate next step in management?

a. Expectant management with analgesics
b. Transvaginal aspiration of the mass
c. Laparoscopic exploration and detorsion
d. Initiate antibiotics for suspected pelvic inflammatory disease

Ans: c. Laparoscopic exploration and detorsion

Q5. A young woman with a history of STIs presents with a fever and a palpable, tender, and fixed mass in the lower abdomen. What is the most likely diagnosis?

a. Ovarian cyst
b. Tubo-ovarian abscess
c. Ectopic pregnancy
d. Uterine fibroid

Ans: b. Tubo-ovarian abscess

Q6. What is the primary concern when a patient presents with a large ovarian cyst, especially in premenopausal women?

a. Malignant transformation
b. Torsion
c. Hemorrhage
d. Infection
e. All of the above

Ans: b. Torsion

Q7. A 60-year-old postmenopausal woman presents with persistent bloating, early satiety, and a palpable abdominal mass. Her CA125 level is significantly elevated, and ultrasound shows a complex ovarian mass with ascites. Which of the following is the most concerning diagnosis?

a. Mature Cystic Teratoma (Dermoid Cyst)
b. Endometrioma
c. Ovarian Malignancy
d. Functional Ovarian Cyst

Ans: c. Ovarian Malignancy

Q8. A 25-year-old woman is being investigated for infertility and is found to have an abdominal lump. Ultrasound reveals a unilocular cyst with low-level internal echoes within the ovary. Which of the following is the most likely diagnosis?

a. Serous Cystadenoma
b. Mature Cystic Teratoma (Dermoid Cyst)
c. Endometrioma
d. Hydrosalpinx

Ans: c. Endometrioma

Q9. Which of the following factors, if present in a reproductive-aged woman with early-stage EOC undergoing fertility-sparing surgery (FSS), would be considered a contraindication or warrant significant caution regarding the FSS approach?

a. FIGO Stage IA disease
b. Grade 1 endometrioid histology
c. Suspected or confirmed BRCA1 mutation
d. Strong desire for future pregnancy

Ans: c. Suspected or confirmed BRCA1 mutation

Q10. Which of the following is a characteristic feature of a mucinous cystadenoma on ultrasound?

a. Thin-walled, unilocular cyst
b. Thick-walled, multilocular cyst with low-level internal echoes
c. Presence of solid components with high vascularity
d. Presence of internal septations and papillary projections

Ans: b. Thick-walled, multilocular cyst with low-level internal echoes

Q11. A 35-year-old woman presents with heavy menstrual bleeding, pelvic pain, and a palpable abdominal mass. Imaging studies reveal multiple uterine masses with well-defined borders. Which of the following is the most likely diagnosis?

a. Adenomyosis
b. Uterine fibroids (Leiomyomas)
c. Endometrial polyps
d. Pelvic inflammatory disease

Ans: b. Uterine fibroids (Leiomyomas)

Q12. A 45-year-old woman presents with a large abdominopelvic mass, heavy menstrual bleeding, and pelvic pain. Imaging studies reveal a significantly enlarged uterus with heterogeneous echotexture. What is the most likely diagnosis?

a. Uterine fibroid
b. Adenomyosis
c. Ovarian cyst
d. Pelvic abscess

Ans: b. Adenomyosis

Q13. A 50-year-old woman presents with a rapidly enlarging pelvic mass, abdominal pain, and vaginal bleeding. Imaging studies reveal a large uterine mass with areas of necrosis and central vascularity. What is the most likely diagnosis?

a. Uterine fibroid
b. Adenomyosis
c. Leiomyosarcoma
d. Endometrial cancer

Ans: c. Leiomyosarcoma

Q14. What is the estimated percentage of uterine fibroids that undergo sarcomatous change (i.e., transform into leiomyosarcoma)?

a. 0.1–0.5%
b. 1–2%
c. 5–10%
d. 20–30%

Ans: a. 0.1–0.5%

Q15. What is the primary purpose of the MUSA (Morphological Uterine Sonographic Assessment) classification system in the context of adenomyosis?

a. To diagnose endometrial cancer
b. To assess the severity of fibroids
c. To standardize the description of adenomyosis features on ultrasound
d. To evaluate the effectiveness of treatment for adenomyosis

Ans: c. To standardize the description of adenomyosis features on ultrasound

Myomectomy

Shikha Singh, Neelansha Varshney

INTRODUCTION

Myomectomy is conservative treatment involving surgical removal of leiomyoma, leaving uterus in place. This can be done by abdominal, laparoscopic, hysteroscopic, or vaginal route.[1,2]

INDICATIONS OF MYOMECTOMY[3,4]

- Symptoms interfering with quality of life
  - Abnormal uterine bleeding
  - Urinary symptoms
  - Pelvic pressure or pelvic pain
- Asymptomatic women with infertility or recurrent pregnancy loss
  - After investigating all other causes
  - Cavity-distorting fibroid
- Previous adverse pregnancy outcome
- Asymptomatic women in presence of moderate or severe hydronephrosis from ureteral compression

CONTRAINDICATIONS OF MYOMECTOMY[4]

Absolute

- Symptomatic leiomyoma in patients who *no longer desire for fertility* or uterine preservation (*hysterectomy* will be the treatment of choice in these patients).
- Possibility of *endometrial or uterine sarcoma* has not been excluded.
- *No* evidence of *prophylactic myomectomy in an asymptomatic* patient.

Relative

- Strong possibility that a *functional uterus could not be reconstructed* after excision of fibroid. Large and multiple fibroids making large uterus defects where closure is compromised leaving future pregnancy at high risk for rupture.
- Myomectomy *during ongoing pregnancy* is not ideally recommended. It is rarely for pedunculated subserosal fibroid undergoing necrosis causing pain not responding to medical therapy.
- Myomectomy *during cesarean section* is generally not performed due to risk of bleeding and difficulty in obliterating fibroid cavity. Generally small intramural, subserosal fibroid can be removed after baby delivery during cesarean section. Sometimes, myomectomy

may have to be performed where uterine defect closure is not possible without removing lower segment fibroid.

PREOPERATIVE PREPARATION FOR MYOMECTOMY

Gynecologists should consider symptoms, size, and location of fibroid, patient preferences, and the patient's health and medical status.

Preoperative Counseling

- Patient selection: A detailed review should be taken of the patient's menstrual symptoms, heavy bleeding, dysmenorrhea, urinary or bowel pressure symptoms. Also enquire about her desire for future fertility. If she desires fertility, myomectomy will be the ideal surgical treatment for fibroids >3 cm in size if symptomatic or if interfering with pregnancy
- Route of surgery—either open, laparoscopic, hysteroscopy, or robotic.

Route of surgery depends on, size, site, type of fibroid, skill and experience of surgeon, and patient preference.

- Open myomectomy is done mostly for large intramural or subserosal fibroids.
- Intracavitary (FIGO grade 0 or 1) (submucosal less than 3 cm) **(Figs. 1 and 2)** are dealt with hysteroscopically; submucosal 4–5 cm type 2 are dealt hysteroscopically by an experienced[4] surgeon (AAGL recommendation).
- Rest are operated by laparoscopy or open route.

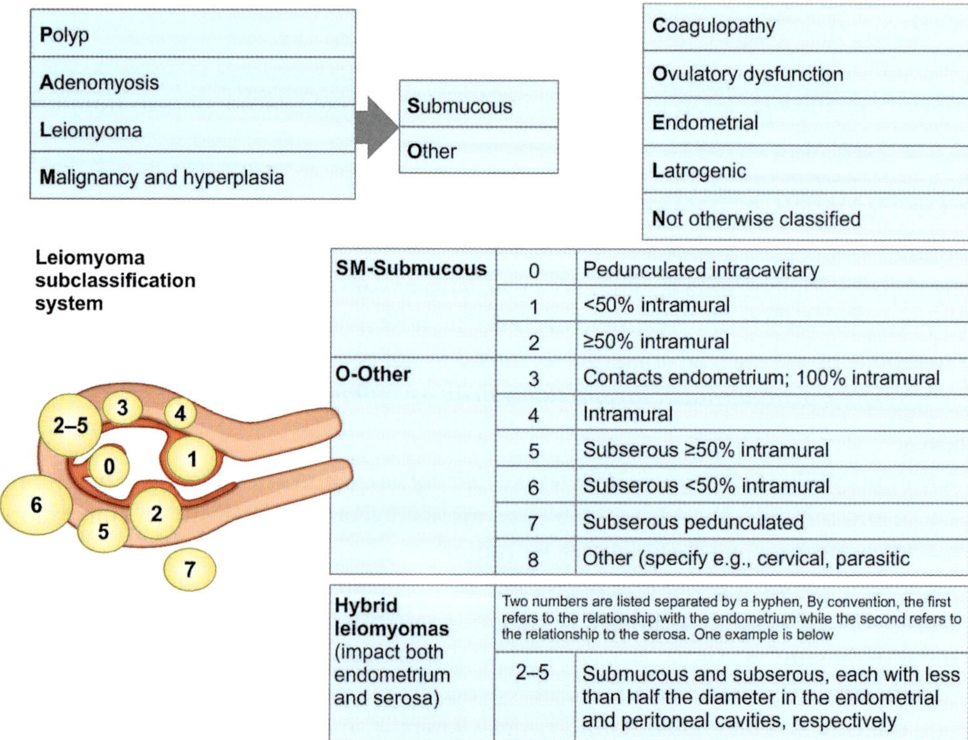

Fig. 1: Classification system including leiomyoma subclassification system.

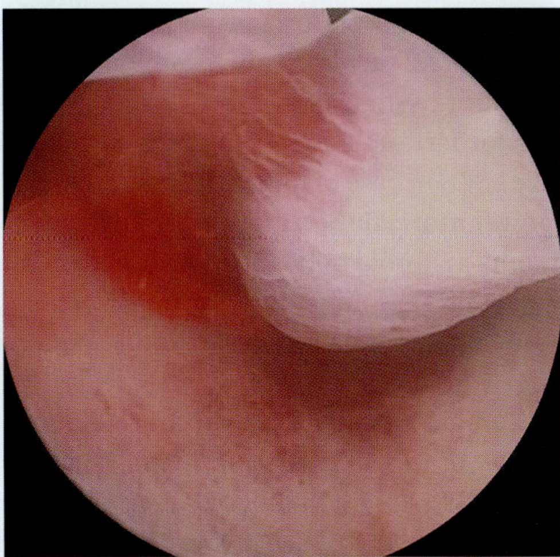

Fig. 2: Hysteroscopic view of submucous fibroid.

Informed consent: After counseling and detailed discussion about the following issues, written consent to be taken.

- *Understanding the disease* and its symptoms
- Treatment options:

  Expectant management (wait and watch)

  Pharmacological options include:
  - Nonhormonal treatment options include tranexamic acid and NSAIDs
  - Hormonal options include LNG-IUS, combined oral contraceptive, or progesterone which may be used if the patient is not planning pregnancy
  - Ulipristal acetate

  Interventions include:
  - Uterine artery embolization
  - Endometrial ablation for fibroids less than 3 cm
  - Myomectomy
  - Hysterectomy are other options for treatment (Not to mention if patient desires fertility)
  - High-frequency magnetic resonance-guided focused ultrasound
- Endometrial ablation may be an option for fibroids less than 3 cm in size
- Surgical management: Discuss need for **myomectomy**, procedure overview, risk and benefits of surgery, route of surgery like laparoscopic, open, robotic or hysteroscopic with its advantages and risks, postoperative recovery, and recurrence of fibroid. Possible complications of the surgery are to be discussed in details.

Surgical Management (Myomectomy in this Case)

Common Risks: Intraoperative *hemorrhage requiring blood transfusion*, postoperative pain, urine infection, inability to pass urine and/or frequency of urination, wound infection, bruising and delayed wound healing.

Uncommon Risks: Damage to the bowel, bladder, ureter (especially broad ligament or cervical fibroid), pelvic abscess or infection, venous thrombosis and pulmonary embolism, complications of distension media in hysteroscopy route, incisional hernia, return to theater because of delayed bleeding, adverse reaction to the anesthetic drugs, conversion to laparotomy in cases of laparoscopy, robotic or hysteroscopy routes, rarely need for hysterectomy

If myomectomy is done for fertility enhancement, then possibility of scar dehiscence, uterine rupture, and elective LSCS in case of future pregnancy is also discussed.

Risks and benefits of power morcellation during fibroid extraction in laparoscopic route.[5]

Risk of malignancy sarcoma in fibroid below 50 years of age is around 1/769–1/1,250 cases. Risk is higher in solitary, large fibroids and rapidly growing fibroids.

Risk of malignancy is much higher above 50 years. After menopause, the risk is reported as 1/166.

Detailed **discussion to be held with patients on morcellation** or **breaching of fibroid capsule** resulting in possibility of *sarcoma dissemination.* Though neither Ultrasound scan nor MRI is able to definitively exclude sarcomatous change in a fibroid, any fibroid that looks *suspicious on imaging or where there is concern of uterine sarcoma* should be considered for discussion at a *multidisciplinary forum* before morcellation is performed. The guiding principle should be that if **sarcoma is suspected**, then *morcellation or breaching of a fibroid capsule* **should not** be undertaken for individuals who **are over 50 years of age** or **postmenopausal** morcellation **not** recommended.

Serious and frequently occurring risks with morcellation are to be discussed with the patient and documented.

- Unintended morcellation of a uterine sarcoma
- Worsening the prognosis of an existing sarcoma
- Disseminated fibroids 1/120–1/1,200 (presence of noncancerous fibroids within the abdominal and pelvic cavity)
- Damage to bowel, bladder, ureters, and blood vessels and need for exploration for treating the same

Preoperative Evaluation

History: Through *medical history* to determine the *symptoms of the fibroid* and its overall effect on *quality of life.*

Detailed medical history to rule out *bleeding disorders* and *medical comorbidity* which may affect the surgery and its outcome.

Pelvic Examination: Through *bimanual pelvic examination* for *size, mobility, contour of uterus,* any adnexal mass, cervical mass, and cervical deviation. **These findings determine the choice of route and surgical incision (transverse or vertical).**

Imaging: USG, MRI, *Saline Infusion Sonography* (for submucosal fibroid) to confirm presence of *uterine fibroid* and also *incidental finding* of other lesions (ovarian cyst) which may affect surgical planning. USG for *fibroid mapping* in which *type, number, and location of fibroid* are done, especially in multiple fibroids, for better planning of surgery. For large fibroid causing ureteral compression and backpressure changes in kidney (hydronephrosis) is documented.

MRI scan is used to differentiate fibroid from adenomyosis (especially posterior wall) and leiomyosarcoma.

Leiomyosarcoma may show solid, inhomogeneous echoes, irregular cystic areas, fan-shaped shadowing, moderate vascularity. These are considered as red flag signs. Other risks include abnormal uterine bleeding, family history of cancer with BRCA1/2 mutation and Lynch syndrome, history of Tamoxifen use, no response to GnRH analogue, and history of pelvic radiation.

For leiomyosarcoma diagnosis with total serum lactate dehydrogenase (LDH) and LDH isoenzyme 3 measurements along with gadolinium-enhanced diethylenetriamine penta-acetic acid (Gd-DTPA) dynamic MRI were reported to be highly accurate. **Sarcomas have increased vascularity and show increased enhancement with gadolinium**, while **degenerating fibroids have decreased perfusion and exhibit decreased enhancement**.

Blood Investigation

- Blood grouping and keep adequate blood ready for intraoperative or postoperative transfusion.
- Complete Blood Count
- Coagulation profile
- Assessment of blood sugars, HbA1c
- Renal function test, Liver function test
- **Pregnancy Test:** For all reproductive-aged women with a uterus and without permanent sterilization, pregnancy should be excluded.

Other Tests

Endometrial sampling for abnormal uterine bleeding with age > 45 years or having risk factor for endometrial carcinoma

ECG, X-ray, 2D echocardiography, and pulmonary function may be done as per patient's age and clinical factors.

Preoperative Correction of Anemia

Preoperative anemia from chronic blood loss is associated with increased postoperative morbidity and mortality. Correction of anemia rather than transfusion is the optimal approach.

Recommend: Complete blood count, possible iron studies, Hemoglobin electrophoresis

Treatment: Oral iron supplementation (with vitamin C to enhance absorption) can increase hemoglobin by 2 g/dL within 2–3 weeks if bleeding is controlled. Occasionally, intravenous iron may be necessary to improve preoperative hemoglobin.

Blood transfusions are usually reserved for perioperative periods.

Option of autologous blood donation can be given if feasible.

Pharmacological Treatment Options

Role of GnRH Analogues

GnRH analogues: Leuprorelin Triptorelin (Dose: 3.75 intramuscularly every 4 weeks for 3–6 months); Goserelin (subcutaneous one implant 3.6 mg for every 4 weeks). These drugs can be started for 3–6 months before surgery is planned.

Mechanism of action: The continuous dosing of GnRH agonists, as opposed to the pulsatile release of GnRH from the pituitary gland, eventually leads to ovarian suppression and decreased estrogen and progesterone production. This ovarian suppression leads to a welcomed decrease in heavy menses and a reduction in the size and volume of fibroids.

Advantages: *Reduction in size of large fibroid making myomectomy accessible through transverse incision or by laparoscopy and avoiding vertical incision*; Temporary amenorrhea giving time to *build up the hemoglobin.*

Disadvantages:

- *Enucleation of fibroid difficult after GnRH treatment.*
- Possibility of persistent fibroid due to further reduction of small fibroid due to GnRH and possibility of *being missed out during surgery*

Adverse effects: Climacteric symptoms of *hot flushes and bone mineral density* loss with long-term use.

GnRH agonists produce menopausal-like effects, which reduce the size of fibroid (in 3 months) and severity of symptoms associated with uterine fibroids. The treatment can be given before myomectomy. It can also be used to reduce symptoms in women who do not want invasive treatment. However, the almost immediate rebound in growth (in 4–6 months) upon therapy cessation further limits the efficacy and use of this medication.

Ulipristal acetate (5 mg/day) is used for intermittent treatment of moderate to severe symptoms if surgery and uterine artery embolization are not suitable. UPA is a selective progesterone receptor modulator. It can be used for premenopausal women.

Mechanism of action**:** It causes apoptosis in fibroid cells. It reduces size of fibroid which is maintained up to 6 months.

Adverse Effects

- It carries a risk of liver injury. However, it has been approved by Medicines and Healthcare products Regulatory Agency, UK (2021). However, the liver function test has to be done before starting UPA and monthly for 2 courses. It has to be done also before each new course. A maximum of 4 courses of 3 months each is allowed. It is recommended for patients with anemia.
- It also carries a risk of endometrial changes seen in 2/3rd of the women.

Other Interventions

Role of uterine artery embolization: UAE is considered in patients with symptomatic fibroids with pressure symptoms. It can be considered if surgery is contraindicated.

Aim is to infarct the fibroid while preserving vascularity of uterus, ovaries, and surrounding tissues. A microcatheter is introduced through the femoral artery into the anterior division of the internal iliac artery. The embolic agent is introduced under fluoroscopic guidance.

Contraindications

- Asymptomatic fibroid
- Pregnancy
- Infection in genital tract
- If patient is unwilling for hysterectomy if need arises

Advantage: Quick recovery, but it is not recommended for patients planning to preserve fertility.

Side Effects: Pain, vaginal discharge

- There is a lower chance of major complications and
- Increased risk of repeat interventions in 2–5 years.

Role of MRI-guided Focused Ultrasound

High-frequency ultrasound produces heat to denature proteins leading to cell death and shrinkage of fibroids. MRI is used to target the fibroids, and treatment is monitored by assessing temperature of tissue

Advantages

- Quick recovery, but it is not recommended for patients planning to preserve fertility.
- It causes significant reduction in fibroid symptoms in 12 months.

Adverse Effects

- Mild skin burn, nausea
- Buttock or leg pain and transient sciatic nerve palsy
- High chance of reintervention in 12 months

Measures to Reduce Intraoperative Blood Loss

Surgical hemorrhage is an important complication of myomectomy done by any route (abdominal, laparoscopic, vaginal). Fibroids have increased arterioles and venules. Arcuate arteries supplying fibroids may run in any axis and can get transected by either vertical or transverse incisions during myomectomy.

Bleeding can be reduced or prevented with mechanical or pharmacologic methods. These methods further prevent anemia, hypovolemia, coagulation abnormalities, and blood transfusions

The measures can be taken as preoperative or intraoperatively.

Preoperative Measures

- **Correction of anemia:** Iron deficiency anemia associated with *menorrhagia* coupled with *dietary deficiency* is important preoperative consideration in the fibroid uterus. Preoperative anemia increases the chances of blood transfusion and also increases the risk of perioperative morbidity and mortality. Preoperative anemia may be treated with oral iron supplementation or intravenous iron.
- **GnRH agonist or GnRH antagonist** preoperatively,
  - GnRH agonists can help correct anemia by temporarily inducing *amenorrhea*. It also further helps in *reducing the fibroid size and vascularity*, thus reducing intraoperative blood loss. Preoperative GnRH agonist also reduces the fibroid size permitting the use of **transverse rather than vertical laparotomy** or **laparoscopic approach feasible**. Disadvantages of GnRH are **difficulty in enucleation** of fibroid as the plane between fibroid and myometrium is obscured and increase risk of **persistent fibroids** as **small myomas would shrink** after GnRH treatment and may not be palpable during surgery.

- GnRH antagonists like oral relugolix also can be used to suppress the GnRH secretion and thus help in reducing size and vascularity of fibroid and intraoperative blood loss, the advantage being faster action compared to GnRH agonist but not widely used as it is expensive and requires daily dose.
- Both GnRH agonist and GnRH antagonist given preoperatively can cause menopausal symptoms like hot flushes, mood disturbances, etc.

- Autologous blood donation: A patient who is scheduled for surgery and is not anemic may bank one or more units of her own blood which then can be used intra- or postoperatively.

Intraoperative Measures

Bleeding can be reduced or prevented with mechanical or pharmacologic methods:

Pharmacologic Interventions

1. **Controlled hypotensive anesthesia** is an important adjunct to decrease surgical bleeding in selected patients. *Hypotensive anesthesia* acts by *reduction of venous tone.* This is achieved by *nitroglycerin or sodium nitroprusside, epidural or spinal anesthesia,* to maintain a *target mean blood pressure of 60 mm Hg.* Modified *Trendelenburg* position further reduces bleeding by increasing venous return from lower extremities and pelvis by gravity and decreasing operative site blood pressure.

   Induced hypotension is contraindicated in patients with cerebrovascular disease, myocardial ischemia, peripheral vascular disease, severe renal or hepatic disease, and hypovolemia.
2. **Vasoconstrictors:**[6]
   a. *Most commonly used* is **intramyometrial dilute vasopressin** into *planned uterine incision sites* for each fibroid that reduces blood loss.

      Randomized trial data show that blood loss during myomectomy with vasopressin is significantly less than with placebo and less than or comparable to use of a uterine artery tourniquet.

      Complications of Vasopressin include intravascular injection with bradycardia, cardiovascular collapse, and death. It can cause anaphylaxis. Water intoxication can also occur as a result of the antidiuretic effect of vasopressin. This effect is potentiated in patients taking tricyclic antidepressants. It causes hyponatremia with nausea, confusion, and seizures. Vasopressin causes vasoconstriction which clinically manifests as global hypotension decreased cardiac output.

      Vasopressin is contraindicated in women with cardiovascular, vascular, or renal disease.

      Dosage: An upper limit of a cumulative total vasopressin dose per procedure of 4–6 units has been proposed. Dilute 1 mL (20 units) in 100 mL normal saline and use 20–30 mL of it. It has a plasma half-life of *10–20 minutes.* It is injected into the *superficial myometrium and serosa* overlying the myoma (subserosa and subcapsule). *The effect usually lasts for 30 minutes.* Hence, repeat injections may be required.

   b. Intramyometrial injection **bupivacaine plus epinephrine** been tried with reduction blood loss.

- **Uterotonics:** Vaginal misoprostol (400 μg, 1 hour before) has been tried.

- **Tranexamic acid:** Use of injection tranexamic acid at the beginning of surgery also shown to reduce blood loss

Mechanical Methods (Tourniquets, Clamps, Sutures, Clips)

Use of tourniquets, clamps and suture clips that occlude the uterine blood supply reduce blood loss during myomectomy

A procedure to apply a tourniquet at uterine vessels is as follows:

- Palpate the broad ligament just above the level of the internal cervical os to identify a space that is free of vessels and the ureter.
- Make a 1 cm incision in this clear space bilaterally.
- Pass the tourniquet through the incisions with the ends protruding anteriorly.
- Pull the tourniquet tight and secure by securing the ends with a Kelly clamp. Take care to avoid enlarging the broad ligament incisions or damaging surrounding structures.

Occlusion of the ovarian arteries is accomplished by placing a tourniquet (or more than one tourniquet) or atraumatic vascular clamp (e.g., sponge holder/bulldog clamp) bilaterally across the infundibulopelvic ligaments. Care must be taken to avoid lacerating the ovarian vessels or compressing the ureter.

Tourniquets can be accompanied by hypotensive anesthesia.

It is very important that the arterial blood flow be occluded. **If the venous flow is occluded while the arterial flow remains intact, blood loss could actually be increased with the tourniquets.**

The **mean blood pressure should be reduced to the target hypotensive level (about 60 mm Hg) before the tourniquets are tightened.** *The higher the blood pressure, the tighter the tourniquets must be* to occlude the uterine circulation.

Once the tourniquets are tightened in place, the myomectomy should proceed expeditiously to prevent ischemic damage to the uterus, tubes, and ovaries. Tourniquet time should be monitored and kept to a minimum.

Intermittent release of the tourniquets should be considered if the operating time becomes excessive. After reconstruction of the uterus is complete, the determination of adequate hemostasis in the uterus cannot be made until all the tourniquets are released and the blood pressure has returned to normal.

Clamps: Boney's myomectomy clamp **(Fig. 3)** is used for temporary occlusion of bilateral uterine vessels at the level of isthmus, including the round ligaments in its jaws, **during open myomectomy with usually single anterior or fundal fibroid of moderate size**. These cannot be used for multiple, large fibroid, cervical or broad ligament fibroid. If the timing of clamp application exceeds 20 minutes, the clamp is released for 5 minutes and uterus is wrapped in a hot water towel. This is done to avoid accumulation of histamine-like substances in the uterine circulation which would cause vasodilation and hypotension.

Sutures: Uterine artery ligation using sutures both at the level of isthmus and at origin from the anterior division of internal iliac artery, before incision on the large, multiple fibroid including cervical and broad ligament fibroid, has shown considerable blood loss reduction during myomectomy through both open and laparoscopic routes.

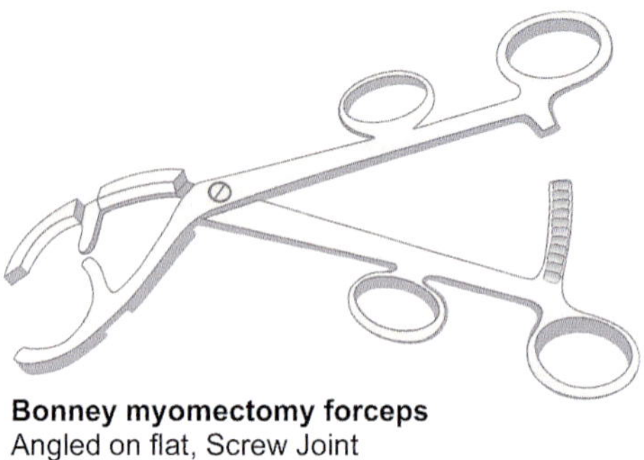

Fig. 3: Bonney's Myomectomy clamp.

The suture can be used as a temporary suture using shoelace technique which can be removed after fibroid bed suture. Even after permanent suturing of the uterine vessels, no effect noted either on uterine vasculature or subsequent fertility.

Clips: Temporary occlusion of dissected **uterine artery at its origin from the anterior division of internal iliac artery,** especially during laparoscopic fibroid, has been tried with good results. The clips are removed after fibroid bed closure. However, cautious removal of clips is suggested as it can cause trauma and bleeding.

Adherence to basic principles is essential for good results. Perhaps the most important of these is careful **planning of the uterine incisions**. Only a *minimal number of single incisions* should be made. If possible, removal of all leiomyomas should be accomplished through an incision in the anterior uterine corpus and in the midline, when feasible, to avoid the vascular areas of the uterus and broad ligaments laterally. Even intramural leiomyoma in the posterior uterine wall can be removed through anterior incisions

Principles of Myomectomy?

Myomectomy by Laparotomy[4]

Position: Lithotomy position which allows uterine manipulation or dye injection to identify uterine cavity.

Incision:
- Pfannenstiel incision (preferred)
- Cherney, Maylard, or midline incision for very large uterus

Procedure:
- After peritoneal entry, a large uterus can be exteriorized, if possible
- Dissect the bladder peritoneum sharply to visualize the parametrium.
- *Various measures to prevent blood loss:*
    - An opening is then made in the posterior leaf of the broad ligament, and a tourniquet (a red rubber catheter) is passed. The ureters are below and lateral. The tourniquet can be tied anteriorly or posteriorly and held in place by a clamp to prevent loosening of the knot.

- Application of a vascular clamp on the ovarian vessels can also be useful in decreasing bleeding.
- Diluted vasopressin is then injected into the pseudocapsule of fibroid.
- Temporary or permanent ligation of uterine vessels using sutures, clips, clamp/ Bonney's clamp at isthmus or at the origin of uterine artery from the anterior division of internal iliac artery.

- *Uterine Incision:*
  - Uterus is palpated for the fibroid. Relationship of round ligament and cornual end of fallopian tube helps in location of fibroid. A transverse or vertical incision is taken on the fibroid and *carried to the pseudocapsule.* The pseudocapsule is identified and cut open, and dissection and coagulation should occur at this level to minimize blood loss. The pseudocapsule has fibroneurovascular fibers. Postoperative myometrial vascularization is crucial in muscle regeneration. Also, neurofibers and neurotransmitters play a role in signaling muscle regeneration. Hence, pseudocapsule should not be damaged. It can affect muscle function subsequently. Hence, it is reasoned that myomectomy should always **be intracapsular myomectomy** which is physiological and biological. The fibroid is removed, sparing as much as possible the pseudocapsule and surrounding neurovascular bundle.
  - *Care should be taken about the cornual end of fallopian tube* and *ascending branch of uterine vessels* while extending the incision laterally.
  - *Anterior uterine incisions are preferred as they are associated with fewer adhesion* compared to posterior incision.
  - Posterior wall leiomyoma be removed by transcavitatory approach. For posterior fundal fibroid anterior, Boney's Hood incision can be taken. A transverse incision is taken just posterior to the line of attachment of the Fallopian tubes.
  - For posterior fibroid, primary posterior incision is preferred for subserous fibroids and low posterior fibroid.
  - *Excision of multiple myomas through a single incision can make effective closure challenging* as *the tunnel created may make access to deep tissue difficult.* Separate incisions can be made directly over each fibroid and sutured separately
- Avoid excessive coagulation in the fibroid cavity and the incised edges of the myometrium as it hampers healing and scar strength.
- A towel clamp, tenaculum. or myoma screw **(Fig. 4)** can be applied to the myoma and with traction/countertraction, the dissection should proceed carefully so as not to accidentally excise the endometrium.
- Dilute methylene transcervical to detect accidental opening of uterine cavity.
- If the cavity is opened during dissection, it is explored to rule out any other fibroid, identify the cervical canal, and *avoid suturing the endometrium* while closing the myometrial layers.
- Entry into the uterine cavity requires a separate repair with fine sutures.
- The principles of repair apply to all surgical approaches, minimally invasive or laparotomy.
- Incision should be closed with braided delayed absorbable sutures (e.g., 0-Vicryl or PolySorb). At least two myometrial layers are required to be closed, avoiding any dead space within the myometrium to prevent the hematoma formation leading to infection,

poor healing of the scar, and increased risk of dehiscence and rupture in subsequent pregnancy. This is followed by a serosal layer of finer suture using baseball technique for minimal suture exposure on the serosal surface to prevent postoperative adhesions.

- Incision can also be closed using barbed sutures with anchors, in a continuous manner in layers with uniform tension on the suture line.
- The clamp, tourniquets, temporary uterine suture, and clips are then removed. Hemostasis is carefully checked again. Deep myometrial sutures are taken if required.
- Antiadhesion barriers can be used if conditions are appropriate.

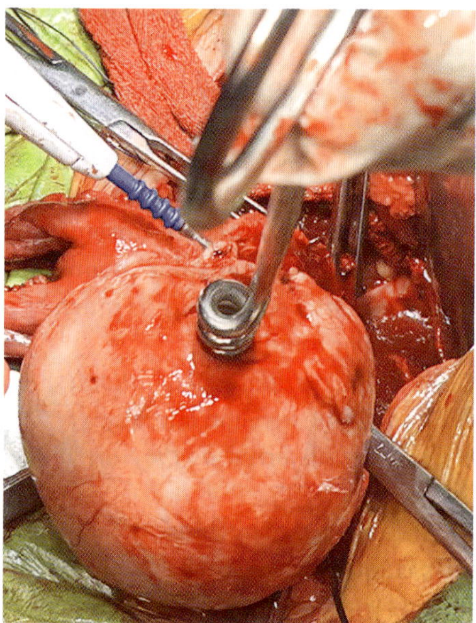

Fig. 4: Myoma screw applied to a myoma during open myomectomy.

Cervical and Broad Ligament Fibroid

Cervical fibroid can be removed from anterior, posterior, or both walls encircling the cervical canal.

Broad ligament fibroid can be primary (originating from the broad ligament) or secondary (originating from the lateral wall of the uterus going into the broad ligaments).

Both cervical and broad ligament fibroids have close proximity to ureter and uterine vessels making it prone to injury.

For cervical fibroid and broad ligament fibroid, make an initial opening of posterior peritoneum and identify the ureter course and its relation with the fibroid.

Anterior cervical fibroid is removed after dissecting the uterovesical fold and dissection of bladder down followed by incision anteriorly on fibroid. Similarly, posterior fibroid is also enucleated after incision is done posteriorly. After removal of the fibroid, check the cervix and the cervical canal. Reconstruct the cervix with careful closure by avoiding the cervical canal and injury to ureters.

Broad ligament fibroid can be accessed by opening the round ligament anteriorly and dissecting all around the fibroid by taking care of uterine vessels and ureters which are displaced laterally in case of secondary broad fibroid and medially in primary broad ligament fibroid. If necessary, uterine vessels can be ligated.

Vaginal Myomectomy[4]

This is performed in a patient presenting with *prolapsing pedunculated submucosal leiomyoma*. Prolapsing vaginal fibroids are the least common.

Diluted vasopressin (20 units mixed in 200 mL normal saline) is slowly injected into the portion of the leiomyoma that is visible until leiomyoma ischemia is detected. The amount of vasopressin given varies and depends on the size of the fibroid. If the myoma is already ischemic, no vasopressin is necessary. If a narrow stalk is palpable, the leiomyoma can generally be twisted off. **Slow downward traction and rotation of the pedunculated leiomyoma will lead to extirpation of the leiomyoma. Avoid pulling on the leiomyoma vigorously** or rapidly as it may lead to uterine inversion.

If brisk bleeding occurs during the procedure, *a 26-Fr, 30-mL Foley catheter can be inserted through the cervix and the balloon distended with 30 mL of sterile water*. It can be *left in place for 12–24 hours and deflated*. If needed, the *cervix can be sutured around the catheter* to keep it in place.

If a large leiomyoma is not able to pull through cervix, then Duhrssen incision can be made on cervix longitudinally at 2, 10, and 6 o'clock positions after injecting dilute pitressin vasopressin intracervically.

Post fibroid removal, an **operative hysteroscope with resectoscope is introduced**. Distention is achieved by putting Allis forces around the hysteroscope. Entire uterine cavity is inspected for any other fibroid or **residual fibroid which can be resected** or **any bleeding from the pedicle is electrocoagulated.**

Laparoscopic Myomectomy[4]

Patient Position: The patient is positioned in lithotomy on egg crate or other devices to avoid slipping during the procedure; arms tucked and padded.

Port Insertion

- An examination is done under anesthesia to plan port placement, as per size and location of fibroid
- **Main Port:** An initial left upper quadrant insertion is done to establish a pneumoperitoneum rather than directly inserting the primary device supraumbilically. After insertion of the left upper quadrant port, the midline trocar should be placed under direct vision.
- **Lateral Ports:** Typically, four ports are placed: An umbilical port, two lateral ports on the side of the principal surgeon, and one on the side of the assistant.
  - 5-mm lateral trocars are placed under direct vision.
  - Placed *at the level of the umbilicus*, either *lateral to the rectus muscle* or in the lower quadrants *lateral to the inferior epigastric vessels.*
  - The lower quadrant ports should be placed *above the anterior superior iliac spine to avoid injuring the ilioinguinal/iliohypogastric nerves*. If not visible (e.g., owing to obesity), the trocars are placed *lateral to the insertion of the round ligament in the deep inguinal ring.*

Procedure

- After a general survey of the peritoneal cavity
- Diluted vasopressin (20 units in 200 mL of normal saline) is injected into the myometrium and pseudocapsule around the myoma.
- An incision is made on the myometrium overlying the myoma, and the dissection then continues until the pseudocapsule is reached.
- Remove as many fibroids as possible from a single incision on the uterus; sometimes, it is necessary to make multiple incisions to achieve rapid hemostasis after enucleation.
- *Horizontal transverse incision is recommended for laparoscopic suturing through the lateral ports.*
- Once the pseudocapsule is reached, a 5-mm tenaculum or myoma screw, grasps the myoma to allow gentle traction–countertraction.
- Dissection can be accomplished with laparoscopic forceps **(Fig. 5)**.
- During the dissection of submucous myomas, there should be minimal pulling but rather dissection of the endometrium off the myoma.
- Judicious use of bipolar electrosurgery for hemostasis.
- Once enucleated, the leiomyoma should be placed in an easily visible area of the pelvic cavity for later retrieval.
- **Myometrial Closure (Fig. 6):** Closure of the myometrial defect is always multilayered. Absorbable polydioxanone, polyglactin, or barbed suture 0 or 00-gauge suture on a curved needle with a tapered tip can be used. Barbed suture may allow less blood loss and faster closure with uniform tension on suture tissue and better approximation. The serosa is approximated with 2/3-O delayed absorbable suture in a running baseball fashion.
- **Endometrial Cavity Closure:** The most critical step is closure of the endometrium. Inadvertent entry into the uterine cavity without separate closure could result in intracavity adhesions. Delayed absorbable 3-0 suture is used to close the endometrium without penetrating the endometrium. There should be no suture in the uterine cavity.

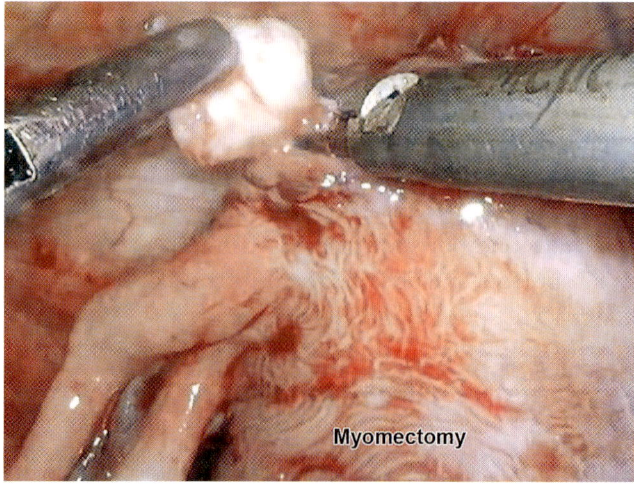

Fig. 5: Laparoscopic myomectomy.

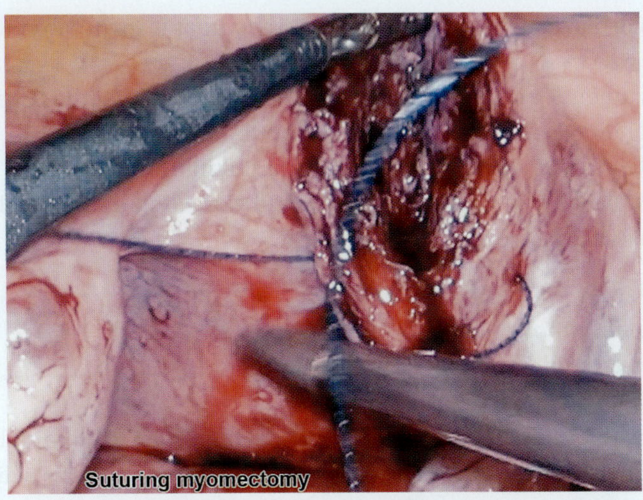

Fig. 6: Laparoscopic suturing of uterus after myomectomy.

- Confirm the hemostasis of myoma bed suturing site, especially after removal of temporary uterine occlusion.
- **Tissue Extraction:** Power/electromechanical morcellators with in-bag morcellation or manual (scalpel) extraction techniques can be used. A containment bag can be introduced through the large trocar in the retractor system allowing extracorporeal morcellation.
- **Advantage of enbag morcellation:** Prevent inadvertent spread of malignancy, and inadvertent missing of fibroid pieces with their subsequent growth in peritoneal cavity at sites like abdominal wall, mesentery, and liver.
- **Adhesion barrier:** Oxidized regenerated cellulose (Surgicel) to be placed on the sutured area to minimize adhesion.

Robot-Assisted Myomectomy[4]

Position: Trendelenburg position

Port Placement: A central port (supraumbilical 12 mm) for the endoscope, two lateral robot ports for the accessory equipment, and a left upper quadrant 5-mm trocar for introduction of a 5-mm tenaculum are placed. The robot tower is side-docked.

Procedure: The surgery proceeds in the same manner as conventional laparoscopy.

- Diluted vasopressin is injected.
- Incision is made with the energy device. The myoma incision *does not have to be made horizontally as robotic suturing with the articulated wrist can be accomplished with any incision direction.*
- Dissection of the myometrium should be continued until reaching the myoma pseudocapsule.
- A tenaculum is used to allow traction–countertraction.
- Enucleation proceeds in a similar manner to conventional laparoscopy.

- Hemostasis is achieved with careful electrosurgery that is focused on the bleeding point only.
- The two instruments are replaced with needle holders. Needles are introduced and removed under direct vision through the suprapubic port.
- The closure of the myometrium is performed in multiple layers.
- The myoma is placed in a containment bag and extraction and morcellated in a similar fashion to conventional laparoscopy.

Complications of Myomectomy

Postoperative Complications[4,7]

- **Intraoperative complications:**
  - *Surgical complications:*
    - Excessive blood loss: Average blood loss from open abdominal myomectomy is approximately 200–800 ml. The blood loss depends on the size of fibroid, number of fibroids, its location, type of fibroid, whether submucosal, intramural, or subserous, whether pedunculated or nonpedunculated, number of incisions on the uterus, whether cavity is entered or not.
    - Myometrial hematoma: This may occur for *deep intramural fibroid* or where cavity is entered as well as in *tunneling incisions* for removal of multiple fibroid through one incision. It also occurs, if the layered suturing of fibroid bed is inadequate. Always press and check for the intramyometrial bed bleeding after closure; if required, few intermittent deep sutures can be taken. Myometrial hematoma is an important cause for infection and postoperative fever with subsequent *poor healing* and *poor scar strength and subsequent uterine dehiscence or rupture* in subsequent pregnancy.
    - Direct Injury to bowel, bladder, ureter, vascular systems: These are uncommon during myomectomy. During cervical or broad ligament fibroid removal, injury to bladder, ureter, and uterine vessels is possible. Bowel injury is uncommon unless associated with pelvic adhesion due to adenomyosis and previous abdominal surgeries including past myomectomies.
    - Risk of conversion to laparotomy in minimally invasive procedures: Laparoscopic myomectomy can be converted into laparotomy if initial evaluation precludes laparoscopic approach or to aid in the management of intraoperative complications, mainly hemorrhage, difficulty in suturing the myoma bed.
    - Risk of conversion to hysterectomy: It is an uncommon complication. Severe uncontrolled hemorrhage has to be tackled by intraoperative blood salvage, uterine artery ligation, internal iliac artery ligation, or conversion to hysterectomy as the last resort.
    - Morcellation injury to bowel, bladder, ureter
  - *Anesthesia-related complications:*
    - Failure to extubate
    - Vasoconstrictor-related complications (e.g., Vasopressin/adrenaline)
    - Abnormal reaction to anesthetic medication

- **Postoperative complications:**
  - Fever: This occurs in about 12–67% of patients. It usually occurs 48 hours of surgery. This fever could be due to intramyometrial hematomas, local surgical site infection, or release of inflammatory mediators. Other causes include respiratory tract infection and urinary tract infection.
  - Infections: Endometritis, cystitis, pelvic infections
  - Morcellation: Disseminated/parasitic fibroids: Careful examination of peritoneal cavity is important to remove all small fibroid pieces after morcellation. This complication is eliminated by doing en-bag morcellation.
- **Long-term complications:**
  - Recurrence of fibroid/persistence of fibroid
  - Intra-abdominal adhesions: Especially after open myomectomy, in paricular posterior incisions.
  - Intrauterine adhesions: When cavity is breached during the fibroid removal, inadvertent partial closure of uterine cavity with sutures in the cavity.
  - Obstetric complications: Rupture during labor
  - Adenomyosis/Endometriosis: Risk increases with cavity breached during fibroid removal and inclusion of endometrium in myometrial bed sutures.

Hysteroscopic Myomectomy

Hysteroscopic myomectomy provides symptomatic relief in 70–90% of cases. Other indications include subfertility, dysmenorrhea, and pelvic pain. As per ASRM fibroid distorting the cavity has to be removed to improve pregnancy rates and decrease risk of early pregnancy loss.

Preoperative Evaluation and Investigation

Preoperative investigation: Submucous fibroids are mapped and evaluated for their number, size, location, and correlation of myometrium and uterine cavity and myometrial mantle which refers to distance between the deepest portion of myoma in myometrium and the serosa. Myometrial mantle is very important in hysteroscopic myomectomy as *transmural myoma reaching the serosa contradicts the hysteroscopic route for myomectomy due to a higher risk of uterine perforation* during the procedure. It is assessed by pelvic ultrasonography, preferably transvaginal, hysterosonography, HSG, MRI pelvis, and by diagnostic hysteroscopy.

HSG is advantageous in cases of infertility with additional information of tubal patency and configuration, but its relation with myometrium is not well appreciated.

Transvaginal sonography is the first investigation to be performed for detailed fibroid mapping for its number, size, location, and correlation of myometrium and uterine cavity and has good accuracy, easy access, and low cost but not suitable for large and multiple fibroids with posterior acoustic shadowing making it difficult to assess and count them.

Hysterosonography is a procedure by which the uterus is distended with saline solution for greater contrast and detailing of uterine cavity and *MRI pelvis* is indicated in uteri with volume greater than 375 cm^3 or with more than 4 fibroids. It is excellent to identify the number, location, and size of nodule, proximity to other fibroids, diagnose adenomyosis and adenomyoma.

Diagnostic hysteroscopy by direct visualization of the uterine cavity offers all possible information about the intracavitary portion of submucous fibroid and also its relation with the tubal ostia. It helps to rule out other intrauterine causes of bleeding, endometrial pathology and sampling.

Preoperative Classification of Submucous Fibroid

Preoperative classification of submucous fibroid indicating degree of difficulty and complexity of the hysteroscopic myomectomy is essential to avoid the complication.

Office Hysteroscopy: For size up to 3 cm, an incision on pseudocapsule during office hysteroscope may allow protrusion of fibroid into uterine cavity for subsequent hysteroscopic myomectomy.

Hysteroscopic Myomectomy[4]

- **Timing:** Surgery during the early proliferative phase may be easier owing to thinner endometrium and less tissue debris.
- **Fluid Management:**
  - Continuous intrauterine distention and fluid is required.
  - Fluids used for uterine distention include ionic or nonionic fluid media administered via a continuous fluid management system.
  - The characteristics of ideal fluid management systems *include instantaneous determination of fluid deficit,* configurable *alarms to alert the surgeon to preset deficit limits,* ability *to vary intrauterine pressure,* technology to facilitate *detection of uterine perforation,* having *automatic flow rate adjustment* and nonpulsatile flow infusion, and *minimizing surgical interruptions* when fluid bags are empty.
  - The lowest intrauterine pressure used for hysteroscopy is 75–100 mm Hg; however, higher pressures may be needed when the uterine size exceeds that of a 12- to 14-week pregnancy, when there are multiple intramural fibroids, and if intracavitary fibroids are greater than 4 cm.
  - Monopolar devices require nonconductive fluid media to complete the electric circuit between the active electrode and dispersive electrode—glycine, sorbitol, and mannitol. Bipolar technology is increasingly used owing to improved safety parameters. It can be used with saline as the distension medium.
- **Instrumentation:**
  - **Operative Resectoscope:** It contains a *working element* through which wire *thermal loops, cutting knife, cold loops, and vaporizing electrodes* (including balls and barrels) can be attached. These instruments include a channel for inflow of distention medium and an outflow channel for the removal of bloody fluid and tissue debris, providing continuous and clear visualization of the endometrial cavity. Further, an element connects the instrument to the electrosurgical generator to activate electrical energy.
  - **Technique:**[4]
    - *Slicing Technique:*
      - Type 0 Fibroid:
        - Using monopolar or bipolar resectoscope repeated and progressive passages of the activated wire loop trough the fibroid. Preferred movement of loop

is cephalad to caudal to avoid uterus perforation. *Continue to slice the leiomyoma until the pink fasciculate myometrial fibers are noted and the whorled appearance of the fibroid is absen*t. Since fundus near tubal ostia is the thinnest portion, care should be taken while resection near these areas to prevent perforation.
    - Divide the type 0 fibroid into two half-spheres and then each half is sliced from the free edge to the base into two to three fragments and retrieved through the cervix with grasping forceps.
- Types 1 and 2: The main objective is to separate the fibroid from its pseudocapsule; *intermittent uterine decompression allows progressive protrusion of the intramural component into the cavity.*
    - Hydromassage: Automatic fluid management system with rapid change in intrauterine pressure achieved via stopping and starting the fluid as well as periodically removing the hysteroscope from the endometrial cavity. It increases myometrial contractions and facilitates migration of the intramural component into the uterine cavity.
    - Manual Massage: It is performed by placing a finger into the uterus and massaging the endocavity to help expel the fibroid into the uterine cavity.
    - Progressive resection can then occur. If the remaining portion is more intramyometrial than intracavitary, postoperative evaluation with a saline infusion sonogram is recommended.

Radiofrequency Ablation
- Myolysis technique, which is applied through ultrasound guidance.
- The system uses a handpiece for radiofrequency ablation, connected to an intrauterine ultrasound probe, forming a single integrated device so that the rods penetrate the myoma.

Laser Technique
- Diode laser device, with 5Fr fiber.
- It leads to myolysis with total destruction of myoma or late expulsion of after volume reduction and ischemia.
- Considered for nodules with greater intramural components.

Mazzon's Cold Loop Technique
- Based on the resection of the submucosal component of the myoma using a resectoscope **(Fig. 7)** with a semicircle loop, with mono- or bipolar energy, until reaching the intramural portion of the myoma.
- Upon reaching the pseudocapsule, the loop is changed to a more rigid one (cold loop), so that the myoma is mechanically mobilized until its enucleation is complete.
- Then, a loop with energy returns to fragment and remove the myoma, which was left free in the uterine cavity.

Cold loop technique may be used rather than diathermy to free fibroid from surrounding myometrium. This minimizes use of energy and there will be less synechia.

It is important in fertility conservation. An intracavitatory balloon tamponade may be used to control the bleeding.

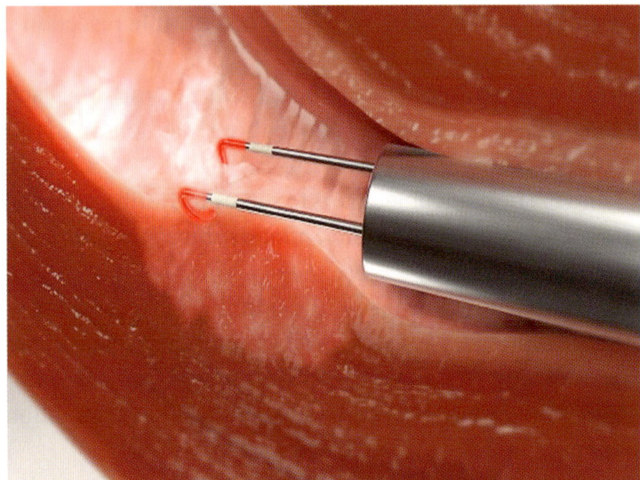

Fig. 7: Hysteroscopic resection of submucosal myoma using a resectoscope.

Complications of Hysteroscopic Myomectomy

Hysteroscopy Complications[4]

Among hysteroscopy surgeries, myomectomy has the highest incidence of complications. It ranges from 0.8 to 2.6%.

Cervical tear or lacerations: They occur at the time of dilatation. They are especially difficult in nulliparous patients, older patients, patients in whom preoperative GnRH is used as well as due to use of vulsellum, tenaculum slippage during the procedure. Tamponed and/or suturing has excellent results.

Uterine Perforation: It can occur during dilatation or during surgery.

Diagnosis: Sudden loss of distention, accelerated negative fluid balance (rapid escape of distending medium into peritoneal cavity), and vision of uterine cavity cannot be established.

Management: Suspend the procedure as further distention is not possible.

If perforation is without the use of energy source, hospitalization with close clinical observation is done. If perforation is done with use of energy, then investigate for damage to bladder and/or bowel either by laparoscopy or by laparotomy. Bladder injury is suspected in anterior wall perforation and in presence of hematuria; then consider cystoscopy. Rectal injury is suspected when the posterior wall is perforated.

Intestinal injury, especially thermal, can have potential consequences as it takes 3–4 days to manifest with fatal peritonitis or sepsis.

MULTIPLE CHOICE QUESTIONS

Q1. Submucous fibroid protruding more than 50% in uterine cavity is classified as fibroid.

a. Type 0
b. Type 1
c. Type 2
d. Type 3

Ans. b. Type 1

Q2. All are complications of power morcellation of fibroid except:

a. Unintended morcellation of sarcoma
b. Dissemination of fibroid
c. Intraoperative hemorrhage
d. Worsening of prognosis of existing sarcoma

Ans. c. Intraoperative hemorrhage

Q3. Following investigations are useful in preoperative diagnosis of leiomyosarcoma except:

a. Total LDH
b. LDH isoenzymes b
c. CT angiography
d. (Gd-DTPA) dynamic MRI

Ans. c. CT angiography

Q4. Regarding imaging of uterine fibroids, all are correct except:

a. Ultrasound is ideal to confirm the diagnosis
b. Saline infusion sonography (SIS) is more sensitive to detect submucosal fibroid
c. MRI is superior to USG to identify exact location of myoma
d. CT scanning is an alternative to MRI

Ans. d. CT scanning is an alternative to MRI

Q5. All of the following are indications for myomectomy in a case of fibroid uterus except:

a. Associated infertility
b. Recurrent pregnancy loss
c. Red degeneration
d. Pressure symptoms

Ans. c. Red degeneration

Q6. All are prerequisites for myomectomy, except:

a. Husband's semen analysis
b. Fibroid mapping by USG
c. Hysterectomy consent
d. Preoperative GnRH agonist

Ans. d. Preoperative GnRH agonist

Q7. All are used intraoperative to reduce the blood loss during myomectomy except:

a. Inj. Vasopressin
b. Vaginal misoprostol
c. Inj. Oxytocin
d. Inj Bupivacaine plus Epinephrine

Ans. c. Inj. Oxytocin

Q8. A 36-year-old female presents with heavy menstrual bleeding with infertility. USG is suggestive of single 5 cm, grade 2 submucosal fibroid. What is the best treatment option?

a. GnRH injection
b. Uterine Artery Embolization
c. Hysteroscopic myomectomy
d. Laparoscopic myomectomy

Ans. d. Laparoscopic myomectomy

Q9. A 42-year-old female arrives with heavy menstrual bleeding. She has a 7-year-old child. Uterus measures 24 weeks with multiple fibroids. Hb is 10 g/dL. What is best treatment option for her?

a. Total Abdominal hysterectomy
b. Myomectomy
c. Total Abdominal hysterectomy with BSO followed by HRT
b. Myomectomy
e. GnRH Inj

Ans. a. Total Abdominal hysterectomy

Q10. Hyponatremia with encephalopathy is a complication of which distention media during hysteroscopic myomectomy?

a. Normal Saline
b. Glycine
c. Ringer Lactate
d. Dextran

Ans. b. Glycine

REFERENCES

1. Baird DD, Dunson DB, Hill MC, et al. High cumulative incidence of uterine leiomyoma in black and white women: ultrasound evidence. Am J Obstet Gynecol. 2003;188:100.
2. Buttram VC Jr, Reiter RC. Uterine leiomyomata: etiology, symptomatology, and management. Fertil Steril. 1981;36:433.
3. Buttram VC Jr, Reiter RC. Uterine leiomyomata: etiology, symptomatology, and management. Fertil Steril. 1981;36:433-45.
4. Handa VL, Van Le L. Te Linde's Operative Gynecology, 12th edition. Philadelphia: Wolters Kluwer; 2019.
5. Royal College of Obstetricians and Gynaecologists. (2019). Morcellation for Abdominal or Laparoscopic Myomectomy or Hysterectomy (Consent Advice No. 13) [online] Available from https://www.rcog.org.uk/guidance/browse-all-guidance/consent-advice/morcellation-for-abdominal-or-laparoscopic-myomectomy-or-hysterectomy-consent-advice-no-13/ [Last accessed December, 2025].
6. Kongnyuy E, Wiysonge CS. Interventions to reduce haemorrhage during myomectomy for fibroids. Cochrane Database Syst Rev 2014;(8):CD005355.
7. Parker WH. Uterine fibroids.

Endoscopy in Gynecology—Laparoscopy

Sandeep Suhas Pophale

LONG QUESTIONS AND ANSWERS

Q1. Natural Orifice Transluminal Endoscopic Surgery in Obstetrics and Gynecology.

DNB Obs and Gyn Paper IV Dec 2022 (10 marks)

The basic concept: Natural Orifice Transluminal endoscopic surgery is a technique that utilizes **natural orifices such as the rectum and vagina. In gynecology**, it refers to the use of **transvaginal endoscopic** exploration to minimize invasiveness while examining the female internal organs, without compromising on safety.[1]

NOTES involves the use of flexible or rigid endoscopes that are advanced through a **natural orifice** and makes **an entry into the peritoneal cavity** by **cutting open that visceral organ.**[2]

Vaginal Natural Orifice Transluminal Endoscopic Surgery (vNOTES) is the most commonly used. This combines **vaginal approach** and **single port** endoscopy.[3]

Advantages

- **Improved precision and accuracy** of the investigation
- It enables convenient and **immediate access** and visualization of the tubo-ovarian structures without the need for additional modification.
- By aligning the endoscope with the tubo-ovarian structures, it becomes convenient to examine the entire **surface of the ovary** and reach the **fossa ovarica.**
- Transvaginal laparoscopy enables the examination of various structures in their **natural position** and normal relationship to one another, without any manipulation.
- This enables the direct monitoring of typical physiological occurrences during **ovulation** and the **retrieval of the ovum**.
- When comparing this treatment to traditional laparoscopy, the majority of patients experienced **minimal pain**, primarily in the lower abdomen.
- It reduces length of hospital stay and blood loss.

Procedure-specific preoperative considerations: Prior to the treatment, it is recommended to perform a routine **vaginal examination** and **vaginal ultrasound** in order to rule out any abnormalities in the pouch of Douglas.

Indications

- Benign **uterine and adnexal pathology**
- **High body mass index** when conventional laparoscopy becomes challenging

Contraindications

- Patient with a narrow vagina/patient is not sexually active
- A fixed and retroverted uterus
- An obliterated cul-de-sac
- An indurated posterior cervix.
- Furthermore, severe clinical problems or sizable ovarian cysts are unequivocal contraindications for the transvaginal approach.
- Severe endometriosis or dense pelvic adhesions with risk of bowel or bladder injury
- Gynecological cancer
- Pelvic radiotherapy
- Stage III or IV uterovaginal prolapse
- Previous rectal surgery
- History of hysterectomy
- History of mesh sacrocolpopexy

Technique of Transvaginal Laparoscopy

An older technique of transvaginal laparoscopy **(TVL)** has been described under local anesthesia or sedation.

With the patient lying on their back, the forceps are used to grab and lift the posterior lip of the cervix.

The pouch of Douglas can be accessed by puncturing the posterior fornix using a specifically designed needle-trocar device.

The access trocar is composed of three components: (1) A needle equipped with a spring mechanism, (2) a device used for dilation, and (3) an outer trocar.

The spring-loaded needle allows for quick and efficient access to the pouch of Douglas. The loaded needle can have a predetermined length ranging from 1 to 2.5 cm. Typically, we choose a predetermined measurement of 1.5 cm for depth.

Once the spring-loaded needle is positioned correctly, it is then released.

The needle is positioned at the back part of the vaginal fornix, directly below the cervix, along the midline, at a depth of approximately 1.5 cm. Vertical movements using the forceps will clearly demonstrate the protrusion of the vaginal fornix, aiding in the identification of the entry location.

By applying gentle pressure, the dilating sheet and outer trocar are advanced while slowly removing the needle, gradually enlarging the entry point to match the diameter of the outer trocar (4 mm). An endoscope is inserted, and precise intra-abdominal localization is verified.

The endoscope utilized is a 2.9 mm endoscope equipped with a 30° angled optical lens, which is identical to the one used during hysteroscopy.

The diameter of the outer trocar is 3.4 mm.

The **posterior aspect of the uterus is assessed** and, in the absence of a comprehensive image, **acts as a reference point**.

Throughout the entire treatment, we utilize a constant stream of preheated Ringer's lactate solution, typically not surpassing 500 cm^3.[4] This distention liquid maintains buoyancy of the organs and facilitates precise detection of lesions on the surfaces of tubes and ovaries.

Transvaginal hydrolaparoscopy **(THL)** has also been described in more recent literature using a fluid medium through a needle in posterior fornix, followed by introduction of a rigid angled endoscope to visualize the POD, pelvis, tubes and adnexa and tube patency with a dye through cervix. Also, minor procedures like adhesiolysis, ovarian drilling, and endometriosis diathermy can be done through this approach. However, there is a significant risk of bowel injury. Salpingoscopy may be done to visualize the endosalpinx of the tube.[5]

After completing the process, the endoscope is taken out, and the distending solution is released through the cannula before it is withdrawn.

Suturing the puncture site is unnecessary unless there is ongoing bleeding.

Operative Procedures

When to do and when not?

For acute problems like intraperitoneal hemorrhage or infection, transvaginal laparoscopy is **NOT** recommended as a panoramic view is not available.

Nevertheless, it provides a precise identification of minor abnormalities on the peritoneal and ovarian surfaces.

The transvaginal operational method is especially beneficial for treating minor or mild peritoneal and ovarian endometriosis, as well as for surgically treating clomiphene-resistant polycystic ovarian syndrome.

Operative interventions are usually performed using general anesthesia or sedation in an ambulatory center.

Potential Complications and Their Treatment

Entry failure:

Failure to gain entry can affect 3–10% of the cases, surgical expertise and experience playing an important role.

The utilization of a small-diameter cannula, along with the needle–trocar combination, enhances the safety of the transvaginal procedure.

Needle injury:

Minor problems may arise during the procedure, such as vaginal hemorrhage, puncture of the posterior uterine wall, and needle perforation of the rectum.

Rectal perforation could have potentially severe consequences.

Injury during ovarian drilling:

Confusing the surface of the intestine with the surface of the ovary has resulted in the unintentional drilling of the intestinal wall via the vagina.

To prevent the intestines from coming in the way, the abdomen can be filled with an adequate amount of Ringer's lactate solution (about 300 mL).

It is essential for the surgeon to have the capability to identify various organs during transvaginal laparoscopy.

Technique of entry for vNOTES

vNOTES is typically performed under general anesthesia with the patient in Trendelenburg position.

vNOTES using Alexis O Retractor

The vaginal mucosa is initially circumscribed around the cervix and mobilized. The uterosacral ligaments are clamped, cut, and ligated. An Alexis O retractor is introduced behind the colpotomy incision and **pneumoperitoneum is created with an insufflation pressure of 10 mm**.

Earlier a home-made device technique has been described by using a surgical glove incising the finger ends to introduce the laparoscope and instruments. Current practice is to use **air-tight seal like Gel Point Vpath to seal the vaginal cuff** to maintain insufflation pressure.

After the surgery, the specimen is retrieved through the vagina and through the colpotomy incision.

The **low-pressure pneumoperitoneum of 6–10 mm versus 12–15 mm** in traditional laparoscopy reduces risk factors like bradycardia and carbon dioxide resorption.[6]

Q2. What is the role of MIS in management of women with infertility?

DNB Obs and Gyn Paper IV Aug 2021 (8 marks)

Introduction

Since the introduction of minimally invasive surgery in the 1980s, surgical procedures have been performed laparoscopically.

This has resulted in several advantages for the patient, including shorter hospital stays, less postoperative discomfort, and for the surgeon, improved visibility and fewer postoperative adhesions.

- Management of clomiphene-resistant PCOS (Ovarian Drilling).
- Management of endometriosis.
- Management of hydrosalpinxes.
- Management of fibroids.
- Management of adenomyomas.
- Hysteroscopic management of B/L tubal block (Hysteroscopic Tubal Cannulation)
- Laparoscopy is also useful for diagnosing infertility issues such as tubal adhesions and mild-to-moderate endometriosis.

Laparoscopic Ovarian Drilling

In patients with polycystic ovary syndrome (PCOS) who are refractory to ovulation induction or do not ovulate or conceive after 3–6 cycles of letrozole, the next step in treatment is either laparoscopic ovarian drilling (LOD) or ovulation induction with gonadotropins.

LOD is recommended in selected anovulatory patients with Polycystic ovaries with normal BMI, as an alternative to ovulation induction. However, it can affect reproductive outcomes.[7]

Laparoscopic ovarian drilling is a single surgery that carries a *lower risk of ovarian hyperstimulation syndrome and multiple pregnancies.*

Technique and Considerations:

- Check tubal patency before starting the surgery.
- The ovary is grasped with a traumatic grasper and 4, 40-watt punctures are done to 4 mm depth.

- Avoid surface coagulation by hitting the ovarian surface at a 90° angle with a monopolar needle.
- Avoid peritubal adhesions by puncturing away from the tubal side of the ovary.
- To avoid postoperative adhesions, allow the ovary to cool before letting it go.
- Choose patients carefully. Prior to ovarian drilling, medical treatment should be fully explored.
- Avoid regularly drilling bulky polycystic ovaries found on diagnostic laparoscopy.

Management of Endometriosis

Approximately 11–13% of women of reproductive age are affected by endometriosis.

Endometriosis commonly presents with progressive dysmenorrhea, dyspareunia, and infertility as the primary symptoms in women.

A 2D/3D transvaginal ultrasound can be used to diagnose endometriosis in people experiencing symptoms.

Laparoscopy, combined with histological confirmation of ectopic endometrial glands and epithelium, is considered the most reliable method, **"The Gold Standard", for definitively diagnosing this condition.**

Techniques and Consideration

- To treat mild-to-moderate peritoneal endometriosis (superficial endometriosis),[8] the lesion can be removed using scissors (excision) or by ablation.
- Deep endometriosis is only treated for symptom relief.[8]
- Normal saline can be infused under a lesion over a crucial structure like the ureter to lift it and protect it.
- For scattered nodules, **cauterize with bipolar forceps** and a brief current burst. Check for endometriotic nodules on the **posterior surface of the ovaries, pouch of Douglas, and uterosacral ligaments.**
- To confirm endometriosis, a biopsy from these nodules is necessary for **histological testing.**
- In endometriotic cyst, incision and drainage or cystectomy have been debated, with the former increasing recurrence rates and the latter potentially reducing ovarian reserve.
- Laparoscopic cyst removal is particularly necessary for cysts larger than 4 cm,[8] those obstructing Oocyte Pick Up (OPU), or multiple implantation failures in young patients.
- Injecting **diluted vasopressin** between the ovarian surface and cyst wall improves planes, reduces bleeding, and reduces cautery usage, preserving ovarian reserve.
- **Before surgery, ovarian reserve tests (AMH, AFC, Day 2 FSH) must be performed**, documented, and conveyed to the patient. **Repeat these tests 3–4 months** following surgery.

Management of Hydrosalpinxes

For hydrosalpinxes. the ideal ultrasound scan timing is mid-cycle, as fluid tends to build during the follicular phase.

Fluid in the endometrial cavity during follicular phase or ET may indicate subclinical hydrosalpinx, requiring laparoscopic investigation.

Hydrosalpinx lowers pregnancy rate and must be addressed before ET. It affects both implantation and the embryo directly.

Embryo toxicity results from fluid leakage from hydrosalpinx into the uterine cavity, negatively impacting the uterine reception and implantation.

Removing the deceased tube not only improves pregnancy rates but also reduces abortion rates in hydrosalpinx patients.

Technique and Considerations

- The tube is completely removed by MIS (salpingectomy).[8] Two ipsilateral ports and a central umbilical port are used.
- Hold the tube with a grasper, cauterize, and cut the mesosalpinx nearest the tube.
- Maintain tight **proximity to the tube** to preserve ovarian reserve.
- Properly **cauterize the stump** following salpingectomy to prevent stump ectopic pregnancy.
- A complete salpingectomy is typically accomplished, although in cases with significant hydrosalpinx and prior procedures, serious bowel adhesions may occur.
- **Intrauterine methylene blue instillation can assist distinguish the dilated tube from the bowel**.
- Consider delinking the isthmic end with bipolar cautery or scissors in such circumstances **(proximal tubal occlusion in complex cases)**.[8]

Management of Fibroids

Fibroids are found in 5–10% of infertile patients. They are only identified as the sole cause in 1–2.4% of infertile patients.[9]

According to Somigliana et al.,[10] myomas negatively impact pregnancy rates, while submucosal fibroids significantly hinder pregnancy.

For patients with fibroid uterus and infertility, it is important to screen out other factors first.

Which fibroids should be removed and which not?

All **submucous fibroids adversely affect the outcome of pregnancy** and should be removed prior to ART.

Subserous fibroids, as anticipated, do not have significant impact on infertility and so need not be removed.

Laparoscopic myomectomy is a suitable treatment for intramural fibroids that cause an **indentation in the uterine cavity** and for **big fibroids that are larger than 5 cm**.

Laparoscopic myomectomy is a potential option for patients who have intramural fibroids and have experienced many failed implantations or recurrent pregnancy loss, even if the fibroid is not causing distortion of the endometrial cavity.[9]

Technique and Considerations

- The surgeon places the port based on the size of the fibroid and her discretion.
- Inject dilute vasopressin 20 units in 200 mL of NS[9] into the subcapsular area after abdominal inspection and fibroid mapping.

- For larger fibroids, hemostatic clips can be placed bilaterally on the uterine arteries and IP ligament and gently removed with the grasper after surgery. Alternatively, a "shoelace" knot using Vicryl (no. 1) may also be placed.
- Transverse incision on myoma bulge using monopolar hook/scissors or harmonic scalpel blade.
- **Stay away from the cornual end** and **continue incision until the cleavage plane is reached.**
- Myometrial and fibroid tissues differ in consistency, making it crucial to select the appropriate dissection plane. **An intracapsular myomectomy is recommended leaving behind the pseudocapsule.**
- Myoma tissue is stabilized for traction using a screw or tenaculum after exposure.
- The myometrium is gently pushed away, and intervening tissue coagulated as needed.
- We can utilize bipolar, scissors, or harmonic scalpel based on surgeon preference.
- If big **intramural fibroids indent into the endometrium**, verify integrity with an **intrauterine injection of methylene blue.**
- If the endometrial cavity is breached, it is important to **avoid including the endometrium in the sutures** due to the **risk of microfistulae formation** leading to a possible scar ectopic pregnancy.
- The myoma bed is closed with **absorbable polyglactin (Vicryl) or barb sutures (V-loc)** based on the surgeon's preference. Barb sutures are tighter with reduced possibility of hematoma formation resulting in a stronger scar.

Management of Adenomyosis

The surgical option is designated for patients with:

- Failed conservative treatment.
- Patient with **chronic pelvic pain** and heavy menstrual blood loss.
- **Recurrent pregnancy loss** and implantation failure.
- Surgery may be necessary for patients with large focal adenomyoma and long-term **infertility** prior to ART cycles.[9]

Technique and Considerations

Vasopressin injection at the adenomyoma bulge minimize intraoperative hemorrhage, but do not provide a definitive plane due to the absence of a capsule.

Incision is made over point of maximum protrusion and wedge-shaped debulking is done.

The **overlapping flap technique is used for suturing to improve scar strength** and reproductive outcomes.

Hysteroscopic management of B/L tubal block (Hysteroscopic Tubal Cannulation): It is performed under laparoscopic supervision, laparoscopic eyesight being essential for this procedure.[9]

Technique and Considerations

- Hysteroscopy and laparoscopy are done simultaneously.
- Initially, inject diluted methylene blue solution into the uterine cavity to conform the cornual block.

- A **5 French catheter with obturator** is introduced through the hysteroscope operating channel to reach the ostia.
- **Push the curved catheter into the ostia and carefully remove the obturator,** *avoiding pushing the obturator beyond the tubal ostia as it may perforate the cornual end of the tube.*
- **Inject diluted methylene blue dye** through the catheter and observe free leak from the fimbrial end laparoscopically.
- Repeat the process on the other side.

SHORT QUESTIONS AND ANSWERS

Q1. Robotic surgery in gynecology. *MD/MS Obs and Gyn Paper IV Jul 2023 (6 marks)*

The da Vinci Surgical System (Intuitive Surgical Inc., Sunnyvale, CA)[11] was approved by the US Food and Drug Administration in 2005, following the first robotic gynecological treatments in 1998.

With **wristed tools**, **three-dimensional imaging**, *and* **ergonomics**, robotic laparoscopy enhances precision and surgeon comfort.

It has a quicker learning curve than conventional laparoscopy, allowing surgeons to overcome that constraint and provide minimally invasive choices to patients.[12]

Port Placement

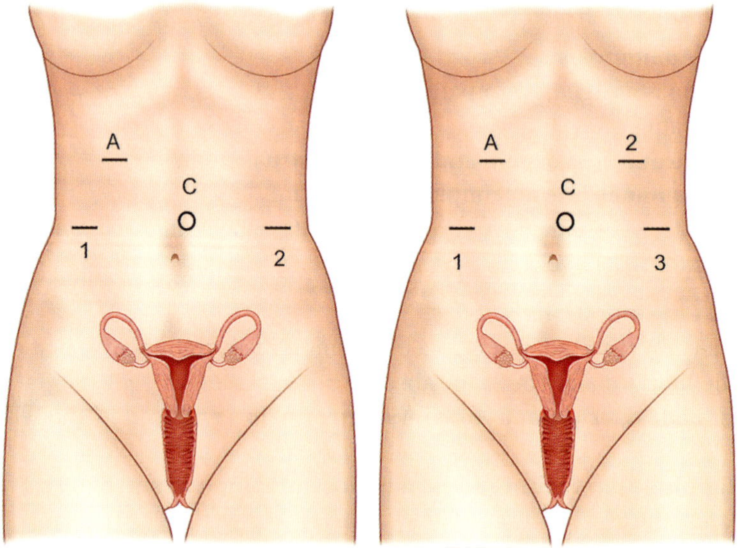

[Robotic port placement in a 3 and 4 port patterns: C: 12 mm camera port, A: 5 mm accessory port, 1, 2, and 3: 8 mm robotic ports]

Robotic Components:

I. Patient Cart (The DaVinci System): The patient cart features three or four interactive robotic arms that dock with the camera and bedside robotic trocars.

These trocars allow the surgeon at the console to handle robotic tools.

In contrast to traditional laparoscopy, these devices **offer 7° of mobility** (4° in traditional MIS), **reduced motion, and tremor filtration**. The degree of movement is higher than the human wrist. There is no autonomous movement of instruments. The movements are surgeon controlled.

Robotic-assisted surgery **alleviates the fulcrum effect** of laparoscopy (instrument moving in opposite direction of hand), **allowing surgeons to operate akin to open surgery**. The da Vinci vision system is loaded through the camera trocar on the patient cart. There is a surgeon-controlled third arm. **There is an intuitive instrument movement which replicates surgeons' hand movements**, in contrast to conventional laparoscopy which is counterintuitive.[13]

II. Vision Tower (HD—3D Vision): The da Vinci system uses two cameras, each with distinct light sources to bring high-definition, three-dimensional views to the surgeon console with better depth perception.

Camera is controlled by surgeon

The *Si system* has 8.5- and 12-mm cameras. Each size has a 0° and 30° lens that can be adjusted up or down based on the surgical incision site.

For the newer *Xi system*, just an 8 mm camera is available.

III. Ergonomic Surgeon Console: The surgeon console is situated away but in line of sight from the robotic cart and operating bed.

The console houses the binocular viewer, camera, and instrument controls, which are controlled by pedals and hand controls.

The surgeon can move instruments and camera and also enlarge the vision up to 15-fold using these settings.

The ability to sit **during surgery offers physical and cognitive ergonomic benefits** compared to traditional laparoscopy. It reduces work-related musculoskeletal symptoms (WMS).[13]

A twin console option is available for the da Vinci Si and Xi systems. Two surgeons can operate at the two consoles simultaneously, which is beneficial for training residents and novice robotic surgeons.

Docking

The **patient cart can be pulled in straight or at an angle to the bed, known as side-docking**.

When "straight" docking (robotic cart between legs of patient) is preferred, it aligns the robotic cart center column and camera port. The patient cart should be brought in between the abducted legs of the patient until the camera arm is comfortably near its port.

Side-docking, which is preferred in Gynecology, affords greater space for an assistant performing uterine manipulation.

A docked operating bed cannot be moved, as it may impact trocar placement and depth, potentially causing abdominal or pelvic injuries.

To access the upper abdomen during gynecologic oncology treatments such as para-aortic lymph node dissections and upper abdominal metastatic excision, the robot may need to be redocked over the patient's head. The recently introduced *Xi system* allows for multiquadrant surgery without redocking.

Disadvantages

- Lack of haptic control
- Positions surgeon away from the patient
- Higher cost of equipment

Advantages

- Ergonomic for surgeon
- Wristed movements
- Intuitive movements
- Three-dimensional view
- Less conversion to laparotomy
- Precise micromovements
- Shorter learning curve
- 6 mm intra-abdominal pressure is feasible and may be advantageous for patients with obesity and poor respiratory compliance.[13]

The Guiding Principles for application of Robotic Surgery

The lack of sufficient level I evidence in the literature about robotic surgery is the reason why one cannot properly determine and define the role of robotics in benign gynecology.

The existing data, albeit predominantly of low quality, broadly agrees on a few key points: Robotic surgery plays a part in noncancerous gynecology. Nevertheless, the precise details of this position are ambiguous. It has been used for endometrial cancer in obese, diabetic, and hypertensive patients.[13]

Robotic surgery provides **a benefit compared to abdominal surgery by offering a less-invasive** surgical option.

Robotic surgery is expensive, and it remains uncertain whether the benefits outweigh the costs.

The **efficacy of robotic surgery compared to laparoscopy has not been substantiated. Robotic surgery should be avoided when vaginal surgery is a viable** alternative.

A **minimally invasive surgical** method is widely recognized as the definitive standard of care. **Vaginal, laparoscopic, and robotic surgery** should always be prioritized and conducted instead of abdominal surgery.

The selection of the minimally invasive surgical approach should be determined by the patient's preference, the surgeon's expertise, and the alternative that is believed to result in the most successful outcome.

Q2. Discuss complications of operative laparoscopy in gynecology practice.

DNB Obs and Gyn Paper III Oct 2023 (5 marks)

The potential benefits of laparoscopic surgery compared to open abdominal surgery are widely recognized. These include decreased blood loss, shorter hospitalization, faster recovery to normal daily activities, lower pain, and improved cosmetic outcomes. Specifically in relation to urogynecologic procedures, it enables a wider and more accurate visualization of the pelvic anatomy for the placement of prosthesis and sutures with utmost precision and safety. In addition, endoscopic techniques have the potential to address all three compartments using a single approach.

However, there are several notable characteristics, such as changes in the physical structure caused by pneumoperitoneum and Trendelenburg positioning, which can make orientation tough. Additionally, there are added challenges owing to a fixed visual axis, a loss of depth perception, and a decrease in magnification when using 2D projection. Three-dimensional optics and robotic methods have the potential to overcome some challenges. Laparoscopic techniques need a more extensive period of study and training compared to other methods and should only be conducted by experienced specialists.[14]

Laparoscopic complications can be classified as follows:

- Positional
- Abdominal entry
- Electrical energy
- Vascular complications
- Bowel complications
- Genitourinary complication

Patient Positioning

Several of nerve group complications due to improper patient positioning may arise.

Prevention

Strategic utilization of padding materials such as fabric, towels, foam mats, and gel pads can effectively reduce the likelihood of nerve damage. Avoid using shoulder restraints to prevent patients from slipping down on the operating room table due to the high frequency of brachial plexus compression injuries. The lower brachial plexus (C8–T1) is injured if the brace is positioned too laterally. This results in Klumpke's paralysis.

Stirrups of the boot type, which provide support to the foot and calf, are favored due to their ability to distribute pressure more uniformly. Common peroneal neuropathy may occur if the peroneal nerve is compressed near the fibular neck in lithotomy.

Sciatic nerve injury may occur due to hyperflexion in lithotomy.[15]

The majority of compression injuries heal on their own without intervention. However, it is important to record and monitor the damage after surgery until it is fully resolved.

Abdominal Entry

The majority (>50%) of difficulties arising from laparoscopy are directly linked to the entrance technique.

The following strategies can enhance safety while doing peritoneal access:

- Entry with the **Verres needle at the base of the umbilicus at 90° to the skin** followed by creation of pneumoperitoneum up to 20–25 mm pressure is recommended. Ensure that the patient is **positioned flat** and centered on the operating table while inserting the primary cannula. Do not employ the Trendelenburg position too early, as it causes the sacral promontory and retroperitoneal vasculature to align more closely with the axis of the umbilicus above.

- By carefully considering the anatomy and selecting the suitable access point and angle (90° to the abdominal wall), there should be **no necessity to utilize longer needles** or trocars.
- Explore **alternative locations** for peritoneal access in patients who may have challenging peritoneal access, such as individuals who are **extremely thin or obese** or those who have already had **abdominal surgery**.

Palmer's point 3 cm below costal margin in the mid-clavicular line is recommended for patients with previous lower abdominal surgery.

Hasson's open entry technique may be considered.

Complications of Electrical Energy

Unintended electrosurgical injuries may arise from **insulation faults** that result in sparking or **direct coupling** with another device. Insulation failures may occur due to overuse of instruments.

Indirect (capacitive) coupling probe activation occurs when the probe **is not in direct contact with the tissue, generating an "open circuit"**. It occurs if the electrosurgical unit is accidentally activated when **close to another metallic instrument**. **Current flows through adjacent instrument through pathway of least resistance** and potentially damages tissues.

Overheating of the active electrode tip can happen when it is covered with dried blood or debris.

Cutting current is a continuous current. Coagulation current is an interrupted current. Coagulation-type current is used to produce the same result as cutting current **depending on tissue contact**.

When utilizing any form of energy in laparoscopy, it is crucial to remember two fundamental concepts:

- Always ensure that the points of the **instruments are positioned at main focus** of **visual field** (screen) while delivering energy.
- It is advisable to refrain from employing two distinct energy sources simultaneously in the abdomen. Mistakenly activating an incorrect energy source can lead to unwanted and catastrophic consequences on the corresponding tissue.

Vascular Complications

The most frequent occurrence of vascular damage happens **during laparoscopic entry**, specifically during inserting the Veress needle or primary trocar.

The **right common iliac artery** and **left common iliac vein** are the veins most frequently harmed during trocar implantation.

In the event of vascular injury, a skilled laparoscopic surgeon may endeavor to do laparoscopic vessel repair. The anesthetist, Operation Theater staff, and blood bank should be alerted.

To halt the ongoing bleeding, the initial procedure involves using a gentle forceps to obstruct the blood vessel.

Following the irrigation with fluids and removal of blood, the bleeding vessels are located and hemostasis is achieved using either **laparoscopic suturing or vascular clamps**.

The optimal selection for suturing the vascular repair is a **durable 6-0 suture**. For minor arterial or venous bleeding, one can employ **bipolar current**, Endoloop, or **mechanical pressure**.

In the case of a minor, widespread hemorrhage, a gauze can be inserted into the abdominal cavity through a 10 mm trocar. The gauze can then be used to **apply pressure** until the bleeding ceases.

Thrombin and gelatin matrix can be utilized as hemostatic agents for managing small-vessel hemorrhage.

If the bleeding is not controlled, **call for help from the vascular surgeon team and resort to laparotomy** in a timely manner.

Bowel Complications

The incidence of intestinal injury after simple laparoscopic procedures is 0.08%, while the incidence for major surgical laparoscopic procedures is 0.3%.

Minor Veress needle injuries in healthy large bowel tissue can be managed conservatively based on clinical assessment.

If little or extensive intestinal injuries are identified during laparoscopic surgery, they can be repaired using laparoscopic techniques. The recommended choice for suturing is 3-0 Vicryl, to be applied in two layers. If necessary, a laparotomy may be undertaken.

A delayed diagnosis of a gut injury can lead to significant sepsis and death rates as high as 20%.

A cautery burn on the bowel with a hot instrument should be examined for blanch and suturing should be considered to avoid delayed perforation.[16]

Genitourinary Complications

Bladder injuries may occur at the time of **suprapubic trocar placement** or **bladder dissection from the lower uterine segment** in women with prior pelvic surgery or cesarean sections. Usually, the injury can be **treated laparoscopically in two layers using absorbable sutures** if diagnosed intraoperatively.

Running stitch with absorbable suture (3-0 Vicryl or 3-0 Monocryl) is recommended. The bladder can be checked for **integrity by filling it with dilute methylene blue** up to 200 cc after repair. For **at least 10 days**, a Foley catheter should be implanted to decompress and drain the bladder, depending on the cystotomy size.

Before withdrawing the catheter, **a retrograde cystogram should be done** to confirm a healthy and defect-free bladder.

Ureteral damage is found in 0.5–1.5% of open gynecological operations and somewhat greater in laparoscopic surgery.

To avoid ureteral injury, **identify the ureters at the start of the surgery** and ascertain their position throughout the procedure by checking peristalsis.

For complex instances with fibrosis and scarring, **pelvic ureter dissection** can clarify their location during surgery.

To treat partial ureteral injuries, pass the stent and repair laparoscopically with 6-0 Vicryl suture. Once the damaged ureter is fully resected, it should be dissected tension-free before passing the stent under laparoscopic guidance. Pass a 3-0 suture through the adventitia and muscularis layer to reattach the ureter cut ends and hold them together during the final surgery.

Four 6-0 or 5-0 absorbable sutures should be inserted consecutively at 6, 9, 3, and 12 o'clock into the wall thickness to reconnect the ureter. The ureteral stent can be withdrawn 14 days following repair.

Q3. What are the criteria and methods for hysteroscopic myomectomy?

DNB Obs and Gyn Paper III Apr 2023 (4 marks)

Abnormal uterine bleeding, dysmenorrhea, and reproductive issues are linked to submucosal myomas. Submucosal myoma is a common indication for hysteroscopic excision. Currently, hysteroscopic excision is the preferred treatment for symptomatic submucosal myomas.

The 2011 FIGO classification identified eight myoma types. FIGO (0-2) kinds are in cavitary: Type 0 is a fibroid pedunculated in the uterine cavity, Type 1 has over 50% of the leiomyoma within the cavity, and Type 2 has less than 50%.

Hysteroscopic myomectomy aims to remove the complete fibroid without harming the surrounding myometrium or endometrium. This alleviates patient symptoms without weakening the myometrium or causing intracavitary synechia. Complete myoma removal reduces the likelihood of regrowth.

Presurgery examination involves TVS, SHG, and office hysteroscopy.[17]

Hysteroscopic submucosal myoma excision significantly improves the prognosis for women experiencing recurrent pregnancy loss and infertility.[18]

Lasmar[19] introduced the Lasmar score system to classify submucosal myomas more precisely. This categorization prioritized surgical aspects, classifying myomas into low and high complexity, and those not amenable to hysteroscopic resection.

Lasmar's Presurgical Classification of Submucous Myomas

Points	Penetration into myometrium	Fibroid size (cm)	Extension of the base of fibroid	Topography	Lateral wall
0	0	≤2	≤1/3	Lower	–
1	≤50%	>2–5	>1/3–2/3	Middle	+1
2	>50%	>5	>2/3	Upper	+

Score	Group	Complexity and therapeutic option
0–4	I	Low-complexity hysteroscopic myomectomy
5–6	II	High-complexity hysteroscopic myomectomy; consider the use of GnRH analog and/or two-stage hysteroscopic myomectomy
7–9	III	Hysteroscopic myomectomy not indicated; consider an alternative nonhysteroscopic technique

Instruments and devices

Leiomyoma resection can be performed hysteroscopically using electrosurgical and mechanical devices. The instruments available are *Mazzon cold loops, Versapoint, MyoSure, Symphion, and TruClear.*

An operative hysteroscope is the tool employed to surgically remove a submucosal myoma while directly observing the procedure.

The working part of this can consist of electrosurgical loops, mechanical cold loops, or morcellator technology.

There are two primary methods used to address submucous myomas: (1) Cold energy and (2) Electrocautery.

The primary method of utilizing cold energy is by the use of 5 Fr hysteroscopic scissors, which are capable of cutting the base of a small submucous myoma and intrauterine morcellators.

The choice of the hysteroscopic myomectomy procedure depends on the individual patient and surgeon, and there are no universally agreed-upon recommendations.[20]

Electrocautery enables the undertaking of more difficult instances, such as myomas with intramural components and bigger diameters. The loop insert is the most appropriate choice for myomas as it enables a secure grip on the myoma and facilitates the division of the fibroid into strips.

Electrosurgical systems can be categorized as either monopolar or bipolar.

Monopolar instruments are characterized by the flow of current from the tip of the resectoscope to a plate. Nonconducting distension fluids, such as sorbitol 5% or glycine 1.5%, are utilized with monopolar electrodes.

The advancement of a more advanced bipolar resectoscope and increasing awareness of the limitations of nonconductive medium have led to the preference for using the bipolar resectoscope as the primary treatment for submucosal myoma types 0-2.

The hysteroscopic mechanical morcellator was later created to address the limitations of the resectoscope. There is a lack of broadly agreed-upon criteria for the preferred usage of different hysteroscopic morcellation techniques. Advocates argue that Type 0 leiomyomas are more suitable for morcellation, whereas Type 2 leiomyomas are more effectively treated using bipolar resectoscopy.

Electrosurgical procedures are more effective than morcellators for completely removing myomas larger than 4 cm that have a considerable intramural component.[21]

Energy Sources in Gynecologic Laparoscopy

In gynecologic laparoscopy, various energy sources are essential for cutting, dissecting, and achieving hemostasis. The primary modalities include monopolar and bipolar electrosurgery, ultrasonic energy, and lasers, each with distinct profiles.

- **Monopolar Electrosurgery**
  - **Mechanism:** An electrical current passes from an active electrode through the patient's body to a distant return electrode pad.
  - **Advantages:**
    - Highly versatile for both cutting and coagulation.
    - Cost-effective and widely available.
  - **Disadvantages:**
    - Risk of lateral thermal spread and unintended injury to adjacent tissues.
    - Potential for alternate site burns at the return electrode.
- **Bipolar Electrosurgery**
  - **Mechanism:** Electrical current is confined between the two jaws of the instrument, affecting only the grasped tissue. Advanced bipolar devices (e.g., LigaSure) integrate tissue feedback for sealing and cutting.

- **Advantages:**
  - Enhanced safety with minimal lateral thermal spread.
  - Effective for sealing blood vessels and reducing instrument changes and operative time.
- **Disadvantages:**
  - Generally, more expensive than basic monopolar instruments.
  - Standard bipolar forceps require a separate instrument for cutting.

- **Ultrasonic Energy**
  - **Mechanism:** High-frequency mechanical vibrations generate heat for coagulation and cutting without electrical current passing through the patient.
  - **Advantages:**
    - Minimal thermal spread and reduced surgical smoke.
    - Precise dissection, ideal for use near delicate structures.
  - **Disadvantages:**
    - High cost of the device and its proprietary instruments.
    - Can require a specific learning curve for effective use.
- **Laser Energy**
  - **Mechanism:** Focused light energy (e.g., CO_2) precisely ablates or vaporizes tissue.
  - **Advantages:**
    - Exceptional precision with very limited lateral damage.
    - Excellent for superficial ablation, such as in endometriosis.
  - **Disadvantages:**
    - Very high cost and requires stringent safety protocols.
    - Limited efficacy for cutting dense tissue or sealing larger vessels.

Conclusion

The choice of energy source is dictated by the surgical task, cost considerations, and the surgeon's preference. While monopolar remains a versatile and economical choice, bipolar and ultrasonic devices are favored for their safety and efficiency in complex dissections and vessel sealing.

MULTIPLE CHOICE QUESTIONS

Q1. All are good practices for prevention of neuropathies in Laparoscopic surgeries *Except*:

a. Boot-type stirrups that support the foot and calf are preferred.
b. The shoulder brace is positioned laterally.[22]
c. Tucking the arms bilaterally with the hands adducted reduces the risk of brachial plexus traction injury from lateral abduction.
d. When the hips and knees are hyperflexed, there is an increased risk of sciatic and femoral neuropathies.

Ans. b. The shoulder brace is positioned laterally.[22]

Q2. All of the following are good practices to prevent injuries during peritoneal access *Except*:

a. Explore alternative locations for needle and trocar insertion in patients who are extremely thin or obese, or who have already undergone abdominal surgery.

b. Early Trendelenburg position for correct angulation.
c. Avoiding multiple re-entry with the Veress needle or the trocar.
d. Always place all secondary ports under direct vision

Ans. b. Early Trendelenburg position for correct angulation.

Q3. The technique of abdominal entry associated with the least rates of complications is:

a. Veress Needle
b. Open Laparoscopy
c. Microlaparoscopy
d. None of the above.[2]

Ans. d. None of the above.[2]

Q4. Vascular injuries are most commonly encountered during:

a. Retroperitoneal lymph node dissection
b. Use of lasers
c. While placing the Veress needle
d. Use of monopolar cautery in ovarian drilling

Ans. c. While placing the Veress needle

Q5. All of the following are advantages of robotic laparoscopy *Except*:

a. Loss of fulcrum effect
b. Ergonomically efficient as surgeon is seated.
c. Greater range of movement of the robotic laparoscopic instrument
d. Loss of depth perception

Ans. d. Loss of depth perception

Q6. All the following anatomical landmarks lie anterior to the Urinary bladder *Except*:

a. Bogros' Space
b. Retzius' Space
c. Santorini's Plexus
d. Latzko's Space

Ans. d. Latzko's Space

The lateral para-rectal space, often referred to as Latzko's space, is a retroperitoneal avascular region that is typically accessed by dissecting between the mesoureter and the pelvic wall, by creating a gap between the internal iliac artery (on the side) and the ureter (toward the middle).

Q7. All of the following are the advantages of Laparoscopic approach in treating endometriosis over laparotomy *Except*:

a. Better long-term pain reduction
b. Decreased immediate post-surgical pain
c. Decreased post-operative recovery time
d. None of the above

Ans. a. Better long-term pain reduction

Comparative nonrandomized trials have demonstrated equally the efficacy of both laparoscopy and laparotomy in achieving long-term pain relief for endometriosis.[23,24]

Q8. The problems associated with untreated ovarian endometriomas include:

a. Gradual replacement of the normal ovarian cortex by fibrosis
b. Lower follicular density in tissue adjacent to the ovarian endometrioma
c. Focal depletion of primordial follicles due to upregulation of follicular recruitment along with demise of early follicles.
d. All of the above.

Ans. d. All of the above.

An ovarian endometrioma (OE) includes significantly higher amounts of proteolytic enzymes, free iron, reactive oxygen species, and inflammatory chemicals compared to other forms of cysts.[25] The fluid components have the potential to cause changes in both the endometriotic cells and the surrounding tissue, where the normal ovarian cortex is replaced by fibrosis. These alterations are linked to the transformation of smooth muscle, damage to blood vessels within the ovary, and the depletion of follicles. The comparative analysis of normal cortical samples from ovaries affected by ovarian endometriosis (OEs) and contralateral normal gonads revealed a decreased follicular density in the tissue surrounding the OE.[26]

Q9. All of the following are disadvantages of the laparoscopic route *Except*:

a. Endoscopic methods in urogynecology do not permit the repair of all three compartments using a single approach.
b. Altered appearance of anatomy due to pneumoperitoneum and Trendelenburg positioning.
c. There is a fixed visual axis and loss of depth perception.
d. None of the above.

Ans. a. Endoscopic methods in urogynecology do not permit the repair of all three compartments using a single approach.

REFERENCES

1. Tulandi T (Ed). Atlas of Laparoscopy and Hysteroscopy Techniques, 3rd edition. London: Taylor & Francis; 2007.
2. Jacobson MT, Osias J, Bizhang R, et al. The Direct Trocar Technique: An Alternative Approach to Abdominal Entry for Laparoscopy. JSLS. 2002;6(2):169-74.
3. Natural Orifice Transluminal Endoscopic Surgery: An Overview. [online] Available from https://www.sciencedirect.com/topics/medicine-and-dentistry/natural-orifice-translumenal-endoscopic-surgery [Last accessed December, 2025]
4. Gordts S, Puttemans P, Gordts Sy, et al. Transvaginal laparoscopy. Best Pract Res Clin Obstet Gynaecol. 2005;(19)5:757-67.
5. Suresh YN, Narvekar NN. The role of tubal patency tests and tubal surgery in the era of assisted reproductive techniques. Obstet Gynaecol. 2014;16(1):37-45.
6. Yoong W, Sampson V, Mwenechanya L. Vnotes (vaginal Natural Orifice Transluminal Endoscopic Surgery): is the future of gynaecological surgery? Obstet Gynaecol. 2023;25(2):97-100.
7. Royal College of Obstetricians and Gynaecologists. (2014). Long-term Consequences of Polycystic Ovary Syndrome (Green-Top Guideline No. 33). [online] Available from https://www.rcog.org.uk/media/qmtlp2b0/gtg_33.pdf [Last accessed December, 2025].
8. Bhandari HM, Choudhary MK, Stewart JA, et al. An overview of assisted reproductive technology procedures. Obstet Gynaecol. 2018;20(3):167-76.
9. Benecke C, Kruger TF, Siebert TI, et al. Effect of fibroids on fertility in patients undergoing assisted reproduction. A structured literature review. Gynecol Obstet Invest. 2005;59(4):225-30.
10. Somigliana E, Vercellini P, Daguati R, et al. Fibroids and female reproduction: A critical analysis of evidence. Hum Reprod. 2007;13(5):465-76.
11. Falcone T, Goldberg JM, Margossian H, et al. Robotic-assisted laparoscopic microsurgical tubal anastomosis: a human pilot study. Fertil Steril. 2000;73:1040-2.
12. Soto E, Lo Y, Friedman K, et al. Total laparoscopic hysterectomy versus da Vinci robotic hysterectomy: is using the robot beneficial? J Gynecol Oncol. 2011;22(4):253-9.
13. Sawan S. What's new in guidance? Obstet Gynaecol. 2024;26(1):16-7.

14. Maher C, Baessler K. Surgical management of anterior vaginal wall prolapse: an evidence based literature review. Int Urogynecol J Pelvic Floor Dysfunct. 2006;17(2):195-201.
15. Kuponiyi O, Alleemudder DI, Latunde-Dada A. Nerve injuries associated with gynaecological surgery. Obstet Gynaecol. 2014;16(1):29-36.
16. El-Sayed M, Mohamed S, Saridogan E. Safe use of electrosurgery in gynaecological laparoscopic surgery. Obstet Gynaecol. 2020;22(1):9-20.
17. Fedele L, Bianchi S, Dorta M, et al. Transvaginal ultrasonography versus hysteroscopy in the diagnosis of uterine submucous fibroids. Obstet Gynecol. 1991;77:745-74.
18. Pritts E. Fibroids and infertility: a systematic review of the evidence. Obstet Gynecol Survey. 2001;56:483-91.
19. Lasmar RB, Barrozo PR, Dias R, et al. Submucous fibroids: a new presurgical classification to evaluate the viability of hysteroscopic surgical treatment–preliminary report. J Minim Invasive Gynecol. 2005;12:308-11.
20. Friedman JA, Wong JMK, Chaudhari A, et al. Hysteroscopic myomectomy: a comparison of techniques and review of current evidence in the management of abnormal uterine bleeding. Curr Opin Obstet Gynecol. 2018;30(4):243-51.
21. Haber K, Hawkins E, Levie M, et al. Hysteroscopic morcellation: review of the manufacturer and user facility device experience (MAUDE) database. J Minim Invasive Gynecol. 2015;22(1):110-4.
22. Garcia-Velasco JA. In vitro fertilization outcome in women with unoperated bilateral endometriomas. Fertil Steril. 2013;99:1714-9.
23. Nezhat CH, Malik S, Nezhat F, et al. Laparoscopic ureteroneocystostomy and vesicopsoas hitch for infiltrative endometriosis. JSLS. 2004;8(1):3-7.
24. Vercellini P, Pisacreta A, Pesole A, et al. Is ureteral endometriosis an asymmetric disease? BJOG. 2000;107(4):559-61.
25. Sánchez AM, Viganò P, Somigliana E, et al. The distinguishing cellular and molecular features of the endometriotic ovarian cyst: from pathophysiology to the potential endometrioma-mediated damage to the ovary. Hum Reprod Update. 2014;20:217-30.
26. Kitajima M, Defrère S, Dolmans MM, et al. Endometriomas as a possible cause of reduced ovarian reserve in women with endometriosis. Fertil Steril. 2011;96:685-91.

Hysteroscopy

Sachin Naiknaware

INTRODUCTION

Hysteroscopy is a minimally invasive surgical procedure for visualization of endometrial cavity with the aid of a hysteroscope inserted through the vagina and into the cervical opening.

It allows for visualization of uterine cavity and openings of fallopian tube as well as direct examination of vagina, cervix, and cervical canal.

In recent times, modern gynecology has witnessed many technical and technological advances, especially in minimally invasive surgery including hysteroscopy due to introduction of small-diameter hysteroscopes, saline use as a distention medium, and use of "Vaginoscopic techniques" which contributed to widespread use of hysteroscopy as a **gold standard technique** for evaluation of uterine cavity.[1]

INDICATIONS

Hysteroscopy is performed for diagnostic and therapeutic indications.

Hysteroscope is used to diagnose intrauterine pathology and to perform surgery within the endometrial cavity.[2] Hysteroscope allows inspection of uterine cavity as whole and allows to take guided biopsies of pathological lesions which could have been missed on doing blind dilatation and curettage. The FIGO classification system adopted in 2011 integrates hysteroscopy findings into the evaluation of abnormal uterine bleeding.[3]

DIAGNOSTIC HYSTEROSCOPY

Hysteroscopy is performed for evaluation of endometrial cavity, endocervix, and tubal ostia. Common diagnostic indications are:

- Abnormal uterine bleeding
- Endometrial polyps—diagnosis and polypectomy
- Pre IVF
- Submucosal fibroids diagnosis
- Endometrial hyperplasia/thickening
- Retained products of conception/persistent bleeding after MTP
- Identification of isthmocele
- Diagnosis of mullerian anomalies
- Abnormal findings as seen on sonography.

OPERATIVE HYSTEROSCOPY[4]

Operative hysteroscopy is commonly used for:

- Endometrial ablation, to destroy the uterine lining
- Uterine septum resection/to treat a vaginal septum
- Hysteroscopic Myomectomy
- Hysteroscopic Polypectomy, to remove any abnormal growth in the uterus.
- Hysteroscopic adhesiolysis in Asherman's syndrome
- Hysteroscopic metroplasty to increase the size of uterine cavity.

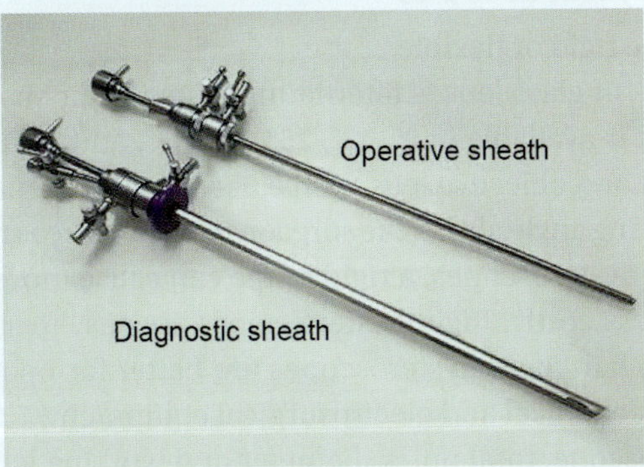

Though laparoscopy has simply modified access into abdominal cavity, hysteroscopy enlightens for the first time the cramped and dark cavity which was not explored till the mid-19th century. During the 1980s, "Traditional Techniques" were used for doing hysteroscopy in which a speculum was inserted and vulsellum was used to hold the cervix and view the uterine cavity but now with the miniaturization of scopes, Vaginoscopic or "no touch technique" is being used for doing hysteroscopy. Vaginoscopic approach to Hysteroscopy was developed by Bettochi et al.

Hysteroscopy offers many benefits to patients requiring evaluation of uterine cavity, especially in a patient presented with abnormal uterine bleeding and also in those patients who had been diagnosed on sonography to have some kind of uterine pathology. It allows a "see and treat" approach.

Traditional operative hysteroscopy has a long learning curve. Th first simultaneous tissue cutting and retrieval system for use in uterine cavity was the TruClear system. It does not use any electrocoagulation. Hemostasis occurred by simultaneous myometrial contraction.

INSTRUMENTATION REQUIRED FOR HYSTEROSCOPY

Though office hysteroscopy can be carried out in an outpatient setting, operative hysteroscopy requiring prolonged time should be carried out in an operation theater. The equipment required are:

- Video camera
- Monitor
- Cold light source
- Light cable

- Suction irrigation pump
- Hysteroscope
- Resectoscope
- Distension media
- Ancillary instruments
- Electrosurgical unit
- Tissue retrieval devices

Types and Sizes of Hysteroscopes

Hysteroscope used can be rigid or flexible,

A rigid scope consists of glass lenses alternating between air spaces to transmit the light to area to be inspected. It is available in 0°, 12°, 25°, 30°, 45°, and 70° as per GTG. It consists of 3 parts—eyepiece, barrel, and objective lens. While 0° scope gives a panoramic view of uterine cavity, increasing the viewing angle allows the surgeon to inspect areas right or left of the midline.

Compared to flexible hysteroscopes, a rigid scope can cause more pain but provide better optical quality and it is less costly. Rigid hysteroscopes are easy to sterilize; the procedure is quicker and less likely to fail. Rigid hysteroscopes are better for operative hysteroscopy and allow use of miniature mechanical and electrosurgical equipment.

While using a hysteroscope, total outer diameter and working length of hysteroscope are considered. Outer diameter of hysteroscope refers to diameter of sheath housing the telescope and instruments. It ranges from 3 to 10 mm. Working length of hysteroscope is measured eyepiece to distal tip and it measures 30–35 cm.

Operative hysteroscopy requires operative sheath with instruments, resectoscopes, and hysteroscopic tissue retrieval system along with distending media **(Table 1)**.

Light Source

Light source with connecting light cable is attached to the eyepiece is used to illuminate the operating field.

Distension Media

Uterine cavity is a potential space between anterior and posterior uterine walls and its lining tends to bleed on contact. Dilatation of uterine cavity is required to provide a global view of endometrial cavity and to clear debris, blood, and tissue fragments.

Distension media used can be gaseous and fluid.

Carbon dioxide is the only gas used in hysteroscopy which was introduced for use during hysteroscopy in 1972 by H J Lindemann, used at an insufflation pressure of 100–120 mm Hg and at a flow rate of 30–60 mL/min to maintain an intracavitary pressure of 40–60 mm Hg.[5]

Three basic distension media used are:

1. High molecular weight dextran
2. Carbon dioxide
3. Low viscosity fluids. Low viscosity fluids can be either **isotonic electrolyte** which includes media such as normal saline and Ringer lactate or **hypotonic electrolyte-free** media such as glycine and sorbitol.

TABLE 1: Hysteroscopic distending media.

Type	*Maximum Fluid Deficit*	*Advantages*	*Disadvantages and Safety Precautions*	*Complications*
Low-Viscosity Fluid Media: Electrolyte-Poor Fluid (e.g., glycine 1.5%; sorbitol 3%; mannitol 5%)	1,000 mL	• Compatible with radiofrequency energy • Monopolar devices require electrolyte-poor fluids	Excessive absorption of these fluids can cause hyponatremia, hyperammonemia, and decreased serum osmolality, with risks of seizures, cerebral edema, and death.	Excessive absorption of these fluids can lead to hyponatremia, hyperammonemia, and decreased serum osmolality, with the potential for seizures, cerebral edema, and death.
Low-Viscosity Fluid Media: Electrolyte-Containing Fluid (e.g., normal saline, sodium lactated solution)	Maximum fluid deficits with isotonic solutions are based on expert opinion; consensus ≈ 2,500 mL	• Readily available • Isotonic • Media of choice during diagnostic hysteroscopy and in operative cases using mechanical, laser, or bipolar energy	Although the risk of hyponatremia and decreased serum osmolality can be reduced by using these media, pulmonary edema and congestive heart failure may still occur. Careful attention to fluid input/output and fluid deficit is required.	Fluid overload causing pulmonary edema and congestive heart failure.

Distension media are used depending on the situation and they have their advantages and disadvantages.

Carbon dioxide

Advantages

- The only gaseous medium used.
- Yields a clear image of endometrial cavity. (However, saline gives a better image.)
- Easy to infuse
- Does not clog essential instrumentation
- Inexpensive
- Readily available
- Well tolerated
- Rapidly absorbed and released.
- Best suited for office diagnostic hysteroscopy

Disadvantages

- May produce bubbling, and bleeding is not lavaged off which is cumbersome and may obscure the view.
- Because CO_2 gas is invisible, a leak in the system may not be noticed for some time.

- A specific machine is required for electronic calibration of the CO_2 flow rate and pressure.
- Finally, use of a laser becomes cumbersome owing to the smoke and fumes.

A high molecular weight (MW)—70,000 MW in a 10% water solution.

Advantages

- Used for both diagnostic and operative hysteroscopy
- Nonelectrolytic
- Nonconductive
- Immiscible with blood
- Minimally leaks through cervix and tubes (viscous)
- Excellent visibility

Disadvantages

- Anaphylactic reaction
- Acute onset respiratory distress syndrome
- Pulmonary edema
- Coagulopathies
- Oliguria
- Acute renal failure

Low molecular weight fluids

Electrolyte free.

- 1.5% Glycine
- 3% Sorbitol
- 5% Mannitol
- Used in operative hysteroscopy while using monopolar resectoscope.

Electrolyte containing

- Normal saline
- Ringer's lactate
- Used in diagnostic hysteroscopy and operative hysteroscopy using bipolar electrode.

Advantages

They can clear debris, mucus, and blood clots from the operative field and continuously wash the uterine cavity, permitting good visualization. Should the mechanism be faulty and leakage of fluid occur, it will be immediately visible. The fluid instilled and recovered can easily be measured.

Procedure

- Surgical planning is the most important part starting from patient selection to choosing a good operative setup.
- Surgery starts with **preoperative evaluation** and preparation of patient starting with explaining and taking **informed consent** of the patient. Patient should be informed about alternative diagnostic and treatment modalities, possible complications, and need to abandon or stop the procedure due to any complication.

- Patient should be evaluated with regard to obstetric and surgical history, medical allergies, or any medical co-morbidities along with complete general examination and abdominal and pelvic examination including bimanual vaginal examination.
- Regarding **timing of hysteroscopy** in premenopausal women, proliferative or follicular phase is good for visualization of uterine cavity and in postmenopausal women it can be done at any time.
- As many cases have difficulty while introducing the scope, it may be prudent to do cervical preparation or dilatation of cervix either by medical pharmacological means or by mechanical methods using dilators. Misoprostol 200–400 µg was given 24–48 hours prior and was found to reduce cervical resistance in a premenopausal patient.
- With all equipment in place, the procedure is started. By positioning the patient in the dorsal lithotomy position, we introduce the speculum and use the tenaculum to hold the cervix. The hysteroscope is then introduced through cervical os under direct endoscopic vision. The speculum is then removed.
- Nowadays, vaginoscopic or "No touch technique" is used while introducing smaller dimeter scopes during office hysteroscopy. Starting from endocervix evaluating its glands, the scope is then advanced to inspect the endometrial cavity in a systematic fashion with both ostia and anterior and posterior uterine walls.

COMPLICATIONS

Complications from hysteroscopy are rare but some are potentially life threatening. Some known complications are

- Uterine perforation
- Cervical laceration
- Urinary tract injury
- Excessive fluid absorption
- Bowel injury
- Hemorrhage
- Embolism
- Electrosurgical injury
- Infection
- Rarely dissemination of tumor.

How to tackle operative challenges.

Sometimes, we may face some operative challenges as:

- Cervical stenosis
- Uterine malposition
- Difficult uterine distention
- Vision blur due to bleeding.
- Cervical trauma
- Uterine perforation

1. **Difficult entry** can be due to cervical stenosis due to conization of cervix, LLETZ, previous curettage, Asherman's syndrome, and Fothergill's repair. Sometimes, it is due to adhesion

and fixed direction of cervix. To prevent this complication, Misoprostol can be used 4–8 hours prior to procedure and mechanical dilatation with Hegar's dilator can be used. Also, risk of false passage can be prevented by entry of hysteroscope under direct vision.

If there is severe stenosis, a scissor can be used in operative channel, advancing the scope while opening jaw of scissor. Sometimes, cruciate incision can be taken on cervix to introduce the scope.

2. **False passage** can sometime occur during insertion of scope. It is recognized by visualization of muscle filers and nonvisualization of tubal ostia. In such a case, move back the scope slowly and try to identify the true cavity.

   If a cavity could not be seen, discontinue the procedure to prevent fluid from being absorbed through the injury.

   False passage can be prevented by dilating the cervix slowly and stop as soon as internal os is seen. Put the scope into external os with inflow open and outflow shut and letting fluid pressure dilating the cervix.
3. **Excessive bleeding** can occur when endomyometrial junction is breached in myomectomy or TCRE (Transcervical resection of endometrium) procedure.

   When the bleeding is excessive, it produces the "JAPANESE FLAG SIGN" obscuring the field of vision. This bleeding can be managed by putting in Foley's catheter with balloon inflation with 15–30 mL of saline, packing with gauze soaked in dilute vasopressin and bipolar coagulation.
4. **Perforation** can also occur during hysteroscopy with approximately 14 perforations per 1,000 operations. Chances of perforation are more in resection of fundal and lateral adhesions. It is diagnosed by collapse of cavity and rapid inflow of fluid. Bowel or omentum can be seen and the scope goes far inside the cavity.

   Management of perforation depends on the instrument that caused it. If perforation is caused by energy source or a hysteroscope more than 5 mm in diameter, then laparoscopy is needed. If perforation occurred by cold scissors, Hegar's dilator patient can be observed. It can be prevented by applying current only when electrode is moving toward the operator and simultaneous use of ultrasound or laparoscopy guidance.
5. **Embolism** is a dreaded complication that may occur when CO_2 is being used as the distention medium but as CO_2 is soluble in blood emboli can resolve rapidly.
   - Embolism can be prevented by purging air from all tubings before introducing scope
   - Intracervical vassopressin
   - Avoiding Trendelenburg position.
   - Remove last dilator just before introducing scope
   - Limit repeated removal and reinsertion
   - Right equipment and setting.

ADVANTAGES OF HYSTEROSCOPY

- A hysteroscopy can be used to: investigate symptoms or problems—such as heavy periods, unusual vaginal bleeding, postmenopausal bleeding, pelvic pain, repeated miscarriages, or infertility. Pathology missed on imaging may be identified under vision.[6]

- After diagnosing conditions such as fibroids and polyps (noncancerous growths in the womb). For these cases a "see and treat" approach may be taken.
- Treat conditions and problems, such as removing fibroids, polyps, displaced intrauterine devices (IUDs), and intrauterine adhesions (scar tissue that causes absent periods and reduced fertility) in a safe manner under vision.
- It can be done as an office procedure with local anesthesia for diagnostic purpose. This is cost effective.

DISADVANTAGES OF HYSTEROSCOPY

- As a diagnostic modality, hysteroscopy is invasive.
- There is a risk of the surgery such as injury, infections and anesthesia risk for operative hysteroscopy.
- Operative hysteroscopy has a long learning curve.
- Rigid hysteroscopy can be painful and requires analgesia.

CONTRAINDICATIONS

- Active pelvic infection including genital herpes infection[7]
- Viable intrauterine pregnancy
- Known Pyometra
- Known cervical cancer.

Coagulopathy, Coronary heart disease, and excessive uterine bleeding are relative contraindications.

Recent advances in technology paved way for outpatient **office hysteroscopy**. Also, introduction of **morcellator and resectoscopes** and tissue retrieval devises makes hysteroscopy a safe, effective alternative to laparoscopic surgery for some intrauterine pathologies, making it a gold standard tool for investigation and treatment of intrauterine pathologies.

From above, we can see that many gynecological operations can be performed with the use of hysteroscope and it will not be wrong to state that hysteroscopy will replace hysterectomy as a therapeutic option in specific cases of heavy menstrual bleeding and menorrhagia and will offer shorter hospital stay and reduced mortality and morbidity along with reduced cost now. "HYSTEROSCOPE IS NOW BEING SEEN AS A STETHOSCOPE OF GYNECOLOGIST".

LONG QUESTIONS AND ANSWERS

Q1. Critically evaluate hysteroscopic tubal sterilization technique.

DNB/2018 (10 marks)

Q2. Critically evaluate hysteroscopic tubal sterilization technique.

RGUHS, 2018 (20 marks) (Add in short equipment, media, preoperative procedure, etc.)

Sterilization

Female sterilization by tubal occlusion or ligation is the most common permanent method for contraception used globally by married women of the reproductive age group. Female sterilization prevents pregnancy by occluding or disrupting the fallopian tube patency and impeding sperm transport to the ampulla of the tube where fertilization of the ovum occurs.

Hysteroscopic Sterilization

Less invasive methods of tubal occlusion have been investigated as potentially safe and effective alternative methods of sterilization. These include hysteroscopic insertion through the vagina into the fallopian tubes of micro-inserts (Essure® system) or substances such as liquid siloxane (Ovabloc) or quinacrine pellets, or application of an electrosurgical technique.

Advantage

The Essure system is indicated for women who desire permanent fertility control by bilateral occlusion of the fallopian tubes. It may also be used in women who desire sterilization and who have comorbidities that are contraindications for laparoscopic tubal sterilization due to a higher surgical risk **(Fig. 1)**.

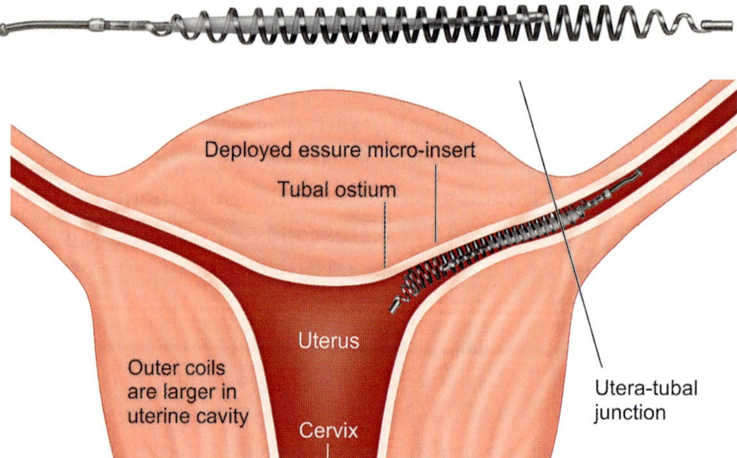

Fig. 1: Essure system.

- The System is comprised of the Essure microinsert, a disposable delivery device, and a disposable split introducer. The Essure microinsert is a spring-like device 40 millimeter (mm) in length and 0.8 mm in diameter that consists of a stainless steel inner coil, a nickel-titanium (Nitinol) expanding outer coil, and polyethylene terephthalate (PET) fibers. The PET fibers are wound in and around the inner coil. The device is placed into the fallopian tube, spanning the uterotubal junction, using a standard 5-mm hysteroscope.
- Patients should be informed that Essure hysteroscopy is irreversible.
- The failure rate of Essure is comparable to laparoscopic sterilization at about 2–3/1,000.

Various agents used for hysteroscopic sterilization with advantages and precautions.

Trans-cervical	*Method*	*Type*	*Advantages*	*Disadvantages*
	Hysteroscopy interval only	Physical occlusion using microinserts (Essure® system)	• Minimally invasive • No incisions, less discomfort • Fast recovery, same day in most cases • Indicated in all women, including those with comorbidities which contraindicate general anesthesia • Can be performed as outpatient procedure • Local rather than general anesthesia	• Women must use another method of birth control until their fallopian tubes are completely blocked (at 3 months) • Relatively new; potential long-term risks are unknown • Irreversible
		Mechanical, formed-in-place silicone plug (Ovaloc®)	• Nonsurgical; high success rate • Silicone conforms to shape of tube • Plug position can be confirmed by X-ray at 3 months after the procedure	• Tubal spasm may require repeat applications in up to 20% of women • Fracture of silicone plug during migration may occur • Expensive delivery equipment • Risk of extravasation of silicone into paratubal or myometrial tissue
		Chemical agents (quinacrine)	• Simple • Nonsurgical • High success rate with two applications • Low cost	• Often requires several applications • Sterilization rate varies • Failure rates depend on dosage and number of insertions • Lack of reliable methods to confirm occlusion (X-ray, HSG, or sonography not consistently accurate) • HSG may increase failure risk • Shown to be mutagenic in vitro, raising safety concerns (not confirmed in large clinical studies
		Thermal electro-coagulation	Ease of access Moderate success rates	Significant complications, including: uterine perforation, bowel damage, and peritonitis

- Contraindications for use of the Essure system listed by manufacturer are:
- Uncertainty about the desire to end fertility
- Prior tubal ligation, pregnancy or suspected pregnancy, delivery or termination of a pregnancy less than 6 weeks before device placement or during menstruation
- Unwillingness to use another method of contraception for at least 3 months after the Essure placement procedure
- Allergy to contrast media or to the microinsert material nickel
- History of tubal surgery (e.g., tubal ligation, ectopic pregnancy, tuboplasty)

- Uterine structural abnormalities that might impede placement of the Essure® microinserts (e.g., bicornuate uterus)
- Women in whom only one microinsert can be placed (e.g., unicornuate uterus)
- Hydrosalpinx
- Active or recent pelvic infection
- Current immunosuppressive therapy (e.g., systemic corticosteroids, chemotherapy)

Confirmation of the success of hysteroscopic sterilization after 3 months is done by X-ray or Ultrasound pelvis. If required, an HSG may be done.

Hysteroscopy is technologically dependent and potentially dangerous, so we should proceed only with good knowledge of procedure and equipment.

Complications

Complications from hysteroscopy are rare but some are potential life-threatening. Some known complications are:

- Uterine perforation
- Cervical laceration
- Urinary tract injury
- Excessive fluid absorption
- Bowel injury
- Hemorrhage
- Embolism
- Electrosurgical injury
- Infection
- Rarely dissemination of tumor

Q3. Write in brief about recent advances in hysteroscopy.

Hysteroscopy is a minimally invasive surgical procedure for visualization of endometrial cavity with the aid of hysteroscope inserted through the vagina and into the cervical opening.

In recent times, modern gynecology has witnessed many technical and technological advances, especially in minimally invasive surgery including hysteroscopy due to introduction of small diameter hysteroscope. Some of the recent advances in hysteroscopic technique and instruments will be discussed here.

Office Hysteroscopy

Also known as "see and treat hysteroscopy" since 1990 because of the small size of scope and less painful procedure, it has gained widespread acceptance in clinical practice and currently office hysteroscopy is considered as gold standard for examination of uterine cavity and overcoming the limitations of dilation and curettage and other blind procedures.[8]

For office hysteroscopy, either rigid or flexible scope of 4 mm/2.9 mm is used. Miniature hysteroscope 2.7 mm (with a 3–3.5 mm sheath) should be used for diagnostic outpatient hysteroscopy **(Fig. 2)**. Flexible scopes are less painful as compared to rigid ones requiring no cervical dilatation, but they have some limitations such as higher cost for purchase and maintenance go equipment, more efforts for cleaning, disinfection, and sterilization, reduced size of image seen on screen, and fragile and difficult to use in use in cases of intrauterine adhesions.

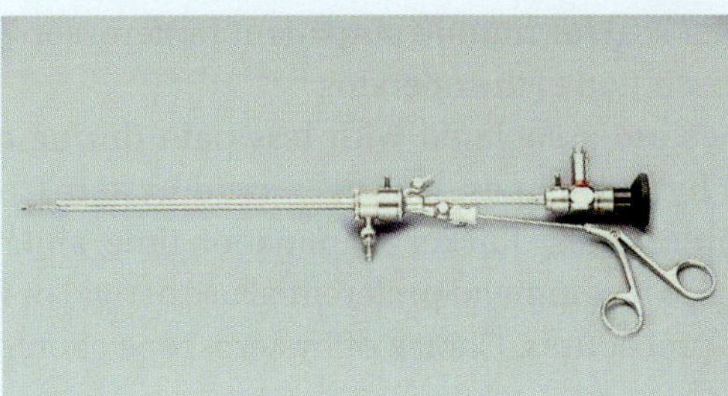

Fig. 2: Hysteroscope.

Saline and CO_2 are the most commonly used distension media used in office hysteroscopy. Now distention with normal saline is preferred due to more patient comfort and its good tolerability. It is more cost effective. It provides good view in cases of intrauterine bleeding and also vaginoscopic or no-touch approach is easier with saline in. Distension pressure is maintained with electronically controlled suction irrigation pump obtaining constant pressure of <70 mm Hg. So nowadays, office hysteroscopy should be the first option to be considered for diagnosing and treating vaginal, cervical, and intrauterine pathologies.

RCOG guidelines for office hysteroscopy recommend the following principles:

- All gynecology units should provide a dedicated outpatient hysteroscopy service to aid management of women with abnormal uterine bleeding. There are clinical and economic benefits associated with this type of service.
- Outpatient hysteroscopy should be conducted outside of the formal operating theater setting in an appropriately sized, equipped, and staffed treatment room with adjoining, private changing facilities and toilet.
- Outpatient hysteroscopy should be performed in an appropriately sized and fully equipped treatment room. This may be a dedicated hysteroscopy suite or a multipurpose facility.
- The healthcare professional should have the necessary skills and expertise to carry out hysteroscopy.
- There should be a nurse chaperone regardless of the gender of the clinician.
- Written patient information should be provided before the appointment and consent for the procedure should be taken.
- Routine use of opiate analgesia before outpatient hysteroscopy should be avoided as it may cause adverse effects.
- Women without contraindications should be advised to consider taking standard doses of **nonsteroidal anti-inflammatory agents (NSAIDs) around 1 hour** before their scheduled outpatient hysteroscopy appointment with the aim of reducing pain in the immediate postoperative period.
- Routine cervical preparation before outpatient hysteroscopy should not be used in the absence of any evidence of benefit in terms of reduction of pain and rates of failure or uterine trauma.
- Miniature hysteroscopes (2.7 mm with a 3–3.5 mm sheath) should be used for diagnostic outpatient hysteroscopy as they significantly reduce the discomfort experienced by the woman. There is insufficient evidence to recommend 0° or fore-oblique optical lenses (i.e.,

12°, 25°, or 30° offset lenses) for routine outpatient hysteroscopy. Choice of hysteroscope should be left to the discretion of the operator.

- Flexible hysteroscopes are associated with less pain during outpatient hysteroscopy compared with rigid hysteroscopes. However, rigid hysteroscopes may provide better images, fewer failed procedures, quicker examination time, and reduced cost. Thus, there is insufficient evidence to recommend preferential use of rigid or flexible hysteroscopes for diagnostic outpatient procedures. Choice of hysteroscope should be left to the discretion of the operator.
- For routine outpatient hysteroscopy, the choice of distension medium between carbon dioxide and normal saline should be left to the discretion of the operator as neither is superior in reducing pain, although uterine distension with **normal saline appears to reduce the incidence of vasovagal episodes**.
- Uterine distension with normal saline allows improved image quality and allows outpatient diagnostic hysteroscopy to be completed more quickly compared with carbon dioxide.
- Operative outpatient hysteroscopy, using bipolar electrosurgery, requires the use of normal saline to act as both the **distension and conducting medium**.
- Blind cervical dilatation to facilitate insertion of the miniature outpatient hysteroscope is unnecessary in the majority of procedures. Routine cervical dilatation is associated with pain, vasovagal reactions, and uterine trauma and should be avoided.
- **Cervical dilatation generally requires administration of local cervical anesthesia**. Standard protocols regarding the type, maximum dosage, and route of administration of anesthesia should be developed and implemented to help both recognize and prevent rare but potentially serious adverse effects resulting from systemic vascular absorption.
- Instillation of **local anesthetic into the cervical canal** does not reduce pain during diagnostic outpatient hysteroscopy but may **reduce the incidence of vasovagal reactions**.
- Topical application of **local anesthetic to the ectocervix** should be considered where **application of a cervical tenaculum** is necessary. Application of local anesthetic into or around the cervix is associated with a **reduction of the pain** experienced during outpatient diagnostic hysteroscopy. However, it is unclear how clinically significant this reduction in pain is. Consideration should be given to the routine administration of **intracervical or paracervical local anesthetic**, particularly in **postmenopausal women**.
- Miniaturization of hysteroscopes and increasing use of the vaginoscopic technique may diminish any advantage of intracervical or paracervical anesthesia. Routine administration of intracervical or paracervical local anesthetic should be used where larger diameter hysteroscopes are being employed (outer diameter greater than 5mm) and where the need for cervical dilatation is anticipated (e.g., cervical stenosis).
- Routine administration of intracervical or paracervical local anesthetic **is not indicated to reduce the incidence of vasovagal reactions**.
- Conscious sedation should not be routinely used in outpatient hysteroscopic procedures as it confers no advantage in terms of pain control and the woman's satisfaction over local anesthesia. Life-threatening complications can result from the use of conscious sedation. Appropriate monitoring and staff skills are mandatory if procedures are to be undertaken using conscious sedation.

- Vaginoscopy reduces pain during diagnostic rigid outpatient hysteroscopy.
- Vaginoscopy should be the standard technique for outpatient hysteroscopy, especially where successful insertion of a vaginal speculum is anticipated to be difficult and where blind endometrial biopsy is not required.[9]

The above are ideal recommendations for office hysteroscopy. However, clinical judgment and availability of resuscitation facilities should be considered for any untoward incidents.

Electronic Suction Irrigation Pump (Hysteromat)

It is an endoscopic automatic system for irrigation during hysteroscopy. It is a pressure-controlled double-roller pump that provides sufficient dilatation of uterine cavity with continuous fluid exchange at all times.

It offers the benefit of ensuring optimal visualization and constant intrauterine pressure allowing a surgeon to perform various intrauterine surgeries with ease **(Fig. 3)**.

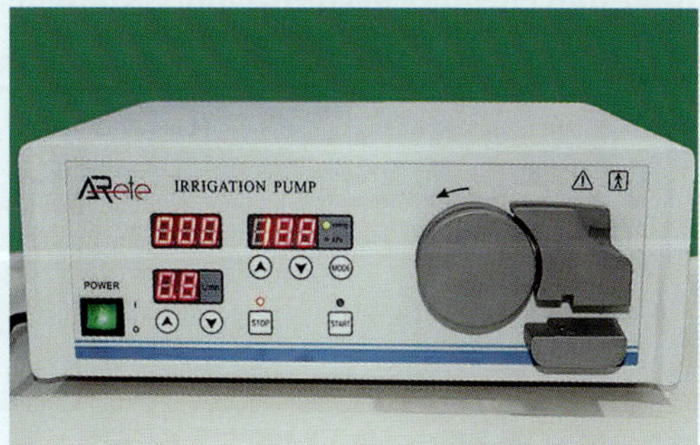

Fig. 3: Hysteromat.

Intrauterine Bigatti shaver was developed as an option for hysteroscopic morcellation with the intention to improve the results of conventional resectoscope by reducing the number of complications **(Fig. 4)**.

- It consists of a 6° angled telescope with an integrated sheath and working channel into which a rigid shaver is introduced. The benefits of using IBS are sustained intraoperative visibility, short procedure time, and definitive management of pathology. It also preserves endometrial integrity.

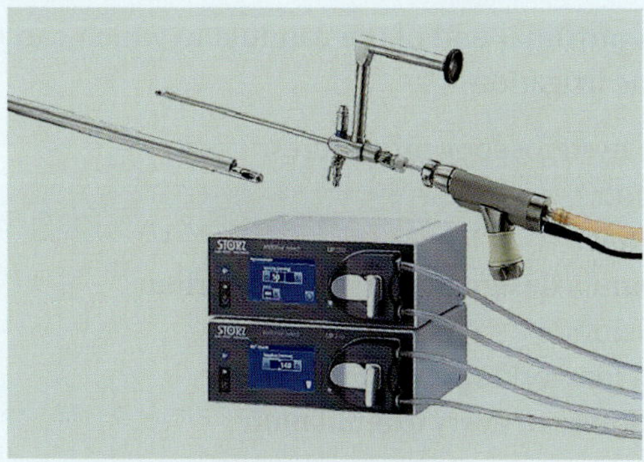

Fig. 4: Intrauterine Bigatti shaving.

Bipolar Resectoscope

- The resectoscope used in hysteroscopy consists of 2.9/4 mm scope with a 12° or 30° viewing angle to always keep the loop under vision.
- Two commonly used resectoscopes are monopolar and bipolar resectoscopes. Conventional hysteroscopy uses a **monopolar resectoscope** in which current passes from the active electrode through the patient's body toward returning electrode, and the distention medium used is glycine. This system is potentially dangerous since the electrons flow through the body outside the surgeon's visual control before they return to the generator.
- To avoid this complication, bipolar resectoscopes are introduced in which the current flows through the tissue are restricted to the area between the two electrode loops that is under visual control of surgeon.

EndoSee (Fig. 5)

It is a **handheld battery-operated cordless hysteroscopy system** that consists of two parts.

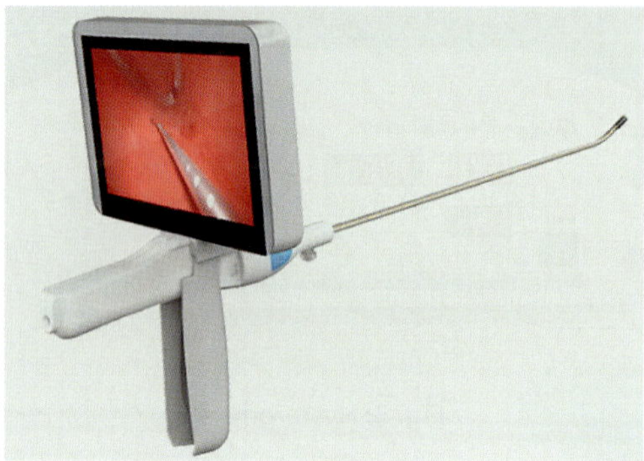

Fig. 5: EndoSee.

- The hand tower contains a 3.5 inch LCD monitor with video and control electronics and a rechargeable battery. The hysteroscopes are a single-use semirigid curved cannula with a diameter of 15 F and length of 287 mm.
- The lens, camera, and light source are placed at the tip and comprises a digital processing chip with CMOS (complimentary metal oxide semiconductor sensor) with integrated LED dual light sources.
- There is a port at the proximal end of the cannula to which can be attached a syringe or inflow tubing for saline irrigation.

Features to help in-office hysteroscopy procedures:

- Clear color visualization.
- Reusable display module.
- Sterile, single-use cannula designed for ease of insertion
- Channel for fluid infusion
- Reusable instruments for working channel
- Still image or video capture of every examination
- The picture that you take can be seen
- Examination data can be transferred to your computer via USB cable.

This device incorporates the benefits of direct visualization without the limitations of traditional hysteroscopy. Its ergonomic, handheld design allows for precise control and ease of use so you can advance patient care and your practice.[10]

Endo-shaft disposable hysteroscopy sheath.

- Endo-shaft **disposable hysteroscopy sheath** is an adjunct to the hysteroscopes that are available, which provides a barrier between the patient and the endoscope so that it can be used with another patient without being re-sterilized.

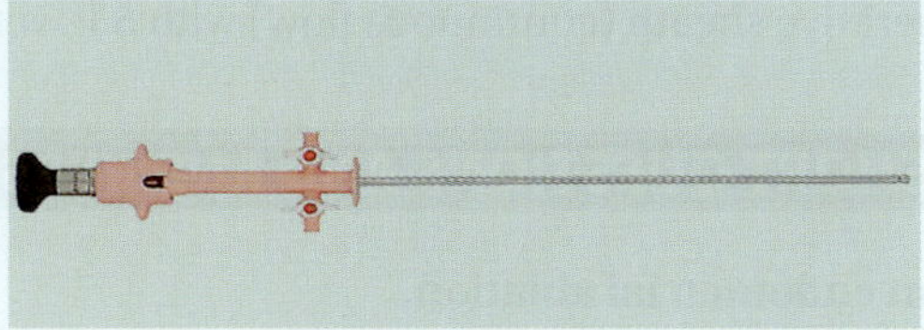

- A single hysteroscope could be used for all patients. This may reduce preparation time, enabling more patients to be seen on a list and without the same capital expenditure.
- Irrigation fluid passes down the outer sheath, and the view at the hysteroscope tip is through a clear window at the distal tip of the sheath.
- The sheath is reported by the company as having smooth rounded surfaces to allow it to easily pass through the cervical canal.
- Endoshaft can be used with the commonly available hysteroscopes.

UBIPack GYN

- The purpose of the UBIPack GYN is to provide a **portable system** for undertaking hysteroscopic procedures.
- It consists of a one CCD (charge-coupled device) camera that has a lower power consumption than the standard CCD camera, with 3 m of cable which can be inserted into a USB port of a laptop or personal computer.
- It can be used with either flexible or rigid endoscopes and the software.
- ICE (Intelligent Control Endoscope) technology provided enables the camera to recognize and adapt to the endoscope in use. Both regular and pendulum heads are available.

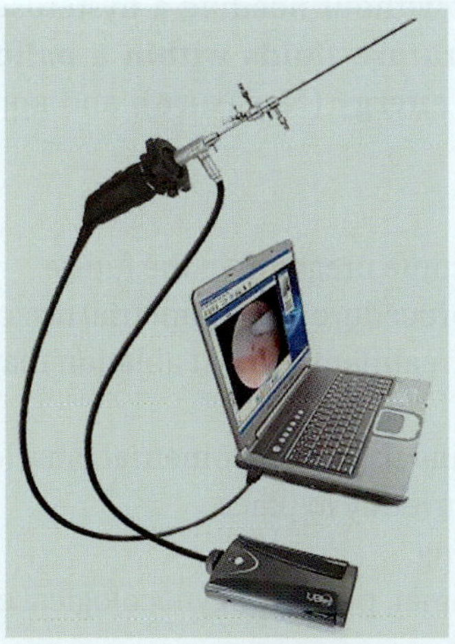

- Light is provided by a compact LED source that has a long duration of use (50,000 h) and with the equivalent light intensity of a 100W Xenon source, but with lower heat emission.

- The computer software provided, Sopro imaging, functions with Windows 7 and provides patient management screens and enables printing of medical reports.
- Conventional diagnostic and operative rigid hysteroscopes are available too; 30° rod lens, 2.7 mm diameter, 300 mm length hysteroscope with a 10-F (3.3-mm) diagnostic sheath and a 14.9-F (5.0-mm) operative sheath (continuous flow) with 5 F working channel.

SHORT QUESTIONS AND ANSWERS

Q1. Write a short note on endometrial ablation.

Q2. Operative hysteroscopy. *MS Obgyn/II/2023. DNB 2007, 2013 (5 marks)*

- **Endometrial ablation** is a procedure for treating abnormal uterine bleeding by destroying the endometrium. It is a minimally invasive surgical procedure used to treat heavy menstrual bleeding. The procedure works by destroying endometrium.
- Abnormal uterine bleeding (AUB) refers to excessive, sustained, or random bleeding from the uterus that occurs without systemic disease of hemostasis, intrauterine contraception, pregnancy, or demonstrable pelvic pathology. It may be ovulatory or anovulatory.
- AUB is a common gynecological condition affecting many premenopausal women, severely disrupting their physical, social, and psychological quality of life. Annually, 1 in 20 women of reproductive age consults their gynecologists concerning heavy menstrual bleeding (AUB).
- Endometrial ablation is broadly classified into the first and second generations. The **first-generation endometrial ablative** techniques are hysteroscopic methods, including **rollerball ablation, laser ablation, and transcervical resection of the endometrium (TCRE)**.
- The **second-generation endometrial ablative** techniques can destroy the endometrium through different methods without needing a hysteroscopy. The most common three methods **use high-temperature fluids within a balloon (Thermachoice), bipolar radiofrequency electrical energy (Novasure),** and application of **microwave energy (Microsulis)**.

Contraindications

- Pregnancy or a desire to become pregnant in the future.
- Prior endometrial ablation procedure or endometrial resection. Currently available devices are not designed for repeat treatment. Repeat ablation may result in serious injury such as internal burns.
- Certain medications that could thin the myometrial muscles such as long-term steroid use.
- Intrauterine device (IUD) currently in place.
- Undiagnosed vaginal bleeding.
- Known or suspected abdominal, pelvic, or gynecological cancer.

- History of previous classical cesarean section or other conditions that could weaken the muscular layer of the uterus.
- Active genital, pelvic, or urinary tract infection, for example, cervicitis, vaginitis, endometritis, salpingitis, or cystitis at the time of treatment.
- Confirmed cases of Endometrial hyperplasia on histopathology

Advantages

- The main benefit of the procedure is the reduction in menstrual bleeding and improvement in quality of life. It has a faster recovery and needs only a short admission.

Adverse Effects

- The most common side effects of endometrial ablation occur during or immediately following the procedure and include pain, cramping, nausea, and vaginal discharge/ bleeding/spotting. You may also have temporary diarrhea or a headache.
- Injury to the organs in the abdomen, such as bowel or bladder perforation or burns, may occur
- Infection
- Need for an additional surgery, including a possible hysterectomy, due to a complication during the procedure.

Polyps

- Polyps increase in incidence with age, and the peak incidence is in the 5th decade of life. They decline after menopause.
- 21–40% of patients with AUB and 10% asymptomatic women may have polyps.
- Symptomatic polyps detected on ultrasound are always removed hysteroscopically.
- Asymptomatic polyps in postmenopausal patients are always removed.
- In premenopausal patients, asymptomatic small polyps of less than 1 cm size may be kept under surveillance. But if the size is more than 1 cm, they are removed hysteroscopically
- Polyps may be avulsed with a pre- and posthysteroscopy. The 2nd hysteroscopy vision may be obscured by bleeding.
- Polyps may be removed hysteroscopically
- It may be removed by cold scissor or bipolar electrosurgical resection may be done.
- Polyps more than 2 cm may be removed piecemeal with a morcellator like TruClear.

Advantages of hysteroscopic polypectomy

- It is safe, simple, and better than blind removal.
- There is lower chance of recurrence.
- There is lower chance of missing a malignancy.

Submucous Fibroids

- Submucous fibroids may cause abnormal uterine bleeding and subfertility.
- They may need hysteroscopic resection. Submucous fibroid FIGO type 1 protrudes into the cavity and is easy to remove hysteroscopically.
  Type 2 (less than 50% intramural) and type 3 (more than equal to 50% intramural) can be resected and fibroid may get extruded into the uterine cavity.

- Larger fibroids which extend into the myometrium may be removed in a 2-step procedure 4–6 weeks apart. The fibroid is shaved to the level of the cavity and left. It then gets extruded. GnRH analog may be used preoperatively.
- Fibroid may be enucleated with a cold loop followed by resection.
- Miniature morcellators like TruClear and MyoCure use mechanical energy followed by suction
- Bipolar resection with Versapoint can be used also.

Complication

- There is a risk of perforation with resection of fibroid. Depth should be carefully assessed.

Q3. Discuss the complications of hysteroscopic surgery.[8]

- Hysteroscopy is a minimally invasive surgical procedure for visualization of endometrial cavity with the aid of a hysteroscope inserted through the vagina and into the cervical opening.
- It allows for visualization of uterine cavity, openings of fallopian tube, and direct examination of vagina, cervix, and cervical canal.

Complications

Complications from hysteroscopy are rare but some are potentially life-threatening. Some known complications are:

- Uterine perforation
- Cervical laceration
- Excessive fluid absorption
- Bowel injury
- Hemorrhage
- Embolism
- Electrosurgical injury
- Infection
- Rarely dissemination of tumor.

Complications tend to occur when contraindications are ignored and when incorrect surgical technique or instruments are used.

Importance of preventing, recognizing, and appropriately managing the complications of hysteroscopy is the need.

Complications can be categorized as complications that occur during surgery, immediate postoperative period, and late complications.

Immediate complications are caused by cervical dilatation and distension media and surgical techniques include uterine perforation, fluid overload-related complications such as in hyponatremia, "transurethral resection of prostate" (TURP) like syndrome and glycine toxicity, hemorrhage caused by cervical or uterine laceration, and electrosurgical burns.

Systemic complications such as arrhythmia and venous gas embolism may occur.

Late complications include intrauterine adhesions, pelvic inflammatory disease, and hematometra. Complications may occur in subsequent pregnancies and in rare cases postablation sterilization syndrome.

Uterine perforation is one of the most common complications of operative hysteroscopy occurring in about 0.8–1.5 % of cases. Most commonly, it occurs during cervical dilatation or during insertion of a hysteroscope. It may lead to vaginal bleeding, visceral organ injury, and sometimes concealed intra-abdominal hemorrhage.

Uterine cavity needs to be distended for visualization and carrying out surgical procedures. **Distension media-related complications** can occur. Commonly used distension media allows continuous irrigation , provides a clear uterine cavity view, and enables to use mechanical and electrosurgical equipment.

Fluid absorption occurs through open sinuses and fallopian tube. Some factors that increase fluid absorption are **duration** of surgical procedure, **pressure of irrigation fluid, presence of trauma to cervix**, **depth of tumor** to be removed.

Complications also depend on the **type of fluid** used. To prevent these complication, the British Society for Gynaecological Endoscopy and ESGE advocated some preventive measures such as:

- Use of sodium chloride 0.9% as irrigation fluid
- **Monitoring the inflow and outflow of fluid** during the procedure.
- Deficit of fluid calculation
- Restricting the intravenous fluids
- Maintaining a normal mean arterial pressure

Distension media-related complications are mostly seen with use of **low viscosity media like 1.5% glycine and 3% sorbitol**. It can cause **hyponatremia, hyperammonemia, and decreased serum osmolality with potential seizures, hypotonic encephalopathy, cerebral edema, permanent neurological damage, and death**. 5% mannitol is less likely to cause hypoosmolality.

Excess absorption in **normal saline** does not cause hyponatremia but can cause **fluid overload**.

Fluid deficit can be estimated by **manual calculation and automated fluid management systems.**

In manual calculation, the volume of fluid collected in the perineal bag is calculated and subtracted from the fluid quantity infused every 15 minutes. Automated fluid management systems use calibrated electronic weighing scales.

The maximum fluid deficit allowed for hypotonic solutions is **1,000 mL for healthy patients and 750 mL for elderly patients**.

For **normal saline**, the fluid deficit allowed is **up to 1,500–2,500 mL for healthy patients and 750 mL for those with cardiovascular disease**.

Fluid absorption is reduced by **preoperative GnRH agonists and intraoperative injection of vasopressin**.

If excess fluid deficit for a hypotonic fluid occurs, **serum electrolytes** need to be measured and the **patient is evaluated for volume overload**.

- Asymptomatic hyponatremia can be treated with **fluid restriction and careful monitoring of urine output**.
- Fluid overload from normal saline can be managed by fluid restriction along with **intravenous diuretic furosemide** (20–40 mg).

- Symptomatic hyponatremia needs management with **hypertonic saline and is done by a multidisciplinary team** including an intensivist.

Venous gas embolism is one of the complications of hysteroscopy when CO_2 is used as a distending medium.

Other complications such as cervical laceration, hemorrhage, and electrosurgical burns can occur; recognizing and managing the complications are of utmost importance.

MULTIPLE CHOICE QUESTIONS

Q1. What is hysteroscopy?

a. Telescopic examination of thorax
b. Telescopic examination of vagina
c. Telescopic examination of abdominal cavity
d. Telescopic examination of uterine cavity

Ans. d. Telescopic examination of uterine cavity

Q2. Can operative hysteroscopy with monopolar cautery be used with this media?

a. Normal saline
b. 3% sorbitol
c. Carbon dioxide
d. Ringer Lactate

Ans. b. 3% sorbitol

Q3. Hypo-osmolality is a complication associated with this distension medium

a. Normal saline
b. Carbon dioxide
c. 1.5% glycine
d. Mannitol

Ans. c. 1.5% glycine

Q4. What size of polyps need to be removed even if asymptomatic?

a. >2 cm
b. >1.5 cm
c. >1 cm
d. Any size

Ans. c. >1 cm

Q5. What size of fibroids may be removed by hysteroscopy by an experienced surgeon?

a. 4 cm
b. 3 cm
c. 2 cm
d. 5 cm

Ans. d. 5 cm

Q6. Which of the following statements is false?

a. Type 1 submucosal fibroids have more than 50% of their volume protruding into the uterine cavity
b. Uterine adhesiolysis for Asherman's syndrome is associated with one of the highest risks for uterine perforation
c. Maintaining good visibility with bipolar resectoscope is more difficult than using monopolar resectoscope
d. Cervical ripening agents should be used for all diagnostic procedures.

Ans. c. Maintaining good visibility with bipolar resectoscope is more difficult than using monopolar resectoscope

Q7. Regarding use of hysteroscopic morcellator, which statement is false?
a. The TruClear system avoids the risk of thermal injury from spread of electrical energy
b. Operative hysteroscopy using traditional electrical resectoscope has a short learning curve
c. Saline solution is used for distention and irrigation
d. Using TruClear system polyps, small fibroids and product of conception can be removed.

Ans. b. Operative hysteroscopy using traditional electrical resectoscope has a short learning curve

Q8. Regarding outpatient hysteroscopy which statement is true?
a. Miniaturization of high-resolution hysteroscope adversely affected optical performance
b. Outpatient hysteroscopy allows accurate diagnosis of submucous fibroid and polyps
c. There is little evidence to suggest that outpatient hysteroscopy avoids complications and allows quicker recovery and lower costs
d. There is clear evidence to support the safety and effectiveness of outpatient endometrial ablation and hysteroscopic cannulation concomitantly.

Ans. b. Outpatient hysteroscopy allows accurate diagnosis of submucous fibroid and polyps

Q9. Mark the false statement.
a. Endometrial thinning agents have no effects on short-term postoperative outcomes.
b. Roller ball ablation in comparison to TCRE shows no difference in reintervention rates in long-term follow-up.
c. Endometrial thinning agents have no effect on long-term postoperative outcomes.
d. All first-generation endometrial ablation techniques have similar complication rates.

Ans. c. Endometrial thinning agents have no effect on long-term postoperative outcomes.

Q10. Regarding diagnostic hysteroscopy, identify the false statement.
a. Diagnostic hysteroscopy is less painful than miniature endometrial biopsy.
b. Hysteroscopy is the gold standard test for focal intrauterine pathologies as polyp and submucous fibroids.
c. Adenomyosis can be reliably detected by hysteroscopic inspection of uterine cavity.
d. Hysteroscopy performed in conjugation with directed endometrial biopsies has high accuracy in diagnosing endometrial hyperplasia and endometrial cancer.

Ans. c. Adenomyosis can be reliably detected by hysteroscopic inspection of uterine cavity.

LONG QUESTIONS

Q1. Discuss indications, advantages, and disadvantages of hysteroscopic surgeries.
DNB II/JUN 2018 (10 marks)

Q2. NOTES Natural Orifice Transluminal Endoscopic Surgery in Obstetrics and Gynecology
DNB/Paper 4/2022 (10 marks)

Q3. Operative hysteroscopy. *MUHS MS Obgy/II/2023, DNB 2007, 2013 (?)*

Q4. Hysteroscopy in gynecology.
DNB/2UY018, 2019. (shorten the same answer for a short note) (5 marks)

Q4. Distension media used in hysteroscopy. *DNB/Paper 4/2023, 2014 (5 marks)*

REFERENCES

1. Bettocchi S,Selvaggi L, A vaginoscopic approach to reduce the pain of office hysteroscopy. J Am Assoc Gynecol Laparosc .1997;4(2):255-8.
2. Orlando MS, Bradley LD. Implementation of office hysteroscopy for the evaluation and treatment of intrauterine pathology. Obstet Gynecol. 2022;140(3):499-513.
3. Munro MG, Critchley HD, Border MS, et al. FIGO classification system (PAL-COEIN) for abnormal uterine bleeding in non gravid women of reproductive age. Int J Gynecol Obstet. 2011;113;3-13.
4. Centini G, Lazzeri L, Petraaglia F, et al. Modern operative hysteroscopy. Minerva Ginecol. 2016; 68(2):126-32.
5. Cooper NA, Smith P, Khan KS, et al. A systematic review of the effect of distention medium on pain during outpatient hysteroscopy. Fertil Steril. 2011;95:264-71.
6. Weinberg S, Pansky M, Burshtein I, et al. A pilot study of guided conservative hysteroscopic evaluation of early miscarriages. J Minim Invasive Gynecol. 2021;28(11):1860-7.
7. Pellicano M, Guida M, Zullo F, et al. Carbon dioxide versus normal saline as a uterine distention media for diagnostic vagianoscopic hysteroscopy in infertile patients: a prospective randomised multi-centre study. Fertil Steril. 2003;79:418-21.
8. Shveiky D, Rojansky N, Revel A, et al. complications of hysteroscopic surgery: Beyond the learning curve. J Minimal invasive Gynecol. 2007;14:218.
9. Royal College of Obstetricians and Gynaecologists. Outpatient Hysteroscopy (Green-top Guideline No. 59). [online] Available from https://www.rcog.org.uk/guidance/browse-all-guidance/green-top-guidelines/outpatient-hysteroscopy-green-top-guideline-no-59/ [Last accessed December, 2025].
10. Sagiv R, Sadan O, Boaz M, et al. A new approach to office hysteroscopy compared with traditional hysteroscopy: a randomised controlled trial. Obstet Gynecol. 2006;108:387.

Contraception

Contraception Combined Hormonal Pill

Ruchika Garg

INTRODUCTION

Contraceptive methods are essential for family planning, enabling individuals to prevent unintended pregnancies and space births. They are broadly classified into modern and nonmodern (traditional) methods, with modern methods further categorized by duration of action and efficacy.[1] In India, 71.8% of women needing contraception use modern methods, predominantly female sterilization (76.1%), followed by condoms (11.8%) and oral contraceptives (8.5%).[2] This chapter outlines the classification, efficacy, types of hormonal contraception, and initiatives to enhance contraceptive access, emphasizing WHO and CDC guidelines.

CLASSIFICATION OF CONTRACEPTIVE METHODS

Contraceptive methods are divided into modern and nonmodern categories, with modern methods further classified by reversibility and duration of action.[3]

TABLE 1: Classification of contraceptive methods.[1,3]

Category	*Modern methods*	*Nonmodern (Traditional) methods*
Methods	• Sterilization (Male: vasectomy; Female: tubal ligation) • Intrauterine devices (IUDs) • Subdermal implants • Oral contraceptives (combined, progestin-only) • Condoms (male, female) • Injectables • Emergency contraceptive pills • Spermicides (gels, foams, creams) • Patches • Diaphragms, cervical caps • Vaginal rings • Sponge	• Fertility awareness methods (standard days, calendar rhythm, two-day, billings ovulation, symptothermal) • Withdrawal • Lactational amenorrhea (modern per WHO) • Abstinence

Table 1 categorizes contraceptive methods, with lactational amenorrhea considered modern by WHO.[1,3]

By Reversibility and Duration.

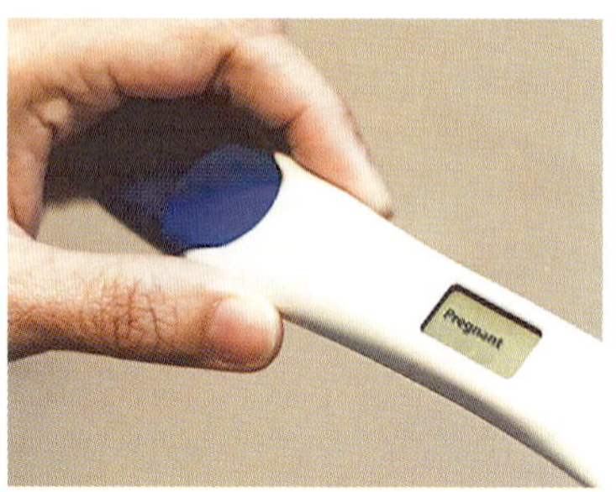

Modern methods are subclassified as:[4]

- **Short-Acting Reversible Contraception (SARC):**
  - Combined hormonal contraceptives (CHCs: pills, patches, vaginal rings).
  - Progestin-only pills (POPs).
  - Injectables [e.g., depot medroxyprogesterone acetate (DMPA)].
  - Condoms, diaphragms, cervical caps, spermicides, emergency contraception.
- **Long-Acting Reversible Contraception (LARC):**
  - IUDs (copper, levonorgestrel-releasing).
  - Subdermal implants (e.g., etonogestrel).
- **Permanent Methods:**
  - Male sterilization (vasectomy).
  - Female sterilization (tubal ligation).

EFFICACY OF CONTRACEPTIVE METHODS

Efficacy is measured by pregnancies per 100 women per year, categorized as:[5]

- **Very Effective:** 0–0.9 pregnancies/100 women.
- **Effective:** 1–9 pregnancies/100 women.
- **Moderately Effective:** 10–19 pregnancies/100 women.
- **Less Effective:** ≥20 pregnancies/100 women.

TABLE 2: Failure rates of modern contraceptives (U.S. Data, First Year).[5,6]

Method	*Perfect use (%)*	*Typical use (%)*	*Percent use (%)*
Top Tier (Very effective)			
LNG-IUD (52 mg)	0.1	0.1	11.8
Etonogestrel implant	0.1	0.1	2.6
Second Tier (Effective)			
Combined oral contraceptive	0.3	7	24.9
Vaginal ring (NuvaRing)	0.3	7	2.4
Transdermal patch (Evra)	0.3	7	0.2
DMPA injectable	**0.2**	**4**	**3.9**
Progestin-only pill	**0.3**	**7**	**0.4**

Table 2 highlights LARC methods as most effective, with higher typical-use failure rates for SARC.[5,6]

Hormonal Contraception

Hormonal contraception uses estrogen and/or progestogen to prevent ovulation, thicken cervical mucus and alter endometrial lining.[7] The first oral contraceptive, Enovid (1960), contained high-dose norethynodrel (10 mg) and mestranol (150 µg), compared to modern low-dose formulations.[8]

Types of Hormonal Contraception

- **Combined Hormonal Contraception (CHC):**

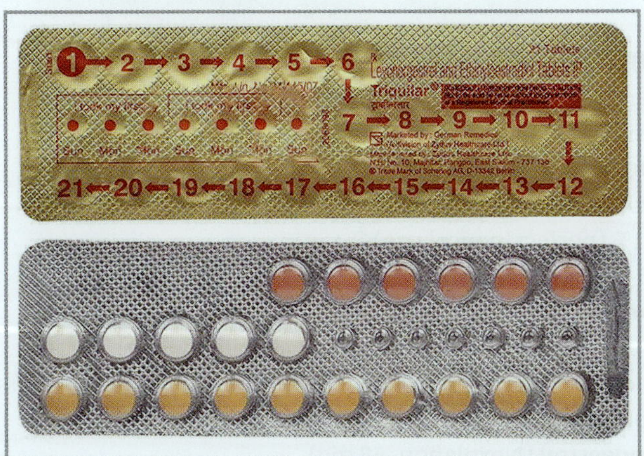

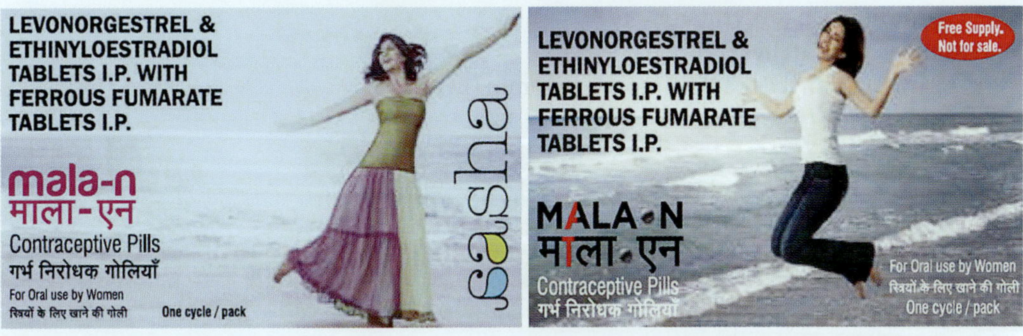

  - **Forms:** Oral pills, transdermal patches (e.g., Evra), vaginal rings (e.g., NuvaRing).
  - **Mechanism:** Estrogen (ethinyl estradiol) + progestin suppress ovulation.
  - **Efficacy:** Perfect use: 0.3%; typical use: 7%.[6]
  - **Considerations:** Contraindicated in women with thrombotic risk (e.g., smoking >35 years).[9]
- **Progestin-Only Pills (POPs):**
  - **Mechanism:** Progestin thickens cervical mucus, inhibits ovulation in ~50% of cycles.
  - **Efficacy:** Perfect use: 0.3%; typical use: 7%.[6]
  - **Advantages:** Safe for women with estrogen contraindications.[9] Cerazette available in India.

- **Injectables:**

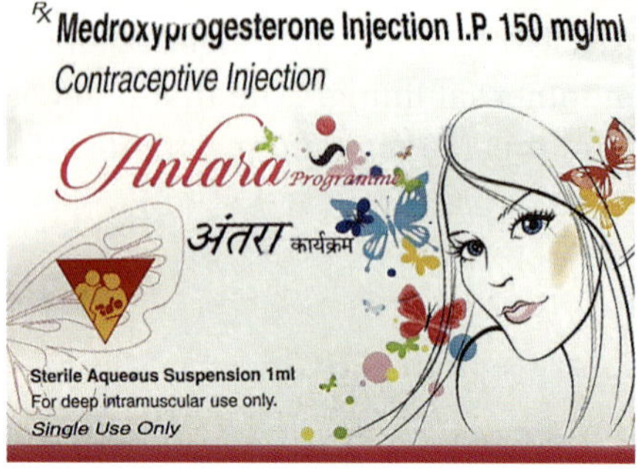

  - **Forms:** DMPA (150 mg IM every 3 months).
  - **Efficacy:** Perfect use: 0.2%; typical use: 4%.[6]
  - **Side Effects:** Weight gain, delayed return to fertility.[10]
- **Intrauterine Devices (IUDs):**
  - **Forms:** Levonorgestrel-releasing (e.g., Mirena, 52 mg).
  - **Efficacy:** 0.1% (perfect/typical use).[6]
  - **Duration:** 5–7 years.
- **Emergency Contraception:**
  - **Forms:** Levonorgestrel (1.5 mg), ulipristal acetate (30 mg).
  - **Efficacy:** Reduces pregnancy risk by 75–89% if taken within 72 hours.
- **Hormonal Implants:**
  - **Forms:** Etonogestrel (Nexplanon, 68 mg).
  - **Efficacy:** 0.1% (perfect/typical use).[6]
  - **Duration:** Up to 3 years.
- **Transdermal Patches:**
  - **Forms:** Ethinyl estradiol + norelgestromin (Evra).
  - **Efficacy:** Perfect use: 0.3%; typical use: 7%.[6]
- **Vaginal Rings:**
  - **Forms:** Ethinyl estradiol + etonogestrel (NuvaRing).
  - **Efficacy:** Perfect use: 0.3%; typical use: 7%.[6]

TABLE 3: Characteristics of hormonal contraceptives.[6,9]

Method	*Hormones*	*Efficacy (Typical use)*	*Duration*
CHC (pill, patch, ring)	Estrogen + progestin	7%	Daily/weekly/monthly
POP	Progestin	7%	Daily
DMPA injectable	Progestin	4%	3 months
LNG-IUD	Progestin	0.1%	5–7 years
Implant	Progestin	0.1%	3 years
Emergency contraception	Progestin/selective progesterone receptor modulator	75–89% (single use)	Single dose

Table 3 summarizes hormonal contraceptive options, with LARC offering superior efficacy.[6,9]

Considerations

- **Benefits:** Effective pregnancy prevention, noncontraceptive benefits (e.g., reduced menstrual pain, acne).[7]
- **Side Effects:** CHC: Nausea, headache, thromboembolism risk; POPs: Irregular bleeding; DMPA: Bone density loss.[10]
- **Counseling:** Tailor method to medical history, lifestyle, and preferences.[9]

CONTRACEPTIVE USE IN INDIA

- **Prevalence:** 71.8% of women needing contraception use modern methods (NFHS-5, 2019–21).[2]
- **Methods:**
  - **Female sterilization:** 76.1%.
  - **Condoms:** 11.8%.
  - **Oral contraceptives:** 8.5%.
  - **IUDs:** 3.2%.[2]
- **Challenges:** Low LARC uptake, reliance on sterilization, limited male involvement.

GOVERNMENT INITIATIVES IN INDIA

To enhance contraceptive access, awareness, and usage, India has implemented:

- **Mission Parivar Vikas (2016):** Targets 13 high-fertility states to increase contraceptive access.
- **Newer Contraceptives:** Introduced DMPA (Antara) and Centchroman (Chhaya) in 2015–16.
- **Compensation Scheme:** Financial support for sterilization acceptors to offset wage loss.
- **Awareness Campaigns:** Annual "World Population Day & Fortnight" and "Vasectomy Fortnight".
- **Post-Pregnancy Services:** Promotes PPIUCD, PAIUCD, and postpartum sterilization.
- **Home Delivery:** Accredited Social Health Activists (ASHAs) deliver contraceptives.
- **Logistics Management:** Family Planning Logistics Management Information System (FP-LMIS) ensures commodity availability.

EMERGING TRENDS AND GUIDELINES

- **Nonhormonal LARC:** Copper IUDs remain cost-effective, with low failure rates.
- **Digital Tools:** Apps for fertility awareness improve traditional method efficacy.
- **Male Contraceptives:** Research on hormonal gels, nonhormonal pills ongoing.
- **WHO/CDC Guidelines (2023):** Emphasize LARC promotion, informed choice, and male engagement.[1,9]
- **NFHS-5 Recommendations:** Expand LARC access, reduce sterilization reliance.[2]

WHO Medical Eligibility Criteria

Category	*Definition*	*With clinical judgement*	*With limited clinical judgement*
1	A condition for which there is no restriction for the use of the contraceptive method	Use method in any circumstance	Yes, use the method
2	A condition where the advantages of using the method generally outweigh the theoretical or proven risks	Generally, use method	
3	A condition where the theoretical or proven risks usually outweigh the advantages of using the method	Use of method not usually recommended unless other more appropriate methods are not available or not acceptable	No, do not use the method
4	A condition that represents an unacceptable health risk if the contraceptive method is used	Method not to be used	

COMBINED HORMONAL CONTRACEPTIVES

Combined hormonal contraceptives (CHCs), including **combined oral contraceptives (COCs; Table 4)** and **vaginal rings**, are widely used for contraception and gynecologic conditions globally and in India. By suppressing ovulation and altering reproductive physiology, CHCs offer high efficacy when used correctly.[1]

Composition

Estrogen component: Ethinyl estradiol, Estradiol, or estetrol
Progesterone component: With varying degrees of androgenic and progestogenic potential
- 1st generation progestin—Norethindrone acetate, Ethynodiol acetate, Lynestrenol and Norethynodrel
- 2nd generation progestin—Levonorgestrel, dl-Norgestrel
- 3rd generation progestin—Norgestimate, Gestodene, Desogestrel
- 4th generation progestin—Drospirenone and Cyproterone acetate

TABLE 4: COC Formulation.

Activity of progestin agents				
Generation	*Progestin*	*Estrogenic activity*	*Progestational activity*	*Androgenic activity*
First	Norethindrone	++	++	++
	Ethynodiol diacetate	++	+++	+
	Norgestrel	–	+++	+++
	Norethindrone acetate	++	++	++
Second	Levonorgestrel	–	++++	++++
Third	Norgestimate	–	++	++
	Desogestrel	+/–	++++	++
Fourth	Drospirenone	–	+/–	–

- +/– indicates *low to no activity*
- – indicates *no activity*

Mechanisms of Action

CHCs combine **ethinyl estradiol (EE)** and a **progestin** to achieve contraception via[2]:

- **Primary Mechanism:** Suppression of ovulation by inhibiting GnRH, LH, and FSH, with EE-driven FSH suppression preventing folliculogenesis.
- **Secondary Mechanisms:**
  - Progestin-induced endometrial decidualization and atrophy, reducing implantation likelihood.
  - Thickened cervical mucus, impeding sperm penetration.
  - Impaired tubal motility and peristalsis.
- **EE Role:** Stabilizes endometrium for regular withdrawal bleeding (cycle control).

Epidemiology

- **Global Use:** ~151 million women use COCs; 8% of reproductive-age women globally.[3]
- **India:**
  - Prevalence: 7.5% among married women (NFHS-5, 2019–21).[4]
  - Urban: 9.1%; rural: 6.3%.[4]
  - Preferred in urban private healthcare settings.[5]
- **Vaginal Rings:** Limited use in India due to cost and awareness; increasing in urban centers.[6]

Formulations and Regimens

COC Regimens:

- **Cyclic:** 21/7 (21 hormone days, 7 placebo) or 24/4 (4 placebo/low-dose EE).[9]
- **Continuous:** Daily hormone pills for 3, 6, 9 months or a year, no withdrawal bleed.[10]
- **Extended-Cycle:** 63 hormone days, 7-day placebo interval.
- **Advantages of Extended or Continuous Contraceptive Regimens:** Advantages
- **Fewer Menstrual-Related Symptoms:** Significantly reduces or eliminates symptoms associated with the withdrawal bleed, such as:
  - Menstrual cramps (dysmenorrhea)
  - Headaches
  - Bloating
  - Mood swings
- **Management of Medical Conditions:** Highly beneficial for managing conditions that are exacerbated by menstruation, including:
  - Endometriosis
  - Heavy menstrual bleeding
  - Anemia (by reducing blood loss)
  - Menstrual migraines
- **Convenience:** Provides control over if and when a bleed occurs, which can be convenient for travel, athletic events, or personal preference.
- **Increased Contraceptive Protection:** Extended hormone exposure reduces the hormone-free interval (HFI), leading to greater suppression of ovarian activity. This minimizes the risk of escape ovulation and contraceptive failure. HFI is 4 days.

- **Decreased Breakthrough Bleeding and Spotting:** Continuous regimens stabilize the endometrium, reducing irregular bleeding compared to traditional cyclic regimens.

Disadvantages/Considerations

- **Breakthrough Bleeding/Spotting:** This is the most common side effect, especially during the first few months. The uterus' lining may still try to shed intermittently, causing unpredictable spotting. This usually decreases over time.
- **Need for Prescription and Guidance:** A healthcare provider must prescribe this regimen. They will determine if it is medically appropriate and can advise on how to manage breakthrough bleeding (e.g., whether to take a short break).
- **Uncertainty for Some:** The absence of a regular monthly bleed can cause anxiety for some users who rely on it as a sign of not being pregnant. Pregnancy risk is very low with perfect use, but this psychological factor is important to consider.
  - **Examples of 24/7 Regimens: Minesse:** 60 μg gestodene + 15 μg ethinyl estradiol
  - **Loestrin 24 Fe:** 1 mg norethindrone acetate + 20 μg ethinyl estradiol, with 4 iron-containing placebo pills.
  - **Yaz:** 3 mg drospirenone + 20 μg ethinyl estradiol.

VAGINAL RINGS

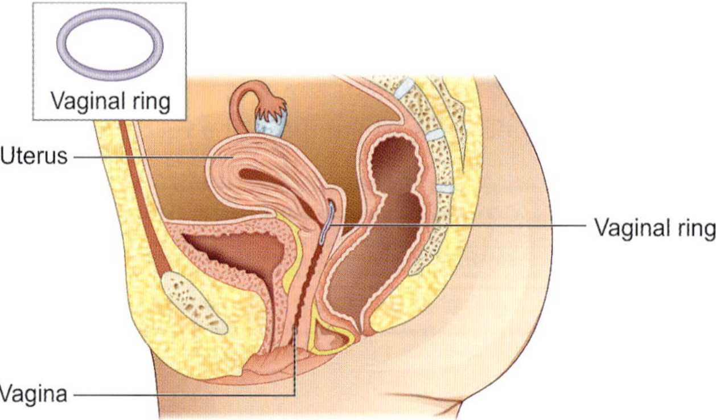

NuvaRing: 3 weeks in, 1 week out; EE/etonogestrel.

Annovera: Reusable, 3 weeks in, 1 week out for 13 cycles; EE/segesterone.

RETURN OF FERTILITY: Majority of woman resume ovulation and regular menses within a month of removal of vaginal rings.[1] In a study conducted on 45 participants using NuvaRing, ovulation was reported to be as early as 13 days after removal of ring and the median time to ovulate was 19 days after removal of vaginal ring.[6] Similarly with Annovera, initial trials reported return of regular menses within 6 months of discontinuation.[2]

Use with other vaginal devices and products

Vaginal rings are known to interfere with other female barrier contraceptive methods such as diaphragm, cervical cap, or female condoms. Hence, female barrier contraceptives cannot be used as backup contraception along with vaginal rings.[7]

Concomitant use of tampons during menses does not affect the hormone absorption from the vaginal ring.[1]

Vaginal rings are compatible with water-based vaginal lubricants and spermicides, but oil-based products including silicone-based lubricants are not compatible with vaginal rings.[1,2]

INTERACTIONS WITH OTHER MEDICATIONS

Interactions of vaginal ring is similar to COCs and most of the information is based on it. Vaginal rings interact with other systemic medications and consequently increase or decrease each other's levels.

- **Decrease in estrogen/progestin levels:** Drugs which increase the activity of liver microsomal enzymes decrease systemic exposure to the estrogen and progestins in contraceptive vaginal rings, and thus contraceptive efficacy is reduced.

  Some such medications are:
  - Antiepileptics such as barbiturate, phenytoin, carbamazepine, oxcarbazepine, topiramate
  - Antifungal like griseofulvin
  - Antitubercular drugs like rifampicin, rifabutin
  - Anti-HIV medications like efavirenz, nelfinavir, ritonavir, darunavir, lopinavir, Nevirapine[1,2]
  - Individuals using the above medications should use an additional form of contraception such as condoms or choose an alternative form of contraception.
- **Altered levels of certain medications:** Plasma levels of Lamotrigine are known to decrease when used along with combined hormonal methods. Hence, seizure control may not be optimal, and a higher dose of Lamotrigine may be needed to attain good seizure control.[8,9]

  Combined hormonal methods are avoided in those women on antiviral medications for hepatitis C (ritonavir, paritaprevir) since ALT levels are significantly elevated.
- **Use with other vaginal medications:** Water-based vaginal drugs used in the treatment of vaginal candidiasis or bacterial vaginosis can be used along with vaginal rings.[1,2]

  Oil-based suppositories such as Miconazole suppositories are associated with increased hormonal levels and hence avoided along with vaginal rings.[1,2]

SPECIAL SITUATIONS

1. If the vaginal ring is out for an unknown duration of time, then pregnancy has to be ruled out before inserting a new ring.[7]
2. **Continuous use of ring for menstrual suppression:** Some women desire fewer days of withdrawal bleed and may prefer using vaginal ring for an extended period. Vaginal ring may be used without ring-free period wherein a new ring is inserted immediately after the removal of old ring. This omits hormone-free interval. Extended use of ring is effective but the woman may suffer from unscheduled bleeding and spotting.[10]
3. Data supporting continuous use of the Annovera are not yet available, but continuous use may be associated with an increase in unscheduled bleeding.
4. **Broken ring:** Very rarely, the contraceptive ring may break at the weld joint.[1] The break does not affect the contraceptive effectiveness, but it is more likely that the ring slips out. Hence, in the event of broken ring, the ring needs to be removed and replaced with a new one.

NON-CONTRACEPTIVE BENEFITS OF VAGINAL RING: SAME AS COC

Initiation and Management

- **Starting CHCs:**
  - **First Day Start:** On day 1 of menses; no backup needed.
  - **>5 Days Postmenses:** Backup contraception (e.g., condoms) for 7 days.
  - **Postpartum:** Avoid <21 days post-delivery (VTE risk); breastfeeding women delay until 30 days.
- **Missed Doses (COCs):**
  - **Single Pill:** Take as soon as noticed; no backup needed.
  - **≥2 Pills:** Take remaining pills; use backup if missed in week 1 or 3; consider emergency contraception if unprotected intercourse.
- **Duration:** Safe until menopause (~50–51 years) in healthy, nonsmoking women.

Contraceptive Effectiveness

- **Perfect Use:** Failure rate 0.3% per year.
- **Typical Use:** Failure rate 9% due to inconsistent use.
- **Factors:** No consistent evidence linking weight/BMI to reduced efficacy.
- **Drug Interactions:**
  - **Enzyme-Inducing Drugs** (e.g., rifampicin): Reduce efficacy; switch to nonhormonal methods (IUD, injectable).
  - **Lamotrigine:** CHCs reduce levels, risking seizures; benefits may not outweigh risks.
  - **Antibiotics:** No additional contraception needed unless vomiting/diarrhea occurs.

Noncontraceptive Benefits (Table 5)

TABLE 5: Noncontraceptive benefits of CHCs.

Condition	*Benefit*	*Evidence*
Heavy menstrual bleeding	Reduces blood loss and dysmenorrhea	RCTs, nonrandomized trials
Endometriosis	Reduces recurrence post-surgery; symptom relief	Meta-analysis
Acne	Decreases lesion counts and severity	Cochrane Review
Premenstrual syndrome (PMS)	Improves symptoms, especially with continuous regimens	RCOG guideline
PCOS	Manages menstrual irregularity, acne, hirsutism	Endocrine society guideline

- **Cancer Risk Reduction:**
  - **Endometrial:** 50% risk reduction with 10–15 years use; persists 30 years post cessation.
  - **Ovarian:** 50% risk reduction with ≥10 years use; benefits in BRCA carriers.
  - **Colorectal:** Reduced risk in ever-users.
  - **Menopause:** Alternative to HRT for symptom relief and bone health until age 50 years.

Risks and Side Effects

- **Early Side Effects:** Nausea, breast tenderness, headaches (<10% of users); resolve within 3–4 months.

- **Unscheduled Bleeding:** 10–18% per cycle; improves over time; higher EE doses reduce risk.
- **Amenorrhea:** Common with continuous regimens; may occur with low-dose cyclic COCs.
- **Serious Risks (Table 6):**
  - **VTE:** 3–3.5-fold increased risk; highest in first year; absolute risk low.
  - **Cardiovascular:** Increased MI (RR 1.6) and stroke risk in smokers, hypertensives, or migraine with aura.
  - **Breast Cancer:** Small increased risk (RR 1.19) with current use; diminishes post-cessation.
  - **Cervical Cancer:** Doubled risk with >5 years use; normalizes 10 years post-cessation.

TABLE 6: Serious risks of CHC use.

Risk	*Relative risk*	*Notes*
VTE	3–3.5	Highest in 1st year; low absolute risk
Myocardial infarction	1.6	Smokers, hypertensives at higher risk
Breast cancer	1.19	Risk reduces post-cessation
Cervical cancer	1.9 (>5 years)	Normalizes 10 years post-cessation

- **No Evidence:** Consistent association with weight gain, depression, or reduced libido.

Medical Eligibility Criteria (Table 7)

TABLE 7: UKMEC category 4 (Unacceptablerisk) and 3 (Risks outweigh benefits)

Category	*Conditions*
UKMEC 4	Age ≥35 years + ≥15 cigarettes/day, severe hypertension (≥160/100 mm Hg), current breast cancer, VTE (unless anticoagulated), migraine with aura
UKMEC 3	Age ≥35 years + <15 cigarettes/day, controlled hypertension, past breast cancer (>5 years disease-free), superficial venous thrombosis

- **Assessment:**
  - **Blood Pressure:** Measure before initiation; avoid if ≥140/90 mm Hg.
  - **BMI:** No routine restriction; counsel obese women on VTE risk.
  - **Breast Exam:** Not required due to low breast cancer prevalence in reproductive age.

BOX 1: Symptoms requiring urgent medical review

- Calf pain/swelling/redness, chest pain/breathlessness, loss of motor/sensory function
- New breast lump, new-onset migraine, persistent unscheduled bleeding
- *New diagnoses:* Hypertension, VTE, breast cancer, liver tumor

RCOG/NICE/FSRH Guidelines (2023)

- **Eligibility:** Use UKMEC criteria; avoid CHCs in UKMEC 4 conditions.
- **Initiation:** First-day start preferred; backup for 7 days if started later.
- **Missed Doses:** Follow FSRH guidance; emergency contraception if ≥2 pills missed in week 1/3.
- **Noncontraceptive Use:** Recommend for HMB, endometriosis, PCOS, PMS; consider continuous regimens.

- **Cancer Risk:** Counsel on small breast/cervical cancer risks versus significant endometrial/ovarian cancer reduction.
- **Follow-Up:** Annual BP check; review if new medical conditions arise.

Indian Context

- **Challenges:** Low awareness (30% rural women unaware per NFHS-5), cultural stigma, and access barriers.
- **Strategies:** Integrate CHC counseling into family planning programs; train ASHAs for distribution.
- **Recent Data:** 2022 study showed 12% COC use in urban Maharashtra; vaginal rings <1%.

Postpartum Contraceptive Eligibility Table

Method CHCs[a]	*Cat.*	*DMPA, POPs, Implants*	*Cat.*	*LNG-IUS*	*Cat.*	*Cu-IUD*	*Cat.*
Breastfeeding <21 days	4	**Breastfeeding** <1 month	2	**±Breastfeeding** <10 mins	2	**± Breastfeeding**[c] <10 mins	1
21 to <30 days	3	≥1 month	1	10 minutes to ≤4 weeks	2	10 minutes to ≥4 weeks	2
30–42 days[b]	2	1		≥4 weeks	1	≥4 weeks	1
>42 days	2	1		Puerperal sepsis	4	Puerperal sepsis	4
Nonbreastfeeding <21 days	4	**Nonbreastfeeding**	1				
Nonbreastfeeding 21–42 days[b]	2						
Nonbreastfeeding >42 days	1						

[a]CHCs include pills, vaginal ring, and patch.
[b]Higher risk category if age ≥35 years, BMI ≥30, transfusion at delivery, postpartum hemorrhage, cesarean delivery, smoking, or preeclampsia.
[c]"±Breastfeeding" means applicable with or without breastfeeding.
(Cat.: category; Cu-IUD: copper-containing intrauterine device; DMPA: depot medroxyprogesterone acetate; LNG-IUS: levonorgestrel-releasing intrauterine system; POPs: progestin-only pills)
Source: Curtis (2016)[1]

Clinical Case Scenario

Case: A 28-year-old nulliparous woman requests contraception. BP: 120/80 mm Hg, BMI: 24 kg/m^2, nonsmoker. She reports heavy menstrual bleeding. No medical history.

Management:

- **Counseling:** Discuss CHC options, efficacy, and noncontraceptive benefits (HMB reduction).
- **Prescription:** Start **EE 30 µg/levonorgestrel 150 µg** COC (21/7 regimen).
- **Initiation:** Begin on day 1 of menses; no backup needed.
- **Education:** Explain missed pill protocol, side effects, and urgent symptoms (e.g., calf pain).
- **Follow-Up:** BP check and symptom review at 3 months.
- **Outcome:** Reduced HMB; no side effects; satisfied with COC.

Exam Tip: Highlight UKMEC criteria, noncontraceptive benefits, and missed dose management in answers.

KEY POINTS

Contraception can also be classified as:

- Short-acting reversible contraception (SARC): Including contraceptive pills, injectables, condoms, diaphragms, spermicidal agents, and emergency contraception
- Long-acting reversible contraception (LARC): Including IUD, hormone patches and implants.
- Permanent methods: Including male and female sterilization.

Types of Hormonal Contraception

- Combined hormonal contraception (CHC)
- Progesterone-only pills (POPs)
- Injectable contraceptives
- Intrauterine Devices (IUDs)
- Emergency contraception
- Hormonal Implants
- Transdermal patches
- Vaginal rings
- **CHC use in India:** 7.5% among married women; higher in urban areas.
- **Efficacy:** 0.3% failure with perfect use; 9% with typical use.
  - Mechanism of Action: E and P inhibit the release of hypothalamic gonadotropin-releasing hormone (GnRH), which in turn suppresses the release of FSH and LH from the pituitary gland leading to disruption of midcycle LH surge and suppression of ovulation.
  - **Changes in endometrial lining:** Rendering it less suitable for implantation. *Endometrial decidualization and eventual atrophy.*
- **Thickening of cervical mucus**
- Can be started at any time if it is reasonably certain that the woman is not pregnant.
- **How to confirm that a woman is not pregnant:** If she has no symptoms or signs of pregnancy and meets any one of the following criteria:
  - Is ≤7 days after the start of normal menses
  - Has not had sexual intercourse since the start of last normal menses
  - Has been correctly and consistently using a reliable method of contraception
  - Is ≤7 days after spontaneous or induced abortion
  - Is within 4 weeks postpartum
  - Is fully or nearly fully breastfeeding [exclusively breastfeeding or the vast majority (≥85%) of feeds are breastfeeds], amenorrheic, and <6 months postpartum
  - The lowest dose of estrogen that preferred is **20–35 μg** ethinyl estradiol ≥**50 μg** not used for contraception

COCs in the public sector can be supplied by ASHA **and** Free supply is there.

In the public sector, available COC pill is Mala-N.

- Mala-N contains Levonorgestrel (0.15 mg) + Ethinyl estradiol (30 µg).
- Is supplied free of cost through government health centers and hospitals.
- Each strip of Mala-N contains 21 hormonal tablets and 7 nonhormonal (iron) tablets.
- **Noncontraceptive Benefits:** Reduces HMB, endometriosis recurrence, acne, PMS, and endometrial/ovarian cancer risk.
- **Risks:** Small increase in VTE, breast, and cervical cancer; no consistent link to weight gain or depression.
- **Guidelines:** Follow UKMEC for eligibility; counsel on serious symptoms.
- **Vaginal Rings:** Alternative for women preferring nondaily methods.
- Combined transdermal patch (CTP) that releases an average of 33.9 µg EE and 203 µg norelgestromin (Progesterone) per 24 hours.

BOX 2: Important points to remember.

- CHCs are contraindicated in women with severe hypertension, current breast cancer, or migraine with aura
- Continuous regimens reduce unscheduled bleeding and are effective for endometriosis/PMS
- Counsel on small VTE risk (3–3.5-fold); absolute risk remains low compared to pregnancy
- Annual BP monitoring is mandatory for CHC users

Extended Regimens (Shortened Hormone Free Interval—HFI): **24/4 Extended cycle** (less frequent HFI)—84/7 formulations: **Provides** active hormone pills for 12 weeks followed by a week for withdrawal menses. **Continuous use** (No HFI)—provides continuous active hormone pills for 365 days. No withdrawal bleeds, e.g., Amethyst containing levonorgestrel (0.09 mg) and ethinyl estradiol (20 µg).

Traditional pills are designed to be taken as a 28-day cycle. Active pills are taken for 21 consecutive days followed by 7-day HFI (placebo pills) before starting the next packet. The first 7 active pills inhibit ovulation and the next 14 active pills maintain anovulation. Monthly withdrawal bleeding during HFI mimics a natural menstrual cycle. However, there is no health benefit from a monthly withdrawal bleeding and the 7 day HFI has the following drawbacks:

- Withdrawal bleeding may be heavy and painful.
- May be associated with symptoms like headache, bloating, pelvic pain, breast tenderness, and mood changes
- Reduced ovarian suppression and follicular development in HFI. Imperfect use of CHC around HFI, may extend the HFI leading to an increased risk of ovulation and pregnancy.

Contraindications for Combined Oral Contraceptive Pills (COCs):

- Current or past history of venous thromboembolism (VTE).
- Recent major surgery with prolonged immobility.
- Known thrombogenic conditions (e.g., Factor V Leiden).
- Hypertension (even if controlled).
- Known ischemic heart disease.
- History of stroke.
- Complicated valvular heart disease (e.g., pulmonary hypertension, risk of atrial fibrillation, history of subacute bacterial endocarditis).

- Current or past history of breast cancer.
- Postpartum:
  - 0–6 weeks if breastfeeding.
  - 0–3 weeks if not breastfeeding.
  - 0–6 weeks with VTE risk factors, regardless of breastfeeding status.
- Migraine with focal aura.
- Age ≥35 years and smoking ≥15 cigarettes per day.
- Hepatocellular adenoma or malignant hepatoma.
- Cirrhosis.

BOX 3: Management of missed pill.

Missed 3 or more pills in the first or second week/started new pack 3 or more days late?	• Take one hormonal pill as soon as possible and continue the scheduled pill • Use a backup method for 7 days • Take emergency pill, if she had sex in the past 72 hours
Missed 3 or more pills in the third week?	Take one hormonal pill as soon as possible and finish all pills in the pack and start a new pack the next day

MULTIPLE CHOICE QUESTION

Q1. Which of the following is true as Benefit of COC?
1. Less mittelschmerz (midcycle ovulation pain)
2. Reduction in hot flashes and other perimenopausal symptoms
3. Lowered incidence of symptomatic endometriosis, adenomyosis, and fibroids
4. Reduction of lifetime risk of ovarian cancer including some hereditary forms, such as those associated with mutations in the BRCA1 or BRCA2 gene
5. All are true.

REFERENCES

1. Curtis KM, Tepper NK, Jatlaoui TC, et al. U.S. medical eligibility criteria for contraceptive use, 2016. MMWR Recomm Rep. 2016;65(3):1-103.
2. Faculty of Sexual and Reproductive Healthcare (FSRH). Combined hormonal contraception. London: Faculty of Sexual and Reproductive Healthcare; 2019.
3. United Nations. Contraceptive use by method 2019. New York: United Nations; 2019.
4. NFHS-5. National Family Health Survey 2019–21. Mumbai: IIPS; 2021.
5. Mogan KA, Sharma R, Khokhar A, et al. Contraceptive preferences in urban India. J Family Med Prim Care. 2020;9(6):2978-83.
6. Gupta S, et al. Vaginal contraceptive rings: awareness and uptake in India. Indian J Community Med. 2022;47(3):401-5.
7. Cooper DB, Patel P. Oral contraceptive pills. StatPearls. Treasure Island (FL): StatPearls Publishing; 2025 Jan.
8. World Health Organization. Medical eligibility criteria for contraceptive use, 2015. Geneva: World Health Organization; 2015.
9. Tepper NK, Krashin JW, Curtis KM, et al. Update to CDC's U.S. medical eligibility criteria for contraceptive use. MMWR Morb Mortal Wkly Rep. 2017;66(29):781-5.
10. Edelman A, Gallo MF, Nichols MD, et al. Continuous vs. cyclic COC regimens: a systematic review. Contraception. 2019;99(2):75-82.

Progestogen-Only Pills and Depot Medroxyprogesterone Acetate

Ruchika Garg, Neelansha Varshney

INTRODUCTION

Progestogen-only pills (POPs) and **depot medroxyprogesterone acetate (DMPA)** are effective contraceptive options, particularly for women unsuitable for estrogen-containing methods. POPs require daily compliance, while DMPA offers long-acting reversible contraception (LARC).[1,2]

EPIDEMIOLOGY

- **India:**
  - POP prevalence: <1% among married women (NFHS-5, 2019–21).[3]
  - DMPA prevalence: 2.3%, higher in rural areas due to accessibility.[4]
  - DMPA, Antra promoted under India's National Family Planning Program free of cost.[5]
- **Trends:** DMPA uptake increasing; POPs underutilized due to bleeding concerns.[6]

PROGESTOGEN-ONLY PILLS (POPS) (FIG. 2)

Progesterone-only pills come under brand name Cerazette.

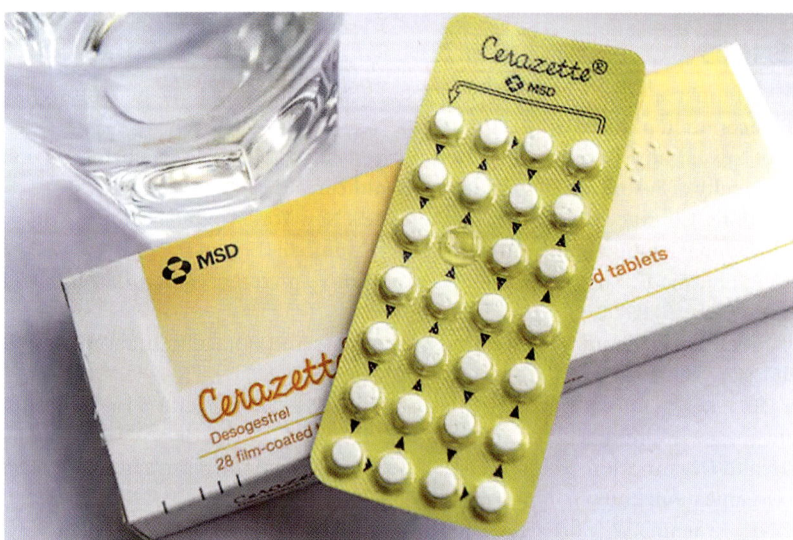

Fig. 1: Progesterone-only pills come under brand name Cerazette.

Types and Formulations

- **Available POPs (Table 1):**[7]
    - Levonorgestrel (LNG): 30 µg
    - Norethisterone (NET): 350 µg
    - Desogestrel (DSG): 75 µg
    - Drospirenone (DRSP): 4 mg

TABLE 1: POP formulations.[7,8]

POP	*Dose*	*Regimen*	*Ovulation suppression*
LNG	30 µg	Daily, no hormone-free interval (HFI)	Partial
NET	350 µg	Daily, no HFI	Partial
DSG	75 µg	Daily, no HFI	Consistent
DRSP	4 mg	24 active pills, 4-day HFI	Consistent

Mechanism of Action

- **Primary:** Thickens cervical mucus, impairing sperm penetration.[9]
- **Secondary:**
    - Thins endometrium, reducing implantation likelihood.
    - Slows tubal motility.
    - DSG/DRSP: Inhibits ovulation via anti-gonadotropic effects.[10]

Effectiveness

- **Perfect Use:** >99% effective; failure rate 0.1–0.3%.
- **Typical Use:** 9% failure rate due to non-compliance.
- **Factors:**
    - Timing: Must be taken same time daily (±3 h for LNG/NET, ±12 h for DSG, ±24 h for DRSP).
    - Vomiting/Diarrhea: Replace pill if within 2 h (LNG/NET) or 3–4 h (DSG/DRSP).
    - Drug Interactions: Enzyme inducers (e.g., rifampicin) reduce efficacy; use DMPA or IUD instead.
    - BMI: No impact on efficacy.

Initiation

- **Standard Start:** Day 1–5 of menses, post-abortion (day 5), or postpartum (day 21).
- **Quick Start:** Any cycle day; use condoms for 2 days (LNG/NET/DSG) or 7 days (DRSP).
- **Post-EC:**
    - LNG-EC: Start POP immediately; condoms for 2–7 days.
    - UPA-EC: Delay POP 5 days; condoms for 2–7 days.

TABLE 2: POP Initiation protocols

POP type	*Standard start*	*Quick start (Backup)*
LNG/NET/DSG	Day 1–5 menses, day 5 abortion, day 21 postpartum	2 days condoms
DRSP	Day 1 menses, day 1 abortion, day 21 postpartum	7 days condoms

Missed Pill Management

TABLE 3: Missed pill protocols.

POP	*Missed pill threshold*	*Management*
LNG/NET	>3 h (>27 h since last)	Take missed pill ASAP; next pill at usual time; condoms for 48 h; consider EC
DSG	>12 h (>36 h since last)	Same as above
DRSP	>24 h (>48 h since last)	Take missed pill ASAP; condoms for 7 days; skip HFI if last 7 pills missed; EC

Contraindications

- **WHO MEC 4 (Unacceptable Risk):** Current breast cancer.
- **WHO MEC 3 (Risks Outweigh Benefits):** Past breast cancer, severe cirrhosis, ischemic heart disease/stroke (continuation only).
- **DRSP-Specific:** Avoid in severe renal failure, hyperkalemia, or with potassium-sparing drugs.

Side Effects

- **Common:** Unscheduled bleeding (20–40%); improves over time, often leading to amenorrhea.
- Management: Rule out pathology; consider NSAIDs, tranexamic acid, or DSG double dose (150 μg, off-label).
- **Others:** Headache, acne, mood changes (no consistent evidence).
- **No Evidence:** Increased VTE, depression, weight gain, or bone loss.

Noncontraceptive Benefits

- **DSG/DRSP:** Reduce heavy menstrual bleeding (HMB) and dysmenorrhea.
- **DRSP:** Potential antiandrogenic effects for acne/hirsutism (unproven).

Follow-up and Discontinuation

- **Follow-up:** Annual review; earlier if side effects or method switch needed.
- **Discontinuation:** Immediate fertility return; offer alternative contraception if needed.

Depot Medroxyprogesterone Acetate (DMPA) (Fig. 2)

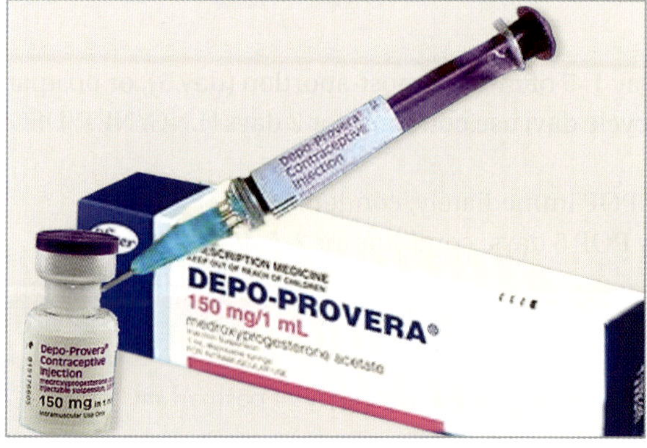

Fig. 2: Depot medroxyprogesterone acetate (DMPA) injection.

Formulation and Administration

- **India:** Depo-Provera (150 mg/1 mL IM every 12 weeks).
- **Sites:** Gluteus maximus, lateral thigh, or deltoid (obese women).
- **Timing:** Every 12 weeks (10–14 weeks acceptable; WHO allows up to 16 weeks).

Mechanism of Action

- **Primary:** Inhibits ovulation via gonadotropin suppression.
- **Secondary:** Thickens cervical mucus; thins endometrium.

Effectiveness

- **Perfect Use:** 0.2% failure rate.
- **Typical Use:** 6% failure rate due to missed injections.
- **Factors:**
- BMI: Effective in obesity (BMI <40 kg/m^2); caution if BMI ≥40 kg/m^2.
- Drug Interactions: Unaffected by enzyme inducers (e.g., antiretrovirals, antiepileptics).

Initiation

- **Standard Start:** Day 1–5 of menses, postabortion, or 21 days postpartum.
- **Quick Start:** Any day; use condoms for 7 days; rule out pregnancy **(Box 1)**.
- **Post-EC:** Same as POPs.

BOX 1: Criteria to rule out pregnancy

- No intercourse since last menstrual period (LMP), abortion, or delivery
- Consistent use of reliable contraception
- Negative urine pregnancy test (>21 days post-UPSI)
- Within 5 days of menses/abortion or 21 days postpartum
- Exclusively breastfeeding, amenorrheic, <6 months postpartum

Switching to DMPA

TABLE 4: Switching to DMPA

From	*Timing*	*Backup needed*
Combined Hormonal	Day 1–2 or weeks 2–3 of cycle	None
POP (LNG/NET)	Any day	7 days
POP (DSG)	Any day (if used correctly)	None
Copper IUD	Day 1–5 of cycle	None
LNG-IUS/Implant	Any day	7 days

Contraindications

- **WHO MEC 4:** Current breast cancer.
- **WHO MEC 3:** Severe hypertension, diabetes with vascular disease, ischemic heart disease/stroke (continuation).

Side Effects

- **Bleeding:** Amenorrhea (50% after 1 year), spotting, or prolonged bleeding; evaluate for pathology.

- **Weight Gain:** 1–3 kg/yr, higher in adolescents with BMI >30 kg/m^2.
- **Bone Mineral Density (BMD):** Reversible loss; greatest in first year; no routine DEXA needed.
- **Others:** Acne, mood changes, headache (unproven).

Noncontraceptive Benefits

- Reduces HMB, endometriosis pain, dysmenorrhea.
- Decreases ovarian/endometrial cancer risk.
- Possible reduction in sickle cell crisis pain.

Health Risks

- **Breast Cancer:** Weak, nonsignificant risk with recent use.
- **Cervical Cancer:** Possible association; screen regularly.
- **VTE/CVD:** No increased risk; safe in thrombophilia.
- **HIV:** No conclusive link to acquisition.

Follow-up and Discontinuation

- **Follow-up:** Every 12 weeks; reassess eligibility, side effects, and BMI.
- **Discontinuation:** Fertility return delayed up to 12 months; offer alternative contraception.

WHO/RCOG/FSRH Guidelines (2023)

- **POPs:**
  - Safe for most women, including breastfeeding; no BMI restrictions.
  - Counsel on bleeding patterns; offer alternatives if unacceptable.
- **DMPA:**
  - Preferred LARC in enzyme-inducer users; safe in obesity (BMI <40 kg/m^2) **(Box 2)**
  - Monitor adolescents/older women for BMD risk; no routine screening.
- **Counseling:** Emphasize noncontraceptive benefits, side effects, and fertility return.
- **Access:** Ensure availability in primary care; train providers for DMPA administration.

Indian Context

- **Challenges:** Low POP use due to bleeding concerns; DMPA preferred for simplicity.
- **Strategies:** Promote DMPA via ASHA workers; address bleeding misconceptions.
- **2022 Study:** DMPA uptake 5% in rural Uttar Pradesh; POPs <0.5%.

Clinical Case Scenario

Case: A 30-year-old breastfeeding mother, 8 weeks postpartum, requests contraception. BMI: 28 kg/m^2, no medical history.

BOX 2: Important points to remember

- POPs are safe in breastfeeding; DSG/DRSP inhibit ovulation
- DMPA is effective in obesity and enzyme-inducer users; monitor BMD in adolescents
- Unscheduled bleeding is common; rule out pathology before attributing to POPs/DMPA
- Fertility return: Immediate for POPs, delayed up to 12 months for DMPA

Management:

- **Counseling:** Discuss POPs (safe in lactation) versus DMPA (long-acting).
- **Prescription: DSG 75 µg** daily (no HFI, ovulation suppression).

- **Initiation:** Start immediately; no backup needed (postpartum day >21).
- **Education:** Explain bleeding patterns, missed pill protocol, and annual follow-up.
- **Outcome:** No bleeding issues; continues DSG; satisfied.

REFERENCES

1. United Nations. Contraceptive use by method 2019. New York: United Nations; 2019.
2. World Health Organization. Family planning: a global handbook. Geneva: World Health Organization; 2022.
3. NFHS-5. National Family Health Survey 2019–21. Mumbai: IIPS; 2021.
4. Sharma V, et al. Contraceptive trends in India: NFHS-5 analysis. Indian J Community Med. 2021;46(3):401–6.
5. MoHFW. Family planning program in India. New Delhi: Government of India; 2020.
6. Gupta A, et al. Barriers to POP and DMPA use in India. J Fam Plann Reprod Health Care. 2020;46(2):89-95.
7. FSRH. Progestogen-only pills. London: Faculty of Sexual and Reproductive Healthcare; 2023.
8. WHO. Medical eligibility criteria for contraceptive use, 5th edition. Geneva: World Health Organization; 22015.
9. Curtis KM, et al. Progestin-only contraception: mechanisms and efficacy. Contraception. 2016;94(5):419-25.
10. Archer DF, et al. Drospirenone-only pill: a new contraceptive option. Eur J Contracept Reprod Health Care. 2019;24(1):4-10.

Emergency Contraception

Anu Chaudhary

INTRODUCTION

Emergency contraception (EC) prevents unintended pregnancies after unprotected sexual intercourse (UPSI) or contraceptive failure, reducing the global burden of unsafe abortions (~20 million annually).[1] In India, unsafe abortions contribute to a maternal death every 2 hours.[2]

EPIDEMIOLOGY

- **Global:**
  - ~42 million abortions yearly; 20 million unsafe.[3]
  - 1 in 10 pregnancies ends in unsafe abortion.[4]
  - EC use: ~5–10% of women aged 15–44 years in high-income countries.[5]
- **India:**
  - Highest number of unsafe abortions globally (~8 million annually).[6]
  - EC use: 11% among women aged 15–49 (NFHS-5, 2019–21).[7]
  - Levonorgestrel (LNG) ECPs dominate; ulipristal acetate (UPA) and IUDs less common.[8]
- **Trends:** Increased EC awareness in urban India; rural access remains limited.[9]

DEFINITION AND INDICATIONS

Emergency contraception: Methods used within days post-UPSI to prevent pregnancy.[10]

- **Indications (Table 1):**
  - No contraception used during UPSI.
  - Contraceptive failure: Condom breakage, missed pills (≥3 combined oral contraceptives), delayed injectables.
  - Incorrect use: Miscalculated fertile days, failed withdrawal.
  - Sexual assault without contraceptive protection.

TABLE 1: Common scenarios requiring EC

Scenario	*Details*
Condom Failure	Breakage, slippage, incorrect use
Missed Pills	≥3 combined pills; >27h for LNG minipill
Delayed Injection	>2 weeks for NET-EN; >4 weeks for DMPA
IUD Expulsion	Partial or complete expulsion
Sexual Assault	No effective contraception used

METHODS OF EMERGENCY CONTRACEPTION (TABLE 2)

TABLE 2: EC methods and regimens

Method	*Regimen*	*Timing post-UPSI*	*Failure rate*
Yuzpe (COC)	100 µg EE + 0.5 mg LNG, 2 doses 12 h apart	Within 72 h	0–2%
LNG ECP	1.5 mg single dose or 0.75 mg 2 doses 12 h apart	Within 72 h	0–1%
UPA	30 mg single dose	Within 120 h	0.9–1.8%
Mifepristone	10 mg single dose	Within 120 h	0.06%
Copper IUD	Insertion (e.g., Cu T 380A)	Within 5 days	0–0.1%

- **Hormonal Methods:**
    - **Yuzpe Regimen:** Combined EE + LNG; less effective, more side effects.
    - **LNG ECP:** Preferred in India; single-dose 1.5 mg most common; shown in **Figure 1**.
    - **UPA:** Selective progesterone receptor modulator; more effective than LNG, especially in obese women; shown in **Figure 2**.
    - **Mifepristone:** Antiprogestin; limited availability in India.

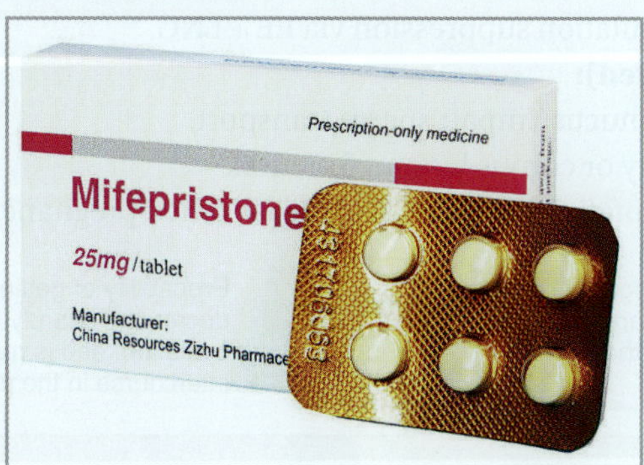

- **Mechanical Method:**
    - **Copper IUD:** Most effective; suitable for ongoing contraception; contraindicated in PID, AUB, pregnancy.

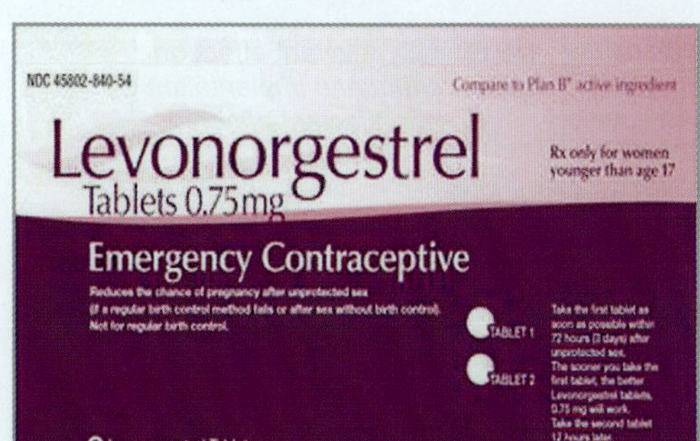

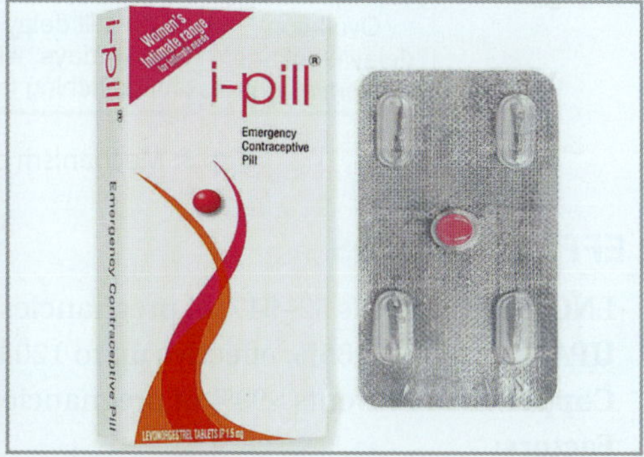

Fig. 1: Levonorgestrel emergency contraceptive.

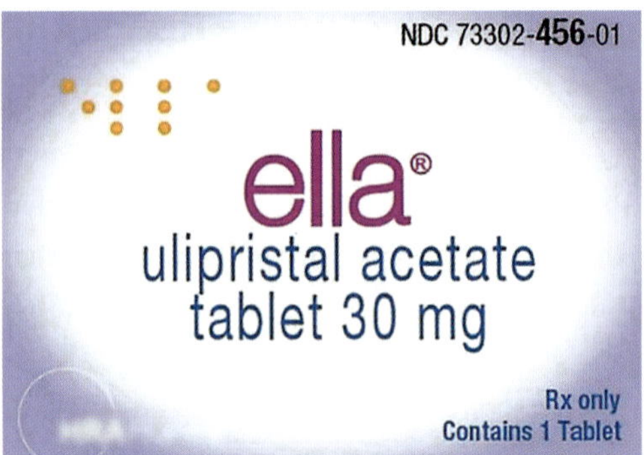

Fig. 2: Ulipristal acetate emergency contraceptive.

MECHANISMS OF ACTION

- **Primary:**
  - **LNG/UPA:** Inhibit or delay ovulation by suppressing LH surge; UPA effective post-LH surge **(Fig. 3)**.
  - **Yuzpe:** Similar ovulation suppression via EE + LNG.
- **Secondary (Postulated):**
  - Thicken cervical mucus, impair sperm transport.
  - Alter tubal motility or corpus luteum function.
- **No Effect:** Postimplantation; do not disrupt established pregnancies or harm fetuses.

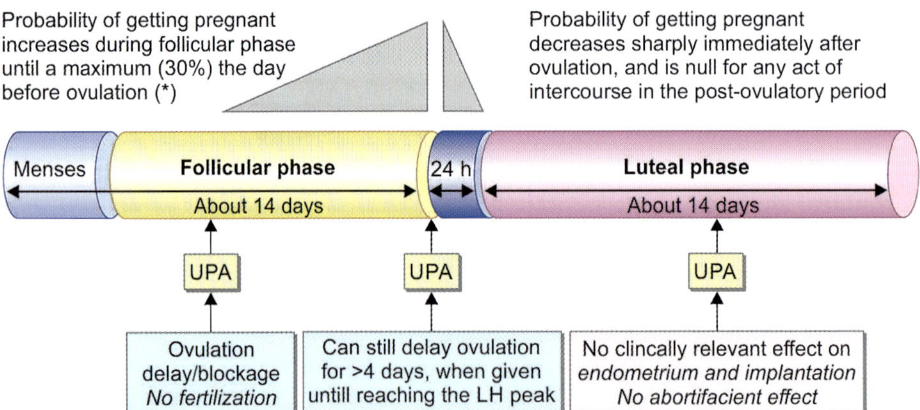

Fig. 3: Mechanism of LNG and UPA ECPs.

EFFECTIVENESS

- **LNG ECP:** Prevents 52–94% of pregnancies; most effective within 24 h.
- **UPA:** Prevents 62–85%; effective up to 120 h.
- **Copper IUD:** Prevents >99% of pregnancies.
- **Factors:**
  - Timing: Efficacy decreases with delay post-UPSI.

- BMI: LNG less effective in BMI ≥30 kg/m^2; UPA or IUD preferred.
- Repeated UPSI: Single ECP dose sufficient if all acts within 120 h.

SIDE EFFECTS

- **Common (Table 3):**
  - Nausea: LNG (20%), UPA (12%).
  - Vomiting: If within 2 h (LNG) or 3 h (UPA), repeat dose.
  - Altered menses: Early (LNG, 1 day) or delayed (UPA, 2 days); resolves spontaneously.
  - Headache, fatigue, breast tenderness: Self-limiting within 24 h.

TABLE 3: Side effects of hormonal ECPs

Side effect	*LNG prevalence*	*UPA prevalence*	*Management*
Nausea	~20%	~12%	Antiemetic if needed
Vomiting	<5%	<5%	Repeat dose if within 2–3 h
Menstrual Changes	Common	Common	Reassure; resolves spontaneously

- **Safety:** No increased risk of miscarriage, ectopic pregnancy, or congenital anomalies.

MEDICAL ELIGIBILITY AND SPECIAL CONSIDERATIONS

- **WHO Medical Eligibility Criteria (MEC):**
  - **Category 1:** No restrictions for LNG, UPA, or Yuzpe; safe in all women, including adolescents.
  - **Category 2:** Breastfeeding women (UPA: avoid breastfeeding for 1 week).
- **Special Populations:**
  - **Adolescents:** Safe; recommended post-rape within 5 days.
  - **Breastfeeding:** LNG preferred; UPA requires milk discard for 1 week.
  - **Obesity:** UPA or IUD preferred; consider double-dose LNG (3 mg).
- **Drug Interactions:**
  - Hepatic enzyme inducers (e.g., rifampicin, efavirenz): Reduce LNG/UPA efficacy; use IUD or double-dose LNG.
  - Recent progestin use: May reduce UPA efficacy.

GUIDELINES

WHO (2023):

- **Preferred Methods:** UPA (120 h), LNG (72 h), or IUD (5 days).
- **Yuzpe:** Alternative if others unavailable.
- **Access:** No prescription needed; ensure availability post-rape.

RCOG/NICE/FSRH (2023):

- **First-Line:** Copper IUD (most effective); UPA if IUD declined/unavailable.
- **LNG:** Use within 72 h; consider double dose in BMI ≥30 kg/m^2.
- **Counseling:** Discuss side effects, follow-up contraception, and STI screening post-rape.
- **Adolescents:** No age restrictions; ensure confidentiality.

India (MoHFW, 2008, updated 2019):

- **Approved:** LNG 1.5 mg single dose or 0.75 mg 12 h apart (72 h); Yuzpe; IUD.
- **Access:** Over-the-counter LNG; IUD requires trained provider.
- **Challenges:** Limited UPA/mifepristone availability; rural access barriers.

Indian Context

- **Burden:** ~26 million pregnancies annually; 30% unintended.
- **EC Use:** LNG dominates (Ezy Pill, i-Pill); 80% of EC market.
- **Issues:**
  - Misconceptions: 40% of women confuse ECPs with abortion pills.
  - Rural uptake: <5% due to stigma and supply chain issues.
- **2022 Study:** EC awareness 65% in urban versus 25% in rural India.

CLINICAL CASE SCENARIO

Case: A 22-year-old nulliparous woman presents 48 h post-UPSI due to condom breakage. BMI: 22 kg/m^2, no medical history, not breastfeeding.

Management:

- **Counseling:** Explain EC options, efficacy, and side effects; discuss ongoing contraception.
- **Prescription: LNG 1.5 mg** single dose (available OTC in India).
- **Advice:** Take immediately; use antiemetic if nausea occurs; expect menses within 7 days.
- **Follow-up:** Return if no menses in 3 weeks; initiate combined oral contraceptive.
- **Outcome:** Menses on day 30; starts COC; no pregnancy.

Exam Tip: Highlight LNG as India's preferred ECP, timing (72 h), and IUD's superior efficacy.

KEY POINTS

- **EC use in India:** 11% among women; LNG dominates.
- **Methods:** LNG (72 h), UPA (120 h), IUD (5 days); IUD most effective.
- **Mechanism:** Delays ovulation; no effect post implantation.
- **Safety:** Safe for all women, including adolescents; no fetal harm.
- **Guidelines:** WHO prefers UPA/IUD; India approves LNG/Yuzpe/IUD.
- **Challenges:** Rural access, misconceptions, limited UPA use.

BOX 1: Important points to remember

- EC prevents pregnancy post-UPSI; not an abortifacient.
- Copper IUD is the most effective EC method (failure rate <0.1%).
- LNG ECP is first-line in India; take within 72 h for optimal efficacy.
- Counsel on side effects and ongoing contraception post-EC.

REFERENCES

1. Leung VWY, Levine M, Soon JA. Mechanisms of action of hormonal emergency contraceptives. Pharmacotherapy. 2016;36(2):158-68.

2. Trussell J, Schwarz EB. Emergency contraception. In: In Hatcher RA, Trussell J, Nelson AL, et al. (Eds). Contraceptive Technology, 20th edition. New York: Ardent Media; 2017.
3. World Health Organization. Emergency contraception. Geneva: World Health Organization; 2018.
4. Guttmacher Institute. (2022). Unintended pregnancy and abortion worldwide. [online] Available from https://www.guttmacher.org/fact-sheet/induced-abortion-worldwide.
5. Haeger KO, et al. Global emergency contraception use: a systematic review. Contraception. 2018;98(4):264-71.
6. Singh S, Shekhar C, Acharya R, et al. The incidence of abortion and unintended pregnancy in India, 2015. Lancet Glob Health. 2018;6(8):e849–59.
7. NFHS-5. National Family Health Survey 2019–21. Mumbai: IIPS; 2021.
8. Sharma P, et al. Emergency contraception trends in India. Indian J Community Med. 2020;45(3):301-5.
9. Gupta R, et al. Barriers to EC access in rural India. J Fam Plann Reprod Health Care. 2019;45(2):112–8.
10. ACOG. Emergency contraception. Practice Bulletin No. 152. Obstet Gynecol. 2017;130(3):e117–24.

Barrier Contraceptives: Condoms, Occlusive Caps, Sponges, and Spermicides

Ruchika Garg

INTRODUCTION

Barrier contraceptives, including male and female condoms, occlusive caps (diaphragms, cervical caps, vault caps, Vimule caps), contraceptive sponges, and spermicides, prevent pregnancy and sexually transmitted infections (STIs) by creating physical or chemical barriers to sperm. These methods are widely used due to their accessibility, nonhormonal nature, and dual protection capabilities. This chapter explores their types, efficacy, mechanisms, indications, contraindications, advantages, disadvantages, and recent advancements, emphasizing WHO and CDC guidelines.[1,2]

MALE CONDOMS

Description

Male condoms are fine latex, polyurethane, or polyisoprene sheaths, typically 15–20 cm long, 3–3.5 cm in diameter, and 0.003–0.007 cm thick. They are closed at one end (plain or teat-ended) with an open rimmed end, available in various shapes, colors, textures, and lubrications.[3]

- **Types:**
  - Material: Latex (most common), polyurethane (non-latex, longer shelf life), polyisoprene (latex-free).
  - Shape: Plain, reservoir tip, contoured.
  - Lubrication: Dry, silicone-based, water-based, spermicidal (nonoxynol-9, N-9).
  - Texture: Smooth, ribbed, studded.
  - Packaging: Hermetically sealed in plastic/aluminum foil (3–12 per pack) or blister packs.

TABLE 1: Characteristics of male condoms.[3]

Feature	*Options*
Material	Latex, polyurethane, polyisoprene
Shape	Plain, reservoir tip, contoured
Lubrication	Dry, silicone, water-based, N-9 spermicidal
Texture	Smooth, ribbed, studded
Failure Rate	Perfect use: 2%; Typical use: 18%

Male condoms vary in material and design, impacting efficacy and user preference **(Table 1)**.[3]

Medical Eligibility Criteria (WHO)[1]

- Category 4 (Contraindications): None.
- Category 3 (Risks outweigh benefits):
  - Latex allergy (use polyurethane/polyisoprene).
  - High-risk pregnancy (if failure occurs).

Efficacy and Effectiveness

- Latex Condoms: Perfect use failure rate: 2%; typical use: 18%.[3]
- Polyurethane Condoms: Higher breakage/slippage rates; similar typical-use failure rates to latex (e.g., Avanti, Tactylon).[4]
- Polyisoprene Condoms: Comparable to latex, though limited contraceptive efficacy data.[5]
- N-9 Spermicidal Condoms: No added efficacy; increased HIV transmission risk due to genital irritation; not recommended.[6]

Mechanism of Action

Condoms act as mechanical barriers, preventing semen and fluid exchange, thus reducing pregnancy and STI risks.

Indications

- Pregnancy prevention.
- STI prevention (HIV, chlamydia, gonorrhea, trichomoniasis).
- Dual protection with another contraceptive method.[1]

Contraindications

- Absolute: None.
- Relative: Latex allergy (use non-latex alternatives).[7]

Advantages[3,7]

- Prescription-free, widely accessible.
- Suitable for infrequent intercourse, lactation, older age, teenagers.
- Effective STI protection (80% HIV reduction with consistent use).[8]
- Harmless, reliable if used correctly.
- May delay premature ejaculation.

Disadvantages[3]

- Higher failure rate than hormonal methods.
- Minor reduction in sexual pleasure due to interruption/sensitivity.
- Rare hypersensitivity reactions.

Noncontraceptive Benefits[8,9]

- Reduces STI transmission (chlamydia, gonorrhea, trichomoniasis, HIV).
- May lower cervical neoplasia risk (inconsistent HPV protection).
- Prolongs ejaculatory latency.

Proper Use and Precautions[3,7]

- Storage: Keep in dry, cool (<37°C) conditions; shelf life up to 5 years.
- Lubricants: Use water/silicone-based only with latex/polyisoprene **(Table 2)**.

- Application **(Table 3)**:
  - Apply on erect penis before contact.
  - Pinch tip to remove air, unroll to base.
  - Hold rim during withdrawal to prevent slippage.
- Precautions:
  - Use new condom per act.
  - Avoid reuse or flushing.
  - Check expiry date.
  - Consider emergency contraception/STI testing if breakage occurs.[10]

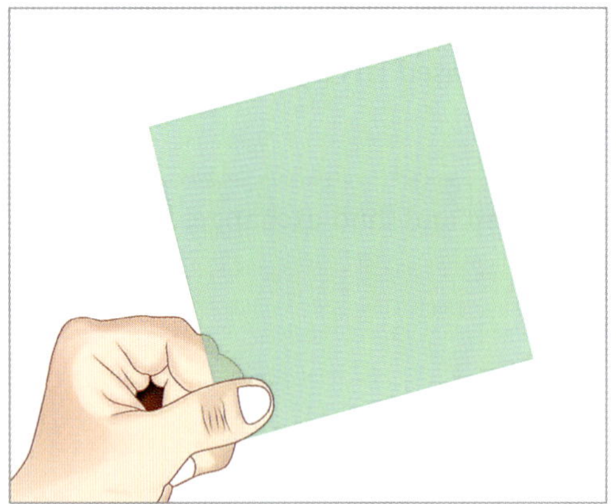

Vaginal contraceptive film.

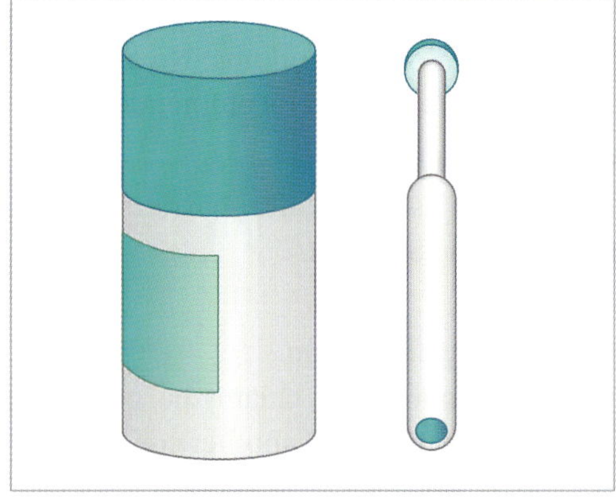

Spermicide Foam.

TABLE 2: Safe and unsafe lubricants for latex condoms.[7]

Safe	*Unsafe*
Water/silicone-based lubricants	Oil-based (baby, mineral, coconut)
Contraceptive foam/film	Butter, margarine
Glycerin, egg white, saliva	Petroleum jelly, vaginal creams

Only water-based lubricants should be used with latex condoms to prevent breakage **(Table 2)**.[7]

TABLE 3: Steps for male condom use.[3]

Step	*Action*
1	Apply lubricant inside condom tip
2	Place rolled condom on erect penis tip
3	Leave 0.5-inch space at tip
4	Pinch air from tip, unroll to base
5	Hold rim during withdrawal
6	Dispose of condom (do not flush)

Correct condom application, as outlined in **Table 3**, maximizes efficacy.[3]

FEMALE CONDOMS

Description

Female condoms (internal condoms) are nitrile polymer sheaths with flexible rings at both ends. The internal ring anchors the closed end vaginally, while the external ring covers the perineum.[11]

- Features:
- Length: ~17 cm; width: ~7.8 cm.
- Lubrication: Silicone-based (inner surface).
- Material: Nitrile (latex-free, oil-based lubricant compatible).
- Types: FC2 (synthetic latex), VA/Reddy (sponge-based), PATH Woman's (dissolving capsule).[12]

Efficacy and Effectiveness

- Perfect use: 5% pregnancy rate at 12 months.
- Typical use: 21% pregnancy rate.[11]
- Comparison: Polyurethane female condoms comparable to synthetic latex (5.24 vs. 4.3% failure).[13]
- Failure Causes: Breakage, slippage, misdirection, invagination.[14]

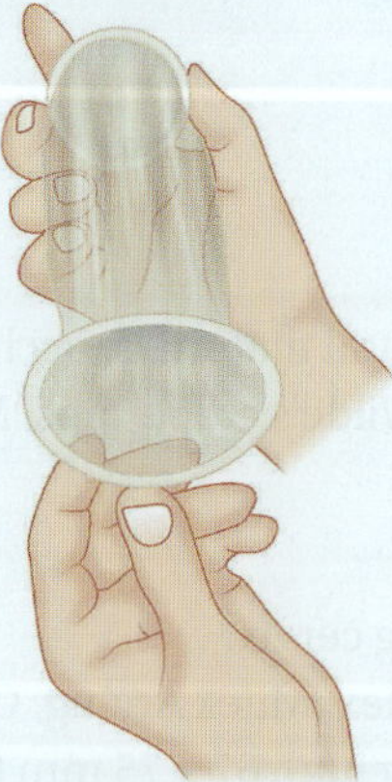

Female condom.

Mechanism of Action

Acts as an intravaginal barrier, lining the vagina to prevent sperm–cervix contact. Not to be used with male condoms due to adherence risks.[11]

Indications

- Dual protection (pregnancy/STI prevention).
- Woman-controlled contraception.[1]

Contraindications[7]

- Absolute: None.
- Relative:
- Nitrile allergy.
- Abnormal vaginal anatomy.
- Inability to master insertion technique.

Advantages[11,12]

- Autonomous female use.
- Insertable up to 8 hours preintercourse.
- Oil-based lubricant compatible.
- Less constricting for males.
- Enhanced stimulation from rings.

Disadvantages[11]

- Requires motivation/training.
- Noisy during intercourse.
- Slippage risk (~10% of uses).
- Potential for incorrect penis placement.
- Higher cost than male condoms.

Method of Use[11]

- Compress inner ring, insert high vaginally to cover cervix.
- Ensure outer ring covers labia.
- Remove by twisting outer ring, dispose of properly.
- Reapply for each act.

OCCLUSIVE CAPS

History

Originating in ancient times with natural materials, occlusive caps evolved into rubber-based devices in the 19th century (e.g., Dr. Wilde's crepe caps, Mensinga's diaphragm).[15]

Types[15]

- Vaginal Diaphragm:
  - Silicone/rubber dome covering cervix.
  - Types: Milex Wide-Seal Omniflex, Milex Arcing, Caya SILCS (one-size-fits-most).
  - Sizes: 65–95 mm (Omniflex/Arcing); 67 × 75 mm (Caya).
- Cervical Cap:
  - Small, thimble-shaped device.
  - Sizes: 22–31 mm; suction-based retention.

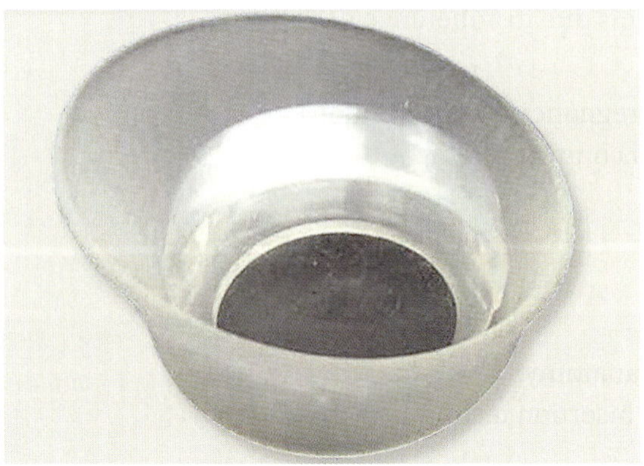

- Vault Cap:
  - Dome-shaped, fits vaginal vault.
  - Sizes: 50–75 mm; largely replaced by diaphragms.
- Vimule Cap:
  - Rigid cervical cap with flanged base.
  - Sizes: 45–51 mm; used in cystocele/prolapse.

Medical Eligibility Criteria (WHO)[1]

- Category 4: None.
- Category 3:
  - History of toxic shock syndrome (TSS).
  - Vaginal/uterine abnormalities (prolapse, poor tone).
  - High HIV risk.
  - Latex/spermicide allergy.
  - Inability to insert correctly.
- Category 2:
  - Recent delivery (6–12 weeks).
  - Parous women.
  - Valvular heart disease.
  - Urinary tract infections (UTIs).

Efficacy and Effectiveness

- Diaphragm: Perfect use: 6%; typical use: 12% (with spermicide).[16]
- Caya SILCS: 6-month perfect use: 7.9%; typical use: 10.4% (extrapolated 12-month: 18.8%).[17]
- Cervical Cap: 6-month pregnancy rate: 13.5% (FemCap) versus 7.9% (diaphragm).[18]

Mechanism of Action

Diaphragms/caps act as physical barriers, retaining spermicides (e.g., N-9, acid-buffering gels) to immobilize/kill sperm. Gels lower vaginal pH, inhibiting motility.[15]

Method of Use[15]

- Diaphragm:
  - Compress rim, insert along posterior vaginal wall.
  - Position anterior rim behind pubic bone, cover cervix.
  - Apply spermicide before insertion; reapply for repeat acts.
  - Leave in place 6–24 hours post intercourse.
- Cervical Cap:
  - Fill half with spermicide, compress, insert to cover cervix.
  - Check position; leave 6–48 hours.
- Vault/Vimule Cap:
  - Similar to diaphragm; fill with spermicide, insert to cover cervix.

Advantages[15]

- Woman-controlled.
- Nonhormonal, minimal side effects.
- Reusable (diaphragms: 1–2 years; caps: longer).
- Partial STI protection.

Disadvantages[15]

- Requires training/motivation.
- Messy spermicide application.
- Limited to motivated, educated users.
- Rare risks: TSS, UTIs, cervical erosion, allergies.
- Ineffective against HIV.

CONTRACEPTIVE SPONGE AND SPERMICIDES

Description

- Sponge: Polyurethane foam device impregnated with N-9, inserted vaginally.[19]
- Spermicides: N-9 or octoxynol-9 in various forms (suppositories, creams, jellies, foams, C-film).[20]

Types:[20]

- Suppositories: Gelatin/wax-based, melt at body temperature (e.g., Orthoforms).
- Creams/Jellies: Gelatinous (jelly) or soap-based (cream) (e.g., Delfen, Orthogynol).
- Foam Tablets: Effervescent, create foam barrier (e.g., Gynomin).
- Aerosols/Foams: Propellant-driven creams (e.g., Emko).
- C-Film: Water-soluble film with N-9.

Medical Eligibility Criteria[1]

- Category 4:
  - High HIV risk, HIV-positive status, AIDS.
- Category 2:
  - High pregnancy risk.
  - N-9 sensitivity.
  - Cervical cancer.

Efficacy and Effectiveness

- Sponge: Perfect use: ~9%; typical use: 12–24%.[19]
- Spermicides Alone: Less effective than combined use; typical use failure rate: ~28%.[20]

Mechanism of Action

- Sponge: Sustained-release N-9 reservoir, absorbs/traps sperm for 24 hours.
- Spermicides: N-9 disrupts sperm cell membranes; carrier ensures vaginal dispersion.[20]

Method of Use[19,20]

- Sponge: Moisten, insert high vaginally to cover cervix; leave 6–24 hours.
- Spermicides:
  - Insert suppositories/foams 10–30 minutes preintercourse.
  - Apply creams/jellies via applicator near cervix.
  - Reapply for repeat acts; avoid douching for 8 hours.

Indications

- Nonhormonal contraception.
- Backup with other barrier methods.
- Suitable for women avoiding hormonal/IUD methods.[1]

Contraindications[7]

- Absolute: High HIV risk (N-9 increases transmission).
- Relative: N-9 allergy, TSS history, abnormal vaginal anatomy, recent delivery/abortion, UTIs.

Risks and Side Effects[6,21]

- Increased HIV transmission risk with frequent N-9 use.
- UTIs associated with spermicides.
- TSS risk with prolonged sponge/diaphragm use.

Emerging Trends and Guidelines

- Non-N-9 Spermicides: Acid-buffering gels (e.g., Contragel) reduce irritation risks.[22]
- Smart Condoms: IoT-enabled devices for usage tracking in research.[23]
- WHO Recommendations (2023): Promote dual protection; discourage N-9 spermicides.[1]
- CDC Guidelines (2021): Emphasize STI counseling and emergency contraception awareness.[2]

CONCLUSION

Barrier contraceptives offer accessible, nonhormonal options for pregnancy and STI prevention. Male condoms are the most effective, followed by female condoms, diaphragms, and sponges/spermicides. Proper use, patient education, and adherence to updated guidelines maximize efficacy and safety, supporting global family planning efforts.

KEY POINTS

- Male condoms: 2% perfect-use failure; effective STI protection; latex-free options available.[3]
- Female condoms: Woman-controlled, 5% perfect-use failure; nitrile-based.[11]
- Diaphragms/caps: Require spermicides, higher failure rates (6–18%); limited STI protection.[15]
- Sponges/spermicides: Less effective alone; N-9 increases HIV risk.[19,20]
- WHO/CDC advocate dual protection and non-N-9 alternatives.[1,2]

REFERENCES

1. World Health Organization. Medical eligibility criteria for contraceptive use, 5th edition. Geneva: World Health Organization; 2015.
2. Centers for Disease Control and Prevention. U.S. selected practice recommendations for contraceptive use. MMWR Recomm Rep. 2021;70(3):1-77.
3. Trussell J, Aiken ARA, Micks E, et al. Efficacy, safety, and personal considerations in contraceptive methods. Contraception. 2018;97(2):86-94.
4. Steiner MJ, Dominik R, Rountree RW, et al. Contraceptive effectiveness of polyurethane vs. latex condoms. Contraception. 2016;94(3):250-6.
5. Gallo MF, Warner L, Bell AJ, et al. Polyisoprene condoms: A review of available evidence. Sex Transm Dis. 2017;44(8):485-90.
6. Wilkinson D, Ramjee G, Tholandi M, et al. Nonoxynol-9 for preventing HIV transmission: A systematic review. Bull World Health Organ. 2019;97(4):287-94.

7. Curtis KM, Tepper NK, Jatlaoui TC, et al. U.S. medical eligibility criteria for contraceptive use. MMWR Recomm Rep. 2016;65(3):1-103.
8. Weller SC, Davis-Beaty K. Condom effectiveness in reducing HIV transmission. Cochrane Database Syst Rev. 2018;5:CD003255.
9. Manhart LE, Koutsky LA. Do condoms prevent HPV and cervical neoplasia? Emerg Infect Dis. 2017;23(6):928-34.
10. Workowski KA, Bachmann LH, Chan PA, et al. Sexually transmitted infections treatment guidelines. MMWR Recomm Rep. 2021;70(4):1-187.
11. Beksinska M, Smit J, Joanis C, et al. Female condom technology: New products and regulatory issues. Contraception. 2016;93(4):293-300.
12. Schwartz JL, Barnhart K, Creinin MD, et al. New female condoms in development. Contraception. 2018;97(2):124-9.
13. Beksinska M, Greener R, Kleinschmidt I, et al. A randomized trial of polyurethane vs. synthetic latex female condoms. Contraception. 2017;96(3):165-71.
14. Farr G, Gabelnick H, Sturgen K, et al. Contraceptive efficacy of the female condom. Am J Public Health. 2019;109(6):849-54.
15. Schwartz JL, Weiner DH, Lai JJ, et al. Diaphragms and cervical caps: Current status and future prospects. Contraception. 2017;96(4):238-45.
16. Trussell J. Contraceptive failure in the United States. Contraception. 2018;97(5):397-404.
17. Schwartz JL, Poindexter A, Schmitz K, et al. SILCS diaphragm: Postcoital testing and 6-month pregnancy outcomes. Contraception. 2016;94(5):498-504.
18. Mauck CK, Lai JJ, Weiner DH, et al. Comparison of FemCap and Ortho All-Flex diaphragm. Contraception. 2018;97(3):205-11.
19. Kestelman P, Trussell J. Efficacy of the contraceptive sponge. Contraception. 2017;95(5):437-43.
20. Grimes DA, Lopez LM, Raymond EG, et al. Spermicide used alone for contraception. Cochrane Database Syst Rev. 2019;12:CD005218.
21. Fihn SD, Boyko EJ, Normand EH, et al. Spermicide use and urinary tract infections. Am J Epidemiol. 2016;183(8):729-36.
22. Thurman AR, Doncel GF. Advances in non-hormonal barrier contraception. Contraception. 2020;101(2):73-9.
23. Gupta SK, Kumar R. Smart contraceptives: The future of barrier methods. J Med Eng Technol. 2022;46(3):189-96.

Intrauterine Contraceptive Device

Ruchika Garg

What is an IUCD?

- Intrauterine Contraceptive Device (IUD/IUCD)
- Highly effective, reversible, long-acting reversible contraception (LARC)
- "Insert once, forget for years" method
- Does NOT interfere with intercourse
- No daily compliance needed → very low user failure

Composition

- Mostly polyethylene plastic
- Barium sulfate added → radiopaque (visible on X-ray/USG)

Types of IUCDs

Generation	*Type*	*Examples*	*Duration*	*Key points*
1st	Inert (nonmedicated)	Lippes Loop, Saf-T-Coil	Obsolete	First introduced in India's family planning program
2nd	Copper-bearing	Cu-T 380A (ParaGard)	10 years	Gold standard in govt programs
		Multiload 375	5 years	
		Cu-T 200, Nova-T	3–5 years	
3rd	Hormonal (LNG-IUS)	Mirena (52 mg LNG)	8 years (FDA approved 2024–2025)	20 → 10 μg/day release
		Liletta, Kyleena, etc.	5–8 years	Therapeutic uses ++
Frameless	GyneFix	Copper cylinders on thread	5 years	Less expulsion in small uterus

Best in public sector (India): Cu-T 380A—free, 10-year efficacy

Best hormonal: LNG IUS—now 8 years approved

Mechanism of Action

- Foreign body reaction → leukocytic infiltration → sperms/blastocyst destroyed
- ↑ Prostaglandins → ↑ tubal peristalsis → fertilized egg reaches uterus too early → cannot implant

Copper IUCDs (additional)

- Copper ions toxic to sperm and oocyte
- ↓ Sperm motility, viability, capacitation
- Enzymatic changes in endometrium → hostile to implantation

LNG-IUS (additional)

- Thickens cervical mucus (main spermicidal effect)
- Endometrial atrophy/decidualization
- Ovulation suppressed in only ~40% cycles in 1st year → most cycles ovulatory later
- Minimal systemic absorption → almost no systemic side effects

WHO Medical Eligibility Criteria (MEC)—Simplified

Category	*Meaning*	*IUCD (Copper and LNG)*
1	Use freely	Most women
2	Advantages > risks	Breastfeeding <6 weeks, nulliparous, HIV on ART
3	Risks > advantages (generally avoid)	Current PID, puerperal sepsis
4	Unacceptable risk (absolute CI)	Pregnancy, distorted cavity, active cervical/endometrial Ca, unexplained bleeding, Wilson's (for Cu)

Ideal Candidates for IUCD

- Wants long-term, reversible method
- Spacing or limiting births
- Completed family but does not want sterilization yet
- Fed up with pills/condoms
- Menorrhagia/dysmenorrhea (for Mirena)

Timing of Insertion

Timing	*When*	*Advantage*
Interval	Anytime (if not pregnant)	Preferably during/after menses (cervix soft + rules out pregnancy)
Post-placental	Within 10 min of placenta delivery	High acceptance in India (PPIUCD program)
Intra-caesarean	During LSCS	Very low expulsion rate
Postpartum PPIUCD	Within 48 hrs	
Post-abortion/MTP	Immediate	Safe if no infection
Emergency contraception	Within 5 days of UPSI	Cu-T only (not Mirena)

Insertion Technique (Withdrawal technique preferred—less perforation)

- Bimanual exam → confirm position and size
- Speculum → clean cervix with povidone-iodine
- Grasp anterior lip with vulsellum
- Sound uterus
- Load Cu-T 380A (no-touch), set blue flange

- Withdrawal technique (preferred):
  - Insert till fundus
  - Withdraw outer sheath → arms open
  - Push inner rod to fundus
  - Withdraw everything
- Cut threads 2–3 cm from os

LNG IUS Mirena insertion slightly different—arms loaded inside tube, release arms first at fundus, then release from inserter. 52 mg levonorgestrel is present.

Complications of IUCD

Timing	*Complication*
Immediate	Pain, vasovagal, failed insertion
Early	Expulsion (2–10%), spotting, cramps
Late	PID (mostly <20 days), actinomycosis, lost threads, perforation, pregnancy (mostly ectopic if fails)

Ectopic pregnancy
- Overall pregnancy risk ↓↓↓
- But if pregnancy occurs → higher chance it is ectopic
- Highest risk: LNG-IUS (Mirena) > Copper IUCDs

Missing Threads—Management Algorithm
- Pregnancy test
- USG → locate IUCD
  - If intrauterine → retrieve with hook/hysteroscopy
  - If extrauterine → X-ray → laparoscopy/laparotomy removal (mandatory for copper—adhesions risk)

Pregnancy with IUCD in situ
- Rule out ectopic (USG + β-hCG)
- If threads visible → remove (↓ miscarriage/sepsis risk)
- If threads not visible → counsel (risk of 2nd trimester miscarriage, chorioamnionitis); many clinicians leave it if patient wants to continue

Advantages of IUCD
- Highly effective (CuT 380A and Mirena <1 pregnancy/100 woman-years)
- Immediate return of fertility after removal
- Cost-effective long term
- No systemic effects (copper)/minimal (Mirena)
- Mirena → ↓ menorrhagia by 90%, ↓ dysmenorrhea, ↓ hysterectomy rates

LNG IUS Mirena Special Points
- Approved for 8 years (2024–2025 update)
- Reduces endometrial hyperplasia in tamoxifen users
- Therapeutic for:
  - Menorrhagia

    - Dysmenorrhea
    - Adenomyosis
    - Endometriosis
    - Part of HRT (estrogen + Mirena)
- Bleeding pattern: Irregular spotting 3–6 months → oligomenorrhea/amenorrhea in 20–50%
- Safe in breastfeeding (after 6 weeks)

Follow-up Schedule

- 1st visit: 4–6 weeks or after next menses
    - Check threads, side effects
- Then: 3 months, 6 months, then yearly
- Teach patient: Monthly thread check after menses

Quick Revision Table

Feature	*Cu-T 380A*	*Mirena (LNG-IUS)*
Duration	10 years	8 years
Failure rate	0.6–0.8%	0.2–0.5%
Menstrual bleeding	↑ (10–20%)	↓↓↓ (amenorrhea 20–50%)
Emergency contraception	Yes (within 5 days)	No
Therapeutic uses	No	Yes (AUB, adenomyosis, etc.)
Ectopic risk if fails	Higher than normal	Highest

Menstrual Abnormalities

Dysmenorrhea

Neelansha Varshney

Dysmenorrhea is defined as painful menstruation of sufficient magnitude so as to incapacitate day-to-day activities.[1,2] Dysmenorrhea pain may be spasmodic (sharp pelvic cramps at the start of menstrual flow) or congestive (deep, dull ache). It is commonly associated with symptoms such as lower backache, vomiting, headache, diarrhea, and fatigue. Prevalence of dysmenorrhea can vary between 16% and 91% in women of reproductive age with severe pain observed in 2–29%.[3] Despite its high prevalence, there is insufficient evidence to support management-seeking practices and their perceived efficacy in females with primary dysmenorrhea.

TYPES OF DYSMENORRHEA

Primary Dysmenorrhea

Dysmenorrhea occurs in the absence of pelvic pathology. It is more common in adolescents and young adult females and usually starts 1–2 days before the onset of menses or just after the menses with pain typically lasting for 1–3 days.

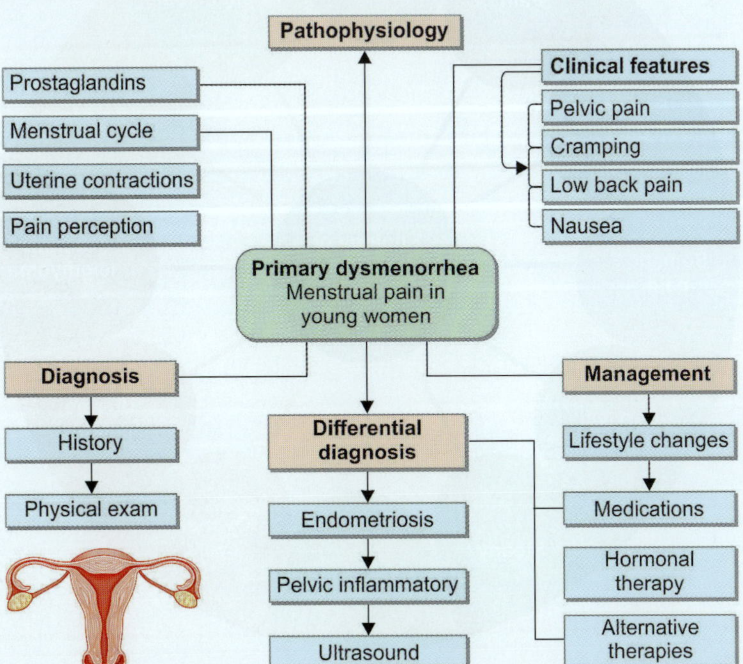

It may be associated with systemic, gastrointestinal, and psychological symptoms. The systemic symptoms include headache, lethargy, fatigue, sleepiness/sleeplessness, tender breasts, heavy lower abdomen, backache, painful knees and inner thighs, myalgia, arthralgia, swollen legs, and sweating. The gastrointestinal symptoms include an increase or decrease in appetite, nausea, vomiting, bloating, constipation, and diarrhea. Psychological symptoms include anxiety, depression, irritability, and nervousness.[4]

Pathophysiology

In ovulatory cycles, during menses endometrial sloughing causes endometrial cells to release prostaglandins PG F2 alpha, PGE2, vasopressin, and leukotrienes which stimulates myometrial contractions and ischemia. Depending upon the levels of prostaglandin release, the degree of dysmenorrhea varies. The secretion of prostaglandins causes uterine contractions along with other ailments such as nausea, vomiting, headache, and tympanites.[5,6]

Secondary Dysmenorrhea

It is defined as painful menstruation due to pelvic pathology or recognized medical condition. It is associated with diffused or constant pain that does not necessarily occur during menstruation.[5] It is usually detected in females with age more than 24 years with no history of dysmenorrhea. They have clinical features that distinguish their condition from primary dysmenorrhea which includes a large uterus, pain during sexual intercourse, and resistance to effective treatment.

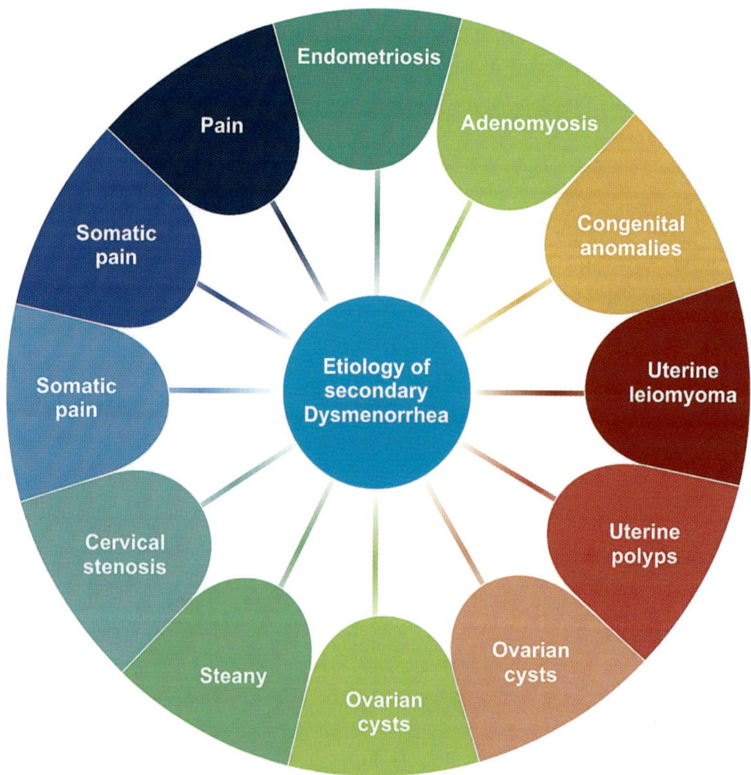

Associated risk factors

Various risk factors are associated with it and enlisted below.

- Age (13–15 years)
- Smoking
- Attempts to lose weight
- MI (less than 17 and more than 30 kg/m^2)
- Depression or anxiety
- Earlier age at menarche
- Nulliparity
- Longer and heavier menstrual flow
- Family history of dysmenorrhea
- Disruption of social network

Treatment of Dysmenorrhea

Treatment of dysmenorrhea depends on the type and severity of dysmenorrhea. In this chapter, we will be discussing case-based medical management approach to treat dysmenorrhea. Drugs which can be used to treat dysmenorrhea will be discussed in different tables along with dosage schedules, side effects, and mechanism of action.

Initial approach: Detailed patient history and clinical examination should be done to rule out pelvic pathology at the first visit. Patients should be educated regarding menstrual cycles, causes, and symptoms of dysmenorrhea and reassurance should be given. Treatment is planned according to age and symptoms.

Nonpharmacological interventions: Pain relief without medication is an important healthcare target and it is safe and inexpensive and easily accepted by patients. Nonpharmacological methods such as acupuncture, heat therapy, psychotherapy, massage therapy, hypnotherapy, physiotherapy, and transcutaneous electrical nerve stimulation (TENS) are used to reduce the primary dysmenorrhea immensity. Several mechanisms are hypothesized to reduce menstrual pain which include increasing pelvic blood supply, inhibiting uterine contractions, stimulating the release of endorphins and serotonin, and altering the ability to receive and perceive pain signs. It will be discussed in detail after pharmacological treatment.

Primary dysmenorrhea pharmacological management (Cases 1 to 9)

Indications: Patients who do not have adequate relief with nonpharmacological interventions or who desire immediate pharmacologic therapy.

Case 1. Adolescent girl (10–18 years) with dysmenorrhea

Most adolescent girls will have primary dysmenorrhea and will respond well to empirical treatment with nonsteroidal anti-inflammatory drugs (NSAIDs) and antispasmodics **(Table 1)** or progesterone oral hormonal preparation **(Table 2)** or both. Progesterone preparation in the form of Norethisterone acetate or medroxyprogesterone acetate 5–10 mg daily is to be used. Dose schedule should be individualized depending upon age and symptoms. Accordingly, a short protocol for the last 10 days before menses or cyclical 21 days regimen can be used.

Duration of treatment will be 6–9 months. Resistant cases can be evaluated by ultrasonography to rule out pelvic pathology.

Medical management:

1. *NSAIDs and antispasmodics:* These drugs are used as the first line of management of dysmenorrhea. It should be started 1 or 2 days prior to menses and to be continued for initial 2–3 days of menses along with antacids. Antispasmodics to be started with initiation of symptoms and can be given for 3–5 days. NSAIDs and antispasmodics which can be used safely in adolescent girls are discussed in detail in **Table 1**.

TABLE 1: NSAIDs and antispasmodics.

Drugs	*Mechanism of action*	*Dosages*	*Max dose*	*Side effect*	*Contraindications*
A. NSAIDs					
Paracetamol (para amino-phenol)	Inhibition of two isoforms of cyclooxygenase, COX-1 and COX-2, which are involved in prostaglandin (PG) synthesis	325 mg to 1 g orally every 4–6 hours	4 g per 24 hours	Nausea, vomiting, **constipation**, hypersensitivity rash, **pruritus**, hepatotoxicity	Hypersensitivity to acetaminophen, severe hepatic impairment, or severe active hepatic disease
Ibuprofen (propionic acid derivative)	Nonselective inhibitor of cyclooxygenase COX-1 and COX-2	200–400 mg orally every 4 hours as needed	3,200 mg/day	Gastritis, ulceration, hemorrhage, perforation, Diminished renal function, rashes	Active GI or cerebrovascular bleeding, uncontrolled heart failure, lupus, renal impairment, and hepatic impairment
Mefenamic acid (anthranilic acid derivative)	Inhibitor of COX-1 and COX-2	250 mg orally every 6 hours as needed	Not to exceed 3 days	• Diarrhea, • Nausea, stomach **bloating** • Swelling of the face, fingers, • Feet,lower legs	History of asthma, urticaria, or other allergic-type reactions after aspirin or other NSAIDs
Naproxen (propionic acid derivative)	Blocks arachidonic acid to inhibit COX-1 and COX-2	275 mg every 6–8 hourly	1,100 mg/day	GI intolerance	Hypersensitivity, liver AND renal impairments
B. Antispasmodics					
Drotaverine (smooth muscle relaxant)	Selective inhibitor of phosphodiesterase-4	80 mg every 12 hourly	240 mg/ day	Heating sensation, dizziness, headache (rarely), insomnia	Liver and kidney failure and in severe heart failure and in children under 12 years of age

Contd...

Contd...

Drugs	*Mechanism of action*	*Dosages*	*Max dose*	*Side effect*	*Contraindications*
Hyoscine Butyl Bromide (antimuscarinic)	Anticholinergic action—binds to muscarinic acetylcholine receptors, blocking their effect	2 tablets (40 mg), taken 4 times a day	160 mg/ day	Side effects may include sleepiness, vision changes, dry mouth, rapid heart rate, triggering of glaucoma, and severe allergies	Myasthenia gravis, mechanical stenosis in the gastrointestinal tract, paralytical or obstructive ileus, megacolon
Dicyclomine + Paracetamol (antimuscarinic)	Dicyclomine is a muscarinic M1, M3, and M2 receptor antagonist as well as a noncompetitive inhibitor of histamine and bradykinin	325–650 mg every 4–6 hours	4 g/day	Liver damage or allergic reactions like swelling of the mouth, face, throat, difficulty in breathing, skin rash, or itching	Hypersensitivity to acetaminophen, severe hepatic impairment, or severe active hepatic disease
Camylofin + Paracetamol	Camylofin is a smooth muscle relaxant with both anticholinergic action	25 mg Camylofin + 300 mg PCM	4 g per 24 hours	Skin rash, headache, granulocytopenia, irregular heart rate	Heart disease, glaucoma (narrow angle)

2. *Hormonal management:* Progesterone preparations (oral formulations): Patients whose dysmenorrhea is not curable by NSAIDs could be given hormone therapy for at least three menstrual cycles. About 75% of patients receiving progestins experience reduction in pain. Combined estrogen-progesterone pills and DMPA use has been associated with smaller gains or loss of bone mass during this critical age period for acquiring bone strength; therefore, they should be averted. Oral progestin formulations are enlisted in **Table 2**.

TABLE 2: Progestin preparations (oral formulations).

Progestin preparation (oral)	*Mechanism*	*Oral dosage*	*Side effects*
Medroxyprogesterone acetate (pregnanes) c-21 progestin	Decidualization and atrophy of endometrium	5 or 10 mg daily for 5–10 days starting on day 16 or daily for 21days (cyclical)	• Irregular bleeding/ spotting • Mood variability • Depression • Bloating • Breast tenderness • Weight gain drowsiness
Norethindrone acetate (estrane) 19-nor-testosterone		5 or 10 mg daily for 5–10 days starting on day 16 or daily for 21days (cyclical)	
Dydrogesterone (gonanes) 19-nor-testosterone		10–30 mg twice/ thrice daily for 6 months	

Case 2. Young unmarried female (age ≥18 years) with dysmenorrhea: Detailed history, clinical examination, pelvic ultrasonography, and if required MRI are to be done. Drugs of choice will be NSAIDs and antispasmodics **(Table 1)** or hormonal suppression or both. Progestin **(Table 2)** or combinations of estrogen and progesterone (low dose or high dose) can be used depending upon USG findings. Duration of treatment will be 6–9 months. If there is any pelvic pathology, then treatment is based on the type of pelvic pathology.

Hormonal management (oral formulations): Progestin preparations or combined estrogen–progesterone: For patients not responding to NSAIDs, start with hormone therapy for at least three menstrual cycles. Continuous combined oral pills for 3 months give excellent results.

Case 3: Married female with dysmenorrhea desiring for contraception: After evaluation if there is no pelvic pathology, different hormonal preparations can be used in the form of oral, injectable, implants, patches, vaginal rings, and intrauterine devices **(Table 3)**. It should be started on day 1–3 of menses and continues for 21 days for 6–9 months or as long as contraception is required. Apart from oral preparation injectables, vaginal rings, transdermal patches, and intrauterine devices are widely available and can also be used safely in these women. Various available formulations of combined estrogen–progesterone and progestin are enlisted in **Table 3**.

TABLE 3: Hormonal preparation: combined estrogen–progesterone and progestin.

Hormonal preparation	*Formulations*	*Dosage*	*Side effects*	*Contraindications*
Combined (Estrogen + Progesterone) Mechanism of action: • Synthetic progestins suppress ovulation and make the endometrium thin which has small amounts of arachidonic acid, the substrate for most prostaglandin synthesis • It reduces both uterine bleeding flow and contractions during menses, which decreases dysmenorrhea	1.OC pills: Low/high dose	Ethinyl estradiol (20 or 30 µg) + LNG (0.15 mg)	Nausea vomiting, weight gain, venous thrombosis, mastalgia	Arterial venous thrombosis Severe hypertension, DM with vascular complications, active liver diseases breast cancers
	Transdermal patch	Ethinyl estradiol (20 µg) + Norelgestromin (0.15 mg)		
	Vaginal ring	Ethinyl estradiol (15 mcg) + Etonogestrel (0.12 mg)		
Progestin Mechanism: Progestins cause endometrial atrophy and inhibit ovulation	Oral progestin	Refer to **Table 2**		
	DMPA: Depot intramuscular	Medroxyproges-terone acetate 150 mg every 3 monthly	Irregular men-ses, amenorrhea, loss of BMD	Unexplained vaginal bleeding, thromboembolic diseases, breast cancer, osteoporosis
	LNG (IUD): Intrauterine device	Levonorgestrel 52-mg (20 µg/day)	Irregular frequent menses, spotting	
	Norplant	Etonogestrel 68 mg	Acne, mastalgia, menstrual irregularities	

Case 4. Patients with continued menstrual pain despite NSAIDs and hormonal treatment: Reassess patients by clinical examination and USG to rule out pelvic pathology. Minimally invasive techniques such as transcutaneous electrical nerve stimulation can be offered to patients who still insist on conservative management.

- Transcutaneous electrical nerve stimulation: Percutaneous tibial nerve stimulation (PTNS). Mechanism:
- It raises the threshold for pain signals from uterine hypoxia and hypercontractility by sending a volley of afferent impulses through the large diameter sensory fibers of the same nerve root, resulting in lower perception of painful uterine signals
- Peripheral nerves and the spinal cord release endorphins. The major limitation: need for continuous treatment for 12 weeks.

Role of Laparoscopy

In the absence of pelvic pathology, diagnostic laparoscopy can be offered. The most common diagnosis is endometriosis as mild grade of endometriosis cannot be detected by USG.

Case 5. Patients with persistent dysmenorrhea who desire to avoid surgery (diagnostic laparoscopy).

Empirical treatment with a GnRH agonist analog or antagonist:

Make an endometriosis presumptive diagnosis and suggest empirical GnRH agonist or antagonist therapy. With either agonist or antagonist medication, if the pain significantly diminishes or goes away, endometriosis is likely present; however, this is not proven. Details of GnRH agonist or antagonist are given in **Table 4**.

TABLE 4: GnRH agonists and antagonists.

Preparation	*Mechanism of action*	*Dosages*	*Side effect*
GNRH agonist	Prolonged activation of GnRH receptors by GnRH leads to desensitization and consequently to suppressed gonadotrophin secretion		
Nafarelin		200 µg intranasal spray twice day	Menopause-like side effects, high cost
Leuprolide acetate depot		3.75 mg intramuscularly every 4 weeks	Loss of bone density with long-term use
GnRH antagonist	It competes with GnRH for receptors on gonadotroph cell membranes, inhibits GnRH-induced signal transduction and consequently gonadotrophin secretion.	Tab 150–200 mg OD for 6 months	Hot flushes, night sweat, nausea, weight gain, vomiting
Elagolix			

Case 6. Patients with persistent pain and negative laparoscopy

If laparoscopy is negative and the patient has previously failed both hormonal contraception and NSAIDs, a 3-month course of a GnRH agonist analog can be tried, since endometriosis may have been missed. Even in the hands of experienced laparoscopists, an accurate diagnosis of endometriosis can be difficult since the disease is often microscopic and presents visually with a variety of atypical lesions. Calcium supplementation 1–2 g daily should be considered with GNRH agonist.

Refractory dysmenorrhea (Cases 7, 8, 9)

Despite the above treatments, a minority of patients will continue to have dysmenorrhea that limits their function. Treatment options for refractory dysmenorrhea should be individualized as per age and future childbearing. Cases 7, 8, and 9 are discussed as below.

Case 7. Patient with abnormal uterine bleeding with dysmenorrhea: Patients who do not desire future childbearing but want to retain uterus: Endometrial ablation can be advised.

Case 8. Patients who have exhausted all treatment options and have completed their childbearing: Hysterectomy is the definitive treatment.

Case 9. Patients with Chronic midline pelvic pain with no organic pathology: Nerve transection procedures like presacral neurectomy can be done.

Nonpharmacological supportive treatment:

- *Exercise:* It functions by enhancing pelvic blood flow and triggering the production of endorphins, which serve to reduce pain. Increasing physical activity is a sensible strategy to lessen dysmenorrhea due to its numerous health advantages and a low risk of injury. Walking, yoga, and cardiovascular exercises should be done for 30–45 minutes.
- *Application of a heat pack to the lower abdomen:* Applying localized heat to the belly can increase circulation, ease muscle tension, and relax the abdominal muscles to lessen pain brought on by muscle spasms. The effectiveness of other treatments may be increased by heat therapy
- *Behavioral counseling:* Behavioral counseling offers patients ways to change how they perceive their pain (such as desensitization-based techniques, hypnotherapy, imagery, and coping mechanisms) and how they react to pain (e.g., biofeedback, electromyographic training, exercises, relaxation training). In motivated patients, it serves as an adjuvant to therapeutic exercise and medication.

Complementary Medicine

- *Acupuncture or acupressure*: Improvements were noted in the worst pain intensity, number of days with pain, and proportion of patients using pain medication.
- *Diet and vitamins*: Dietary advice to avoid food that causes bloating and water retention, e.g., fatty foods, carbonated beverages, caffeine, and salty foods. A variety of dietary changes and vitamin therapies have been reported to reduce the severity of menstrual pain, which includes:
  - Low fat vegetarian diet
  - Increased dairy intake
  - Vitamin E (500 units per day or 200 units twice per day, beginning 2 days before menses and continuing through the first 3 days of bleeding)
  - Vitamin B1 (100 mg daily), vitamin B6 (200 mg daily), fish oil supplement, and vitamin D3
  - Ginger powder consumption: 750–2,000 mg on days 1–3 of the menstrual cycle
  - Chinese herbs

Unproven Treatment

- *Nerve transection procedures:* Laparoscopic uterosacral nerve ablation (LUNA) and presacral neurectomy (PSN) involve transection of (uterosacral ligaments or pelvis) afferent nerve fibers causing interruption of cervical sensory pain fibers in patients with chronic midline pelvic pain associated with endometriosis.
- *Tocolytics:* Nitric oxide, calcium channel blockers, and nitroglycerin all have tocolytic effects and are under investigation as potential therapies of dysmenorrhea.
- *Magnesium-Phosphodiesterase inhibitors:* By inhibiting phosphodiesterase, sildenafil enhances the vasodilatory effects of nitric oxide, facilitating myometrial blood flow, and thus reducing primary dysmenorrhea.

Secondary Dysmenorrhea

It is defined as dysmenorrhea due to pelvic pathology. Along with accompanying pelvic disease, prostaglandin release and anatomical mechanisms are also responsible for secondary dysmenorrhea. Various causes of secondary dysmenorrhea, their diagnosis, and management are discussed in **Table 5**.

TABLE 5: Causes of secondary dysmenorrhea.

Causes of secondary dysmenorrhea	*Signs: Dysmenorrhea with*	*Diagnosis*	*Management*
Gynecological causes			
Endometriosis	Dyspareunia, infertility	Clinical examination/USG/ Laparoscopy	Medical/surgical/ combined
Adenomyosis	Abnormal uterine bleeding	Clinical examination/USG/ MRI	Medical/surgical/ combined
Fibroid	Large uterus	Clinical examination/USG	Medical/surgical
Endometrial polyp	Abnormal uterine bleeding	Clinical examination/USG/ hysteroscopy	Polypectomy
Pelvic inflammatory syndrome	Vaginal discharge	Clinical examination/USG	Antibiotics and anti-inflammatory drugs
Obstructive mullerian anomalies:	Large uterus	Clinical examination/USG/ MRI/laparoscopy	Surgery
Use of IUCD	Noncyclical pain	Clinical examination/USG	NSAIDs/removal
Pelvic congestion syndrome	Noncyclical pain	USG/ Doppler	NSAIDs
Other causes			
Gastrointestinal: Inflammatory and Irritable bowel syndrome	Constipation/ diarrhea	USG/gastrointestinal endoscopy	Medical
Renal: Ureteropelvic obstruction	Loin to groin pain	USG/CT scan	Medical/surgical
Psychogenic	Pain at Multiple site	Detailed history by specialist	Counseling/medical

Gynecological pathologies: Most common pelvic pathologies which are associated with secondary dysmenorrhea are discussed below.

- **Endometriosis:** Among the various gynecological pathologies, endometriosis is the most common benign disorder defined as the presence of functional endometrium outside the uterine mucosa. It is seen in around 8–10% of reproductive age group females, affecting 20–50% infertile population and chronic pain (3–80%). It is usually diagnosed based on symptoms/physical examination and confirmed on ultrasonography or laparoscopy but finally proven by histopathology of the specimen.
- **Fibroid uterus:** It is the second most common pelvic pathology. Fibroids vary in number, size, and location. It gives rise to different types of pain patterns like dull to sharp pain, menstrual cramping pelvic pain, low back pain, abdominal pressure, dyspareunia, rectal and bladder pressure (uncomfortable pressure leads to pain). It can also compress sciatic nerves leading to leg pain. Causes of acute pain in the abdomen are twisted pedunculated fibroid, submucosal fibroid, and red degeneration of fibroid. Posterior fibroids may cause low backache and anterior fibroid can contribute to anterior pelvic pain, pressure, and urinary complications.
- **PID (pelvic inflammatory disease):** It involves infection and inflammation of the upper genital tract including uterus, cervix, ovary, and fallopian tube. Outpatient and inpatient management depends upon severity of disease. Patients may complain of continuous dull, aching, lower abdomen pain with or without fever. Oral or parenteral antibiotics are required to treat this condition. For chronic pelvic pain, the possibility of tuberculosis should be ruled out.

Treatment for Secondary Dysmenorrhea

It varies depending upon the type of pelvic pathology, age of patient, severity of symptoms, and child-bearing status. For mild-to-moderate grades of above-mentioned pathology, medical management is preferred whereas moderate-to-severe grades of pelvic pathologies may require surgical interventions. **Table 6** enlists different drugs used in various pelvic pathologies.

TABLE 6: Medical management for secondary dysmenorrhea.

Gynecological pathology	*Drugs used*	*Mechanism of action*	*Dosages*	*Side effects*
Endometriosis/ adenomyosis	Dienogest	Atrophy of endometrium	2 mg one or twice a day for 3–6 months	• Irregular bleeding, spotting • Mood variability
	Androgens: • Danazol • Gestrinone	Inhibits steroidogenesis and atrophy of lesion	• 400–800 mg orally in 4 divided doses for 6–9 months • 1.25/2.5 mg twice a week for 6–9 months	Acne, hirsutism, voice changes, diminished breast size, decreased libido
	Progesterone (New) Drospirenone	Decidualization of endometrium	4 mg once a day for 21 days for 3 cycles	

Contd...

Contd...

Gynecological pathology	*Drugs used*	*Mechanism of action*	*Dosages*	*Side effects*
	Aromatase inhibitors: • Letrozole • Anastrozole	Reduces estrogen synthesis with lesion atrophy	• 2.5 mg daily for 6 months • 1 mg daily for 6 months	Headache, nausea, vomiting, skin changes, vasomotor symptoms, arthralgia, osteoporosis
	SERMs: • Tamoxifen • Raloxifene	Inhibit estrogen receptors	40–60 mg/day for 6 months	Fatigue, hot flushes, night sweats, vaginal discharge, mood swings
Fibroid	SPRMs: Ulipristal Mifepristone	Antiproliferative effects in the endometrium	• 5 mg/day for 6 months • 25 mg/day for 3 months	Dizziness, hot flushes, fatigue, headache, nausea, vomiting
PID	Antibiotics and anti-inflamma-tory drugs	Cap. Doxycycline Tab metro-nidazole	• 100 mg BD for 14 days • 400 mg TDS for 7 days	Nausea, vomiting

CONCLUSION

Due to the vast range of physical and psychological symptoms, dysmenorrhea has a detrimental impact on quality of life and decreases attendance at work and school. The primary focus of treatment for this illness is pain reduction, whether achieved pharmaceutically or through the use of complementary therapies. Treatment should be individualized depending upon age of patient and severity of symptoms.

Algorithm: Management of dysmenorrhea.

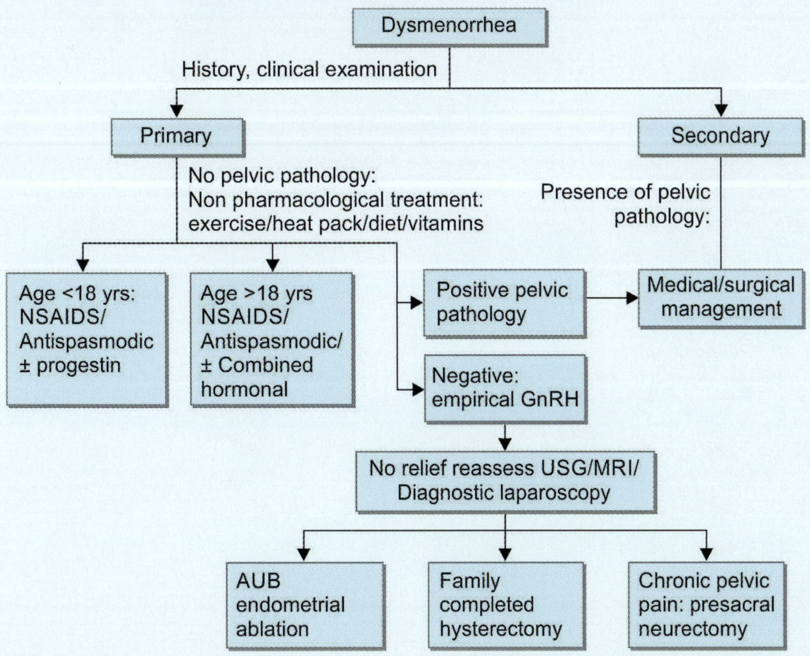

REFERENCES

1. Kulkarni A, Deb S. Dysmenorrhoea. Obstet Gynecol Reprod Med. 2019;29(10):286-91.
2. Bernardi M, Lazzeri L, Perelli F, et al. Dysmenorrhea and related disorders. F1000Res. 2017;6:1645.
3. Ju H, Jones M, Mishra G. The prevalence and risk factors of dysmenorrhea. Epidemiol Rev. 2014:36:104-13.
4. Itani R, Soubra L, Karout S, et al. Primary Dysmenorrhea: Pathophysiology, Diagnosis, and Treatment Updates. Korean J Fam Med. 2022;43(2):101-8.
5. Mendiratta V, Lentz GM. Primary and secondary dysmenorrhea, premenstrual syndrome, and premenstrual dysphoric disorder. In: Lobo RA, Gershenson DM, Lentz GM (Eds). Comprehensive Gynecology, 7th edition. Philadelphia (PA): Elsevier Inc; 2017. pp. 815--28.
6. Bernardi M, Lazzeri L, Perelli F, et al. Dysmenorrhea and related disorders. F1000Res. 2017;6:1645.

Premenstrual Syndrome

Ruchika Garg

PREMENSTRUAL SYNDROME (PMS)

- **Definition:** A collection of physical, emotional, and behavioral symptoms occurring cyclically during the luteal phase (1–2 weeks before menstruation) and resolving with menstruation onset.
- **Common Symptoms:** Bloating, breast tenderness, headaches, irritability, mood swings, fatigue, food cravings, and mild anxiety.
- **Pathophysiology:** Related to cyclical hormonal changes (estrogen/progesterone fluctuations) affecting neurotransmitters such as serotonin.
- **Diagnosis:** Based on symptom diary tracking for at least two menstrual cycles; absence of other medical or psychiatric conditions.

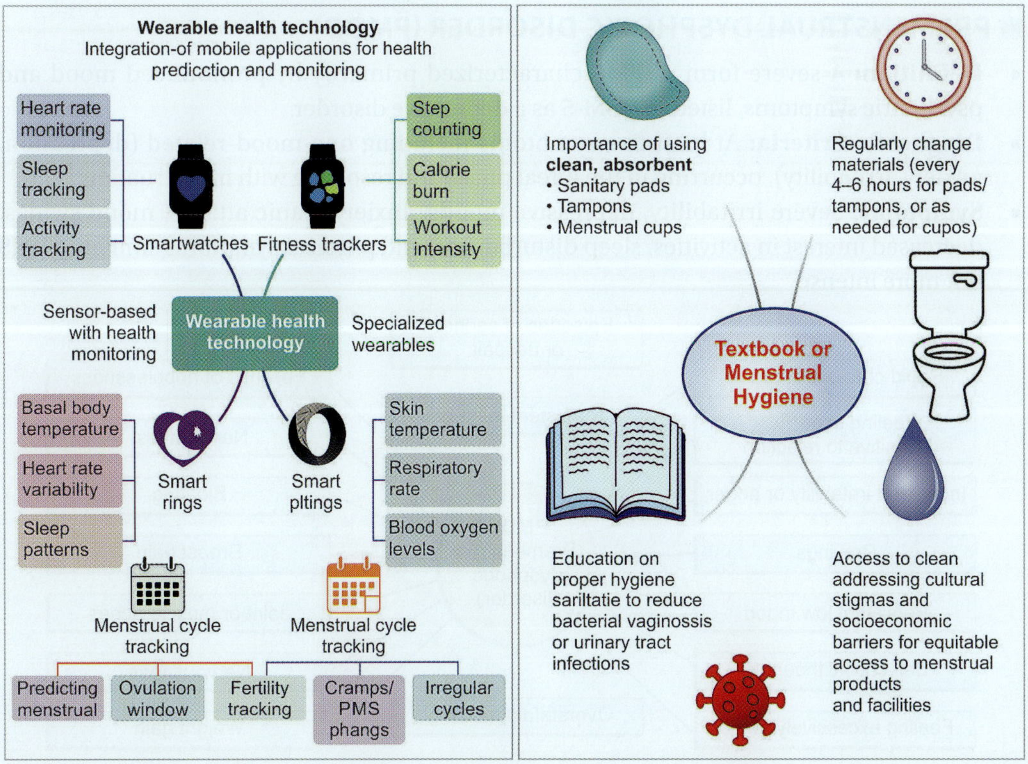

- **Management:** Lifestyle modifications, stress reduction, dietary changes, NSAIDs for pain, and hormonal therapies in selected cases.

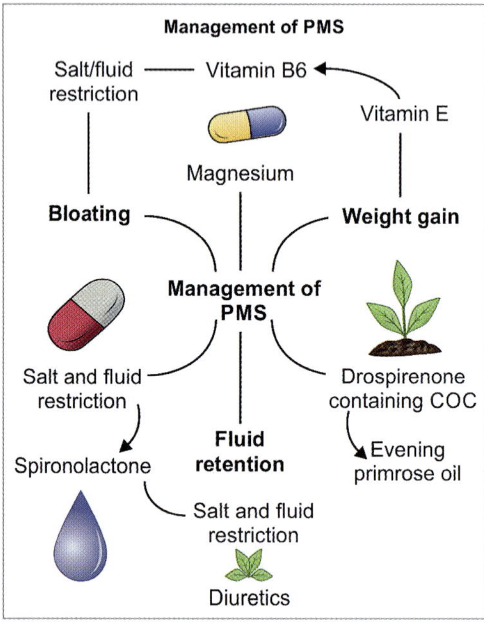

PREMENSTRUAL DYSPHORIC DISORDER (PMDD)

- **Definition:** A severe form of PMS characterized primarily by pronounced mood and psychiatric symptoms, listed in DSM-5 as a depressive disorder.
- **Diagnostic Criteria:** At least five symptoms including one mood-related (depression, anxiety, irritability), occurring in the luteal phase and resolving with menstruation.
- **Symptoms:** Severe irritability, depressive moods, anxiety, panic attacks, mood swings, decreased interest in activities, sleep disturbances, and physical symptoms similar to PMS but more intense.

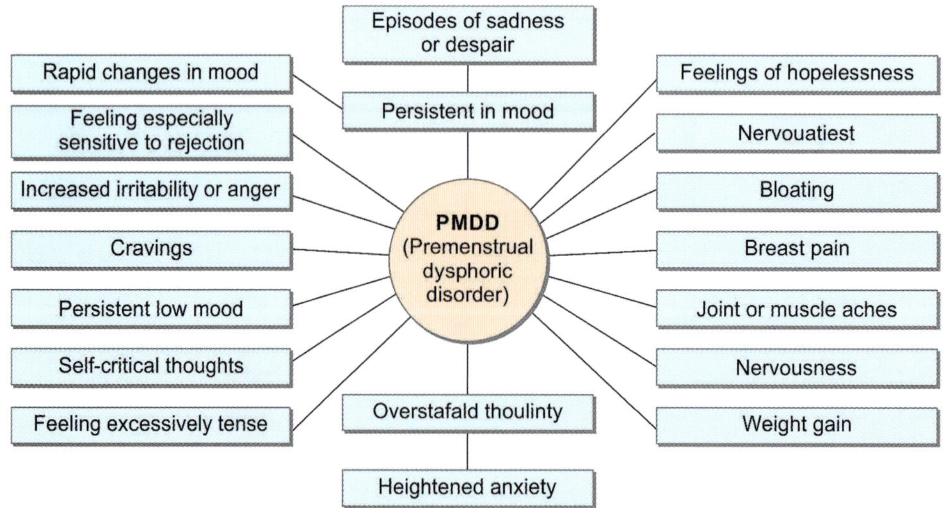

- **Etiology:** Hypersensitivity to normal hormonal fluctuations leading to serotonin dysregulation.
- **Diagnosis:** Requires prospective symptom charting over two cycles and exclusion of other psychiatric disorders.
- **Treatment:** Selective Serotonin reuptake Inhibitors (SSRIs), cognitive behavioral therapy, lifestyle modification, hormonal suppression (e.g., GnRH analogs or hormonal contraceptives), and supportive counseling.

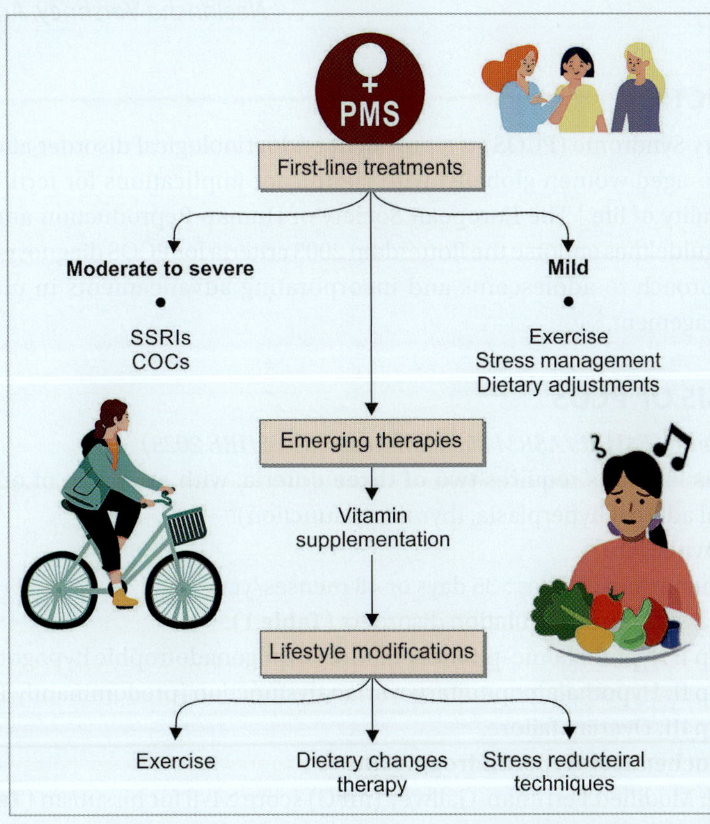

Polycystic Ovary Syndrome: Diagnosis, Pathophysiology, and Management

Neelansha Varshney, Anu Chaudhary

INTRODUCTION

Polycystic Ovary Syndrome (PCOS) is a prevalent endocrinological disorder affecting 10–13% of reproductive-aged women globally, with significant implications for fertility, metabolic health, and quality of life.[1] The European Society of Human Reproduction and Embryology (ESHRE) 2023 guidelines endorse the Rotterdam 2003 criteria for PCOS diagnosis, emphasizing a nuanced approach to adolescents and incorporating advancements in ultrasound and metabolic management.[2]

DIAGNOSIS OF PCOS

Rotterdam Criteria (ESHRE/ASRM 2003, Endorsed by ESHRE 2023)

PCOS diagnosis in adults requires **two of three** criteria, with exclusion of other etiologies (e.g., congenital adrenal hyperplasia, thyroid dysfunction):[2]

- **Oligo-/Anovulation:**
  - Oligoamenorrhea: Cycles >35 days or <8 menses/yr.
  - WHO classification of ovulation disorders **(Table 1)**:
    - Group I: Hypothalamic-pituitary failure (hypogonadotrophic hypogonadism).
    - Group II: Hypothalamopituitaryovarian dysfunction (predominantly PCOS).
    - Group III: Ovarian failure.[3]
- **Clinical/Biochemical Hyperandrogenism:**
  - **Clinical:** Modified Ferriman-Gallwey (mFG) score ≥4–8 for hirsutism **(Table 2)**.[4]
  - **Biochemical:** Elevated total/free testosterone or free androgen index (FAI = Total Testosterone/SHBG × 100).
- **Polycystic Ovarian Morphology (PCOM):**
  - Ovary volume ≥10 cc and/or ≥20 follicles (2–9 mm) per ovary on transvaginal ultrasound (TVS) with ≥8 MHz transducer[5] as shown in **Figures 1A and B**.

TABLE 1: WHO classification of ovulation disorders.[3]

Group	*Description*	*Example*
I	Hypothalamic–pituitary failure	Hypogonadotrophic hypogonadism
II	Hypothalam opituitary ovarian dysfunction	PCOS
III	Ovarian failure	Premature ovarian insufficiency

TABLE 2: Modified Ferriman-Gallwey scoring system for hirsutism (9 areas, score 0–4 per area, total ≥4-8 indicates hirsutism).[4]

Site	*Grade 1*	*Grade 2*	*Grade 3*	*Grade 4*
Upper lip	Few hairs at the outer margin	Small moustache at outer margin	Moustache extending halfway from outer margin	Moustache extending to mid-line
Chin	Few scattered hairs	Scattered hairs with small concentrations	Complete cover, light	Complete cover, heavy
Chest	Circumareolar hairs	Circumareolar hairs with mid-line hair	Fusion of circumareolar hairs with mid-line hair giving three-quarter cover	Complete cover
Upper back	Few scattered hairs	More than a few scattered hairs but still scattered	Complete cover, light	Complete cover, heavy
Lower back	Sacral tuft of hair	Sacral tuft of hair with some lateral extension	Three-quarter cover	Complete cover
Upper abdomen	Few mid-line hairs	Rather more but still mid-line	Half cover	Complete cover
Lower abdomen	Few mid-line hairs	Mid-line streak of hair	Mid-line band of hair	An inverted V-shaped growth
Upper arm and thigh	Sparse hair growth affecting not more than a quarter of limb surface	More than a quarter coverage but still incomplete	Complete cover, light	Complete cover, heavy
Forearm and legs	–	–	–	Complete cover, heavy

Note: Forearm and hand, lower leg, and feet are **not included** in the "hormonal" score and only single value is added even when hirsutism involves these extremities bilaterally. Minimum score is **0** and maximum score is **36**. A score of **<8** = No hirsutism, **8–16** = Mild hirsutism,**17–25** = Moderate hirsutism, **>25** = Severe hirsutism. Values may vary across different ethnic groups.

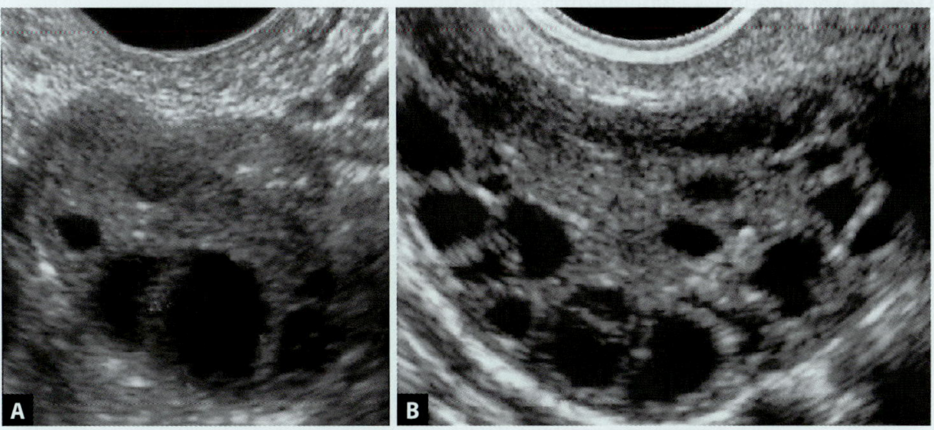

Figs. 1A and B: Difference between (A) normal ovary and (B) polycystic ovary.[60]

Adolescent PCOS Diagnosis (ESHRE 2023)

Adult criteria may overdiagnose PCOS in adolescents due to pubertal overlap (e.g., irregular cycles, multifollicular ovaries). Diagnosis requires:[6]

- **Irregular Menstrual Cycles** (based on years post-menarche):
  - *90 days for any cycle (>1 year post-menarche).*
  - Cycles <21 or >45 days (1–3 years post-menarche).
  - Cycles <21 or >35 days (>3 years post-menarche).
  - Primary amenorrhea by age 15 or >3 years post-thelarche.
  - <1 year post-menarche: Normal pubertal transition, no diagnosis.
- **Hyperandrogenism:** Hirsutism (mFG ≥4–8), severe acne, or biochemical hyperandrogenemia (high-quality assays). Hirsutism is a stronger marker than acne, which may be transient.[7]
- **Ultrasound:** Not recommended <8 years post-menarche due to a high incidence of multifollicular ovaries.[8]
- **Anti-Müllerian Hormone (AMH):** Not used for diagnosis due to lack of standardized cutoffs.[9]
- **Consensus:** Diagnosis deferred until 2 years post-menarche; all Rotterdam criteria (anovulation, hyperandrogenism, PCOM) required for confirmation.[10]

Historical Diagnostic Criteria

The Rotterdam criteria remain the gold standard, superseding earlier frameworks **(Table 3)**.[11]

TABLE 3: Evolution of PCOS diagnostic criteria.[11]

Criteria	*Year*	*Requirements*
NIH	1990	Hyperandrogenism + anovulation
AE-PCOS	2006	Hyperandrogenism + one of anovulation/PCOM
Rotterdam	2003	Two of: Hyperandrogenism, anovulation, PCOM
NIH 2012	2012	Rotterdam + phenotype identification

Phenotypes and BMI in PCOS

PCOS phenotypes reflect clinical heterogeneity, influencing management **(Tables 4 and 5)**:[12]

- **Type A:** Anovulation + Hyperandrogenism + PCOM (classic PCOS).
- **Type B:** Anovulation + Hyperandrogenism.
- **Type C:** Hyperandrogenism + PCOM.
- **Type D:** Anovulation + PCOM (nonhyperandrogenic).

Mnemonic: Type **A** for **All** (all three are present)

1. Type **B** for **B** mode ultrasound (USG criteria is absent)
2. Type **C** for **C**ycles (cycles are normal)
3. Type **D** for an**D**rogenic (androgenic feature is not there)

TABLE 4: PCOS phenotypes.[12]

Phenotype	*Features*	*Prevalence*
A	Anovulation + Hyperandrogenism + PCOM	60–70%
B	Anovulation + Hyperandrogenism	15–20%
C	Hyperandrogenism + PCOM	10–15%
D	Anovulation + PCOM	5–10%

TABLE 5: Different PCOS phenotypes.

Feature	*Phenotype A*	*Phenotype B*	*Phenotype C*	*Phenotype D*
Hyperandrogenism and hirsutism	✓	✓	✓	X
Ovulatory dysfunction	✓	✓	X	✓
Polycystic ovarian morphology	✓	X	✓	✓

- **BMI:**
  - **Lean PCOS:** Elevated luteinizing hormone (LH), normal insulin sensitivity.
  - **Obese PCOS:** Insulin resistance, hyperandrogenemia; insulin amplifies LH effects.[13]

Pathophysiology of PCOS (Fig. 2)

PCOS arises from complex interactions of hyperinsulinemia, hyperandrogenism, and genetic predisposition, perpetuating a cycle of anovulation and metabolic dysfunction.[14]

- **Genetic Variation in Gonadotropin Secretion:**
  - Increased LH pulse frequency/amplitude, low-normal follicle-stimulating hormone (FSH), LH:FSH ratio 2:1 or 3:1.
  - No progesterone feedback (due to anovulation) sustains high LH.
  - Reduced FSH from:
    - Rapid gonadotropin-releasing hormone (GnRH) pulses.
    - Elevated estrone (E1) from peripheral aromatization of androstenedione.
    - Inhibin B from small antral follicles.[15]
- **Insulin Secretion and Action:**
  - Insulin sensitivity reduced by 35–40%; insulin resistance in 65–80% of PCOS women.
  - Impaired glucose tolerance (IGT) in 35%; type 2 diabetes mellitus (T2DM) in 7–10%.
- **Insulin promotes:**
  - Ovarian androgen synthesis.
  - Reduced sex hormone-binding globulin (SHBG), increasing free androgens.
  - Anovulation via synergistic LH effects.[16]
- **Androgen Synthesis and Action:**
  - Hyperandrogenism (from ovaries, adrenals, or peripheral tissues) disrupts GnRH feedback, increasing LH and intraovarian androgens.
  - Continuous LH stimulation and stromal hyperplasia cause follicular atresia, forming PCOM.
  - *Cycle:* Hyperandrogenism → anovulation → stromal hypertrophy → hyperandrogenism.[17]

Clinical Features[18]

- **Anovulation:** Oligomenorrhea due to inhibited FSH-induced LH receptor formation, preventing dominant follicle development.
- **Hyperandrogenism:** Hirsutism, acne, androgenic alopecia.
- **Infertility:** Anovulation is the primary cause.

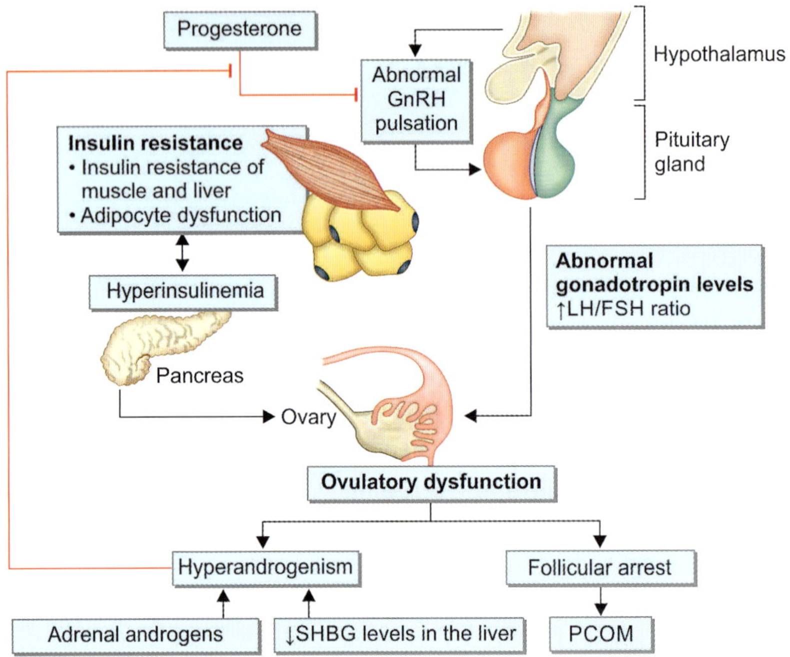

Fig. 2: Pathophysiology of PCOS (cycle of hyperandrogenism, insulin resistance, and anovulation).[14]

Q1. Assessment and Treatment of Infertility in PCOS. *(UP 2011, 2019, 5 + 5 Marks)*

Assessment of Infertility in PCOS

Infertility in PCOS primarily stems from anovulation, but other female, male, or combined factors must be excluded. A comprehensive evaluation includes history, examination, and investigations.[19]

- **History:**
  - **Couple:**
    - Duration of marriage, contraception use, fertile window knowledge.
    - Sexual history: Frequency, dyspareunia, erectile dysfunction, premature/retrograde ejaculation.
    - Past medical/surgical history (e.g., diabetes, hypertension, tuberculosis).
    - Occupation, substance abuse (smoking, alcohol).
  - **Female-Specific (PCOS):**
    - Menstrual history: Age at menarche, cycle length, flow, dysmenorrhea.
    - Onset/duration of androgenic features (hirsutism, acne, alopecia).
    - Hoarseness of voice, weight gain, sleep disturbances, galactorrhea, headache.
    - Obstetric history, prior infertility treatments.[20]
- **Examination:**
  - **General:**
    - Height, weight, BMI (obese: ≥30 kg/m^2).
    - Waist circumference (>80 cm indicates visceral fat), waist-hip ratio (>0.8).
    - Blood pressure, thyroid palpation, pallor.

- Acne, hirsutism (mFG score ≥4–8), androgenic alopecia, acanthosis nigricans [shown in **Fig. 3**].
- Signs of other disorders (e.g., Cushing's: purple striae, buffalo hump).

- **Pelvic:**
  - Tanner staging, clitoral enlargement, uterine size, adnexal masses.[21]

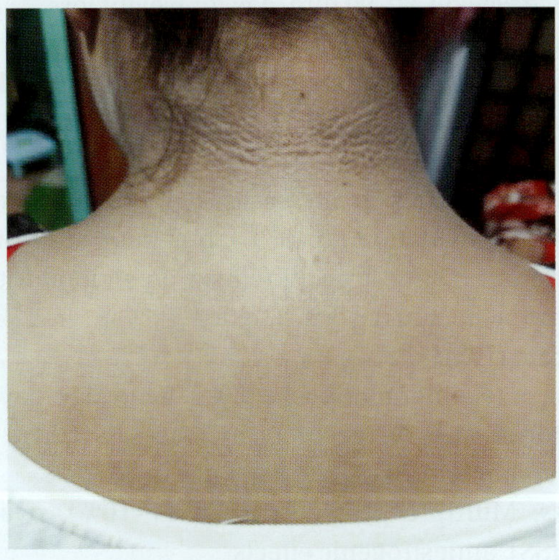

Fig. 3: Acanthosis nigricans.

- **Investigations (Table 6):**
  - **Blood:** Complete blood count, fasting blood sugar/oral glucose tolerance test (OGTT), thyroid profile, prolactin, testosterone, FAI.
  - **Semen Analysis:** Mandatory for male partner.
  - **Ultrasound:** Day 2 TVS for uterus, ovaries, endometrial thickness, antral follicular count (AFC). Follicular monitoring (day 9–18) for ovulation.
  - **Tubal Patency:** Hysterosalpingography (HSG) on day 8–9 if tubal pathology suspected (e.g., history of pelvic inflammatory disease).[22]
  - **Preconception Risk:** Assess blood pressure, OGTT, lipid profile for IGT, T2DM, dyslipidemia, hypertension.[23]

TABLE 6: Investigations for infertility in PCOS.[22]

Test	*Purpose*	*Timing*
OGTT	Detect IGT/T2DM	Preconception
Thyroid/Prolactin	Rule out endocrine causes	Day 2–3
TVS	Assess PCOM, ovulation	Day 2, 9–18
Semen analysis	Male factor	Anytime
HSG	Tubal patency	Day 8–9

Treatment of Infertility in PCOS

Management addresses anovulation, metabolic risks, and long-term complications, guided by ESHRE 2023, RCOG, and NICE NG197 (2023).[2,24]

- **Lifestyle Modification** (First-Line, Nonpharmacological):
  - **Diet:** Energy deficit of 500–750 kcal/day (1,200–1,500 kcal/day), low sugar/fat.
  - **Weight Loss:** 5-10% loss improves ovulation (30–40%), reduces visceral fat (30% with 10% loss). BMI <30 kg/m^2 targeted.[25]
  - **Exercise:** 150 min/week moderate or 75 min/week vigorous activity, plus muscle-strengthening twice weekly. 60–90 min/day for weight loss.[26]
  - **Folic Acid:** 400 μg/day (5 mg/day if obese) preconception.[27]
- **Ovulation Induction** (First-Line, Pharmacological) **(Tables 6 and 7)**:
  - **Letrozole** (Preferred):
    - Aromatase inhibitor; 2.5–7.5 mg/day, day 3–7 of cycle.
    - Mechanism: Reduces estrogen, increases FSH/LH, promotes follicular growth.
    - Advantages: Higher ovulation (70–85%), pregnancy (20–30%), and live birth rates versus clomiphene; no antiestrogenic effects on endometrium/cervix.
    - Side Effects: Headache, hot flashes, fatigue.[28]
  - **Clomiphene Citrate (CC):**
    - Selective estrogen receptor modulator; 50–150 mg/day, day 3–7.
    - *Mechanism:* Blocks estrogen receptors, increases FSH/LH.
    - *Advantages:* Ovulation in 70–85%, pregnancy in 60–70%.
    - *Disadvantages:* Multiple pregnancy risk (7–10%), ovarian hyperstimulation syndrome (OHSS), antiestrogenic effects.
    - *Side Effects:* Hot flashes, mood swings, visual disturbances.[29]
  - **Monitoring:** TVS follicular monitoring (day 9–18); hCG trigger (5,000–10,000 IU) when follicle ≥17 mm.[30]

TABLE 7: Comparison of Letrozole versus Clomiphene citrate.[28,29]

Parameter	*Letrozole*	*Clomiphene citrate*
Class	Aromatase inhibitor	Selective estrogen receptor modulator
Dose	2.5–7.5 mg/day	50–150 mg/day
Ovulation rate	70–85%	70–85%
Pregnancy rate	20–30%	15–20%
Multiple pregnancy	Low (1–2%)	High (7–10%)
Side effects	Headache, fatigue	Hot flashes, visual disturbances

- **Second-Line Pharmacological Treatment:**
  - **Gonadotrophins:**
    - Low-dose FSH (37.5–75 IU/day) step-up protocol for monofollicular development.
    - *Success rate:* 65–70% pregnancy in 6 months.
    - *Risks:* OHSS (5–10%), multiple pregnancy (20–30%). Cancel cycle if ≥2 follicles >14 mm.
    - *Indication:* CC resistance.[31]
  - **Metformin:**
    - 500–2,500 mg/day (TDS or 850 mg BD).

    - Improves insulin sensitivity, ovulation (30–40%), and pregnancy rates in CC-resistant cases.
    - Less effective than letrozole/CC; no follicular monitoring needed.
    - NICE NG197: CC, metformin, or combination for WHO Group II anovulation.[24]
- **Laparoscopic Ovarian Drilling (LOD):** Shown in **Figure 4**
    - Second-line for CC-resistant anovulation.
    - *Technique:* 4 punctures/ovary, 40W, 4 mm deep, 4 seconds each.
    - *Benefits:* Ovulation (73%), pregnancy (72%) within 2 years; reduced LH/androgens, lower OHSS/multiple pregnancy risk.
    - *Risks:* Adhesions, reduced ovarian reserve.[32]

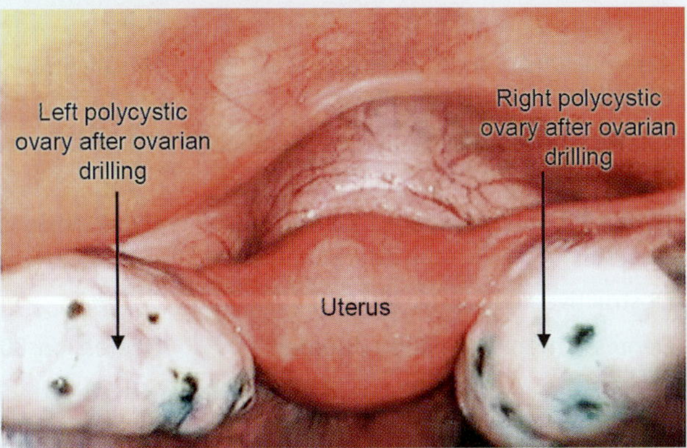

Fig. 4: Completion of laparoscopic ovarian drilling.

- **In Vitro Fertilization (IVF):**
    - *Indication:* Failure of ovulation induction (6 cycles if <25 years, 12 cycles if ≥25 years), or additional factors (e.g., tubal/male infertility).
    - *Protocol:* GnRH antagonist with GnRH agonist trigger preferred (lower OHSS risk vs. hCG trigger). Frozen embryo transfer improves pregnancy rates.
    - *Outcomes:* No increased risk of miscarriage, preterm birth, or fetal growth restriction versus non-PCOS.[33]
    - **Adjunct Metformin:** Improves ovulation, reduces early miscarriage, but limited evidence for routine use. Concerns for childhood obesity with in utero exposure.[34]
- **Other Therapies:**
    - **Antiobesity Drugs:** Orlistat, liraglutide discontinued preconception.
    - **Bariatric Surgery:** For BMI ≥35 kg/m^2 or 30–34.9 kg/m^2 with comorbidities. Delay pregnancy 1 year post surgery to avoid prematurity, small for gestational age (SGA).[35]
- **Risks of Ovulation Induction:**
    - **Multiple Pregnancy:** Increased perinatal mortality, maternal risks (e.g., preeclampsia).
    - **OHSS:** PCOS patients at high risk (5–10%). Symptoms: Nausea, ascites, pleural effusion. Management: Fluid balance, colloids, heparin for thromboembolism prevention.[36]

SHORT QUESTIONS

Q1. Long-Term Complications and Management of PCOS. *(DNB 2023, Paper 3, 5 Marks)*

Long-Term Complications

PCOS increases risks of metabolic, reproductive, and psychological complications due to hyperandrogenism and insulin resistance **(Table 8)**.[37]

TABLE 8: Long-term complications of PCOS.[37]

Category	*Complications*	*Prevalence*
Anovulation	Infertility, endometrial cancer	Infertility: 70–80%; Cancer: 2-6-fold risk
Hyperandrogenism	Acne, hirsutism, androgenic alopecia, psychological distress	Hirsutism: 60–70%; Acne: 15–30%
Insulin Resistance	IGT, T2DM, gestational diabetes, metabolic syndrome	IGT: 35%; T2DM: 7–10%
Metabolic	Hypertension, dyslipidemia, cardiovascular disease	Hypertension: 20–30%
Sleep	Obstructive sleep apnea (OSA)	5–10%
Psychological	Depression, anxiety, eating disorders	Depression: 30–40%
Pregnancy	Miscarriage, gestational hypertension, preeclampsia, preterm delivery, SGA	Miscarriage: 20–40%

- **Anovulation**:
  - **Endometrial Cancer:** Unopposed estrogen increases risk 2-6-fold. Risk factors: Prolonged amenorrhea, abnormal uterine bleeding (AUB), obesity.[38]
- **Insulin Resistance:**
  - IGT (35%), T2DM (7-10%), gestational diabetes (20-30%).
  - Metabolic syndrome: Hypertension, dyslipidemia, central obesity.[39]
- **Cardiovascular:**
  - Increased risk of hypertension (20-30%), dyslipidemia, and stroke.[40]
- **Obstructive Sleep Apnea (OSA):**
  - 5-10% prevalence; symptoms: Snoring, daytime fatigue. Exacerbated by androgens/ insulin resistance.[41]
- **Psychological:**
  - Depression (30-40%), anxiety, body image issues due to hirsutism, infertility, obesity.[42]
- **Pregnancy:**
  - Miscarriage (20-40%), gestational hypertension, preeclampsia, preterm delivery, SGA.[43]

Management

- **Endometrial Protection:**
  - Induce ≥4 menses/year with progestins (e.g., medroxyprogesterone 10 mg for 12 days) or combined oral contraceptives (COCs).

- Levonorgestrel intrauterine device (LNG-IUD) for endometrial protection.
- TVS/endometrial biopsy for AUB or endometrial thickness >7 mm.[38]

- **Metabolic Screening:**
  - **OGTT:** At diagnosis, every 1–3 years (annually if BMI ≥25 kg/m^2, family history of T2DM, GDM, or age >40 years).
  - **Lipid Profile/BP:** At diagnosis, annually if abnormal or high risk.[24]
  - **Metformin:** 500–2,500 mg/day for IGT/T2DM, improves insulin sensitivity.[44]
- **OSA Screening:** Berlin Questionnaire for snoring, fatigue; refer for polysomnography if positive.[41]
- **Psychological Support:**
  - Cognitive behavioral therapy (CBT) first-line.
  - Lifestyle and cosmetic interventions (e.g., laser hair removal) improve quality of life.
  - Antidepressants/antianxiety medications for moderate-to-severe cases.[42]
- **Pregnancy Monitoring:**
  - Early OGTT, BP monitoring at antenatal visits to detect gestational diabetes/hypertension.[43]

Q2. Clinical Features, Evaluation, and Management of Hyperandrogenism/Hirsutism

(DNB 2023, Paper 3, 5 Marks)

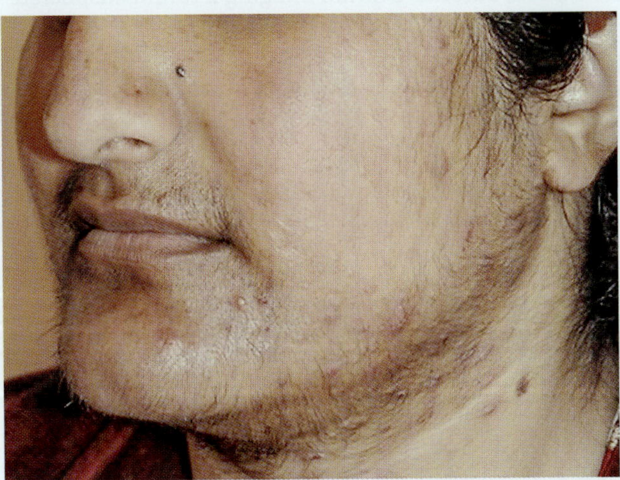

Fig. 5: Features of hirsutism.

Clinical Features of Hyperandrogenism

- **Hirsutism:** Excessive terminal hair in male-pattern areas (60–70% of PCOS women) as shown in **Figure 5**.
- **Acne:** Inflammatory lesions, often severe (15–30%).
- **Androgenic Alopecia:** Male-pattern hair loss (5–10%).
- **Anovulation/Oligomenorrhea:** Due to ovarian androgen-induced follicular atresia (70–80%).
- **Virilization (Rare):** Deepening voice, clitoromegaly, temporal balding; suggests tumors or congenital adrenal hyperplasia (CAH) (45).

Causes of Hirsutism

- PCOS (70–80%).
- Nonclassical CAH (raised 17α-hydroxyprogesterone).
- Androgen-secreting tumors (ovary/adrenal).
- Cushing's syndrome, acromegaly, severe insulin resistance.
- *Drug-induced:* Testosterone, danazol, phenytoin, minoxidil (46).

Clinical Evaluation

- **History:** Onset, progression, AUB, weight gain, virilization symptoms, drug use.
- **Examination:**
  - mFG score (9 areas, score 0–4; ≥4–8 indicates hirsutism).
  - *Acne:* Count active lesions/scars (no validated scale).
  - *Alopecia:* Ludwig/Olsen scales **(Fig. 6)**.
  - Signs of CAH (e.g., hyperpigmentation), Cushing's (striae), or tumors (rapid virilization).[47]
- **Biochemical:**
  - Total/free testosterone, FAI; androstenedione, DHEAS if normal testosterone.
  - 17α-hydroxyprogesterone for CAH (>200 ng/dL or ACTH stimulation test).
  - Stop COCs 3 months prior for accurate androgen assessment.[48]
- **Imaging:** TVS for PCOM; adrenal/ovarian imaging if tumor suspected.[49]

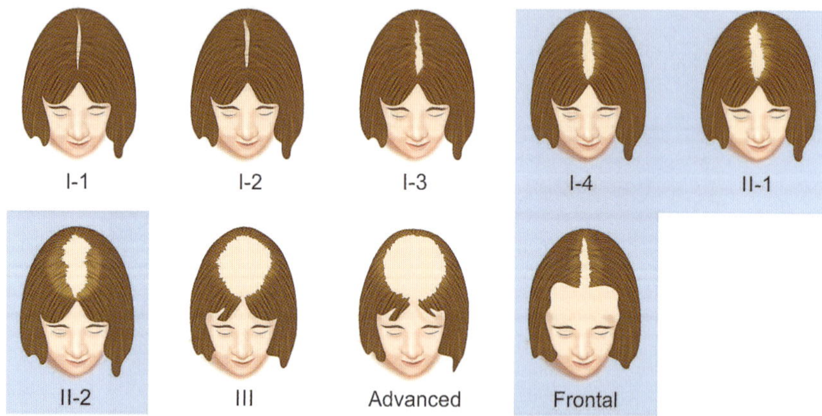

Fig. 6: *Placeholder:* Ludwig's classification of female hair loss.[47]

Management of Hirsutism

- **Lifestyle:** 5–10% weight loss reduces hirsutism by 50% in obese patients.[25]
- **Cosmetic:**
  - Photoepilation (laser): 30% hair reduction.
  - Electrolysis: Effective but painful, 18–24 months.
  - Waxing, shaving, depilatory creams.[50]
- **Pharmacological:**
  - **COCs** (First-Line): Reduce LH, increase SHBG, decrease free testosterone. Effect in 9–12 months (50% hirsutism reduction).

- Preferred: 20–30 µg ethinyl estradiol with desogestrel, norgestimate, or drospirenone (lower DVT risk).
- Avoid 35 µg ethinyl estradiol + cyproterone acetate as first-line due to DVT risk (51) as shown in **Figure 7**.

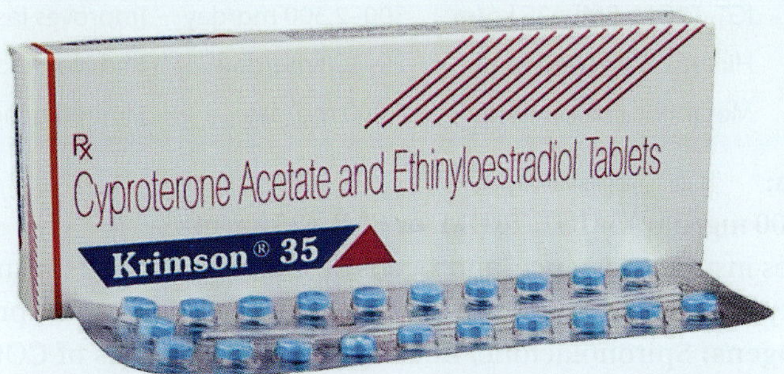

Fig. 7: OCP having ethinyl estradiol and cyproterone acetate.

- **Antiandrogens** (After 6 Months of COCs if Suboptimal):
  - Spironolactone (25–100 mg/day): Low side effects, requires contraception.
  - Cyproterone acetate, finasteride: Effective but higher risks (e.g., hepatotoxicity with flutamide).
  - Eflornithine cream: Topical, reduces hair growth, may cause rash.[52]
- **Metformin:** Reduces androgens by 20%, useful in obese/nonobese patients.[44]

Q3. Recent Guidelines in Management of PCOS.

(DNB 2023, Paper 3; UP 2015, Paper 4, 5 Marks)

ESHRE 2023, RCOG, and NICE NG197 Guidelines

Management of PCOS is multidisciplinary, addressing anovulation, hyperandrogenism, metabolic risks, and psychological effects.[2,24]

- **Lifestyle Management:**
  - **Diet:** Energy deficit (500–750 kcal/day) for weight loss (BMI <30 kg/m^2).
  - **Exercise:**
    - *Prevention:* 150–300 min/week moderate or 75–150 min/week vigorous activity, plus muscle training twice weekly.
    - *Weight loss:* 250 min/week moderate or 150 min/week vigorous activity.[26]
  - **Behavioral Support:** SMART goals (Specific, Measurable, Achievable, Realistic, Timely).[25]
- **Pharmacotherapy (Table 9):**
  - **COCs** (First-Line for Hirsutism/Irregular Cycles):
    - 20–30 µg ethinyl estradiol with third-/fourth-generation progestins (e.g., drospirenone).
    - Cyproterone acetate for severe hirsutism/acne (not first-line).
    - Progestin-only pills or LNG-IUD for endometrial protection.[51]

TABLE 9: Pharmacotherapy for PCOS.[2,24]

Drug	*Indication*	*Dose*	*Effect*
COCs	Hirsutism, irregular cycles	20–30 μg ethinyl estradiol	Reduces androgens, cycle control
Metformin	IGT, T2DM, BMI ≥25 kg/m^2	500–2,500 mg/day	Improves insulin sensitivity
Spironolactone	Hirsutism (second-line)	25–100 mg/day	Reduces androgens
Myo-Inositol	Metabolic (experimental)	4,000 mg/day	Limited benefit

- **Metformin:**
    - 500–2,500 mg/day for IGT, T2DM, or BMI ≥25 kg/m^2.
    - Improves insulin resistance, androgens; less effective for hirsutism versus COCs.[44]
- **Antiobesity Drugs:** Liraglutide, orlistat, semaglutide (discontinue preconception).[35]
- **Antiandrogens:** Spironolactone, finasteride after 6 months of COCs; contraception mandatory.[52]
- **Inositol:** Myo-inositol (4,000 mg/day) experimental for metabolic benefits; metformin preferred for hirsutism/obesity.[53]

- **Cosmetic Interventions:**
    - Laser/photoepilation, electrolysis for hirsutism; combined with COCs/metformin improves psychological outcomes.[50]
- **Bariatric Surgery:**
    - Indication: BMI ≥35 kg/m^2 or 30–34.9 kg/m^2 with comorbidities.
    - Improves ovulation, hirsutism, metabolic profile; delay pregnancy 1 year.[35]
- **Psychological Interventions:**
    - CBT for depression/anxiety; lifestyle/cosmetic measures enhance quality of life.[42]

Q4. Place of Ovarian Surgery for PCOS. *(DNB 2023, Paper 3, 5 Marks)*

Ovarian surgery is not first-line for PCOS but is a second-line option for clomiphene-resistant anovulatory infertility **(Table 10)**.[32]

- **Ovarian Wedge Resection:**
    - Historical technique; reduces androgens and restores ovulation (85% pregnancy rate initially reported).
    - Disadvantages: High risk of adhesions, premature ovarian failure, infertility.
    - Obsolete due to safer alternatives.[54]
- **Laparoscopic Ovarian Drilling (LOD):**
    - **Technique:** 4 punctures/ovary, 40W, 4 mm deep, 4 seconds each (Rule of 4).
    - **Benefits:**
        - Ovulation rate: 73%; pregnancy rate: 72% within 2 years.
        - Reduces LH, androgens, OHSS, multiple pregnancy risk.
        - Sustained hirsutism improvement (9 years).
    - **Complications:**
        - Adhesions, periadnexal cysts, reduced anti-Müllerian hormone (AMH), ovarian reserve loss.
        - Higher risks in obese patients, requires expertise.[55]

- **Indications:** CC-resistant anovulation, no other infertility factors.

TABLE 10: Comparison of ovarian surgery techniques.[54,55]

Technique	*Ovulation rate*	*Pregnancy rate*	*Complications*
Wedge Resection	70–80%	50–85%	Adhesions, ovarian failure
LOD	73%	72%	Adhesions, reduced AMH

Q5. Role of Inositol in PCOS Management.

(DNB 2021, Paper 4, 3 Marks; DNB 2016, 3 + 3 + 4 Marks)

What are Inositols?

Inositols are polyalcohols acting as second messengers in insulin and FSH signaling. Two isomers are relevant: [53]

- **Myo-Inositol (MI):** Most abundant, enhances glucose uptake, FSH-mediated granulosa cell proliferation, and aromatase synthesis (reduces androgens) **(Table 11)**.
- **D-Chiro-Inositol (DCI):** Converted from MI under insulin stimulation; improves insulin sensitivity.
- **MI:DCI Ratio:** Normal women: 100:1; PCOS: 0.2:1, indicating impaired conversion.

TABLE 11: Clinical effects of Myo-Inositol in PCOS.[57]

Effect	*Improvement*	*Evidence level*
Insulin Resistance	30–40%	Moderate
Ovulation	50–60%	Limited
Androgens	20–30%	Limited
IVF Outcomes	Better oocyte quality	Emerging

Physiological Role

- **Insulin Signaling:** MI/DCI improve glucose uptake, reduce insulin resistance.
- **Ovarian Function:** MI enhances folliculogenesis, reduces androgen production.
- **Metabolic Health:** Lowers cardiovascular risk by improving lipid profile.[56]

Clinical Utility

- **Effects:**
    - Improves insulin resistance (30–40%), androgen levels (20–30%), ovulation frequency (50–60%).
    - Enhances egg/embryo quality, reduces FSH dose/days in IVF.
    - Regularizes cycles, accelerates weight loss.[57]
- **Dosage:** 4,000 mg/day (MI, or MI + DCI) in two divided doses.
- **Sources:** Fruits, nuts, beans, whole wheat.
- **Side Effects:** Safe up to 10 weeks; rare diarrhea, nausea.
- **ESHRE 2023:** Experimental therapy; limited evidence for ovulation, hirsutism, or weight loss. Metformin preferred for hirsutism/obesity.[2]
- **IVF:** Reduces stimulation dose, improves oocyte quality, but more studies needed.[58]

Guidelines

- **RCOG Green-top Guideline No. 33 (2023):** Recommends lifestyle modification as first-line, letrozole over CC for ovulation induction, and annual metabolic screening (OGTT, lipids, BP).[59]
- **NICE NG197 (2023):** Advocates CC, metformin, or combination for WHO Group II anovulation; LOD for CC-resistant cases; and psychological support for quality of life.[24]
- **ESHRE 2023:** Endorses Rotterdam criteria, restricts ultrasound in adolescents, and considers inositol experimental.[2]

Key Points

- PCOS affects 10–13% of women, diagnosed by Rotterdam criteria (2/3: anovulation, hyperandrogenism, PCOM).
- Adolescent diagnosis requires irregular cycles and hyperandrogenism; ultrasound avoided <8 years post-menarche.
- Pathophysiology involves hyperinsulinemia, hyperandrogenism, and gonadotropin dysregulation.
- Infertility management: Lifestyle (5–10% weight loss), letrozole (first-line), gonadotrophins/LOD (second-line), IVF (third-line).
- Long-term complications: Endometrial cancer, T2DM, cardiovascular disease, psychological distress.
- Hirsutism management: COCs, anti-androgens (second-line), cosmetic therapies.
- Inositol: Experimental, improves metabolic parameters but limited for ovulation/hirsutism.
- RCOG/NICE/ESHRE emphasize lifestyle, metabolic screening, and patient-centered care.

Monitoring of Antiandrogen Therapy

Monitoring response to treatment can be done objectively using Ferriman-Gallwey system, scoring at baseline and, if possible, at each visit.

Treatment can be continued as long as the patient desires and should be discontinued if planning for pregnancy.

Monitoring testosterone levels after instituting pharmacologic therapy is generally unnecessary because hirsutism scores correlate poorly with serum androgen levels.

Other useful pharmacologic therapies can be advised based on symptoms related to hyperandrogenism like:

- Antibiotics, topical retinoids, or isotretinoin for acne
- Minoxidil topical solution to be applied on area of desired hair growth. Max: 2 mL/day.
- Eflornithine for hirsutism

  Topical eflornithine slows growth of unwanted facial hair in 4–8 weeks. Inhibits hair growth (potentially by inhibiting ornithine decarboxylase)
- Bicalutamide (≤50 mg daily)

  There is emerging data to support use with oral contraceptives in PCOS.[8]

Nonpharmacologic cosmetic therapies for hirsutism include shaving, depilating, hair bleaching, electrolysis, and laser hair removal.

Imeglimin used in diabetes is in trial phase.

Drugs to Aid Weight Loss in PCOS[14]

Orlistat

It assists in weight loss by inhibiting intestinal fat absorption (inhibits gastric and pancreatic lipases). There are various studies in PCOS obese patients with good results.

Bupropion/Naltrexone

It is a new antiobesity medication which suppresses appetite. Its use and safety in PCOS needs further studies.

Glucagon-like peptide-1 (GLP-1) receptor agonists

This new group of medication promotes weight loss in PCOS. Liraglutide has been shown to be superior to placebo, as well as to metformin and orlistat in head-to head comparisons. The efficacy of Liraglutide in promoting weight loss in PCOS patients is proven.

Medical management may be needed for other associated problems in PCOS:[15]

- **Dyslipidemia:** Approximately 70% of patients with newly diagnosed disease have abnormal lipid levels, including increased total cholesterol level, high triglyceride levels, high LDL-C level, and decreased HDL-C level.
- **Hypertension:** Women with PCOS have a risk of developing hypertension which if untreated may accelerate atherosclerotic cardiovascular disease
- Nonalcoholic fatty liver disease is frequently seen in patients with polycystic ovary syndrome, likely as a result of insulin resistance as well as obesity
- Depression and anxiety
  Increased incidence and prevalence over lifetime

Special Populations

Adolescents

Diagnosis can be difficult in adolescents owing to overlap between normal pubertal development and characteristic features of polycystic ovary syndrome. **Suggested criteria include demonstration of chemical and/or biochemical hyperandrogenism and presence of persistent oligomenorrhea for at least 2 years after menarche.**[16]

Hormonal contraceptives: In early adolescence, using hormonal contraceptives is controversial. Ideal hormonal contraceptive regimen and appropriate duration of therapy for adolescents are uncertain. **The standard practice is to wait for 2 years after menarche to prevent reduction in peak bone mass.**[3]

Metformin therapy: Small, short-term studies have found that metformin restores menstrual regularity and improves hyperandrogenemia, insulin resistance, and glucose intolerance in obese and nonobese adolescents with PCOS.

Postmenopausal Women

After menopause, two of the key diagnostic criteria of PCOS (irregular menses and polycystic ovaries on transvaginal ultrasonography) are no longer applicable.

Most women who had polycystic ovary syndrome during their reproductive years continue to manifest both metabolic phenotype and unfavorable cardiovascular risk factors. Androgen levels are still higher than in postmenopausal women without history of PCOS.

It is advisable to maintain vigilance for monitoring lipid levels, blood pressure, and glycemia in accordance with standards of care in this population of women.

CONCLUSION

PCOS is a heterogeneous endocrinopathy affecting adolescent girls. The exact etiology is unknown; however, hyperinsulinemia and hyperandrogenism form the main pathological basis of this syndrome. In adolescents, it may be difficult to differentiate irregular cycles of PCOS from physiologic anovulation. However, persistence of menstrual irregularity for >2 years post menarche is a strong predictor of long-term ovulatory dysfunction. COC pills are the first line of medical management for menstrual disturbances and acne, metformin for weight reduction and dysglycemia, and a combination of both in addition to other treatment modalities for treatment of hirsutism.

Clinical Case Scenario

Case: A 28-year-old woman presents with irregular menses (4–5 cycles/year), hirsutism, and BMI 32 kg/m^2.

USG: Polycystic ovaries.

Labs: Elevated testosterone, fasting insulin 20 μIU/mL.

Management

- **Diagnosis:** PCOS (Rotterdam: Oligo-anovulation, hyperandrogenism, polycystic ovaries).
- **Counseling:** Explain PCOS, lifestyle benefits, and fertility implications.
- **Treatment:**
    - *Lifestyle:* 5–10% weight loss, low-GI diet, 150 min/week exercise.
    - *Inositol:* MI 2 g + DCI 50 mg twice daily for 3 months.
    - *Metformin:* Start 500 mg daily, titrate to 1500 mg/day.
- **Follow-Up:** Reassess menses, insulin, lipids at 3 months.
- **Outcome: Menses regularize in 4 months; BMI drops to 30 kg/m^2; ovulation confirmed.**
  Exam Tip: Emphasize lifestyle as first-line, MI/DCI 40:1 ratio, and metformin's metabolic role.

Key Points

- **Prevalence in India:** 20–26%; obesity-driven, high IR burden.
- **Inositol:** MI/DCI (40:1) improves IR, ovulation, lipids; GI side effects at high doses.
- **Metformin:** Enhances insulin sensitivity, ovulation; less effective than clomiphene for fertility.
- **Thiazolidinediones:** Limited use due to safety concerns in pregnancy.
- **Guidelines:** Lifestyle first; inositol/metformin for IR; clomiphene for ovulation induction.

BOX 1: Important points to remember.

- *Rotterdam Criteria:* 2/3 (oligo-anovulation, hyperandrogenism, polycystic ovaries)
- *MI/DCI Ratio:* 40:1 optimal; excess DCI worsens androgens
- *Metformin:* Start 500 mg/day, titrate to 1,500–2,000 mg; monitor GFR annually
- *Lifestyle:* 5–10% weight loss restores ovulation in 60% of obese PCOS patients

REFERENCES

1. ESHRE. International evidence-based guideline for PCOS: 2023 update. Hum Reprod Open. 2023;2023(3):hoad024.
2. Balen AH, Rutherford AJ. WHO classification of ovulation disorders. Hum Reprod. 2017;32(6):1131-6.
3. Ferriman D, Gallwey JD. Modified scoring for hirsutism. Clin Endocrinol. 2019;91(3):401-7.
4. Balen AH, Laven JS. Ultrasound criteria for PCOM. Ultrasound Obstet Gynecol. 2018;51(6):821-7.
5. Peña AS, Witchel SF. Adolescent PCOS diagnosis. J Clin Endocrinol Metab. 2020;105(12):e4567-75.
6. Ibáñez L, Oberfield SE. Hyperandrogenism in adolescents. Endocr Rev. 2018;39(5):685-709.
7. Dewailly D, Lujan ME. PCOM in adolescents. Hum Reprod Update. 2016;22(6):687-708.
8. Fauser BC, Tarlatzis BC. AMH in PCOS diagnosis. Fertil Steril. 2017;108(6):933-9.
9. Teede HJ, Norman RJ. Adolescent PCOS consensus. Lancet Child Adolesc Health. 2018;2(4):295-304.
10. Rotterdam ESHRE/ASRM-Sponsored PCOS Consensus. Revised 2003 criteria. Hum Reprod. 2016;31(12):2841-7.
11. Lizneva D, Suturina L. PCOS phenotypes. Fertil Steril. 2016;106(1):6-15.
12. Diamanti-Kandarakis E, Dunaif A. Insulin resistance in PCOS. Endocr Rev. 2017;38(4):378-99.
13. Escobar-Morreale HF. PCOS pathophysiology. Nat Rev Endocrinol. 2018;14(5):270-84.
14. Goodarzi MO, Dumesic DA. Gonadotropin dysregulation in PCOS. J Clin Endocrinol Metab. 2016;101(12):4315-23.
15. Dunaif A. Insulin resistance and PCOS. J Clin Endocrinol Metab. 2019;104(11):5337-46.
16. Rosenfield RL, Ehrmann DA. Hyperandrogenism in PCOS. Endocr Rev. 2016;37(5):467-520.
17. Azziz R, Carmina E. Clinical features of PCOS. Lancet Diabetes Endocrinol. 2018;6(8):659-69.
18. Practice Committee of ASRM. Evaluation of infertility in PCOS. Fertil Steril. 2018;110(4):605-15.
19. Legro RS, Arslanian SA. Infertility workup in PCOS. N Engl J Med. 2017;377(13):1267-76.
20. Martin KA, Anderson RR. Hirsutism evaluation. J Clin Endocrinol Metab. 2019;104(8):2873-83.
21. NICE. Fertility problems: Assessment and treatment. NG197 2023.
22. Bozdag G, Mumusoglu S. Preconception risks in PCOS. Hum Reprod Update. 2016;22(5):557-71.
23. RCOG. Green-top Guideline No. 33: PCOS management. 2023.
24. Moran LJ, Norman RJ. Lifestyle interventions in PCOS. Lancet Diabetes Endocrinol. 2017;5(12):986-96.
25. Harrison CL, Lombard CB. Exercise in PCOS. Obstet Gynecol. 2018;131(6):1102-11.
26. Czeizel AE, Dudás I. Folic acid in PCOS. Hum Reprod. 2016;31(10):2357-63.
27. Legro RS, Brzyski RG. Letrozole vs. clomiphene for PCOS. N Engl J Med. 2017;376(6):548-57.
28. Thessaloniki ESHRE/ASRM-Sponsored PCOS Consensus. Ovulation induction in PCOS. Hum Reprod. 2018;33(4):577-88.
29. Franik S, Eltrop SM. Ovulation induction monitoring. Cochrane Database Syst Rev. 2018;10:CD011163.
30. Farquhar C, Brown J. Gonadotrophins for PCOS. Cochrane Database Syst Rev. 2017;7:CD010290.
31. Abu Hashim H, Al-Inany H. Laparoscopic ovarian drilling. Cochrane Database Syst Rev. 2018;6:CD005122.
32. Yu Y, Cai H. IVF in PCOS. Hum Reprod. 2019;34(6):1015-24.
33. Tso LO, Costello MF. Metformin in PCOS pregnancy. Cochrane Database Syst Rev. 2018;12:CD012214.
34. Sha T, Wang X. Bariatric surgery in PCOS. Fertil Steril. 2020;113(4):707-14.
35. Mourad S, Brown J. OHSS in PCOS. Cochrane Database Syst Rev. 2017;8:CD011084.
36. Dokras A, Stener-Victorin E. Long-term complications of PCOS. Fertil Steril. 2017;108(3):428-36.
37. Barry JA, Azizia MM. Endometrial cancer risk in PCOS. Hum Reprod Update. 2016;22(4):412-20.
38. Glueck CJ, Goldenberg N. Metabolic syndrome in PCOS. J Clin Endocrinol Metab. 2019;104(7):2641-50.
39. Osibogun O, Ogunmoroti O. Cardiovascular risks in PCOS. J Am Coll Cardiol. 2020;75(18):2349-58.

40. Kahal H, Kyrou I. Obstructive sleep apnea in PCOS. Sleep Med Rev. 2018;37:104-11.
41. Dokras A, Sarwer DB. Psychological issues in PCOS. Fertil Steril. 2017;108(3):437-43.
42. Palomba S, de Wilde MA. Pregnancy complications in PCOS. Lancet Diabetes Endocrinol. 2017;5(8): 651-61.
43. Sam S, Ehrmann DA. Metformin in PCOS. J Clin Endocrinol Metab. 2017;102(11):3943-51.
44. Azziz R, Sanchez LA. Hyperandrogenism evaluation. Endocr Rev. 2018;39(2):157-91.
45. Martin KA, Chang RJ. Hirsutism causes. J Clin Endocrinol Metab. 2016;101(12):4383-91.
46. Escobar-Morreale HF, Carmina E. Hirsutism evaluation. Fertil Steril. 2018;110(3):380-7.
47. Goodman NF, Cobin RH. Biochemical hyperandrogenism. Endocr Pract. 2017;23(7):876-94.
48. Rosenfield RL. Ultrasound in hyperandrogenism. Ultrasound Obstet Gynecol. 2016;47(6):683-91.
49. Deplewski D, Rosenfield RL. Cosmetic therapies for hirsutism. J Clin Endocrinol Metab. 2019; 104(4):1209-19.
50. Spritzer PM, Lisboa TC. COCs in PCOS. Cochrane Database Syst Rev. 2016;10:CD010071.
51. van Zuuren EJ, Fedorowicz Z. Anti-androgens for hirsutism. Cochrane Database Syst Rev. 2015;4: CD010334.
52. Facchinetti F, Orrù B. Inositol in PCOS. Hum Reprod Update. 2020;26(4):552-67.
53. Flyckt RL, Goldberg JM. Ovarian wedge resection. Fertil Steril. 2016;106(3):519-25.
54. Bordewijk EM, Ng KY. Laparoscopic ovarian drilling. Cochrane Database Syst Rev. 2020;2:CD005122.
55. Unfer V, Nestler JE. Inositol physiology. J Clin Endocrinol Metab. 2017;102(9):3111-9.
56. Pundir J, Psaroudakis D. Inositol for PCOS. Cochrane Database Syst Rev. 2018;3:CD012378.
57. Mendoza N, Pérez L. Inositol in IVF for PCOS. Gynecol Endocrinol. 2019;35(10):833-7.
58. Royal College of Obstetricians and Gynaecologists (RCOG). Long-term Consequences of Polycystic Ovary Syndrome (Green-top Guideline No. 33). [online] Available from https://www.rcog.org.uk/guidance/browse-all-guidance/green-top-guidelines/ovarian-cysts-in-postmenopausal-women-green-top-guideline-no-34/ [Last accessed December, 2025].
59. Role of Artificial Intelligence in PCOS Detection - Scientific Figure on ResearchGate. [online] Available from https://www.researchgate.net/figure/Ultrasound-image-of-normal-ovary-and-polycystic-ovary_fig1_369491657 [Last accessed December, 2025].
60. Azziz R, Carmina E, Chen Z, et al. Polycystic ovary syndrome. Nature Rev. 2016;2:1-18.

Puberty and Amenorrhea

Ruchika Garg

PHYSIOLOGY OF PUBERTY

Definition: Puberty is the process of physical maturation leading to sexual maturity and reproductive capability, occurring during adolescence (ages 10–19 years, per WHO). It involves rapid physical, cognitive, and psychosocial growth.

Physiological Mechanisms

- **Hypothalamic–Pituitary–Gonadal (HPG) Axis Activation:**
  - Hypothalamus increases pulsatile gonadotropin-releasing hormone (GnRH) secretion.
  - GnRH stimulates pituitary to release luteinizing hormone (LH) and follicle-stimulating hormone (FSH), initially during sleep and then 24/7 as puberty progresses.
- **Ovarian Hormone Production:**
  - FSH promotes ovarian follicle growth.
  - LH triggers ovulation and corpus luteum formation, producing progesterone.
  - Estrogen (estradiol) drives secondary sexual characteristics (e.g., breast development, menstrual cycle regulation).
  - Progesterone prepares the endometrium for pregnancy.
- **Adrenal Androgens (Adrenarche):**
  - Adrenal glands secrete dehydroepiandrosterone (DHEA/DHEAS), contributing to pubic/axillary hair and growth.

Physical Changes

- **Thelarche:** Breast development (ages 8–13 years), driven by estrogen, progresses through Tanner stages.
- **Pubarche:** Pubic hair appears post-thelarche, followed by axillary hair, advancing through Tanner stages.
- **Growth Spurt:** Estrogen and growth hormone increase height (ages 9–14 years), peaking before menarche.
- **Menarche:** First menstruation (ages 12–13 years), 2–3 years after thelarche; initial cycles may be irregular (50% anovulatory in the first year).
- **Other:** Increased body fat (hips/thighs), vaginal secretions, and mucosal changes.

Tanner Staging

- **Breast Development:**
  - Stage 1: Prepubertal, no glandular tissue.
  - Stage 2: Breast bud formation.

- Stage 3: Enlarged breast/areola, no separation.
- Stage 4: Secondary mound of areola/nipple.
- Stage 5: Mature breast, nipple raised.

- **Pubic Hair:**
  - Stage 1: None.
  - Stage 2: Sparse, downy hair.
  - Stage 3: Darker, curlier, sparse spread.
  - Stage 4: Adult-like, smaller area.
  - Stage 5: Adult quantity, extends to thighs.

Psychosocial Changes

- Cognitive advancement enables abstract thinking.
- Emotional shifts include mood swings, identity formation, and independence.
- Socially, peer relationships, social status, and romantic exploration intensify.

Causes of Delayed Puberty

Definition: Absence or incomplete secondary sexual characteristics by age 13 years (girls, no thelarche) or 14 years (boys, no testicular enlargement), or no menarche by age 15 years (girls).

Classification

- **Hypergonadotropic Hypogonadism (Primary Gonadal Failure):**
  - Elevated LH/FSH due to gonadal dysfunction.
  - **Causes:**
    - **Turner Syndrome:** 45,XO, ovarian failure.
    - **Klinefelter Syndrome:** 47,XXY, testicular dysfunction.
    - **Gonadal Dysgenesis:** Abnormal gonad development (e.g., Swyer's syndrome).
    - **Autoimmune Disorders:** Oophoritis/orchitis.
    - **Chemotherapy/Radiation:** Gonadal damage.
- **Hypogonadotropic Hypogonadism (Central Causes):**
  - Low/normal LH/FSH due to hypothalamic/pituitary dysfunction.
  - **Causes:**
    - **Constitutional Delay of Growth and Puberty (CDGP):** Most common, familial, temporary delay.
    - **Kallmann Syndrome:** GnRH deficiency, anosmia.
    - **Prader-Willi Syndrome:** Obesity, delayed milestones.
    - **Chronic Illnesses:** Cystic fibrosis, celiac disease, inflammatory bowel disease.
    - **Nutritional Deficiencies:** Malnutrition, anorexia nervosa.
    - **Hypopituitarism:** Inadequate LH/FSH production.
    - **Excessive Exercise:** Common in athletes.

Management of Delayed Puberty

Diagnostic Evaluation:

- **History:**
  - Timing of secondary sexual characteristics.
  - Medical/drug history (chronic illness, medications).

- Lifestyle (eating disorders, exercise, stress).
- Symptoms (headaches, visual changes, anosmia, galactorrhea).
- Family history of delayed puberty.
- Sexual/pregnancy history.

- **Physical Examination:**
  - Weight/BMI (low in hypothalamic amenorrhea, TB).
  - Height (short in Turner syndrome, gonadal dysgenesis).
  - Tanner staging for pubertal progress.
  - Thyroid, breast (galactorrhea, widely spaced nipples), genitalia (virilization, outflow issues).
  - Systemic exam for chronic illness.
  - Turner syndrome features: webbed neck, low hairline.
- **Investigations:**
  - **Hormonal Tests:** LH, FSH (high in gonadal failure, low in central causes), estradiol/testosterone, thyroid function, prolactin.
  - **Pregnancy Test:** Rule out pregnancy.
  - **Imaging:** Pelvic ultrasound (uterus/ovaries), brain MRI/CT (hypothalamus/pituitary), bone age X-ray.
  - **Other:** CBC, ESR, Mantoux (TB), IGF-1 (growth hormone deficiency).
  - **Karyotyping:** For Turner/Klinefelter syndromes.
  - **Genetic Testing:** For Kallmann syndrome, if suspected.

Management

- **Observation:**
  - For CDGP, monitor with reassurance; puberty often progresses naturally.
- **Medical Management:**
  - **Hormone Replacement Therapy (HRT):**
    - Estrogen (girls): Low-dose (estradiol 100 mcg transdermal or conjugated estrogen 0.625 mg oral) to initiate puberty, gradually increased.
    - Progestin: Added after months of estrogen to induce menstrual cycles, protect endometrium.
    - Monitor for pubertal signs (e.g., breast development); may pause HRT to assess spontaneous progression.
    - Calcium (1,200 mg) and vitamin D (1,000 IU) with weight-bearing exercise for bone health.
  - **Nutrition:** Optimize diet/weight for hypothalamic amenorrhea (e.g., eating disorders, exercise-induced).
  - **Treat Underlying Conditions:** Thyroid disorders, hyperprolactinemia, chronic illnesses (TB, celiac disease).
- **Lifestyle/Psychological Support:**
  - Address stress, overexercise, or eating disorders.
  - Psychological counseling for emotional impact (isolation, low self-esteem).
  - Cognitive behavioral therapy (CBT) for eating disorders/stress.
  - Family education for supportive environment.
- **Follow-Up:** Regular monitoring to adjust therapy and track pubertal progress.

PRIMARY AMENORRHEA

Definition: Absence of menarche by age 15 years with normal secondary sexual characteristics, or by age 13 years without secondary sexual characteristics.

Etiology

- **Hypothalamic/Pituitary Disorders:**
    - Functional hypothalamic amenorrhea (stress, exercise, weight loss, eating disorders).
    - Tumors (prolactinomas, craniopharyngiomas).
    - Kallmann syndrome, Prader-Willi syndrome, empty sella syndrome.
    - Hyperprolactinemia.
- **Ovarian Causes:**
    - Chromosomal: Turner syndrome (45,XO), gonadal dysgenesis, androgen insensitivity syndrome (46,XY).
    - Ovarian damage: Radiation, chemotherapy, autoimmune oophoritis.
    - Iatrogenic: Surgical removal.
- **Anatomic Abnormalities:**
    - Müllerian agenesis (MRKH syndrome).
    - Cervical/vaginal agenesis, transverse vaginal septum, imperforate hymen.
    - Androgen insensitivity syndrome.
- **Chronic Medical Conditions:**
    - TB, celiac disease, Crohn's disease, cystic fibrosis.
    - Congenital adrenal hyperplasia.
- **Endocrine Disorders:**
    - Hypothyroidism, hyperthyroidism, PCOS.
- **Systemic Conditions:**
    - Malnutrition, extreme exercise, stress.

Turner Syndrome

- **Definition:** Chromosomal disorder (45,XO or variants) causing ovarian failure in females.
- **Features:**
    - Short stature, webbed neck, low hairline, high-arched palate, widely spaced nipples.
    - Primary amenorrhea, absent/incomplete puberty (due to ovarian dysgenesis).
    - Normal external genitalia, underdeveloped uterus/ovaries.
    - *Associated:* Cardiac anomalies (coarctation of aorta), renal abnormalities, hearing loss.
- **Diagnosis**: Karyotyping (45,XO), low estradiol, high LH/FSH, pelvic ultrasound (streak ovaries).
- **Management**:
    - HRT: Estrogen/progestin to induce puberty, maintain bone health.
    - Growth hormone for height.
    - Monitor cardiac/renal issues.
    - Psychological support for infertility and body image.

Diagnostic Evaluation (Same as delayed puberty):

- History, physical exam, hormonal tests (LH, FSH, estradiol, thyroid, prolactin), pregnancy test.
- *Imaging:* Pelvic ultrasound, brain MRI/CT, bone age X-ray.
- Karyotyping, genetic testing, TB screening (CBC, ESR, Mantoux).

Management of Primary Amenorrhea:

- **Observation:** For constitutional delay, monitor with reassurance.
- **Medical Management:**
    - **HRT:** Estrogen (100 µg estradiol transdermal or 0.625 mg conjugated estrogen oral), gradually increased; add progestin for menstrual cycles, endometrial protection.
    - **Nutrition:** Optimize weight/diet for hypothalamic amenorrhea.
    - **Treat Underlying Conditions:** Thyroid disorders, hyperprolactinemia, chronic illnesses (TB, celiac disease).
    - **Bone Health:** Calcium (1,200 mg), vitamin D (1,000 IU), weight-bearing exercise.
- **Surgical Intervention:**
    - Correct anatomic issues: Imperforate hymen, transverse vaginal septum.
    - Vaginoplasty/dilators for MRKH syndrome, androgen insensitivity syndrome (if vaginal coitus desired).
    - Gonadectomy for androgen insensitivity syndrome, gonadal dysgenesis (cancer risk).
- **Lifestyle/Psychological Support:**
    - Address stress, exercise, eating disorders.
    - Counseling for emotional impact (isolation, low self-esteem).
    - CBT for eating disorders/stress.
    - Family education for support.
- **Follow-Up:** Monitor pubertal progress, adjust therapy, assess prognosis based on cause.

Flowchart for management of primary amenorrhea

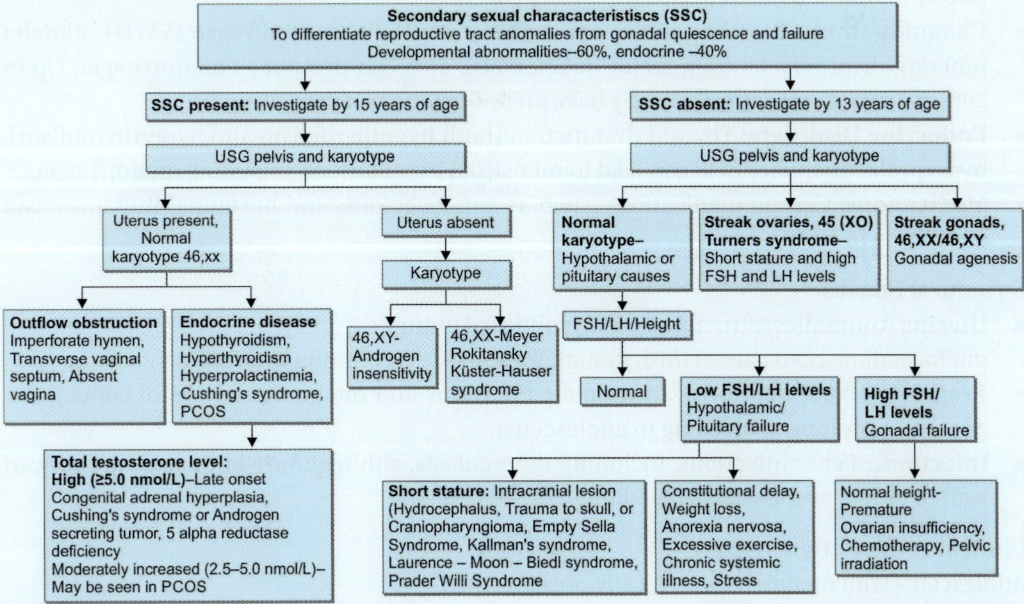

Precocious puberty is defined as the onset of secondary sexual characteristics before age 8 years in girls and before age 9 years in males. Discussed in detail in Chapter Precocious puberty.

LONG QUESTIONS AND ANSWERS

Q1. What is Puberty Menorrhagia? Discuss etiology, diagnosis, and management of puberty menorrhagia. *(10 marks)*

Abnormal uterine bleeding (AUB) is one of the most common indications for gynecological visits in adolescent girls. Almost 20–25% of adolescent girls will experience heavy menstrual bleeding (HMB) within the first few years of menarche.

The normal cycle of an adolescent female occurs every 21–45 days with bleeding lasting between 2 and 7 days with an average blood loss of 30–40 mL. Puberty Menorrhagia is defined as excessive menstrual blood loss in adolescent girls that interferes with her physical, social, emotional, or material quality of life.

Quantitatively, any menstrual bleeding lasting more than 7 days or involving the loss of more than 80 mL of blood per menstrual cycle signifies puberty menorrhagia.

Etiology

The causes of puberty menorrhagia can be categorized into nonstructural and structural causes. The most common cause of puberty menorrhagia is anovulation followed by bleeding disorders. Structural causes are uncommon and account for only a small percentage of puberty menorrhagia.

Nonstructural Causes

- **Anovulation:** Anovulatory cycles are the most common cause of menorrhagia in adolescents. The immature hypothalamic-pituitary-ovarian axis results in irregular and often prolonged bleeding.
- **Coagulopathies:** Bleeding disorders such as von Willebrand disease (VWD), platelet function disorders, clotting factor deficiencies, etc., can present as menorrhagia. Up to 20% of adolescents with HMB may have an underlying bleeding disorder.
- **Endocrine Disorders:** Thyroid dysfunction (both hypothyroidism and hyperthyroidism), hyperprolactinemia, PCOS can lead to menstrual irregularities, including menorrhagia.
- **Medications:** Certain medications, such as anticoagulants and hormonal therapies, can contribute to HMB.

Structural Causes

- **Uterine Anomalies:** Structural abnormalities of uterus, e.g., polyps, fibroids, or congenital malformations, can cause HMB, though these are less common in adolescents.
- **Pregnancy complications:** Incomplete abortions and retained products of conception can cause prolonged bleeding in adolescents.
- **Infections:** Pelvic infections, including tuberculosis, although rare in this age group, can lead to excessive menstrual bleeding.

Clinical Presentation

Adolescents with menorrhagia typically present with:

- **Excessive Menstrual Bleeding:**
  - Prolonged periods lasting more than 7 days.

- Heavy bleeding that soaks sanitary protection every 1–2 hours.
- Passing large clots.

- **Symptoms of Anemia:** Fatigue, pallor, shortness of breath, and dizziness due to significant blood loss.
- **Impact on Daily Life:** Menorrhagia can affect school attendance, participation in sports and social activities, leading to significant distress and decreased quality of life.
- **Symptoms of other disorders:**
  - History symptomatic of bleeding disorders: Bleeding gums, petechiae, epistaxis, family history, etc.
  - History of other medical conditions—weight loss/ weight gain, chronic cough,
  - History symptomatic of pelvic infections—fever, vaginal discharge, lower abdominal pain, etc.

Diagnostic Approach

- **History and Physical Examination:**
  - Detailed menstrual history, including cycle length, variability over time, duration and volume of bleeding.
  - Assessment for signs of anemia (pallor, tachycardia, hypotension) and coagulopathies (petechiae, bleeding gums, etc.).
  - Sexual and contraception history
  - Family history of bleeding disorders.
  - Clinical examination
  - General examination to assess vitals
  - Pelvic examination, especially in cases of suspected structural causes, infections, pregnancy complications, etc.
- **Laboratory Tests:**
  - UPT to r/o pregnancy
  - CBC to assess for anemia.
  - Blood grouping and cross matching in c/o severe anemia.
  - Coagulation profile—prothrombin time (PT), activated partial thromboplastin time (aPTT), fibrinogen and specific tests for von Willebrand factor.
  - Thyroid function tests.
  - Hormonal profile if an endocrine disorder is suspected.
  - ESR, Chest X-ray, Mantoux test to r/o tuberculosis
  - Vaginal swabs, screening for STIs to r/o infection
- **Imaging Studies:** Pelvic USG, especially in cases where an underlying structural cause is suspected or if there is failure of initial management.

Treatment: Most girls can be managed on an outpatient basis with medical management alone. They should be reassured that their cycles will regularize and become ovulatory over time. Admission is required only in cases of acute heavy bleeding with severe anemia.

Medical Management: Medical management is the first line of therapy.

Management of Mild to Moderate Bleeding

- **Nonhormonal Therapy:**
    - *Nonsteroidal anti-inflammatory drugs (NSAIDs):* Mefenamic acid and ibuprofen reduce menstrual blood loss by inhibiting prostaglandin synthesis. NSAIDs should be avoided in patients with bleeding disorders.
    - *Tranexamic acid:* Antifibrinolytic agent that significantly reduces menstrual blood loss.
- **Hormonal Therapy:**
    - Hormonal therapy can be considered if bleeding is not controlled by nonhormonal therapy, in irregular cycles or those needing contraception.
    - Monophasic combined oral contraceptive pills (COCPs) are first-line treatment. They regularize the menstrual cycle, reduce menstrual flow, and provide contraception.
    - Progestin-only therapies:
        - Oral progestins (e.g., medroxyprogesterone acetate, nor ethisterone acetate for at least 12 days a cycle) or
        - Levonorgestrel intrauterine system (LNG-IUS) is another effective management of menorrhagia.
- **Iron Supplementation:** In patients with anemia, oral iron supplementation is essential to replenish iron stores and improve hemoglobin levels to above 12 g%.

Management of Severe Bleeding

- Patients with active heavy bleeding (soakage of >1 pad/hour) with signs of hypovolemia and hypotension should be admitted.
- In the absence of contraindications of estrogen, monophasic COCPs containing 30–50 μg ethinyl estradiol can be used every 6–8 hours until bleeding stops and then tapered gradually to one pill daily.
- If the patient does not tolerate oral COCPs or if bleeding persists after COCPs, intravenous 25 mg conjugated estrogen every 4–6 hours should be considered until bleeding stops.
- Intravenous tranexamic acid can be given to control bleeding. However, concomitant use of COCPs and tranexamic acid should be avoided to reduce risk of thrombosis.
- Blood transfusion with packed cell volume (PCV) may be required in the presence of hemodynamic instability or the presence of symptoms of severe anemia.
- In extreme cases, when bleeding does not get controlled with medical management, surgical treatment in the form of dilatation and curettage, intrauterine balloon tamponade, and uterine artery embolization may be required to control intractable bleeding.

Management of Underlying Causes

- **Treatment of Coagulopathies:** In patients with bleeding disorders, factor replacement therapy or desmopressin in VWD may be required.
- **Management of endocrine diseases:** Appropriate treatment of thyroid disorders, hyperprolactinemia, and PCOS should be started to normalize menstrual cycles.
- **Psychological Support:** Adolescents with menorrhagia may experience significant stress and anxiety. Counseling and support from healthcare providers, school personnel, and family are essential.

Q2. What is Turner Syndrome? Describe the clinical features, investigations, and management of Turner Syndrome.

Turner Syndrome (TS) is a chromosomal disorder affecting females, characterized by the partial or complete absence of one X chromosome. (45 XO).

It is also called Congenital Ovarian Hypoplasia syndrome. TS affects approximately 1 in 2,500 live female births and is the most common sex chromosomal abnormality in women.

Etiology and Pathophysiology

- TS results from the complete or partial absence of one X chromosome (45 X karyotype) or mosaicism (45 X/46,XX or other variants).
- The loss of genetic material from X chromosome disrupts normal development, leading to the characteristic features of TS.
- The *SHOX* gene, important for bone growth and development, is often implicated in the short stature observed in TS.

Clinical Features

- **Physical Characteristics:**
  - **Short Stature:** Growth failure is a hallmark, with adult height typically below the 5th percentile.
  - **Webbed Neck:** Excess skin folds extending from the top of the shoulders to the sides of the neck.
  - **Low Hairline and Low-Set Ears:** These features are commonly observed in TS.
  - **Skeletal Abnormalities:**
    - Cubitus valgus (increased carrying angle of the arms)
    - Broad chest with widely spaced nipples.
    - Osteoporosis due to estrogen deficiency
    - Scoliosis
- **Ovarian Insufficiency:**
  - "Streak gonads" are a characteristic feature of TS which consist of mainly connective tissue with only a few atretic follicles.
  - Girls with TS often experience delayed puberty or primary amenorrhea secondary to premature ovarian failure.
  - Some patients with mosaicism may have spontaneous menarche followed by secondary amenorrhea after a few cycles and infertility.
- **Cardiovascular Abnormalities:**
  - **Congenital Heart Defects:**
    - Bicuspid aortic valve, coarctation of the aorta, and other structural heart anomalies.
    - Patients are at an increased risk of aortic dissection.
  - **Hypertension:** Women with TS have an increased risk of high blood pressure.
- **Renal and Urinary Abnormalities:**
  - **Horseshoe Kidney:** Abnormal fusion of the kidneys, occurring in about 30% of TS cases.
  - **Nonstructural Kidney Defects:** Increased susceptibility to urinary tract infections and renal dysfunction.

- **Other Features:**
  - Lymphedema (swelling of hands and feet, particularly in infancy), high-arched palate.
  - **Hearing Loss:** Conductive or sensorineural hearing loss, increased risk of middle ear infections
  - **Autoimmune Disorders:** Increased risk of autoimmune thyroiditis, celiac disease, and diabetes mellitus.
  - **Vision Problems:** Possible vision problems such as strabismus, ptosis, hypertelorism, etc.
- **Cognitive and Psychological Aspects:**
  - Most patients with TS have normal intelligence but may have specific learning difficulties involving spatial reasoning and calculations.
  - Increased risk of social adjustment difficulties and anxiety

Diagnosis of TS

Diagnosis of TS is based on detailed clinical examination with laboratory and imaging studies and confirmed by karyotyping.

Clinical Evaluation

- Detailed assessment of characteristic physical features and growth patterns.
- Hearing and vision assessment.

Laboratory investigations

Hormone Levels:

- Measurement of FSH, LH, AMH, and estradiol to assess ovarian function.
- Thyroid function tests

Imaging studies

- Echocardiogram: To identify congenital heart defects.
- Pelvic ultrasound: To assess uterine size and ovarian tissue
- Renal Ultrasound: To evaluate kidney structure and function.

Karyotyping

Chromosomal analysis to confirm the diagnosis and identify the specific karyotype (45 XO, mosaicism, or structural abnormalities).

Prenatal diagnosis:

- TS is suspected when antenatal ultrasound shows features like cystic hygroma, hydrops fetalis, or cardiac defects.
- Turner syndrome is diagnosed by doing chorionic villus sampling or amniocentesis and sending cells for karyotyping.

Management of TS

Early diagnosis and management are important for optimizing outcomes and quality of life for individuals with TS. Management should be multidisciplinary with involvement of specialists in endocrinology, cardiology, genetics, and psychology.

Endocrine Therapy

- *Growth Hormone Therapy:*
  - It is indicated in girls with short stature where the height is less than the 5th centile.
  - Although TS does not cause growth hormone deficiency, girls with short stature respond well to growth hormone therapy.
  - Recombinant human growth hormone enhances growth and helps achieve a better adult height.
  - Treatment should begin in early childhood and continue until growth plates close.
- **Hormonal Replacement Therapy:**
  Estrogen Therapy:
  - Estrogen replacement therapy should start if no breast development begins at around 11–12 years of age with elevated levels of FSH, LH, and low levels of AMH.
  - Initiation of low-dose estrogen therapy around the age of puberty (11–12 years) is critical
    - To initiate puberty
    - To induce and maintain secondary sexual characteristics
    - To allow uterine development
    - To maintain bone health.
  - Transdermal patches or oral estrogen can be used. The dose of estrogen should be gradually stepped up.

  Cyclical Progesterone therapy: Progesterone therapy is added after 1–2 years of estrogen therapy or once breakthrough bleeding occurs to promote regular menstrual cycles and prevent development of endometrial hyperplasia.

Cardiovascular Monitoring

- *Regular Cardiac Evaluations*
  - Annual Echocardiograms and MRIs should be considered to monitor structural heart abnormalities and aortic dilation.
  - Corrective surgery may be offered for coarctation of aorta.
  - BP should be monitored in both upper and lower extremities and treatment initiated.

Fertility options

- Most women with TS experience infertility due to ovarian insufficiency.
- In vitro fertilization (IVF) with donor eggs may be considered in women desirous of pregnancy.
- In women with functioning ovarian tissue, fertility preservation options, including oocyte or ovarian tissue cryopreservation, should be considered.

Bone Density Monitoring: Regular DEXA scans should be offered to assess bone health and manage risk of osteoporosis secondary to estrogen deficiency.

Psychosocial Support:

- *Counseling and Support Groups:*
  - Women with TS should be offered psychological counseling to address emotional and social challenges associated with TS like delayed puberty, body image, premature ovarian failure, and infertility.
  - Referral to suitable support groups.

- *Educational Support:*
  - Women with learning disabilities should be offered training in social skills and vocational training to help achieve their full potential.
  - ther Associated Conditions:
  - Early assessment and management of thyroid diseases.
  - Management of visual and hearing problems.

Q3. What is Imperforate Hymen? Describe the clinical features, investigations, and management of imperforate hymen. *(10 Marks)*

The hymen is a thin membrane made of stratified squamous membrane covering the vaginal introitus. Imperforate hymen is a congenital disorder in which the hymen completely covers the vaginal orifice, preventing the normal outflow of menstrual blood. This condition is commonly diagnosed in adolescence when menstrual blood accumulates behind the hymen, leading to various symptoms.

Etiology and Pathogenesis:

- Imperforate hymen is a result of abnormal embryological development of the female reproductive tract.
- The exact cause is not well understood but is considered a sporadic congenital anomaly.
- During fetal development, the hymen develops from the urogenital sinus and typically perforates around 22 weeks' gestation.
- In imperforate hymen, this process does not occur, resulting in a membrane that obstructs the vaginal opening.
- As the hymen is not a Müllerian structure, it is usually not associated with urinary tract anomalies.

Clinical Features:

- In newborn and infants, accumulation of vaginal secretions behind the hymen may lead to a bulging introitus (mucocolpos/hydrocolpos). It is often detected during routine neonatal examination.
- Adolescents may present with primary amenorrhea.
- There is usually a history of cyclic lower abdominal pain due to the accumulation of menstrual blood (hematocolpos) behind the imperforate hymen.
- Menstrual blood accumulates behind the hymen, loses its water contents over a period of time, and eventually becomes tarry or dark brown in color.
- A palpable lower abdominal mass due to distended vagina and uterus filled with blood (hematometra) may be the presenting complaints.
- Patients may present with urinary retention or difficulty due to pressure from the distended vagina and uterus on the ureter and the bladder neck.
- In long-standing untreated cases, patients may present with endometriosis, infertility, and hydronephrosis.

On physical Examination:

- Bulging hymen: Hymen appears bulging and bluish due to accumulation of blood.
- Absence of visible vaginal opening: The vaginal orifice is completely covered by the hymenal membrane.
- Rectal examination may reveal a bulging tense mass in the midline.

Diagnosis:

Clinical Evaluation:

- *History and clinical examination:*
  - Detailed history of cyclic pelvic pain, primary amenorrhea, and urinary symptoms.
  - Inspection of the external genitalia revealing a bulging, blueish hymen without a visible vaginal opening.

Imaging:

- *Ultrasound:*
  - Ultrasound is usually sufficient to confirm diagnosis of imperforate hymen.
  - Ultrasound reveals a distended vagina and uterus filled with fluid.
  - Hydroureter and hydronephrosis due to pressure by the distended uterus and vagina.
  - Ovaries are usually normal. In long-standing cases, hematosalpinges may be seen.

MRI: MRI can provide detailed anatomical information, especially in complex cases.

Management: The mainstay of management is surgical. There is no role of conservative or medical management.

Hymenotomy or Hymenectomy:

- Hymenotomy involves making a small cruciate incision on the hymen to allow drainage of accumulated blood followed by suturing the four corners of the flaps created to the vestibule, to prevent re-epithelization.
- During and after the procedure, the patient should be given head-low position to allow drainage of accumulated blood.
- Hymenectomy is the complete removal of the hymenal tissue.
- The procedure can be done in regional anesthesia, general anesthesia, or local anesthesia.

Postoperative Care

- Analgesics and anti-inflammatory medications should be given to manage postoperative pain.
- Antibiotics may be prescribed to prevent infection.
- Regular follow-up should be done to ensure proper healing, ensure patency of the outflow tract, and look for any complications such as infection, stenosis, etc.

MULTIPLE CHOICE QUESTIONS

Q1. According to WHO, what age range defines adolescence?

a. 8–16 years
b. 10–19 years
c. 12–21 years
d. 15–25 years

Ans. b. 10–19 years

Q2. What initiates puberty through the hypothalamic–pituitary–gonadal (HPG) axis?

a. Increased cortisol secretion
b. Pulsatile release of gonadotropin-releasing hormone (GnRH)
c. Continuous thyroid hormone production
d. Adrenal androgen surge

Ans. b. Pulsatile release of gonadotropin-releasing hormone (GnRH)

Q3. Which hormone primarily drives breast development (thelarche) during puberty in girls?

a. Progesterone
b. Estradiol
c. Dehydroepiandrosterone (DHEA)
d. Follicle-stimulating hormone (FSH)

Ans. b. Estradiol

Q4. At which Tanner stage of breast development do the areola and nipple form a secondary mound?

a. Stage 2
b. Stage 3
c. Stage 4
d. Stage 5

Ans. c. Stage 4

Q5. What is the typical age range for menarche in girls?

a. 8–10 years
b. 12–13 years
c. 15–17 years
d. 18–20 years

Ans. b. 12–13 years

Q6. Which factor is most likely to delay the onset of puberty?

a. High carbohydrate diet
b. Chronic illness
c. Moderate exercise
d. Genetic predisposition to early puberty

Ans. b. Chronic illness

Q7. What is the most common cause of delayed puberty in both genders?

a. Turner syndrome
b. Constitutional delay of growth and puberty (CDGP)
c. Kallmann syndrome
d. Hypothyroidism

Ans. b. Constitutional delay of growth and puberty (CDGP)

Q8. Which condition is characterized by hypergonadotropic hypogonadism in females?

a. Kallmann syndrome
b. Turner syndrome
c. Functional hypothalamic amenorrhea
d. Prader-Willi syndrome

Ans. b. Turner syndrome

Q9. What is a key diagnostic criterion for delayed puberty in girls?

a. No menarche by age 12 years
b. No breast development by age 13 years
c. No pubic hair by age 11 years
d. No growth spurt by age 10 years

Ans. b. No breast development by age 13 years

Q10. Which investigation differentiates hypergonadotropic from hypogonadotropic hypogonadism?

a. Thyroid function tests
b. LH and FSH levels
c. Prolactin levels
d. Bone age X-ray

Ans. b. LH and FSH levels

Q11. What is the initial treatment for delayed puberty in girls with hypogonadotropic hypogonadism?

a. Progesterone monotherapy
b. Low-dose estrogen therapy
c. Growth hormone injections
d. Surgical correction

Ans. b. Low-dose estrogen therapy

Q12. Primary amenorrhea is defined as the absence of menarche by what age with normal secondary sexual characteristics?

a. 13 years
b. 15 years
c. 17 years
d. 19 years

Ans. b. 15 years

Q13. Which condition causing primary amenorrhea is associated with Müllerian agenesis?

a. Turner syndrome
b. Mayer-Rokitansky-Küster-Hauser (MRKH) syndrome
c. Kallmann syndrome
d. Polycystic ovary syndrome (PCOS)

Ans. b. Mayer-Rokitansky-Küster-Hauser (MRKH) syndrome

Q14. Which feature is characteristic of Turner syndrome?

a. Tall stature and anosmia
b. Short stature and webbed neck
c. Obesity and delayed milestones
d. Normal puberty with irregular menses

Ans. b. Short stature and webbed neck

SUGGESTED READING

1. Breehl L, Caban O. Physiology, Puberty. In: StatPearls [Internet]. Treasure Island (FL): StatPearls Publishing; 2024 Jan-. [online] Available from https://www.ncbi.nlm.nih.gov/books/NBK534827/ [Last accessed December, 2025]
2. https://www.who.int/health-topics/adolescent-health/#tab=tab_1
3. Klein DA, Emerick JE, Sylvester JE, Vogt KS. Disorders of Puberty: An Approach to Diagnosis and Management. Am Fam Physician. 2017;96(9):590-9.
4. Tang C, Zafar Gondal A, Damian M. Delayed Puberty. In: StatPearls [Internet]. Treasure Island (FL): StatPearls Publishing; 2024 Jan-. Available from: https://www.ncbi.nlm.nih.gov/books/NBK544322/

Amenorrhea: A Clinical Approach to Diagnosis and Management

Shivani Singh Bundela

Amenorrhea is absence or abnormal cessation of menstruation in a woman of reproductive age group. It may be primary or secondary.

- Primary amenorrhea is defined as failure to attained menarche by the age of 15 years. (ACOG)
  - Absence of menses by 13 years of age when there is no visible development of secondary sexual characteristics **OR** Absence of menses by 15 years of age in the presence of normal secondary sexual characteristics or within 5 years after breast development if that occurs before the age of 10 years (ASRM 2024).
  - Secondary amenorrhea is the absence of menstruation for 3 or more months in a woman who previously had regular menstrual cycles or for 6 or more months in a woman with previously irregular cycles. (ACOG, ASRM)

Primary Amenorrhea

- **When to evaluate:**
  - Failure to attain menarche by 15 years of age in the presence of secondary sexual characters.
  - No thelarche by age 13 years
  - Absence of onset of menses by age 13 years in the absence of secondary sexual characters
  - Failure to attain menarche within 3 years of breast development if it starts before age 13 years.
- Pubertal changes **(Table 1)**
  Sequence of events: Thelarche → Pubarche → Adrenarche → Menarche

TABLE 1: Puberty changes.

Growth spurt	8–14 years (10.5 years)
Breast growth (thelarche)	9–11 years
Pubic hair (pubarche)	9–13 years
Axillary hair (adrenarche)	9.5–15 years
Menstruation (menarche)	10–16 years (13 years)

- **Causes of primary amenorrhea** (ASRM 2024)
  - Hypothalamic **10–21%**
  - Anterior pituitary **1–4%**
  - Ovarian **24–52%**
  - Genital outflow tract and uterine **15–43%**
  - Others (Cushing's, complete androgen insensitivity, and medication) **2–8% (Table 2)**

TABLE 2: Common causes of amenorrhea.

Primary amenorrhea	• Hypothalamic and pituitary causes – Constitutional Delay/functional hypothalamic amenorrhea, hyperprolactinemia • Anatomic abnormalities: – Imperforate hymen – Transverse vaginal septum – MRKH (Mayer-Rokitansky-Kuster-Hauser) syndrome • Ovarian – Gonadal dysgenesis • Others – Complete androgen insensitivity – Medication – Cushing's syndrome
Secondary amenorrhea	• Functional hypothalamic amenorrhea • PCOS • Hyperprolactinemia • Hypothyroidism • Cushing's syndrome • Sheehan's syndrome • Primary ovarian insufficiency (chemotherapy/radiation) • Exogenous hormonal suppression (DMPA Inj.) • Asherman syndrome/Intrauterine adhesion

- Classification of primary amenorrhea
  - Hypergonadotropic hypogonadism
    High FSH >40 mIU/mL, absence of secondary sexual characteristics
    - Turner syndrome
    - Pure gonadal dysgenesis
    - Sawyer's syndrome
    - Savage syndrome
    - Klinefelter syndrome
  - Eugonadotropic primary amenorrhea
    Normal FSH, normal secondary sexual characteristics
    - *Mullerian agenesis (46,XX):* MRKH syndrome → absence of vagina, absent/hypoplastic uterus, normal ovaries, renal anomalies, skeletal malformations
    - Androgen Insensitivity syndrome (46,XY) (inactivating mutation in gene encoding androgen receptor) → phenotypically females, absent cervix and uterus (AMH action), vagina is short and ends blindly (urogenital sinus), breast development (peripheral conversion of testosterone to estrogen), sparse pubic and axillary hair (androgen insensitivity)
    - Normal mullerian development
      - Transverse vaginal septum
      - Imperforate hymen
      - Female intersex
      - Adult-onset congenital adrenal hyperplasia
      - Cushing's syndrome
      - Thyroid diseases

- Hypogonadotropic hypogonadism
  Low FSH, absence of secondary sexual characteristics
  - Constitutional delayed puberty
  - Functional hypothalamic amenorrhea
  - Pituitary lesion/Hyperprolactinemia
  - Kallmann syndrome
  - Cushing syndrome
  - Drugs (opiate/anabolic steroids)
- **Evaluation of primary amenorrhea (Flowchart 1):**
  - History:
    - Cyclical abdominal pain → Imperforate hymen, Transverse vaginal septum
    - History related to time of appearance and development of secondary sexual characters.
    - Family history of time of menarche and puberty in siblings and mother → Constitutional delay
    - History of eating disorder, extreme weigh loss/weight gain
    - Strenuous exercise/athletic training
    - History of Anosmia (Kallman syndrome), galactorrhea, headache, or visual changes indicates CNS or pituitary disorder.
    - Family history of complete androgen insensitivity syndrome (CAIS), Constitutional delay of growth and puberty.
    - Medical history and current medication (antipsychotics, antidepressants, anticonvulsants, opiates, chemotherapy/radiotherapy)
  - Examination:
    - Height, weight, and BMI (indicates hormonal or developmental issues, particularly in hypothalamic amenorrhea)
    - Short stature without secondary sexual character development: A sign of gonadal dysgenesis.
    - Low body weight: Functional Hypothalamic amenorrhea (malnutrition, physical or psychological stress)
  - General examination:
    - Low hairline, high arched palate, webbed neck. (Suggestive of Turner syndrome.)
    - Moon fancies and buffalo hump: Cushing's syndrome.
    - Presence of hirsutism, deepening of voice—Skin, hair, and nail changes: Thyroid disorder
    - A blind or absent vagina with breast development usually indicates Mullerian agenesis, Transverse vaginal septum, or AIS.
  - Investigations:
    - USG Pelvis
    - Serum FSH, LH and estradiol, prolactin, TSH
    - Bone age radiography for physiological delay
    - Testosterone levels and DHEAS for hyperandrogenism
    - CT head (pituitary tumor, if prolactin >100)
    - Karyotyping in gonadal dysgenesis cases

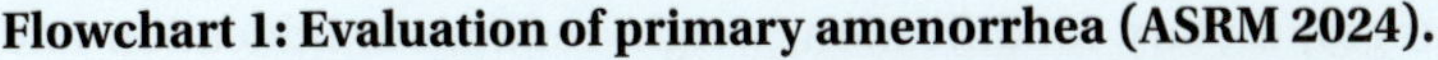

Flowchart 1: Evaluation of primary amenorrhea (ASRM 2024).

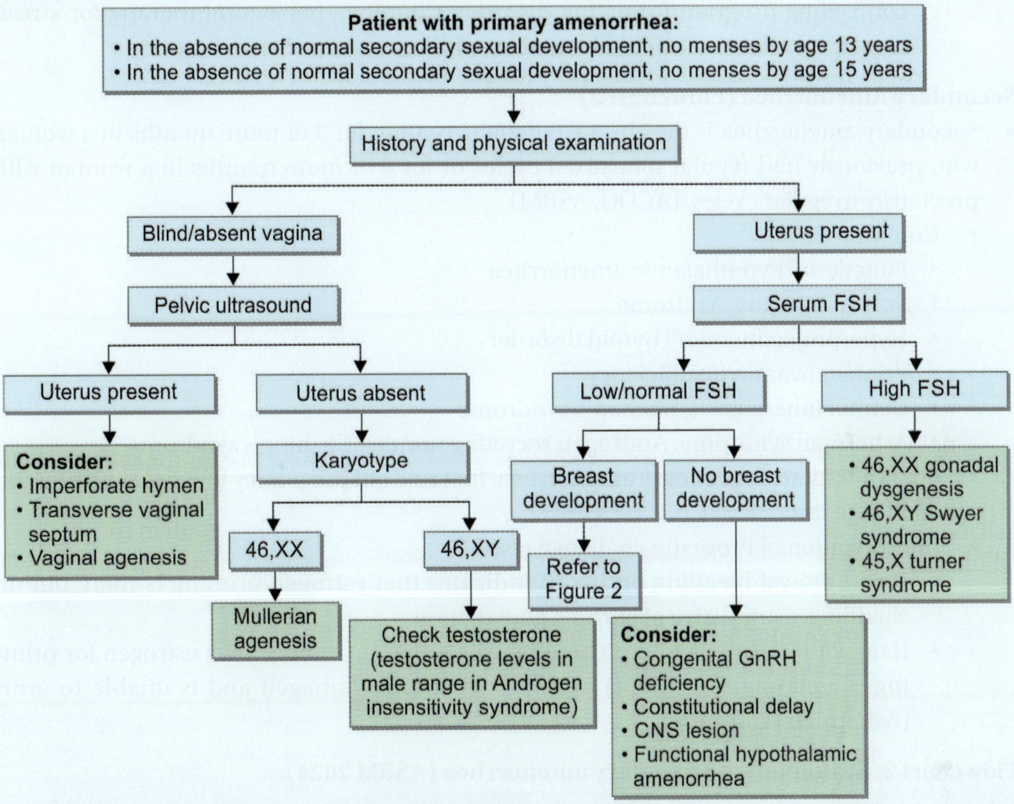

Patient with primary amenorrhea:
- In the absence of normal secondary sexual development, no menses by age 13 years
- In the absence of normal secondary sexual development, no menses by age 15 years

→ History and physical examination

- Blind/absent vagina → Pelvic ultrasound
  - Uterus present → **Consider:** Imperforate hymen; Transverse vaginal septum; Vaginal agenesis
  - Uterus absent → Karyotype
    - 46,XX → Mullerian agenesis
    - 46,XY → Check testosterone (testosterone levels in male range in Androgen insensitivity syndrome)
- Uterus present → Serum FSH
  - Low/normal FSH
    - Breast development → Refer to Figure 2
    - No breast development → **Consider:** Congenital GnRH deficiency; Constitutional delay; CNS lesion; Functional hypothalamic amenorrhea
  - High FSH → 46,XX gonadal dysgenesis; 46,XY Swyer syndrome; 45,X turner syndrome

- **Androgen Insensitivity** syndrome (46,XY) (inactivating mutation in gene encoding androgen receptor) → phenotypically females, gonads testis, uterus and cervix absent, vagina is short and ends blindly, normal breast development, sparse pubic and axillary hair
- **Kallmann syndrome** (Defect in KAL- GENE), X-LINKED RECESSIVE DISORDER (46,XX)
  - GONADS: Ovary, Hypogonadotropic hypogonadism
  - Presents with primary amenorrhea, infertility, anosmia, secondary sexual character absent, phenotypically female, infantile Uterus, cervix and vagina.
- **Turner Syndrome (45,XO)**
  - Streak ovaries, short stature, High LH and FSH, Estrogen low, poor breast development, infantile uterus
- **Management**
  - Outflow tract obstruction:
    - Imperforate hymen—surgical correction
    - Blind vagina—vaginoplasty
      - In patients with Y chromosome and streak gonads—gonadectomy as there is risk of malignancy
      - Hypothalamic/pituitary/gonadal dysgenesis
    - POI/Kallman syndrome
      - Endocrinologist opinion for HRT, calcium, and vitamin D supplementation, weight bearing exercises for bone health, Screening for hypothyroidism

- FHA: lifestyle changes, dietary modification, weight reduction, Education and counseling program for eating disorder. Cognitive behavioral therapy for stress. Hyperprolactinemia should be treated with bromocriptine.

Secondary Amenorrhea (Flowchart 2)

- Secondary amenorrhea is the absence of menstruation for 3 or more months in a woman who previously had regular menstrual cycles or for 6 or more months in a woman with previously irregular cycles. (ACOG, ASRM)
  - Common Causes:
    - Functional hypothalamic amenorrhea
    - Polycystic ovary syndrome
    - Hyperprolactinemia/Thyroid disorder
    - Primary ovarian insufficiency
    - Genital tuberculosis, Shehan's syndrome
    - Asherman syndrome, Androgen secreting tumors, Cushing's syndrome
  - For evaluation of secondary amenorrhea, first rule out pregnancy followed by progestin challenge test.
  - Interpretation of Progestin challenge test:
    - If withdrawal bleeding occurs, it indicates that estrogen priming is there but no shedding—suggestive of chronic anovulation.
    - If no withdrawal bleeding: There may be either no endogenous estrogen for priming of endometrium (POI) or endometrium is damaged and is unable to grow (Asherman syndrome).

Flowchart 2: Evaluation of secondary amenorrhea (ASRM 2024).

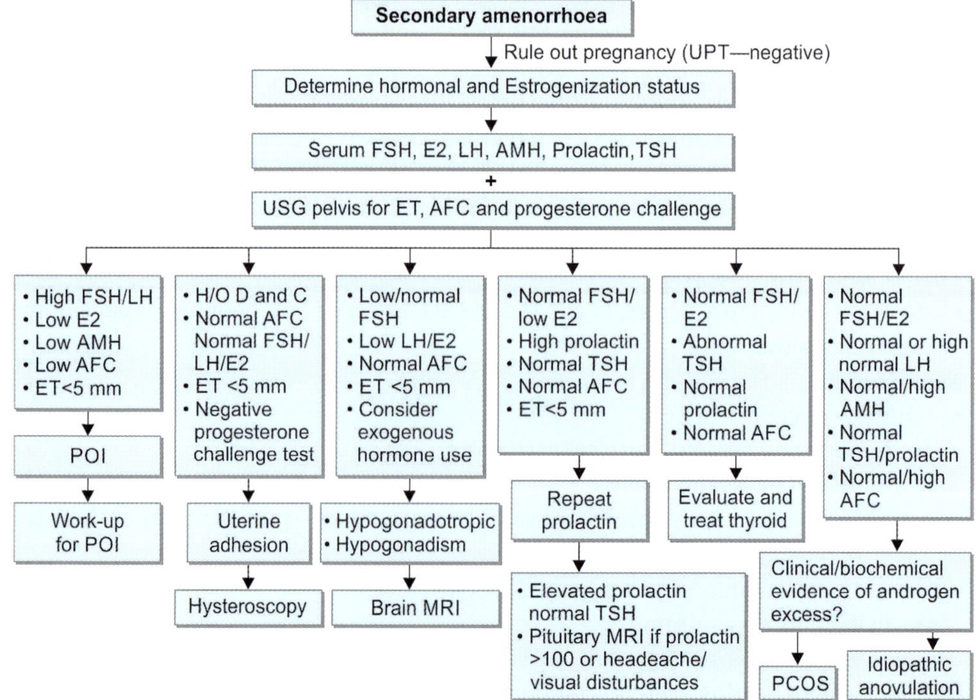

- **Management:** Depends on the underlying etiology.
- **Functional hypothalamic amenorrhea (FHA):** Patient education, counseling, nutritional support, oral contraceptive pills
- **PCOS:** Weight loss, metformin, nutrition counseling, OCPs
- **POI:** HRT
- **Hyperprolactinemia:** Cabergoline, bromocriptine
- **Hypothyroidism:** Thyroxin replacement
- **Asherman syndrome:** Hysteroscopic adhesiolysis **(Flowcharts 1 and 2)**

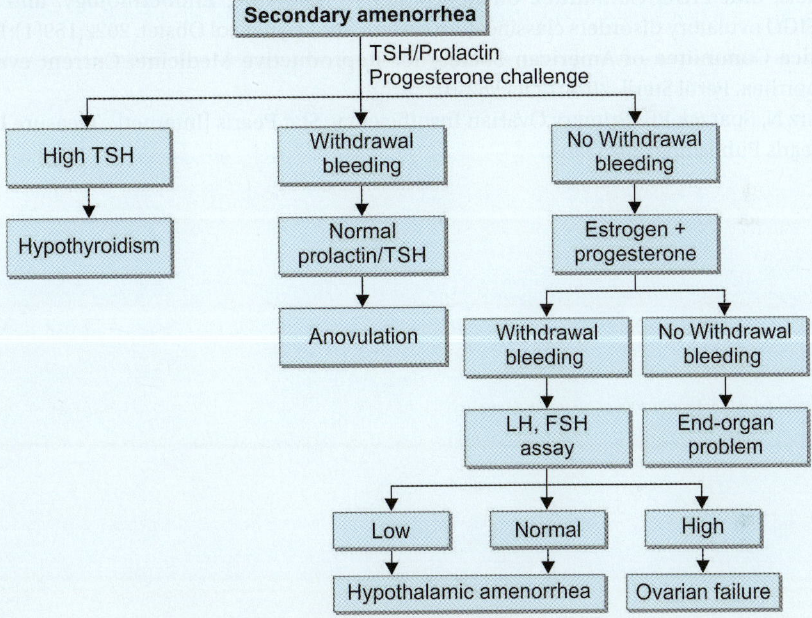

QUESTIONS

Q1. a. Define primary amenorrhea.
b. Enlist various etiologies of primary amenorrhea.
c. Describe workup of a case of primary amenorrhea in a methodical manner.
(DNB June 2022)

Q2. a. Define primary amenorrhea.
b. Enumerate causes of primary amenorrhea.
c. Turner syndrome *(DNB June 2019)*

Q3. Discuss the management of primary amenorrhea in an 18-year-old girl. *(Oct 2022)*

Q4. A 35-years old multiparous woman presents with amenorrhea of 1-year duration. Discuss causes, evaluation, and management of same. *(Aug 2021)*

SUGGESTED READING

1. American Society for Reproductive Medicine (ASRM). (2024). Current evaluation of amenorrhea: a committee opinion. [online] Available from https://www.asrm.org/practice-guidance/practice-committee-documents/current-evaluation-of-amenorrhea/ [Last accessed December, 2025].

2. Fraietta R, Zylberstejn DS, Esteves SC. Hypogonadotropic Hypogonadism Revisited. Clinics (Sao Paulo). 2013;68 Suppl 1(Suppl 1):81-8.
3. Kalkanli A, Akdere H, Cevic G, et al. Hypergonadotropic Hypogonadism: Management of Infertility. Curr Pharma Des. 2021;27(24):2790-5.
4. Layman LC. Hypogonadotropic hypogonadism. Endocrinol Metab Clin North Am. 2007;36(2): 283-96.
5. Lord M, Jenkins SM, Sahni M. Secondary amenorrhoea. Stat Pearls [Internet]. Treasure Island (FL): StatPearls Publishing; 2025 Jan-.
6. Munro MG, Balen AH, Cho S, et al. FIGO Committee on Menstrual Disorders and Related Health Impacts, and FIGO Committee on Reproductive Medicine, Endocrinology, and Infertility. The FIGO ovulatory disorders classification system. Int J Gynaecol Obstet. 2022;159(1):1-20.
7. Practice Committee of American Society for Reproductive Medicine. Current evaluation of amenorrhea. Fertil Steril. 2024;122(1):52-61.
8. Sopiarz N, Sparzak PB. Primary Ovarian Insufficiency. Stat Pearls [Internet]. Treasure Island (FL): StatPearls Publishing; 2025 Jan-.

CHAPTER 37

Fibroid

Neelansha Varshney, Ruchika Garg

INTRODUCTION

Uterine fibroids are benign monoclonal tumors of the myometrium, affecting 20–25% of women of reproductive age and up to 70–80% by age 50 years. They are the most common pelvic tumors in women, contributing significantly to gynecological morbidity, including heavy menstrual bleeding (HMB), pelvic pain, bulk symptoms, and infertility. Management is individualized based on symptom severity, fibroid characteristics (size, number, location), patient age, fertility desires, and comorbidities. Options range from expectant management for asymptomatic cases to medical, nonsurgical, and surgical interventions for symptomatic fibroids. Myomectomy, a uterus-preserving surgical procedure, is a cornerstone for women desiring fertility preservation. This chapter provides a detailed overview of fibroid management, emphasizing evidence-based approaches and recent advancements.

PATHOPHYSIOLOGY OF UTERINE FIBROIDS

Uterine fibroids originate from myometrial smooth muscle cells and are driven by complex interactions between hormonal, genetic, and molecular pathways. Key factors include:

- Hormonal Influence: Estrogen and progesterone play critical roles in fibroid growth. Estrogen promotes cellular proliferation, while progesterone enhances extracellular matrix production, contributing to fibroid size. Fibroids express higher levels of estrogen and progesterone receptors compared to normal myometrium.
- Genetic Alterations: Recurrent genetic mutations, such as those in the *MED12* gene, are identified in up to 70% of fibroids. Other mutations involve HMGA2 overexpression and chromosomal translocations.
- Molecular Pathways: Growth factors (e.g., TGF-β, VEGF), cytokines, and extracellular matrix remodeling contribute to fibroid development and growth.

CLASSIFICATION OF FIBROIDS

Fibroids are classified by their location within the uterus, which guides management decisions **(Table 1; Fig. 1)**. The International Federation of Gynecology and Obstetrics (FIGO) classification is widely used.

TABLE 1: FIGO Classification of uterine fibroids.

Type	*Description*	*Clinical implications*
0	Pedunculated intracavitary	HMB, infertility; suitable for hysteroscopic resection
1	Submucosal, <50% intramural	HMB, infertility; amenable to hysteroscopic myomectomy
2	Submucosal, ≥50% intramural	HMB, possible bulk symptoms; may require combined approach
3	Intramural, in contact with endometrium	Infertility, possible HMB; laparoscopic/abdominal approach
4	Intramural	Bulk symptoms; laparoscopic or abdominal myomectomy
5	Subserosal, ≥50% intramural	Bulk symptoms; laparoscopic or abdominal approach
6	Subserosal, <50% intramural	Bulk symptoms; often laparoscopic
7	Subserosal pedunculated	• Pain if torsion occurs; Clinical presentation: Patient presents with *acute pain in abdomen, vomiting, tachycardia*. On per abdominal examination, there will be *tenderness, guarding and rigidity* • Laparoscopic resection
8	Other (e.g., cervical, parasitic)	Variable symptoms; tailored approach

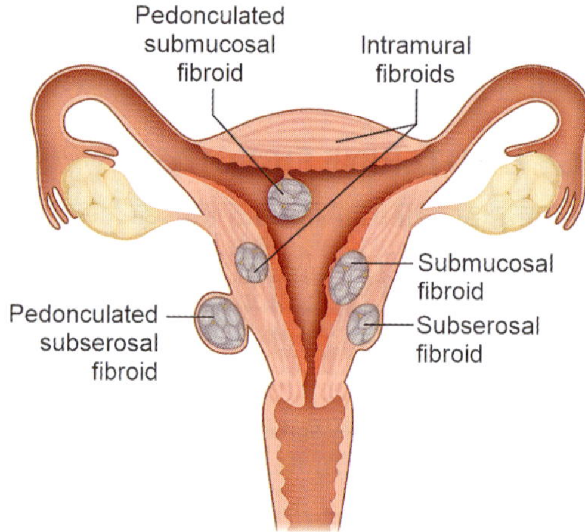

Fig. 1: Location of fibroids.

CLINICAL PRESENTATION AND DIAGNOSIS

Symptoms (Fig. 2)

- *Heavy Menstrual Bleeding (HMB):* Common with submucosal fibroids, leading to anemia.
- *Pelvic Pain/Pressure:* Associated with intramural or subserosal fibroids, causing urinary frequency, constipation, or dyspareunia.
- *Infertility:* Submucosal and intramural fibroids may distort the endometrial cavity, impairing implantation or increasing miscarriage risk.
- *Obstetric Complications:* Increased risk of preterm labor, placental abruption, and cesarean delivery in pregnancy.
- *Asymptomatic:* Up to 50–60% of fibroids are asymptomatic, detected incidentally.

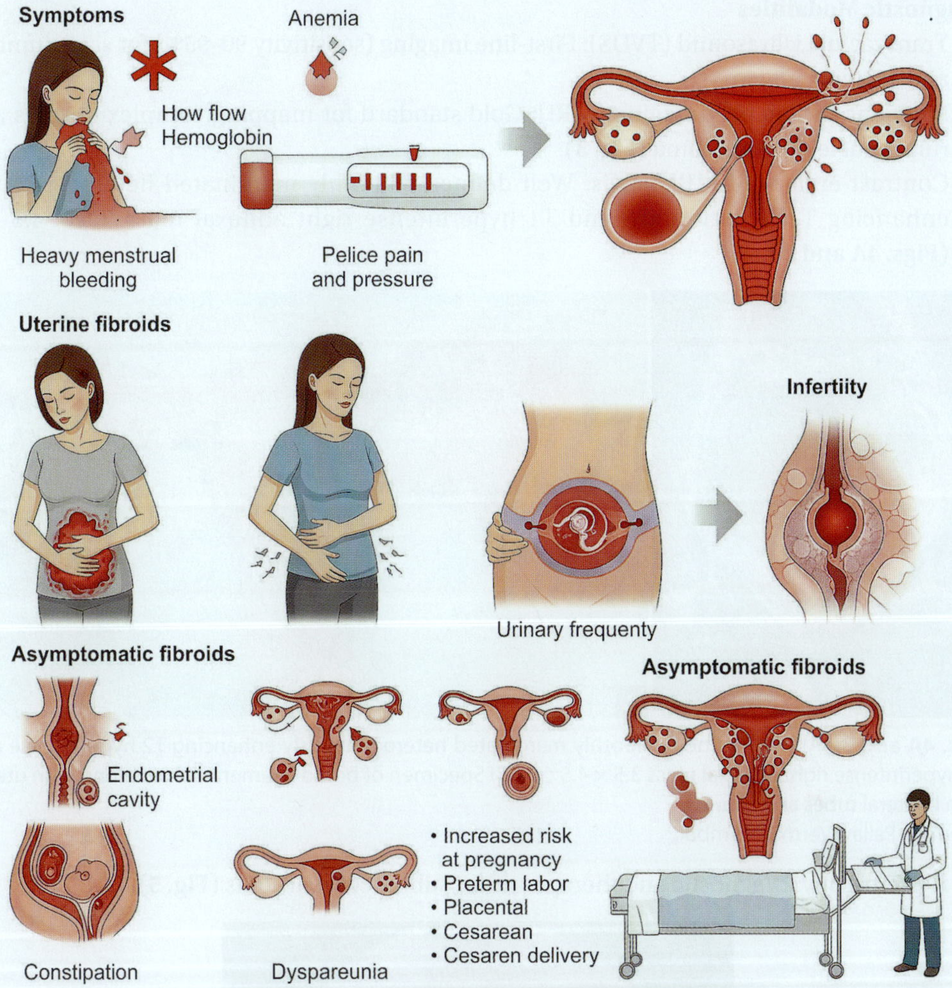

Fig. 2: Symptoms of fibroids.

Placental Abruptio

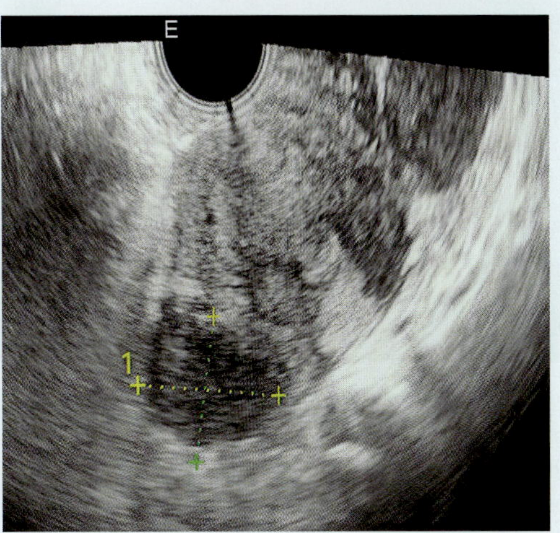

Fig. 3: B-mode ultrasound showing fundal fibroid.

Diagnostic Modalities

- Transvaginal Ultrasound (TVUS): First-line imaging (sensitivity 90–95%) for size, number, and location.
- Magnetic Resonance Imaging (MRI): Gold standard for mapping complex fibroids and ruling out leiomyosarcoma **(Fig. 3)**.
- Contrast-enhanced MRI Pelvis: Well-defined smoothly marginated heterogeneously enhancing T2 hyperintense and T1 hyperintense right adnexal mass 3.5 × 4.5 cm **(Figs. 4A and B)**.

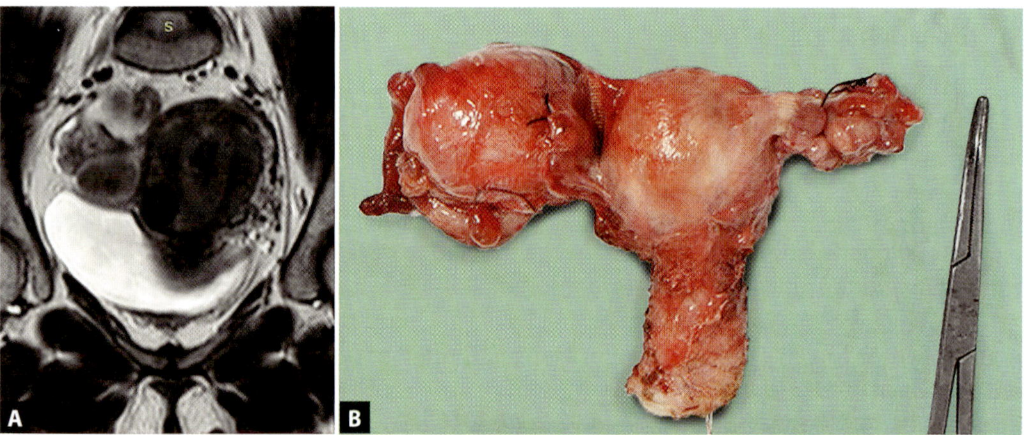

Figs. 4A and B: (A) Well-defined smoothly marginated heterogeneously enhancing T2 hyperintense and T1 hyperintense right adnexal mass 3.5 × 4.5 cm; (B) Specimen of broad ligament fibroid along with uterus with bilateral tubes and ovaries.
Courtesy: Pallavi Verma, Mumbai.

- Hysteroscopy: Diagnostic and therapeutic for submucosal fibroids **(Fig. 5)**.

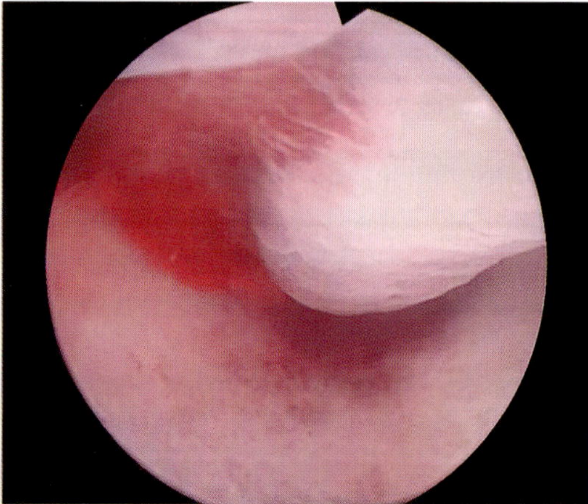

Fig. 5: Hysteroscopic view of submucous fibroid.

- Saline Infusion Sonography (SIS): Enhances visualization of submucosal fibroids.
- Laboratory Tests: Complete blood count for anemia; rule out coagulopathies in HMB.

Differential diagnoses include adenomyosis, endometrial polyps, and, rarely, leiomyosarcoma (incidence <0.5%).

Step-W classification

The STEP-W (or STEPW) classification is a scoring system for submucous fibroids that was originally proposed by Lasmar and is recommended in international hysteroscopic myomectomy guidelines. It evaluates five features of a submucous leiomyoma: Size (S), Topography in the cavity (T), Extension of the base (E), depth of myometrial Penetration (P), and involvement of the lateral Wall (W), each assigned a score; the total score stratifies fibroids into groups that predict surgical complexity, likelihood of complete hysteroscopic resection, operative time, fluid overload, and complication risk.

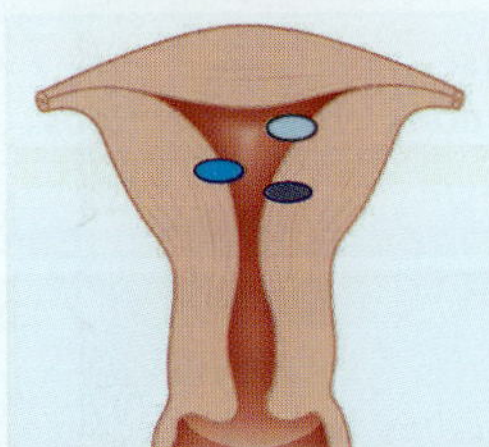

Degree of penetration of the myoma into myometrium

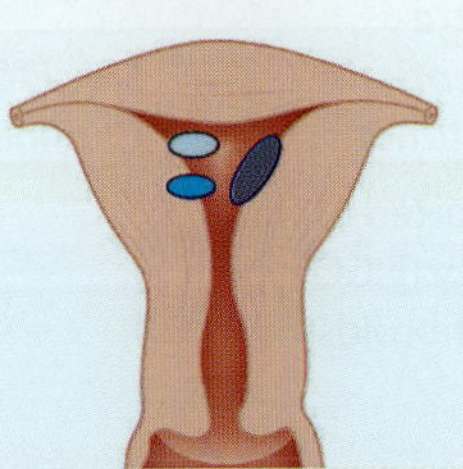

The extension of the base of the nodule with respect to the wall of the uterus

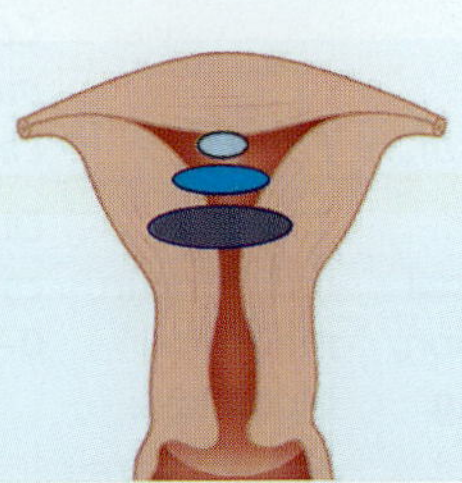

Size of the nodule up to 2 cm, between 2 cm and 5 cm and more than 5 cm

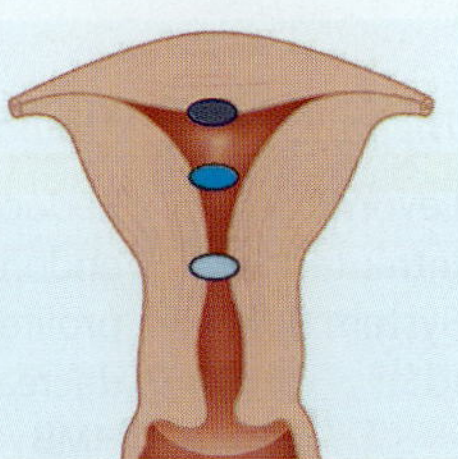

Topography in the lateral wall an extra point is added

Source: Hysteroscopy Newsletter. Adapted from Lasmar et al., 2005, with permission.

Total score guides surgical planning

Parameter	*Score 0*	*Score 1*	*Score 2*	*Score 3*
Size (cm)	<2	2–3	3–4	>4
Topography	Fundal	Posterior/anterior	Lateral	–
Extension (% base/diameter)	>90%	75–90%	50–75%	<50%
Penetration (mm into myometrium)	0	≤5	5–10	>10
Wall	Half thickness	Full thickness	–	–

MANAGEMENT OPTIONS

Fibroid management is tailored to patient symptoms, reproductive goals, and fibroid characteristics. Options include expectant management, medical therapy, nonsurgical interventions, and surgical approaches.

Expectant Management

- Indications: Asymptomatic fibroids, mild symptoms, or perimenopausal women where fibroids may regress post menopause.
- Monitoring: Annual or biennial ultrasound to assess growth or new symptoms.
- Rationale: Fibroids are benign, and many remain stable or asymptomatic. Growth is rare postmenopause due to reduced estrogen levels.
- Considerations: Regular follow-up is essential, especially in younger women or those with risk factors (e.g., African ancestry).

Medical Management

Medical therapies aim to alleviate symptoms (HMB, pain) or reduce fibroid size, often as a bridge to surgery or for women unsuitable for invasive procedures. Options include:

- **Nonhormonal Therapies**
    - Tranexamic Acid: Antifibrinolytic agent (1–1.3 g orally every 8 hours during menstruation) reduces HMB by 40–50%. Safe for women desiring fertility.
    - Nonsteroidal Anti-Inflammatory Drugs (NSAIDs): Reduce dysmenorrhea but less effective for HMB. Example: Ibuprofen 400–800 mg every 6–8 hours.
    - Iron Supplementation: Corrects anemia secondary to HMB.
- **Hormonal Therapies**

Therapy	*Mechanism*	*Efficacy*	*Contra-indications/ Limitations*	*Side Effects/ Considerations*	*Use/Indications*
Levonorgestrel Intrauterine System (LNG-IUS)	Reduces endometrial proliferation, decreasing HMB	70–90% reduction in menstrual blood loss; less effective for large or submucosal fibroids	Distorted uterine cavity (FIGO type 0–2 fibroids)		
Combined Oral Contraceptives (COCs)	Regulate menstrual cycles, reduce HMB	Moderate reduction in bleeding; not effective for fibroid size reduction	Contraindications (e.g., smoking, hypertension)		Suitable for women without contraindications
Gonadotropin-Releasing Hormone (GnRH) Agonists	Induce hypoestrogenic state, reducing fibroid size by 30–50% within 3–6 months		Limited use to 6 months without add-back therapy	Menopausal symptoms (hot flashes, vaginal dryness), bone density loss. Add-Back Therapy: Low-dose estrogen/ progestin to mitigate side effects	Preoperative use to reduce fibroid size, blood loss, and operative time. Examples: Leuprolide (3.75 mg monthly IM), Goserelin (3.6 mg monthly SC)
GnRH Antagonists	Rapid suppression of gonadotropins, reducing fibroid size and HMB			Fewer side effects than agonists	Preoperative or short-term symptom control. Examples: Relugolix (oral, 40 mg daily), Elagolix

Contd...

Contd...

Therapy	Mechanism	Efficacy	Contra-indications/ Limitations	Side Effects/ Considerations	Use/Indications
Selective Progesterone Receptor Modulators (SPRMs)	Inhibits progester-one-driven fibroid growth, induces amenorrhea	Reduces HMB in 90% of patients, fibroid size by 20–30%	Rare risk of liver toxicity (requires monitoring); suspended in some regions		Example: Ulipristal acetate (5–10 mg daily for up to 3 months)

TABLE 2: Medical therapies for fibroid management.

Therapy	Mechanism	Indications	Efficacy	Side effects
Tranexamic Acid	Antifibrinolytic	HMB	40–50% HMB reduction	GI upset, rare thrombosis
LNG-IUS	Endometrial suppression	HMB	70–90% HMB reduction	Expulsion, irregular bleeding
GnRH Agonists	Hypoestrogenic state	Preoperative, HMB	30–50% size reduction	Hot flashes, bone loss
GnRH Antagonists	Gonadotropin suppression	Preoperative, HMB	20–40% size reduction	Mild menopausal symptoms
Ulipristal Acetate	Progesterone receptor modulation	HMB, size reduction	20–30% size reduction	Liver toxicity (rare), headache

Relugolix GnRh Antagonist has demonstrated a robust ability to manage symptoms associated with uterine fibroids, particularly heavy menstrual bleeding and fibroid size reduction. Research shows that short-term use of relugolix prior to surgical intervention, such as myomectomy, can effectively shrink fibroids, improve anemia, and ease uterine reconstruction. When administered as part of a combination therapy (with estradiol and norethisterone acetate), relugolix exhibits both safety and efficacy over periods up to a year, with notable improvements in hemoglobin levels, fatigue, and overall quality of life. This therapy also helps prevent bone mineral density loss, making it suitable for prolonged treatment. Overall, evidence supports relugolix as a valuable option for nonsurgical and presurgical management of symptomatic uterine fibroids, improving patient outcomes without severe adverse effects

Nonsurgical Interventions

Nonsurgical options are suitable for women seeking minimally invasive treatments or those unsuitable for surgery.

1. Uterine Artery Embolization (UAE)

Parameter	*Details*
Procedure Name	Uterine Artery Embolization
Type of Procedure	Minimally invasive, image-guided interventional radiology
Indications	Symptomatic uterine fibroids, adenomyosis, postpartum hemorrhage (PPH)
Access Site	Femoral artery or radial artery puncture
Procedure Description	Catheter-based occlusion of uterine arteries using embolic agents
Embolic Agents Used	Polyvinyl alcohol (PVA) particles, tris-acryl gelatin microspheres, etc.
Mechanism of Action	Blocks arterial blood supply to fibroids → ischemia → shrinkage
Anesthesia	Conscious sedation or regional anesthesia
Duration	30–90 minutes
Postprocedure Effects	Cramping, pain, postembolization syndrome (fever, malaise, leukocytosis)
Expected Outcome	Reduction in fibroid size, symptom relief (bleeding, pressure symptoms)
Advantages	Uterus-sparing, shorter recovery than surgery, outpatient in many cases
Limitations	Not suitable for large pedunculated subserosal fibroids or malignancy
Follow-up	Imaging (USG/MRI) after 3–6 months to assess fibroid shrinkage

2. MRI-Guided Focused Ultrasound Surgery (MRgFUS)

- Procedure: Noninvasive thermal ablation using high-intensity ultrasound under MRI guidance.
- Indications: Symptomatic subserosal or intramural fibroids (<10 cm).
- Efficacy: 60–80% symptom improvement; variable size reduction.
- Advantages: No incision, outpatient procedure.
- Limitations: Limited by fibroid location (deep intramural or pedunculated fibroids unsuitable), high cost, limited pregnancy outcome data.
- Complications: Skin burns, nerve injury (rare).

3. Radiofrequency Ablation (RFA)

- Procedure: Transcervical or laparoscopic delivery of radiofrequency energy to ablate fibroids.
- Indications: Intramural/subserosal fibroids causing HMB or bulk symptoms.
- Efficacy: 70–80% symptom relief; 20–40% size reduction.
- Advantages: Minimally invasive, preserves fertility in select cases.
- Complications: Pain, infection, uterine wall damage.

Surgical Management

Surgical options are indicated for large, symptomatic, or fertility-impacting fibroids. They include myomectomy and hysterectomy.

Myomectomy

Myomectomy is the surgical removal of fibroids with uterine preservation, ideal for women desiring fertility or wishing to avoid hysterectomy.

Indications

- Symptomatic fibroids (HMB, pelvic pain, bulk symptoms).
- Infertility or recurrent miscarriage due to submucosal/intramural fibroids.
- Large or rapidly growing fibroids in women desiring uterine preservation.

Types of Myomectomy

TABLE 3: Types of myomectomy.

Approach	*Indications*	*Technique*	*Advantages*	*Complications*
Hysteroscopic	FIGO 0–2, <3 cm	Resectoscope, fluid distension	No incision, rapid recovery	Fluid overload, perforation
Laparoscopic	Intramural/ subserosal, <15 cm	Laparoscope, vasopressin, suturing	Less pain, shorter recovery	Morcellation risks, rupture in pregnancy
Robotic-Assisted	Complex/multiple fibroids	Robotic system, 3D visualization	Precision, ergonomic	High cost, longer operative time
Abdominal	Large/multiple fibroids	Open incision, direct enucleation	Handles complex cases	Blood loss, adhesions

Preoperative Preparation

- Imaging: MRI or TVUS for fibroid mapping.
- Medical Therapy: GnRH agonists/antagonists (3–6 months) to reduce fibroid size and improve hemoglobin.
- Anemia Correction: Iron supplementation or transfusion.
- Counseling: Discuss risks (bleeding, adhesions, recurrence) and fertility outcomes.

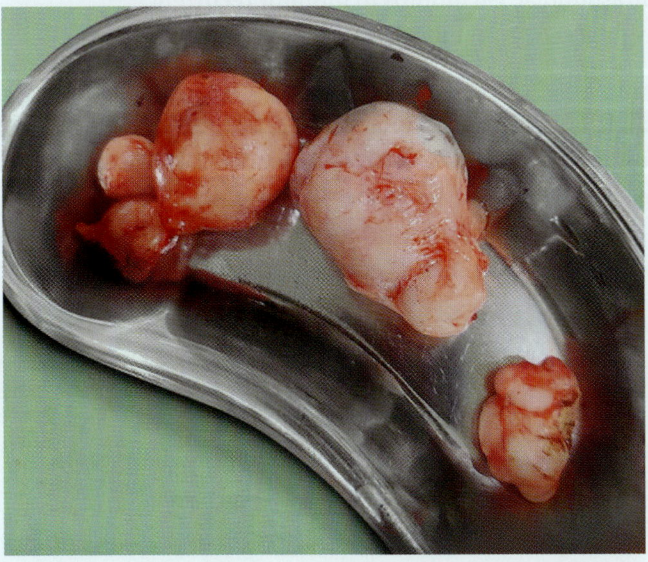

Fig. 6: Fibroids removed by abdominal myomectomy.

Surgical Techniques

Approach	*Key points*
Hysteroscopic Myomectomy	• Performed under general/regional anesthesia using a resectoscope with saline or glycine • Fibroid resected in layers; fluid balance closely monitored to prevent overload (TURP syndrome risk <1%) • Ideal for FIGO type 0–2 submucous fibroids <3 cm
Laparoscopic Myomectomy	• 3–4 small incisions; vasopressin used to minimize bleeding • Fibroids enucleated; multilayer myometrial suturing to prevent uterine rupture • Contained morcellation preferred to reduce risk of occult malignancy spread
Robotic-Assisted Myomectomy	• Similar technique to laparoscopy, but with enhanced robotic precision • Beneficial in anatomically challenging or recurrent cases • May have longer operative time but improved ergonomics and reduced tremor
Abdominal (Open) Myomectomy **(Fig. 5)**	• Performed via low transverse or vertical midline incision • Suitable for large, multiple, or deeply embedded fibroids • Higher intraoperative blood loss (200–800 mL) and risk of postoperative adhesions

Intraoperative Considerations

- Hemostasis: Vasopressin, tourniquets, or hemostatic agents.
- Adhesion Prevention: Antiadhesion barriers (e.g., Interceed, Seprafilm).
- Morcellation: Contained morcellation to minimize risk of sarcoma spread.

Postoperative Management

- Recovery: Hysteroscopic (1–2 days), laparoscopic (2–4 weeks), abdominal (4–6 weeks).
- Pain Control: NSAIDs, opioids as needed.
- Follow-Up: Ultrasound at 3–6 months to monitor recurrence.
- Fertility: Delay pregnancy 3–6 months to ensure uterine healing.

Outcomes

- Symptom Relief: 80–90% improvement in HMB; 50–60% fertility improvement for submucosal fibroids.
- Recurrence: 15–33% within 5 years, higher with multiple fibroids or younger age.
- Pregnancy: Improved implantation rates post myomectomy; cesarean delivery recommended for deep intramural fibroids due to rupture risk (<1%).

Complications

TABLE 4: Complications of myomectomy.

Complication	*Incidence*	*Management*
Bleeding	5–10%	Transfusion, hemostatic agents
Adhesions	10–15%	Anti-adhesion barriers
Uterine rupture	<1%	Cesarean delivery
Recurrence	15–33%	Repeat myomectomy or hysterectomy

2. Hysterectomy

- Indications: Definitive treatment for women not desiring fertility, with severe symptoms or large/multiple fibroids **(Fig. 7)**.

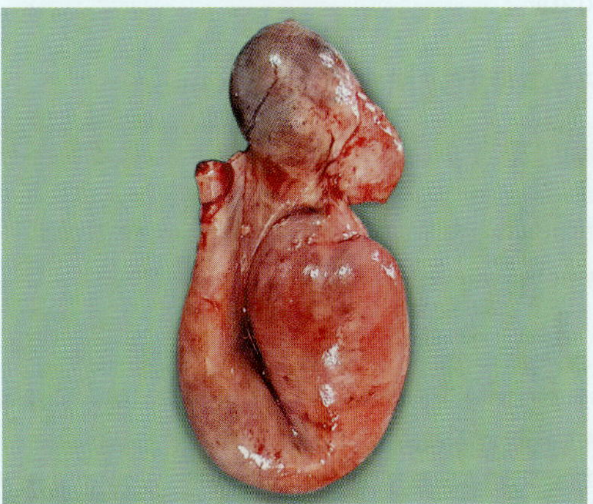

Fig. 7: Hysterectomy specimen with subserosal fibroid.

- Approaches: Vaginal, laparoscopic, robotic, or abdominal.
- Advantages: Eliminates recurrence risk, resolves all symptoms.
- Disadvantages: Loss of fertility, longer recovery for abdominal approach.

Special Considerations

1. Fibroids and Infertility

- Submucosal fibroids (FIGO 0–2) significantly impair fertility by distorting the endometrial cavity.
- Intramural fibroids may reduce pregnancy rates if >4 cm or distorting the cavity.
- Myomectomy improves pregnancy rates in submucosal fibroid cases (RR 1.5–2.0); evidence for intramural fibroids is less clear.

2. Fibroids in Pregnancy

- Most fibroids remain stable; 10–30% increase in size due to hormonal stimulation.
- Complications: Pain (red degeneration), preterm labor, placental abruption.
- Management: Conservative (analgesics for pain); myomectomy rarely performed due to risks of miscarriage or bleeding.

3. Risk of Leiomyosarcoma

- Incidence: <0.5% of presumed fibroids.
- Risk Factors: Rapid growth, postmenopausal status, atypical imaging (MRI).
- Management: Avoid morcellation in high-risk cases; preoperative MRI and biopsy if malignancy suspected.

Emerging Therapies

- Irreversible Electroporation (IRE): Nonthermal ablation targeting fibroid cells, preserving surrounding tissues. Under investigation.

- Novel SPRMs: Safer progesterone receptor modulators to replace ulipristal acetate.
- Gene Therapies: Targeting *MED12* or other genetic drivers of fibroid growth.
- High-Intensity Focused Ultrasound (HIFU): Expanding applications with improved pregnancy outcome data.

COMPARISON OF MANAGEMENT OPTIONS

TABLE 5: Comparison of fibroid management options.

Option	*Indications*	*Fertility preservation*	*Efficacy*	*Risks*
Expectant	Asymptomatic	Yes	N/A	Symptom progression
Medical (LNG-IUS, GnRH analogues)	Heavy menstrual bleeding (HMB), pain	Yes	40–90% symptom relief	Hormonal side effects, temporary
Uterine Artery Embolization (UAE)	HMB, bulk-related symptoms	Uncertain	85–90% symptom relief	Ovarian dysfunction, infection
MRI-guided Focused Ultrasound (MRgFUS)	HMB, bulk symptoms	Uncertain	60–80% symptom relief	Limited access, not for all types
Myomectomy	HMB, infertility, bulk symptoms	Yes	80–90% symptom relief	Bleeding, adhesions, recurrence
Hysterectomy	Severe symptoms, no fertility desire	No	100% symptom relief	Surgical risks, loss of fertility

CONCLUSION

Uterine fibroids present a spectrum of clinical challenges, requiring individualized management based on symptoms, fertility goals, and fibroid characteristics. Expectant management is suitable for asymptomatic cases, while medical therapies offer symptom relief for mild cases or preoperative optimization. Nonsurgical interventions like UAE and MRgFUS provide minimally invasive options but have limitations for fertility preservation. Myomectomy remains the gold standard for women desiring fertility, with laparoscopic and robotic approaches reducing morbidity compared to abdominal myomectomy. Hysterectomy is reserved for definitive treatment in nonfertility-seeking patients. Advances in ablation techniques and molecular therapies promise to further refine fibroid management, emphasizing the need for ongoing research and surgical expertise.

SUGGESTED READING

1. American College of Obstetricians and Gynecologists. Management of symptomatic uterine leiomyomas: ACOG practice bulletin no. 228. Obstet Gynecol. 2021;137(6):e100-15.
2. Donnez J, Dolmans MM. Uterine fibroid management: from the present to the future. Hum Reprod Update. 2016;22(6):665-86.
3. Gupta JK, Sinha A, Lumsden MA, Hickey M. Uterine artery embolization for symptomatic uterine fibroids. Cochrane Database Syst Rev. 2014;2014(12):CD005073.
4. Stewart EA, Laughlin-Tommaso SK. Uterine fibroids. N Engl J Med. 2015;372(17):1646-55.
5. Vilos GA, Allaire C, Laberge PY, et al. The management of uterine leiomyomas. J Obstet Gynaecol Can. 2015;37(2):157-78.

Abnormal Uterine Bleeding

Ruchika Garg, Shaifali Singh

INTRODUCTION

Abnormal uterine bleeding (AUB) is a common gynecological condition characterized by any deviation from normal menstrual bleeding patterns in terms of volume, frequency, duration, or regularity. AUB affects 10–30% of women of reproductive age and up to 50% of perimenopausal women, significantly impacting quality of life, causing anemia, and necessitating medical or surgical intervention.[1] The condition encompasses a broad spectrum of etiologies, ranging from structural abnormalities (e.g., fibroids, polyps) to nonstructural causes (e.g., coagulopathies, ovulatory dysfunction). The International Federation of Gynecology and Obstetrics (FIGO) introduced the PALM-COEIN classification system to standardize terminology and guide management.[2] This chapter provides a detailed overview of AUB, including its pathophysiology, diagnostic approach, and management strategies, tailored for postgraduate medical students.

DEFINITION AND CLASSIFICATION

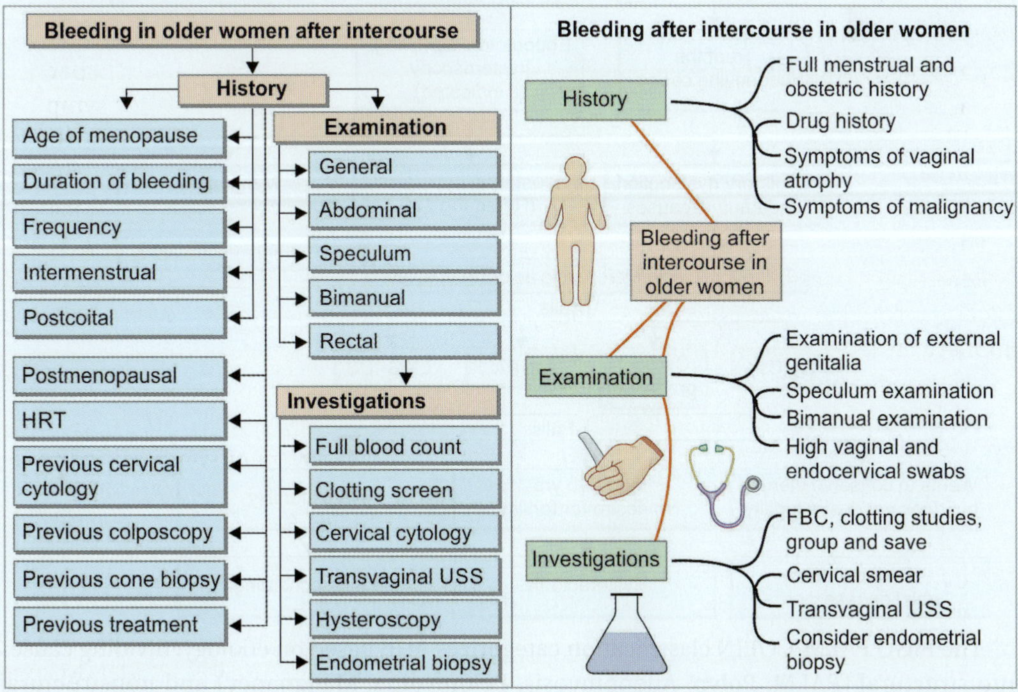

AUB is defined as bleeding from the uterine corpus that is abnormal in volume, frequency, duration, or regularity. Normal menstrual parameters are:

- Frequency: 24–38 days.
- Duration: 4–8 days.
- Volume: 5–80 mL per cycle.
- Regularity: Variation of ≤20 days between cycles.[2]

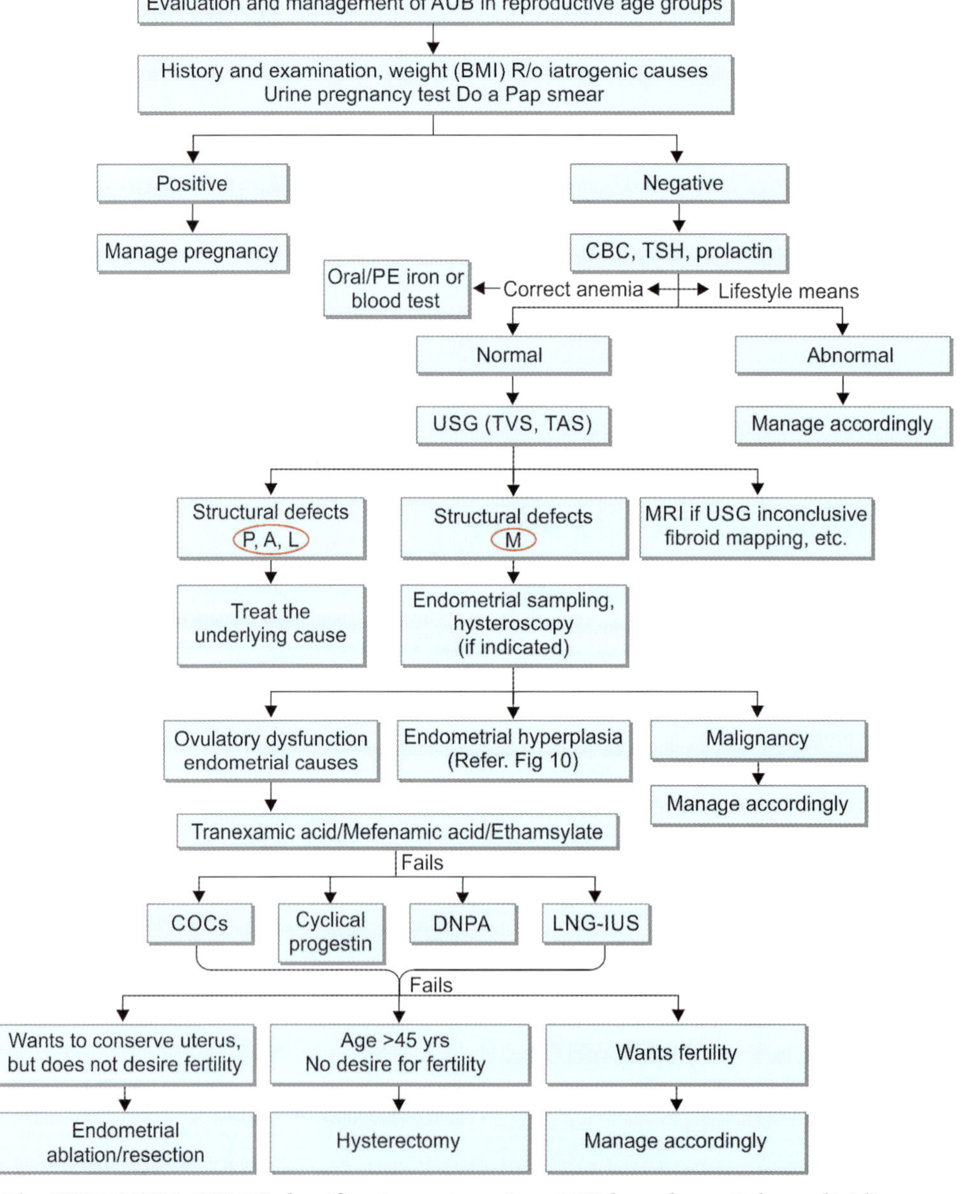

The FIGO PALM-COEIN classification categorizes AUB based on etiology, dividing causes into structural (PALM: Polyp, Adenomyosis, Leiomyoma, Malignancy) and nonstructural (COEIN: Coagulopathy, Ovulatory dysfunction, Endometrial, Iatrogenic, Not yet classified) components **(Table 1)**.[2]

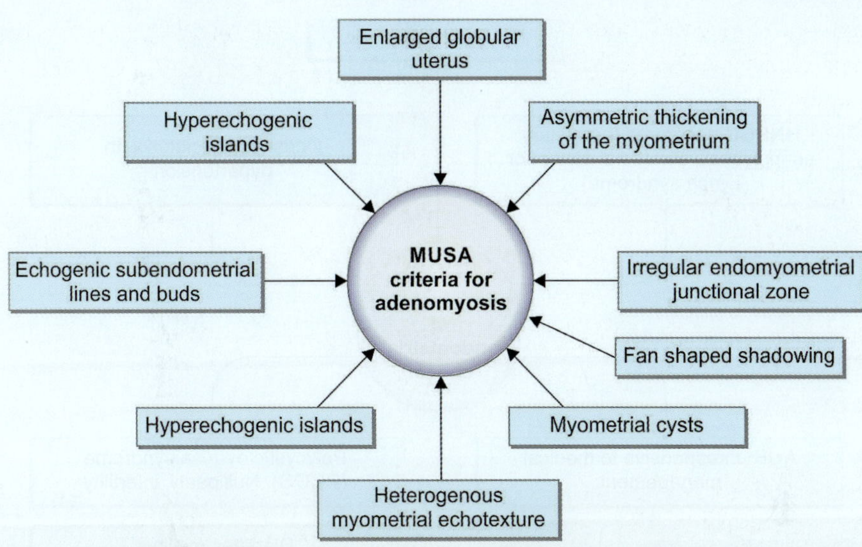

TABLE 1: FIGO PALM-COEIN classification of AUB.[2]

Category	*Description*	*Structural/ Nonstructural*	*Diagnosis*
P—Polyp	Endometrial or cervical polyps; benign growths of epithelial and stromal tissue	Structural	Confirmed by ultrasound, saline infusion sonography (SIS), or hysteroscopy
A—Adenomyosis	Endometrial glands and stroma within the myometrium, causing uterine enlargement and heavy bleeding	Structural	Diagnosed via transvaginal ultrasound (TVUS), MRI, or histopathology
L—Leiomyoma	Uterine fibroids; benign tumors of the uterine muscle (submucosal, intramural, or subserosal)	Structural	Identified by TVUS, MRI, SIS, or hysteroscopy; subcategorized by location
M—Malignancy and hyperplasia	Endometrial or cervical malignancy or hyperplasia (precancerous changes)	Structural	Diagnosed via endometrial biopsy, histopathology, or imaging
C—Coagulopathy	Bleeding disorders (e.g., von Willebrand disease) causing excessive bleeding	Non-Structural	Diagnosed via coagulation tests (e.g., PT, aPTT, von Willebrand factor)
O—Ovulatory dysfunction	Irregular or absent ovulation (e.g., PCOS, thyroid disorders, hyperprolactinemia)	Nonstructural	Diagnosed via history, hormonal profiles (e.g., prolactin, TSH), or ultrasound
E—Endometrial	Primary endometrial disorders affecting hemostasis (e.g., defective endometrial vasoconstriction)	Nonstructural	Diagnosed by exclusion; may involve endometrial biopsy or hysteroscopy
I—Iatrogenic	Bleeding caused by medical interventions (e.g., IUDs, hormonal contraceptives, anticoagulants)	Nonstructural	Identified via history of medication use or procedures
N—Not yet classified	Causes not fitting other categories (e.g., arteriovenous malformations)	Nonstructural	Diagnosed via specialized imaging or exclusion of other causes

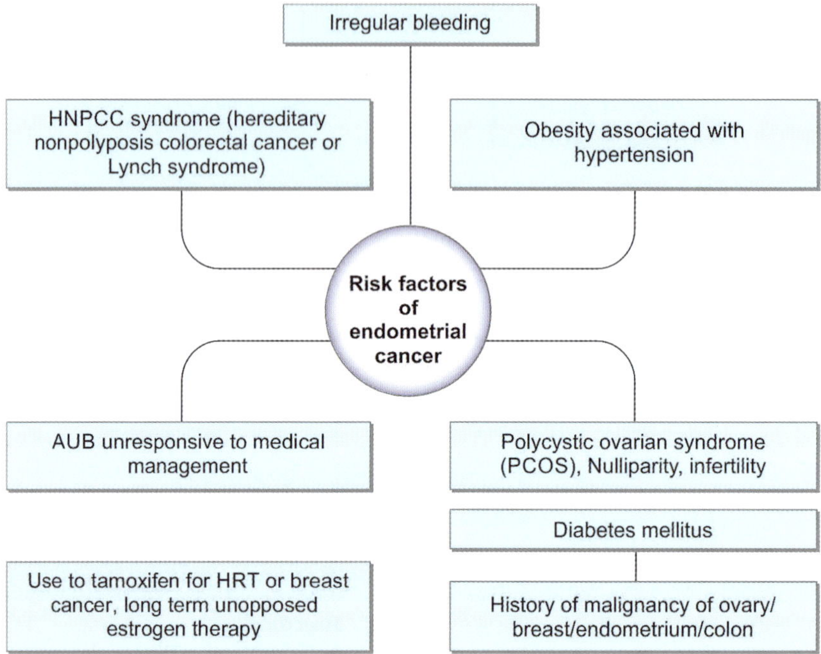

- **Structural Causes (PALM)**: Typically identified through imaging (e.g., ultrasound, MRI) or histopathology.
- **Nonstructural Causes (COEIN)**: Diagnosed through clinical history, laboratory tests, or exclusion of structural abnormalities.
- The system allows for multiple causes to coexist (e.g., AUB-L and AUB-O).
- AUB is defined as bleeding abnormal in frequency, regularity, duration, or volume in nonpregnant women.
- Common in perimenopause, with leiomyoma (AUB-L) and ovulatory dysfunction (AUB-O) often reported as leading causes in studies.

ETIOLOGY AND PATHOPHYSIOLOGY

AUB results from disruptions in the hypothalamic-pituitary-ovarian (HPO) axis, endometrial homeostasis, or structural integrity of the uterus. The pathophysiology varies by etiology, as outlined below.

Structural Causes (PALM)

- Polyps: Benign growths of endometrial or cervical tissue, causing irregular bleeding due to vascular fragility or ulceration. Prevalence: 10–40% in women with AUB.[3]
- Adenomyosis: Invasion of endometrial tissue into the myometrium, leading to heavy menstrual bleeding (HMB) and dysmenorrhea. Associated with increased prostaglandin production and estrogen-driven endometrial proliferation.[4]
- Leiomyomas (Fibroids): Benign myometrial tumors, particularly submucosal, disrupt endometrial vasculature, causing HMB. Mechanisms include increased endometrial surface area, altered angiogenesis (VEGF overexpression), and impaired hemostasis.[5]

- Malignancy/Hyperplasia: Endometrial hyperplasia or carcinoma, often linked to unopposed estrogen exposure (e.g., obesity, PCOS), causes irregular or heavy bleeding due to abnormal endometrial proliferation.[6]

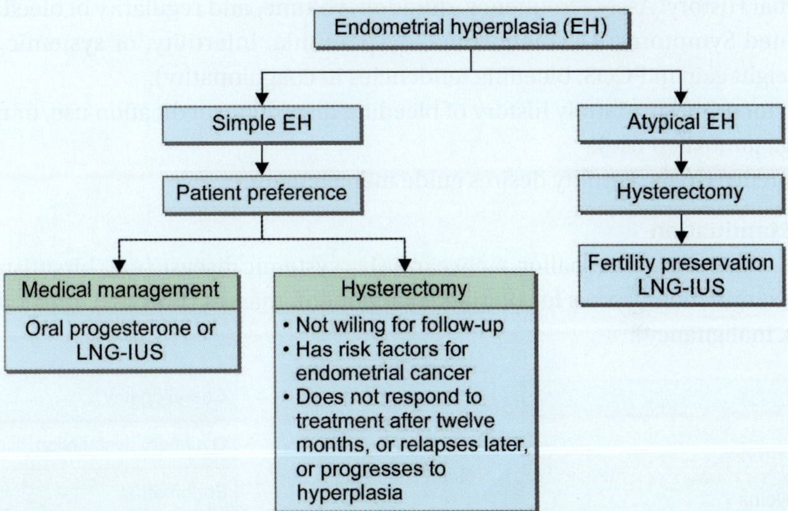

Nonstructural Causes (COEIN)

- Coagulopathy: Bleeding disorders (e.g., von Willebrand disease, factor deficiencies) impair endometrial hemostasis, leading to HMB. Prevalence: 10–20% in women with HMB.[7]
- Ovulatory Dysfunction: Anovulation (e.g., PCOS, hypothyroidism) results in unopposed estrogen, causing endometrial overgrowth and irregular bleeding. Common in adolescents and perimenopausal women.[8]
- Endometrial: Primary endometrial dysfunction (e.g., defective hemostasis, increased fibrinolysis) causes HMB in the absence of structural or systemic causes. Associated with altered prostaglandin metabolism.[9]
- Iatrogenic: Medications (e.g., hormonal contraceptives, anticoagulants) or intrauterine devices may disrupt normal bleeding patterns.[10]
- Not Yet Classified: Rare causes, such as arteriovenous malformations or chronic endometritis, may contribute to AUB.[2]

CLINICAL PRESENTATION

AUB presents as:

- Heavy Menstrual Bleeding (HMB): Excessive bleeding (>80 mL/cycle) or prolonged bleeding (>8 days).
- Intermenstrual Bleeding (IMB): Bleeding between menstrual cycles.
- Irregular Bleeding: Unpredictable cycle frequency or duration.
- Associated Symptoms: Dysmenorrhea, pelvic pain, infertility, or symptoms of anemia (fatigue, pallor).

The clinical impact varies, with HMB often leading to iron-deficiency anemia, reduced quality of life, and significant healthcare costs.

DIAGNOSTIC APPROACH

Diagnosis of AUB involves a systematic approach to identify the underlying cause, guided by history, physical examination, and investigations.

History

- Menstrual History: Assess frequency, duration, volume, and regularity of bleeding.
- Associated Symptoms: Dysmenorrhea, dyspareunia, infertility, or systemic symptoms (e.g., weight gain in PCOS, bleeding tendencies in coagulopathy).
- Risk Factors: Obesity, family history of bleeding disorders, medication use, or malignancy risk (e.g., tamoxifen use).
- Reproductive Goals: Fertility desires guide management.

Physical Examination

- General: Signs of anemia (pallor, tachycardia) or systemic disease (e.g., hirsutism in PCOS).
- Pelvic Examination: Assess for uterine enlargement, masses (fibroids), or cervical lesions (polyps, malignancy).

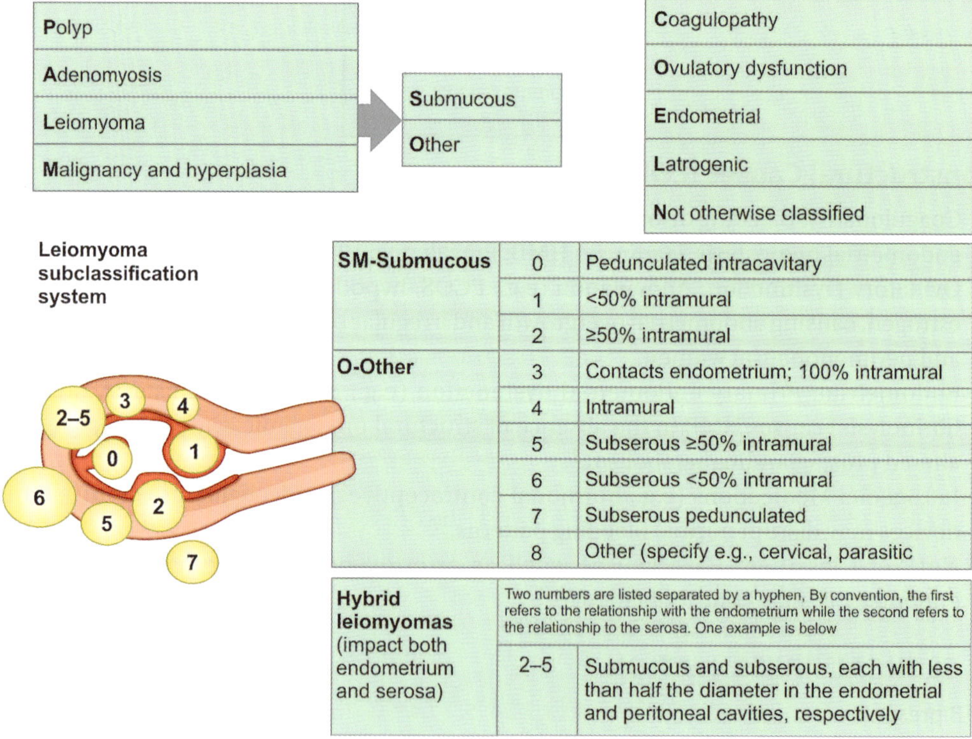

Fig. 1: PALM COEIN.

Investigations

- **Laboratory Tests:**
  - Complete blood count (CBC): Detect anemia.

- Coagulation profile: Screen for coagulopathies (e.g., von Willebrand factor, platelet function).
- Thyroid function tests: Rule out hypothyroidism.
- Serum ferritin: Assess iron stores.

- **Imaging:**
    - Transvaginal Ultrasound (TVUS): First-line imaging to detect polyps, fibroids, or adenomyosis (sensitivity 90–95%)[11] **(Figs. 2)**.

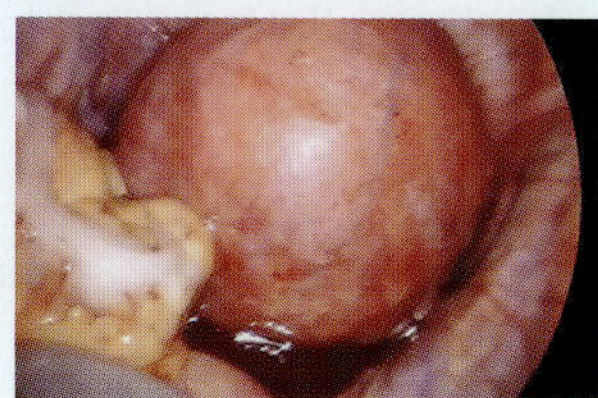

Fig. 2: Adenomyosis.

Saline Infusion Sonography (SIS): Enhances detection of submucosal fibroids or polyps.

- Magnetic Resonance Imaging (MRI): Used for complex cases (e.g., adenomyosis, deep fibroids).
- Endometrial Sampling: Indicated in women >45 years, those with risk factors for endometrial hyperplasia/cancer (e.g., obesity, unopposed estrogen), or persistent AUB.[6]
- Hysteroscopy: Diagnostic and therapeutic for endometrial polyps or submucosal fibroids.

MANAGEMENT OF AUB

Management is tailored to the underlying cause, symptom severity, fertility desires, and patient preferences. Options include expectant management, medical therapy, nonsurgical interventions, and surgical procedures.

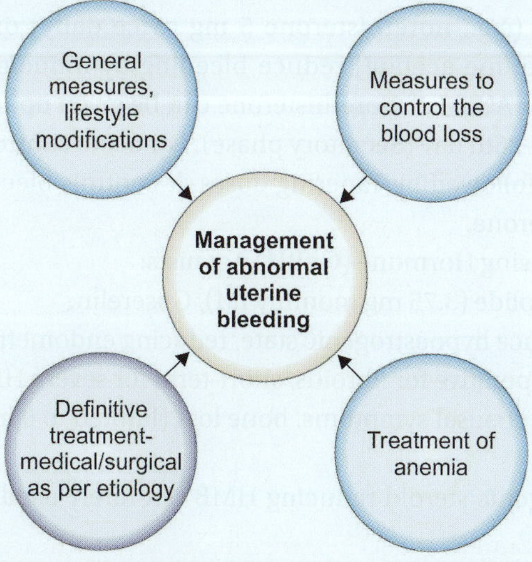

Expectant Management

Indications: Mild, self-limiting AUB in adolescents or perimenopausal women with no structural abnormalities.

Approach: Monitor symptoms, provide iron supplementation for anemia, and reassess periodically.

Medical Management

Medical therapies aim to reduce bleeding, alleviate symptoms, and preserve fertility where desired **(Table 3)**.

Nonhormonal Therapies

Tranexamic Acid: Antifibrinolytic (1–1.3 g orally every 8 hours during menstruation) reduces HMB by 40–50%. Safe for women desiring fertility.[12]

Nonsteroidal Anti-Inflammatory Drugs (NSAIDs): Reduce prostaglandin-mediated bleeding and dysmenorrhea (e.g., mefenamic acid 500 mg every 8 hours). Efficacy: 20–30% reduction in HMB.[13]

Iron Supplementation: Corrects anemia secondary to HMB.

Hormonal Therapies

- Levonorgestrel Intrauterine System (LNG-IUS):
  - Mechanism: Reduces endometrial proliferation, inducing amenorrhea in 20–40% of users.
  - Efficacy: 70–90% reduction in HMB; first line for AUB-C and AUB-E.[14]
  - Contraindications: Distorted uterine cavity, active pelvic infection.
- Combined Oral Contraceptives (COCs):
  - Mechanism: Regulate cycles, reduce endometrial growth.
  - Efficacy: 50–60% reduction in HMB; effective for AUB-O.[15]
  - Progestins: Oral (e.g., norethisterone 5 mg twice daily) or injectable (e.g., depot medroxyprogesterone acetate) reduce bleeding by inducing endometrial atrophy. Used in AUB-O or AUB-E.[16] Norethisterone can be given up to 30 mg from 5th to 25th day of cycle or 15-26th day (Secretory phase). For acute control of bleeding, 2 tabs TDS FOR FEW DAYS followed by Tapering doses. It controls bleeding better compared to medroxyprogesterone.
- Gonadotropin-Releasing Hormone (GnRH) Agonists:
  - Examples: Leuprolide (3.75 mg monthly IM), Goserelin.
  - Mechanism: Induce hypoestrogenic state, reducing endometrial growth.
  - Indications: Preoperative for fibroids, short-term for severe HMB.
  - Side Effects: Menopausal symptoms, bone loss (limited to 6 months without add-back therapy).[17]
  - Danazol: Androgenic steroid reducing HMB but rarely used due to side effects (e.g., virilization).

TABLE 2: Diagnostic investigations for AUB.[11]

Test	*Indication*	*Findings*
CBC	All patients with HMB	Anemia, thrombocytopenia
Coagulation profile	Suspected coagulopathy	Von Willebrand disease, factor deficiencies
TVUS	Structural causes	Fibroids, polyps, adenomyosis
SIS	Suspected endometrial lesions	Submucosal fibroids, polyps
Endometrial biopsy	Age >45 years, risk factors	Hyperplasia, carcinoma
Hysteroscopy	Abnormal imaging, persistent AUB	Polyps, submucosal fibroids

TABLE 3: Medical therapies for AUB.[12-17]

Therapy	*Mechanism*	*Indications*	*Efficacy*	*Side Effects*
Tranexamic acid	Antifibrinolytic	AUB-C, AUB-E	40–50% HMB reduction	GI upset, rare thrombosis
NSAIDs	Prostaglandin inhibition	AUB-E, dysmenorrhea	20–30% HMB reduction	GI irritation
LNG-IUS	Endometrial suppression	AUB-C, AUB-E	70–90% HMB reduction	Irregular bleeding, expulsion
COCs	Cycle regulation	AUB-O	50–60% HMB reduction	Nausea, thromboembolism risk
GnRH agonists	Hypoestrogenic state	Preoperative, severe HMB	70–80% HMB reduction	Hot flashes, bone loss

Nonsurgical Interventions

- **Uterine Artery Embolization (UAE):**
  - Indications: AUB-L (fibroids), unsuitable for surgery.
  - Mechanism: Occludes uterine arteries, reducing fibroid vascularity.
  - Efficacy: 85–90% symptom improvement; not recommended for fertility preservation.[18]
  - Complications: Postembolization syndrome, ovarian dysfunction.
- **Endometrial Ablation:**
  - Indications: AUB-E, completed childbearing.
  - Mechanism: Destroys endometrial lining via thermal, radiofrequency, or microwave energy.
  - Efficacy: 80–90% reduction in HMB; 20–40% achieve amenorrhea.[19]
  - Contraindications: Desire for fertility, endometrial hyperplasia/cancer.

Surgical Management

Surgical options are indicated for structural causes, failed medical therapy, or malignancy.

Hysteroscopic Procedures

- **Polypectomy:** Removal of endometrial/cervical polyps via hysteroscopy. Effective for AUB-P.[20]

- **Myomectomy:** Removal of submucosal fibroids (FIGO types 0–2) via hysteroscopy or laparoscopy for AUB-L. Improves HMB in 80–90% of cases and fertility in 50–60%.[21]

Hysterectomy

- **Indications:** AUB-M, failed medical/nonsurgical therapy, no fertility desire.
- **Approaches:** Vaginal, laparoscopic, robotic, or abdominal.
- **Efficacy:** Definitive treatment, 100% symptom resolution.[22]
- **Complications:** Infection, bleeding, loss of fertility.

Myomectomy (Detailed)

- **Indications:** Symptomatic fibroids (AUB-L), fertility preservation.
- **Approaches:**
    - Hysteroscopic: For submucosal fibroids (<3 cm, FIGO 0–2). Uses resectoscope with saline/glycine. Recovery: 1–2 days.
    - Laparoscopic/Robotic: For intramural/subserosal fibroids (<15 cm). Uses vasopressin to reduce bleeding; contained morcellation for large fibroids. Recovery: 2–4 weeks.
    - Abdominal: For large/multiple fibroids. Higher blood loss (200–800 mL) and adhesion risk. Recovery: 4–6 weeks.
    - Preoperative Preparation: GnRH agonists (3-6 months) reduce fibroid size; iron supplementation for anemia.
    - Outcomes: 80–90% HMB improvement; 15–33% recurrence within 5 years.[21]
    - Complications: Bleeding (5–10%), adhesions (10–15%), uterine rupture in pregnancy (<1%).[21]

SPECIAL CONSIDERATIONS

- **Adolescents:** AUB-O is common due to immature HPO axis. LNG-IUS or COCs are first-line; screen for coagulopathies.[8]
- **Perimenopause:** AUB often due to anovulation or hyperplasia. Endometrial sampling is critical to rule out malignancy.[6]
- **Fertility Preservation:** Myomectomy or UAE preferred for AUB-L; LNG-IUS for AUB-E/C.[14,21]
- **Malignancy Risk:** Endometrial biopsy mandatory in women > 45 years or with risk factors (e.g., obesity, PCOS).[6]

EMERGING THERAPIES

- **Selective Progesterone Receptor Modulators (SPRMs):** Ulipristal acetate reduces HMB and fibroid size but is limited by liver toxicity concerns.[23]
- **GnRH Antagonists:** Oral agents (e.g., Relugolix) offer rapid symptom control with fewer side effects than agonists.[24]
- **Antiangiogenic Agents:** Under investigation for fibroid-related AUB, targeting VEGF pathways.

CONCLUSION

AUB is a prevalent gynecological condition with diverse etiologies, classified by the FIGO PALM-COEIN system. Diagnosis requires a thorough history, physical examination, and targeted investigations to identify structural or nonstructural causes. Management ranges from expectant and medical therapies to nonsurgical and surgical interventions, tailored to the patient's symptoms, reproductive goals, and underlying pathology. Myomectomy is a key option for fertility preservation in AUB-L, while LNG-IUS is highly effective for AUB-E and AUB-C. Advances in hormonal and noninvasive therapies continue to improve outcomes, emphasizing the need for individualized care and ongoing research.

REFERENCES

1. Fraser IS, Critchley HO, Broder M, Munro MG. The FIGO recommendations on terminologies and definitions for normal and abnormal uterine bleeding. Semin Reprod Med. 2011;29(5):383-90.
2. Munro MG, Critchley HO, Fraser IS; FIGO Menstrual Disorders Working Group. The FIGO classification of causes of abnormal uterine bleeding in the reproductive years. Fertil Steril. 2011;95(7):2204-8.
3. Lieng M, Istre O, Qvigstad E. Treatment of endometrial polyps: a systematic review. Acta Obstet Gynecol Scand. 2010;89(8):992-1002.
4. Benagiano G, Brosens I. The pathophysiology of uterine adenomyosis: an update. Fertil Steril. 2012;98(3):572-9.
5. Stewart EA. Uterine fibroids. N Engl J Med. 2015;372(17):1646-55.
6. Clarke MA, Long BJ, Del Mar Morillo A, et al. Association of endometrial cancer risk with obesity and related factors. J Natl Cancer Inst. 2018;110(9):926-35.
7. Kadir RA, Economides DL, Sabin CA, et al. Frequency of inherited bleeding disorders in women with menorrhagia. Lancet. 1998;351(9101):485-9.
8. ACOG Committee Opinion No. 814: Management of abnormal uterine bleeding in adolescents. Obstet Gynecol. 2020;136(5):e79-e91.
9. Critchley HO, Maybin JA, Armstrong GM, et al. Physiology of the endometrium and regulation of menstruation. Physiol Rev. 2020;100(3):1149-79.
10. Schreiber CA, Creinin MD. Unscheduled bleeding patterns in women using contraception. Contraception. 2019;100(4):260-5.
11. Dueholm M, Hjorth IM. Structured imaging in the evaluation of abnormal uterine bleeding. Best Pract Res Clin Obstet Gynaecol. 2016;34:48-63.
12. Lukes AS, Moore KA, Muse KN, et al. Tranexamic acid treatment for heavy menstrual bleeding: a randomized controlled trial. Obstet Gynecol. 2010;116(4):865-75.
13. Lethaby A, Augood C, Duckitt K, et al. Nonsteroidal anti-inflammatory drugs for heavy menstrual bleeding. Cochrane Database Syst Rev. 2013;2013(1):CD000400.
14. Lethaby A, Hussain M, Rishworth JR, et al. Progesterone or progestogen-releasing intrauterine systems for heavy menstrual bleeding. Cochrane Database Syst Rev. 2015;2015(4):CD002126.
15. Farquhar C, Brown J. Oral contraceptive pill for heavy menstrual bleeding. Cochrane Database Syst Rev. 2009;2009(4):CD000154.
16. Fraser IS, McCarron G. Randomized trial of progestogens in the treatment of menorrhagia. Med J Aust. 1987;147(6):278-81.
17. Stovall TG, Muneyyirci-Delale O, Summitt RL Jr, et al. GnRH agonist and iron versus placebo and iron in the anemic patient before surgery for leiomyomas: a randomized controlled trial. Obstet Gynecol. 1995;86(1):65-71.

18. Gupta JK, Sinha A, Lumsden MA, et al. Uterine artery embolization for symptomatic uterine fibroids. Cochrane Database Syst Rev. 2014;2014(12):CD005073.
19. Lethaby A, Penninx J, Hickey M, et al. Endometrial resection and ablation techniques for heavy menstrual bleeding. Cochrane Database Syst Rev. 2013;2013(8):CD001501.
20. Nathani F, Clark TJ. Hysteroscopic polypectomy for women with abnormal uterine bleeding. Eur J Obstet Gynecol Reprod Biol. 2010;149(2):119-24.
21. Donnez J, Dolmans MM. Uterine fibroid management: from the present to the future. Hum Reprod Update. 2016;22(6):665-86.
22. Marjoribanks J, Lethaby A, Farquhar C. Surgery versus medical therapy for heavy menstrual bleeding. Cochrane Database Syst Rev. 2016;2016(1):CD003855.
23. Donnez J, Tatarchuk TF, Bouchard P, et al. Ulipristal acetate versus placebo for fibroid treatment before surgery. N Engl J Med. 2012;366(5):409-20.
24. Al-Hendy A, Lukes AS, Poindexter AN 3rd, et al. Treatment of uterine fibroid symptoms with relugolix combination therapy. N Engl J Med. 2021;384(7):630-42.

CHAPTER 39

Endometriosis

Ruchika Garg

ETIOPATHOGENESIS

Endometriosis involves the presence of endometrial-like glands and stroma outside the uterine cavity, primarily on pelvic peritoneum, ovaries, and rectovaginal septum, driven by a multifactorial process.

Sampson's retrograde menstruation theory remains central, positing viable endometrial fragments reflux through fallopian tubes during menses, implanting on peritoneal surfaces amid impaired immune clearance and heightened adhesion/invasion via matrix metalloproteinases.

Complementary mechanisms include coelomic metaplasia (peritoneal transformation into endometrial tissue), embryonic Müllerian/Wolffian rests activated by estrogen, lymphatic/hematogenous spread, stem cell involvement, genetic predisposition (e.g., KRAS mutations), epigenetic changes, and environmental endocrine disruptors exacerbating estrogen dependence, inflammation, angiogenesis, fibrosis, and progesterone resistance.

Symptoms and Signs

Patients typically present with dysmenorrhea (progressive, debilitating), deep dyspareunia, chronic non-menstrual pelvic pain, dyschezia (painful defecation), cyclical dysuria or hematuria, infertility (30–50% cases), and fatigue; extrapelvic manifestations include cyclical hemoptysis, shoulder pain, or pneumothorax.

Physical exam reveals pelvic tenderness, uterosacral ligament nodularity, reduced organ mobility, adnexal masses (endometriomas), or visible vaginal/rectal lesions; however, normal findings do not exclude disease.

Symptoms correlate poorly with lesion extent or rASRM stage, underscoring chronic neuroinflammation and central sensitization

INTRODUCTION

Endometriosis is characterized by the presence of endometrial-like tissue outside the uterus, commonly affecting the pelvic peritoneum, ovaries **(Figs. 1 and 2)**, and rectovaginal septum **(Fig. 3)**.[1] This chronic, recurrent condition impacts approximately 10% of reproductive-age women, 50% of those with infertility, and 30–80% of women with chronic pelvic pain (CPP).[2-4] Its pathogenesis remains elusive, with retrograde menstruation, where endometrial cells implant on peritoneal surfaces triggering inflammation, it being a leading theory.[5] Other mechanisms include cellular proliferation, invasion, angiogenesis, fibrosis, adhesion formation, and immune dysregulation.[5] Symptoms typically include dysmenorrhea, dyspareunia, dyschezia, and infertility, driven by chronic inflammation, scarring, and adhesions.[6] Infertility management depends on patient's age, infertility duration, and disease stage, often requiring assisted reproductive techniques (ART).[6] Ultrasound showing ground-glass appearance of endomrtrioma **(Fig. 3)**.

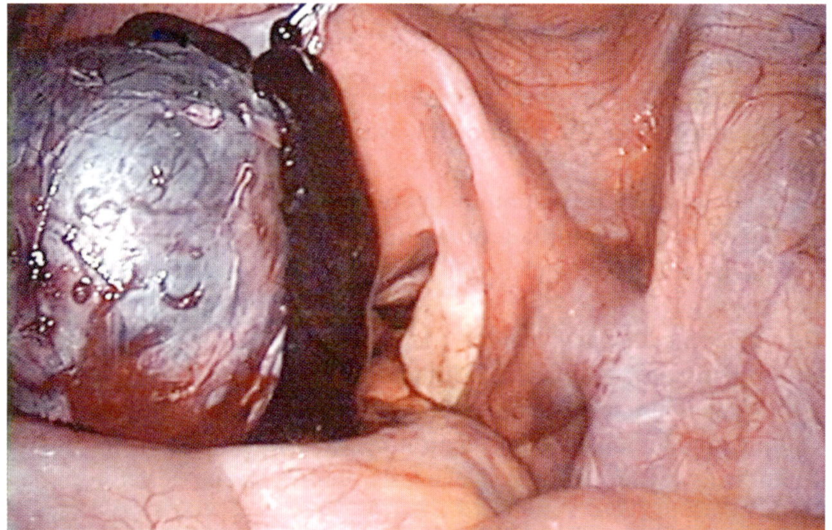

Fig. 1: Laparoscopic endometrioma cystectomy.

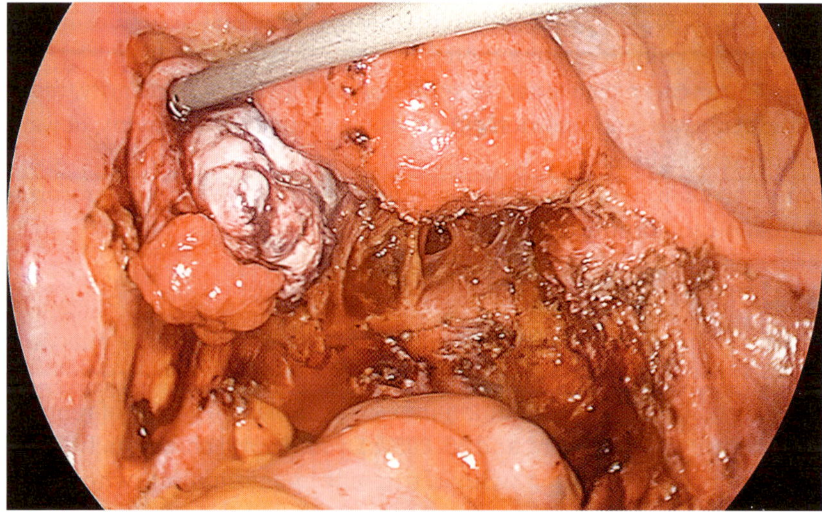

Fig. 2: Laparoscopic view of deep infiltrating endometriosis.

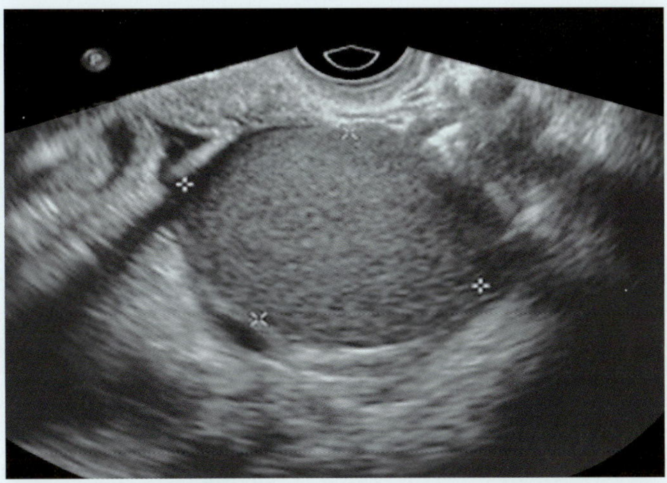

Fig. 3: Ground-glass appearance of endometrioma.

CURRENT MEDICAL MANAGEMENT OF ENDOMETRIOSIS-ASSOCIATED PAIN

Endometriosis management encompasses conservative or radical surgery and medical therapies. Pain often recurs post surgery, necessitating medical treatment as a first-line approach to alleviate symptoms or prevent recurrence.[7] Pharmacological options include nonsteroidal anti-inflammatory drugs (NSAIDs), combined hormonal contraceptives (CHCs), progestins, GnRH agonists, and newer agents like GnRH antagonists and aromatase inhibitors (AIs).[7] Treatment choice depends on efficacy, side effect profile, patient preferences, and cost **(Table 1)**. Most hormonal therapies reduce estrogen levels, inducing atrophy of endometriotic implants and alleviating pain **(Flowchart 1)**.[7]

TABLE 1: Overview of pharmacological treatments for endometriosis.

Drug class	*Examples*	*Mechanism*	*Efficacy*	*Side effects*
NSAIDs	Ibuprofen	Anti-inflammatory	Limited evidence[8]	GI upset, renal risks
CHCs	Ethinyl estradiol + progestins	Decidualization, atrophy	Reduces pain in most[9]	Thromboembolic risk[15]
Progestins	Dienogest, NETA, MPA	Anovulation, atrophy	70–100% pain reduction[17]	Menstrual irregularities, weight gain[17]
GnRH agonists	Leuprolide, Goserelin	Hypoestrogenism	Effective, comparable to LNG-IUS[37]	Hot flushes, bone loss[17]
GnRH antagonists	Elagolix	Dose-dependent estrogen suppression	Reduces dysmenorrhea, pelvic pain[42]	Hot flushes, lipid changes[43]
Aromatase inhibitors	Letrozole, Anastrozole	Estrogen suppression	Reduces pain, lesion size	Bone loss, follicular growth[41]

Source: Compiled from referenced studies 8, 9, 15, 17, 36, 42, 43.

Flowchart 1: Management of endometriosis.

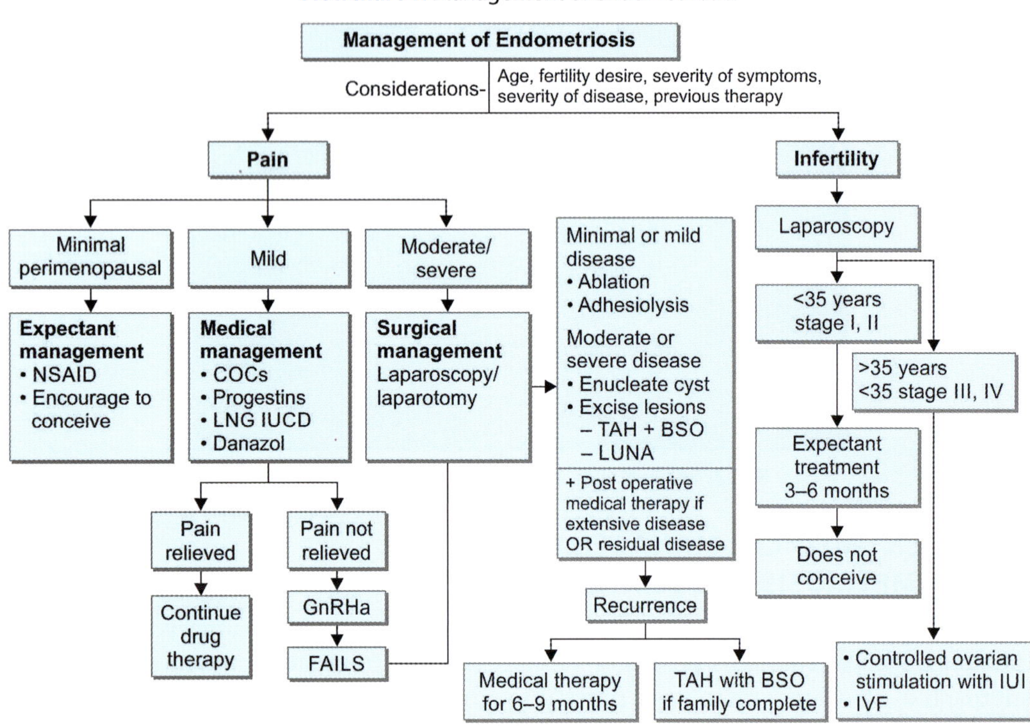

Nonsteroidal Anti-Inflammatory Drugs (NSAIDs)

NSAIDs are frequently used as initial treatment for endometriosis-related pain. However, a Cochrane review found insufficient evidence to confirm their efficacy, limiting their role as a primary therapy.[8]

Combined Hormonal Contraceptives (CHCs)

CHCs, including combined oral contraceptives (COCs), are a cornerstone for managing endometriosis-associated pain due to their affordability and efficacy.[9] They induce decidualization, mimicking a pseudopregnancy state, followed by endometrial atrophy.[11,12] COCs containing androgenic progestins (e.g., 19-nortestosterone derivatives) or newer progestins like desogestrel are effective.[10] Continuous administration, which may lead to amenorrhea, is more effective than cyclic use.[9,13] A 2018 systematic review by Jensen et al. confirmed that CHCs significantly reduce dysmenorrhea, pelvic pain, and dyspareunia, with comparable or lesser efficacy than progestins or GnRH agonists.[9] Despite their widespread use, concerns about long-term effects on fertility and thromboembolism risk question their first-line status.[15]

Progestins

Progestins are preferred over CHCs due to evidence of progesterone resistance in endometriotic implants, which express low progesterone receptor levels.[6] They act by reducing GnRH pulse frequency, suppressing follicle-stimulating hormone (FSH) and luteinizing hormone (LH), causing anovulation, and inducing endometrial atrophy.[16] Progestins also inhibit matrix metalloproteinases and angiogenesis, key to endometriotic growth.[10,14] Common progestins include medroxyprogesterone acetate (MPA), norethisterone acetate (NETA), dienogest (DNG), desogestrel (DSG), and levonorgestrel-releasing intrauterine systems (LNG-IUS).[17]

- **Medroxyprogesterone Acetate (MPA):** Available as oral (10–100 mg/day) or depot injections (150 mg every 3 months), MPA reduces pain with efficacy comparable to GnRH agonists.[15] Side effects include menstrual irregularities, weight gain, and bone mineral density (BMD) loss with prolonged use.[16]
- **Norethisterone Acetate (NETA):** Effective at 2.5–5 mg/day for dysmenorrhea, dyspareunia, and rectovaginal endometriosis, NETA offers better uterine bleeding control and less impact on cholesterol compared to COCs.[19,20]
- **Dienogest (DNG):** A 19-nortestosterone derivative (2 mg/day), DNG combines potent progestogenic and antiandrogenic effects, reducing endometriotic cell proliferation and inflammation.[21-23] It maintains sufficient estradiol (E2) levels to minimize bone loss, offering better tolerability than GnRH agonists.[24-26] Long-term studies show sustained pain relief up to 24 weeks post-treatment.[27] DNG is effective for deep infiltrating endometriosis (DIE) and bladder endometriosis, reducing lesion size.[28-30]
- **Desogestrel (DSG):** A prodrug converted to etonogestrel, DSG is effective for rectovaginal endometriosis, with higher patient satisfaction than vaginal rings.[32] Data on its efficacy are limited.[32]
- **Levonorgestrel-Releasing Intrauterine System (LNG-IUS)** shown in **Figure 5**: LNG-IUS delivers levonorgestrel locally, inducing endometrial atrophy and reducing pain with efficacy comparable to GnRH agonists.[33]. It is particularly effective post surgery and for rectovaginal endometriosis, with minimal hypoestrogenic side effects.[34,] Irregular bleeding is a drawback, though many patients achieve amenorrhea over time.[20,35]

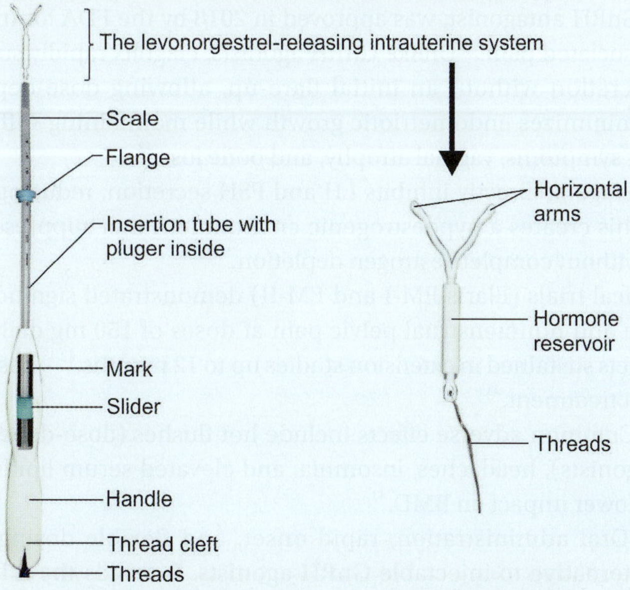

Fig. 5: Levonorgestrel-releasing intrauterine system.

GnRH Agonists

GnRH agonists (e.g., leuprolide, goserelin, nafarelin) induce hypoestrogenism by down-regulating the pituitary-ovarian axis, causing amenorrhea and endometrial atrophy.[17] A Cochrane review of 41 RCTs confirmed their efficacy over placebo and equivalence to LNG-IUS and danazol.[36] Hypoestrogenic side effects (hot flushes, bone loss) necessitate add-back therapy with norethindrone or estrogen-progestin combinations.[37] They are typically second-line for nonresponders to first-line therapies.[16]

Danazol

Danazol (400–800 mg/day), a synthetic steroid, induces endometrial atrophy via hypoestrogenic and hyperandrogenic effects.[16] Its use is limited by androgenic side effects (hirsutism, acne) and risks like fetal virilization if used during pregnancy.[38,47]

Cyproterone Acetate (CPA)

CPA (10–12.5 mg/day), an anti-androgen with progestational activity, shows comparable pain relief to COCs but is limited by side effects like depression and hot flushes.[16,48]

Aromatase Inhibitors (AIs)

AIs (e.g., letrozole 2.5 mg/day, anastrozole 1 mg/day) inhibit estrogen production in endometriotic implants, ovaries, and adipose tissue, suppressing lesion growth.[16,17] A systematic review showed that AIs, when combined with COCs, progestins, or GnRH agonists, reduce pain and lesion size.[39] Due to follicular stimulation and BMD loss, AIs require concomitant ovarian suppression and are used off-label for severe pain.[40,41]

GnRH Antagonists: Elagolix (Table 2)

Elagolix, an oral GnRH antagonist, was approved in 2018 by the FDA for moderate-to-severe endometriosis-associated pain.[42] Unlike GnRH agonists, elagolix rapidly suppresses pituitary gonadotropin secretion without an initial flare-up, allowing dose-dependent estrogen reduction.[5] This minimizes endometriotic growth while maintaining sufficient E2 levels to reduce vasomotor symptoms, vaginal atrophy, and bone loss.[42]

- **Mechanism:** Elagolix directly inhibits LH and FSH secretion, reducing ovarian estrogen production. This creates a hypoestrogenic environment that suppresses endometriotic proliferation without complete estrogen depletion.[5]
- **Efficacy:** Clinical trials (Elaris EM-I and EM-II) demonstrated significant reductions in dysmenorrhea and nonmenstrual pelvic pain at doses of 150 mg daily or 200 mg twice daily, with effects sustained in extension studies up to 12 months.[42,43] Response persistence was noted post treatment.[43]
- **Side Effects:** Common adverse effects include hot flushes (dose-dependent, less severe than GnRH agonists), headaches, insomnia, and elevated serum lipids. Unlike agonists, elagolix has a lower impact on BMD.[43]
- **Advantages:** Oral administration, rapid onset, and flexible dosing make elagolix a convenient alternative to injectable GnRH agonists. It avoids the initial gonadotropin surge, enabling faster symptom relief.[5]

- **Clinical Role:** Elagolix is a promising first- or second-line option for women with moderate-to-severe pain, particularly those seeking noncontraceptive therapy or avoiding surgery.[42]

TABLE 2: Elagolix vs. GnRH agonists.

Feature	*Elagolix*	*GnRH Agonists*
Administration	Oral	Injectable (daily/monthly)
Onset	Immediate	7–14 days (flare-up)
Estrogen Suppression	Dose-dependent	Profound
Side Effects	Mild hot flushes, lipid changes	Severe hot flushes, bone loss
BMD Impact	Minimal	Significant
Efficacy	Reduces dysmenorrhea, pelvic pain[42]	Comparable[36]

Source: Compiled from references 36, 42.

Other GnRH Antagonists

Cetrorelix (3 mg/week subcutaneously) showed symptom improvement in a small study ($n = 15$) without estrogen withdrawal side effects, but further RCTs are needed.[44]

- **First-Line Medical Therapy:** State clearly that **NSAIDs, Combined Hormonal Contraceptives (CHCs), and Progestins (including Dienogest and the LNG-IUS)** are all first-line options. The choice depends on patient preference, contraindications, and side-effect profile.
- **GnRH Antagonists (Elagolix, etc.):** ESHRE recommends them as an effective option for women with confirmed endometriosis who do not respond to or tolerate first-line hormonal treatments. They are **not necessarily second-line after GnRH agonists** but an alternative.
- **Add-Back Therapy (ABT):** Emphasize strongly that **add-back therapy (e.g., low-dose estrogen/progestin or progestin alone) SHOULD be offered concomitantly with GnRH agonists or antagonists to reduce hypoestrogenic side effects and protect bone mineral density, without reducing efficacy (Table 3). Antagonist are second line for pain, Dienogest is first line.**

TABLE 3: Treatment algorithm for endometriosis-associated pain.

Line	*Therapy*	*Indication*
First-line	COCs, Progestins (DNG, NETA, LNG-IUS)	Mild-to-moderate pain, contraception desired
Second-line	GnRH Agonists, Elagolix	Nonresponders, severe pain
Adjunctive	NSAIDs	Short-term pain relief
Off-Label	AIs + COCs/Progestins	Severe, refractory pain
Investigational	SPRMs, SERMs, Immunomodulators	Future therapies, fertility preservation

Source: Adapted from reference 16.

Based on a systematic history and clinical examination, a diagnosis of endometriosis can be made to initiate empirical medical treatment, even without imaging or surgical confirmation.

Primary role of TVUS/MRI is to assess for deep infiltrating endometriosis (DIE) and ovarian endometriomas, not to rule out superficial disease

INFERTILITY

- GnRH agonist prior to ART treatment to improve live birth rate not recommended.
- **Do not use ovulation suppression (e.g., CHCs, progestins, GnRH agonists) to improve fertility in women with endometriosis.** This is a strong ESHRE recommendation.
- For minimal-to-mild endometriosis, **offer controlled ovarian stimulation (COS) with intrauterine insemination (IUI)**.
- For all stages of endometriosis-associated infertility, **In Vitro Fertilization (IVF) is effective**.
- **Surgical excision of endometriomas >3–4 cm may be considered before IVF** to improve access to follicles, but the potential impact on ovarian reserve must be discussed. (ESHREE 2022).

SURGERY

- Laparoscopy is no more the gold standard for endometruiosis ESHRE 2022. Imaging TVS, MRI if not able to reach diagnosis laparoscopy might be done.
- **Surgery is indicated for:** Diagnostic confirmation, treatment of pain refractory to medical therapy, removal of endometriomas, and treatment of DIE.
- **For pain:** Surgical excision of endometriotic lesions is more effective than diagnostic laparoscopy alone.
- **Postoperative suppression:** To reduce pain recurrence, **offer long-term post-operative hormonal suppression** (e.g., CHCs, progestins, LNG-IUS). (ESHREE 2022)

Endometriosis is a chronic medical condition and requires long-term therapy. Various treatment options available have varying degrees of success in symptom control. Many are limited by long-term use, side effects of prolonged hypoestrogenism and high rates of recurrence after therapy is discontinued. Also, endometriosis predominantly is a disease of young reproductive age women and most of the commonly available therapeutic agents interfere with fertility. Due to these drawbacks, there is a constant search for newer therapies that could offer cure and which can be safely used with fewer side effects.

Emerging and Experimental Medical Therapies

Selective progesterone modulators (SPRM): SPRM can have a variable effect from different tissues from pure agonist to mixed agonist and antagonist to pure antagonist. Mifepristone has shown to have dose-dependent inhibitory effect on endometriotic implants. It was shown to have positive effects on endometriosis-related pain. It induced amenorrhea without causing hypoestrogenism.

Ulipristal acetate and asoprisnil also have shown to cause regression of endometriotic lesions. However, in the endometrium, SPRM associated changes closely mimicked hyperplasia which developed after less than 3 months of treatment and resolved after discontinuation of ulipristal and induction of withdrawal bleed. Feasibility of SPRMs is yet to be determined.

Selective estrogen receptor modulators (SERMS): SERMs have different effects in different tissue types makes them interesting agents for further endometriosis research, for example, blocking estrogen-mediated growth of endometriotic lesions and at the same time supporting bone-mass remediation.

Bazedoxiphene, a third-generation SERM, approved for use in menopausal symptoms, has demonstrated to regress endometriotic lesions. Combined with conjugated estrogens, it has better tolerability and reduced side-effect profile. It represents a potential treatment option for endometriosis. The feasibility and effectiveness of BZA are yet to be evaluated.

Antiangiogenesis factors: Angiogenesis is crucial for growth and survival of endometriotic lesions. Studies have shown that these lesions secrete angiogenic factors like vascular endothelial growth factor (VEGF). Therefore, antiangiogenic factors could stop growth of new lesions and regress older ones. This forms the basis of use of antiangiogenic factors in the treatment of endometriosis. These are still in the early development phase. TNP-470, endostatin, anginex and anti-VEGF antibody (Avastin) have been successful in decreasing the size of endometriotic lesions in animal models; however, no data is available in humans.

Dopamine Receptor 2 Agonists, cabergoline and quinagolide, reduce angiogenesis by dephosphorylation of VEGF2. Cabergoline has shown better results compared to LHRH agonist, in reducing the size of endometrioma. It has no major side effects, is easy to administer, and is cheaper than LHRH agonists. In a study comparing cabergoline and medroxyprogesterone acetate, both were found to be equally effective in decreasing chronic pelvic pain due to endometriosis. Cabergoline had a better acceptance and compliance due to lesser side effects and less frequent dosing. It can be a better alternative to medroxyprogesterone acetate, though enough data is not available to recommend its routine use.

Peroxisome proliferator-activated receptor gamma ligands (PPAR-γ): PPARs are ligand activated nuclear receptors. PPAR-γ ligands have anti-inflammatory properties and reduce estrogen production by inhibiting aromatase enzyme. In experimental models, they have been shown to inhibit cell proliferation, increase apoptosis, and inhibit the growth of the endometriotic lesions through angiogenic factor VEGF. In animal models, rosiglitazone and pioglitazone reduce the volume, weight, and size of the endometriotic lesions. Human studies are underway; however, there are concerns about the possible cardiovascular risk.

TNFα blockers: TNFα is a proinflammatory cytokine and its levels have been found to be elevated in the peritoneal fluid of women with endometriosis with a direct correlation with the stage of the disease. Infliximab, a monoclonal antibody against TNFα, has shown to reduce the size and number of the endometriotic implants and decrease in the levels of inflammatory cytokines in animal models. In a study on infliximab versus placebo in women with endometriosis, no improvement was reported in the severity of pain. There is lack of evidence in humans regarding the efficacy of these agents.

Statins: These drugs, e.g., atorvastatin, simvastatin, lovastatin, etc., lower cholesterol levels by blocking the conversion of 3-hydroxy-3-methylglutaryl-coenzyme A into mevalonate, which is a precursor of cholesterol. Their anti-inflammatory, antiangiogenic, and antioxidant properties have provoked interest in their use for endometriosis. Only lipid-soluble statins were effective in inhibition of growth and invasiveness of human endometrial cells in an in vitro study. Though evidence support statins as the potential therapeutic agent for conservative treatment of endometriosis, yet the uncertainties regarding their impact on gonadal function may deter its use as an appropriate therapy for all young fertile women.

Romidepsin: Romidepsin, an anticancer drug used in cutaneous T-cell lymphoma, targets VEGF at the transcriptional level, which cause reduction in secretion of VEGF from human immortalized epithelial cells. Therefore, romidepsin may be a potential therapeutic agent against angiogenesis in endometriosis. Unlike other antiangiogenic treatments that can only target developing angiogenesis, romidepsin eliminates preexisting pathologic vessels. Consequently, romidepsin could serve as a novel, fertility-preserving, and effective treatment for endometriosis.

Pentoxifylline: Pentoxifylline is a methylxanthine with anti-inflammatory property, acting as a phosphodiesterase inhibitor, which has been proposed for treating endometriosis. In a prospective RCT designed to test the effect of oral pentoxifylline combined with laparoscopic surgery on pelvic pain, reduction in pain scores was documented most significantly. Feasibility for clinical use requires Phase 3 RCTs; monitor ESHRE 2025 updates.

Nanotechnology: Some fundamental principles of cancer nanomedicine can potentially be used for the development of novel nanoparticle-based strategies for treatment and imaging of endometriosis. Finding of nanoparticles that can predominantly accumulate in endometriotic lesions without toxic effect on the body, while preserving their imaging and heating properties, is a challenge. The heat generated ablates the endometrial lesions completely within a day or two. Strategy can eventually shift the current paradigm for endometriosis detection and treatment.

SUMMARY

ESHREE 2022 Danazol and anti-progestogens, laparoscopic uterosacral nerve ablation (LUNA), presacral neurectomy (PSN) and anti-adhesion agents are no longer included in recommendations, but still covered in the text.

For the treatment of endometriosis, diverse therapeutic approaches, including no treatment, medical treatment, surgical treatment, and a combination of medical and surgical treatment, have been used. Medical treatment consists of hormonal therapy that most commonly includes combination oral contraceptives, high-dose progestins, danazol, and GnRH agonists. The basis of pharmacologic therapy is that endometriosis implants are capable of responding to hormones. NSAIDs may be considered in patients with mild symptoms and can be combined with hormonal therapy. However, none of these treatments eradicates the disease; they are associated with side effects. Sometimes, endometriosis-related symptoms reappear after therapy is discontinued. GnRH analogs, danazol, and depot progestagens[45] are associated with a higher incidence of adverse events. Hormonal management is not suitable for woman suffering from endometriosis[46] who wish to get pregnant and severe symptoms or severe disease (stages III and IV). AIs can be given in intractable cases along with COCs or progestins.

As long-term treatment and repeated treatment are required, the choice of treatment depends on efficacy, adverse side effects, long-term safety, cost, and availability of the drug.

KEY POINTS

- Endometriosis, a chronic condition, requires long-term management. COCs and progestins (e.g., dienogest, NETA, LNG-IUS) are first-line therapies, effectively reducing pain in most patients with good tolerability.[9,17]
- GnRH agonists, used as second line, are effective but limited by hypoestrogenic side effects, mitigated by add-back therapy.[36]
- NSAIDs lack robust evidence,[8] and danazol's use has declined due to androgenic effects.[37]
- Elagolix, a novel oral GnRH antagonist, offers rapid, dose-dependent pain relief with fewer side effects, making it a promising option.[42]

REFERENCES

1. Burney RO, Giudice LC. Pathogenesis and pathophysiology of endometriosis. Fertil Steril. 2012;98(3):511-9.
2. Giudice LC, Kao L. Endometriosis. Lancet. 2004;364:1789-99.
3. Ilangavan K, Kalu E. High prevalence of endometriosis in infertile women with normal ovulation and normospermic partners. Fertil Steril. 2010;93:e10.
4. Guo SW, Wang Y. The prevalence of endometriosis in women with chronic pelvic pain. Gynecol Obstet Invest. 2006;62:121-30.
5. Rocha AL, Reis FM, Petraglia F. New trends for the medical treatment of endometriosis. Expert Opin Investig Drugs. 2012;21(7):905-19.
6. Bedaiwy MA, Alfaraj S, Yong P, Casper R. New developments in the medical treatment of endometriosis. Fertil Steril. 2017;107(3):555-65.
7. Shakiba K, Bena JF, McGill KM, et al. Surgical treatment of endometriosis: a 7-year follow-up on the requirement for further surgery. Obstet Gynecol. 2008;111(6):1285-92.
8. Allen C, Hopewell S, Prentice A, et al. Nonsteroidal anti-inflammatory drugs for pain in women with endometriosis. Cochrane Database Syst Rev. 2009;2:CD004753.
9. Jensen JT, Schlaff W, Gordon K. Use of combined hormonal contraceptives for the treatment of endometriosis-related pain: a systematic review of the evidence. Fertil Steril. 2018;110(1): 137-152.e1.
10. Razzi S, Luisi S, Ferretti C, et al. Use of a progestogen-only preparation containing desogestrel in the treatment of recurrent pelvic pain after conservative surgery for endometriosis. Eur J Obstet Gynecol Reprod Biol. 2007;135:188-90.
11. Olive DL. Medical therapy of endometriosis. Semin Reprod Med. 2003;21:209-22.
12. Aznaurova YB, Zhumataev MB, Roberts TK, et al. Molecular aspects of development and regulation of endometriosis. Reprod Biol Endocrinol. 2014;12:50.
13. Harada T, Momoeda M, Taketani Y, et al. Low-dose oral contraceptive pill for dysmenorrhea associated with endometriosis: a placebo-controlled, double-blind, randomized trial. Fertil Steril. 2008;90:1583-8.
14. Menakaya U, Infante F, Condous G. Consensus on current management of endometriosis. Hum Reprod. 2013;28:3162-3.
15. Casper RF. Progestin-only pills may be a better first-line treatment for endometriosis than combined estrogen-progestin contraceptive pills. Fertil Steril. 2017;107:533-6.

16. Ferrero S, Barra F, Maggiore ULR. Current and Emerging Therapeutics for the Management of Endometriosis. Drugs. 2018;78(10):995-1012.
17. Practice Committee of the American Society for Reproductive Medicine. Treatment of pelvic pain associated with endometriosis: a committee opinion. Fertil Steril. 2014;101(4):927-35.
18. Harrison RF, Barry-Kinsella C. Efficacy of medroxyprogesterone treatment in infertile women with endometriosis: a prospective, randomized, placebo-controlled study. Fertil Steril. 2000;74(1):24-30.
19. Vercellini P, Pietropaolo G, De Giorgi O, et al. Treatment of symptomatic rectovaginal endometriosis with an estrogen-progestogen combination versus low-dose norethindrone acetate. Fertil Steril. 2005;84(5):1375-87.
20. Buggio L, Somigliana E, Barbara G, et al. Oral and depot progestin therapy for endometriosis: towards a personalized medicine. Expert Opin Pharmacother. 2017;18(15):1569-81.
21. Harada T, Taniguchi F. Dienogest: a new therapeutic agent for the treatment of endometriosis. Women's Health. 2010;6(1):27-35.
22. Schindler AE. Dienogest in long-term treatment of endometriosis. Int J Women's Health. 2011;3:175-84.
23. Bizzarri N, Remorgida V, Maggiore ULR, et al. Dienogest in the treatment of endometriosis. Expert Opin Pharmacother. 2014;15:1889-902.
24. Momoeda M, Taketani Y. Dienogest inhibits aromatase and cyclooxygenase-2 expression and prostaglandin E_2 production in human endometriotic stromal cells in spheroid culture. Jpn Pharmacol Ther. 2007;35:769-83.
25. Strowitzki T, Faustmann T, Gerlinger C, et al. Dienogest in the treatment of endometriosis-associated pelvic pain: a 12-week, randomized, double-blind, placebo-controlled study. Eur J Obstet Gynecol Reprod Biol. 2010;151:193-8.
26. Strowitzki T, Marr J, Gerlinger C, et al. Dienogest is as effective as leuprolide acetate in treating the painful symptoms of endometriosis: a 24-week, randomized, multicentre, open-label trial. Hum Reprod. 2010;25(3):633-41.
27. Petraglia F, Hornung D, Seitz C, et al. Reduced pelvic pain in women with endometriosis: efficacy of long-term dienogest treatment. Arch Gynecol Obstet. 2012;285(1):167-73.
28. Harada M, Osuga Y, Izumi G, et al. Dienogest, a new conservative strategy for extragenital endometriosis: a pilot study. Gynecol Endocrinol. 2011;27(9):717-20.
29. Yamanaka A, Hada T, Matsumoto T, et al. Effect of dienogest on pain and ovarian endometrioma occurrence after laparoscopic resection of uterosacral ligaments with deep infiltrating endometriosis. Eur J Obstet Gynecol Reprod Biol. 2017;216:51-5.
30. Angioni S, Nappi L, Pontis A, et al. Dienogest. A possible conservative approach in bladder endometriosis. Results of a pilot study. Gynecol Endocrinol. 2015;31(5):406-8.
31. Morotti M, Sozzi F, Remorgida V, et al. Dienogest in women with persistent endometriosis-related pelvic pain during norethisterone acetate treatment. Eur J Obstet Gynecol Reprod Biol. 2014; 183:188-92.
32. Leone Roberti Maggiore U, Remorgida V, Scala C, et al. Desogestrel-only contraceptive pill versus sequential contraceptive vaginal ring in the treatment of rectovaginal endometriosis infiltrating the rectum: a prospective open-label comparative study. Acta Obstet Gynecol Scand. 2014;93:239-47.
33. Lan S, Ling L, Jianhong Z, et al. Analysis of the levonorgestrel-releasing intrauterine system in women with endometriosis. J Int Med Res. 2013;41(3):548-58.
34. Vercellini P, Frontino G, De Giorgi O, et al. Comparison of a levonorgestrel-releasing intrauterine device versus expectant management after conservative surgery for symptomatic endometriosis: a pilot study. Fertil Steril. 2003;80:305-9.
35. Gomes MK, Rosa-e-Silva JC, Garcia SB, et al. Effects of the levonorgestrel-releasing intrauterine system on cell proliferation, Fas expression and steroid receptors in endometriosis lesions and normal endometrium. Hum Reprod. 2009;24:2736-45.

36. Brown J, Pan A, Hart RJ. Gonadotrophin-releasing hormone analogues for pain associated with endometriosis. Cochrane Database Syst Rev. 2010;12:CD008475.
37. Kiesel L, Schweppe KW, Sillem M, et al. Should add-back therapy for endometriosis be deferred for optimal results?Br J Obstet Gynaecol. 1996;103(Suppl 14):15-7.
38. Brunskill PJ. The effects of fetal exposure to danazol. Br J Obstet Gynaecol. 1992;99(3):212-5.
39. Almassinokiani F, Almasi A, Akbari P, et al. Effect of Letrozole on endometriosis-related pelvic pain. Med J Islam Repub Iran. 2014;28:107.
40. Pavone ME, Bulun SE. Aromatase inhibitors for the treatment of endometriosis. Fertil Steril. 2012;98:1370-9.
41. ACOG Committee Opinion No. 663. Obstet Gynecol. 2016;127:1187-8.
42. Taylor HS, Giudice LC, Lesse BA, et al. Treatment of Endometriosis-Associated Pain with Elagolix, an Oral GnRH Antagonist. N Engl J Med. 2017;377(1):28-40.
43. Surrey E, Taylor HS, Giudice L, et al. Long-Term Outcomes of Elagolix in Women With Endometriosis: Results From Two Extension Studies. Obstet Gynecol. 2018;132(1):147-60.
44. Kupker W, Felberbaum RE, Krapp M, et al. Use of GnRH antagonists in the treatment of endometriosis. Reprod Biomed Online. 2002;5(1):12–6.
45. Brown J, Kives S, Akhtar M. Progestagens and anti-progestagens for pain associated with endometriosis. Cochrane Database Syst Rev. 2012;3:CD002122.
46. Prentice A. Regular review: Endometriosis. BMJ. 2001;323:93-5.
47. Rafique S, DeCherney AH. Medical Management of Endometriosis. Clin Obstet Gynecol. 2017; 60(3):485-96.
48. Gezer A, Oral E. Progestin therapy in endometriosis. Womens Health (Lond). 2015;11(5):643-52.

Adenomyosis

Ruchika Garg

LONG ANSWER QUESTIONS (LAQS)

Q1. Direct and Indirect Features of Adenomyosis.

Adenomyosis is characterized by the presence of endometrial tissue within the myometrium, leading to distinct ultrasound features classified by the Morphological Uterus Sonographic Assessment (MUSA) group as direct (indicating ectopic endometrial tissue) and indirect (secondary to myometrial changes).[1,2]

TABLE 1: MUSA features of adenomyosis.

Feature type	*Feature*	*Description*
Direct	Myometrial cysts	Rounded, anechoic, or mixed echogenicity lesions in myometrium; may have hyperechoic rim
	Hyperechogenic islands	Hyperechoic areas within myometrium; regular, irregular, or ill-defined margins
	Echogenic subendometrial lines/buds	Hyperechoic lines/buds perpendicular to endometrium, disrupting junctional zone
Indirect	Globular uterus	Spherical uterus with equal length/width/depth; serosa diverges from cervix
	Asymmetrical myometrial thickening	Anterior/posterior wall thickness ratio ≠ 1, indicating asymmetry
	Fan-shaped shadowing	Hypoechoic linear stripes, sometimes with hyperechoic bands, in myometrium
	Translesional vascularity	Blood vessels perpendicular to uterine cavity/serosa; common in diffuse adenomyosis
	Irregular junctional zone	Ill-defined or thickened junctional zone; no specific thickness cutoff
	Interrupted junctional zone	Discontinuous junctional zone on 2D/3D ultrasound, not visible in all planes

- **Direct Features:** Reflect ectopic endometrial tissue invasion into the myometrium, causing cystic or hyperechoic changes.
- **Indirect Features:** Result from myometrial hypertrophy, distortion, or imaging artifacts due to adenomyosis.

Recent Advances: The 2022 MUSA consensus refined definitions, emphasizing 3D ultrasound for junctional zone assessment.[2]

Q2. Detailed Diagnosis of Adenomyosis.

Overview: Adenomyosis diagnosis relies on clinical suspicion and imaging, as there are no specific biomarkers. Advances in transvaginal ultrasound (TVUS) and magnetic resonance imaging (MRI) have improved diagnostic accuracy.[3]

Diagnostic Approach:

- **Clinical Suspicion:**
  - **Symptoms:** Heavy menstrual bleeding (HMB), dysmenorrhea, chronic pelvic pain, dyspareunia.
  - **Examination:** Symmetrically enlarged, globular uterus (10–12 weeks size), often tender (Halban's sign).
  - **Challenges:** Symptoms overlap with fibroids or endometriosis, necessitating imaging.
- **Imaging Modalities:**
  - **Transvaginal Ultrasound (TVUS):**
    - **Primary Tool:** Cost-effective, widely available, with MUSA criteria for standardization.[1]
    - **Findings** (see **Table 1**):
      - Globular uterus, asymmetrical thickening.
      - Myometrial cysts, hyperechoic islands, subendometrial lines/buds.
      - Fan-shaped shadowing, irregular/interrupted junctional zone.
    - **Sensitivity/Specificity:** 83.8%/63.9%.[4]
    - **3D TVUS:** Enhances junctional zone visualization, improving diagnostic precision.[2]

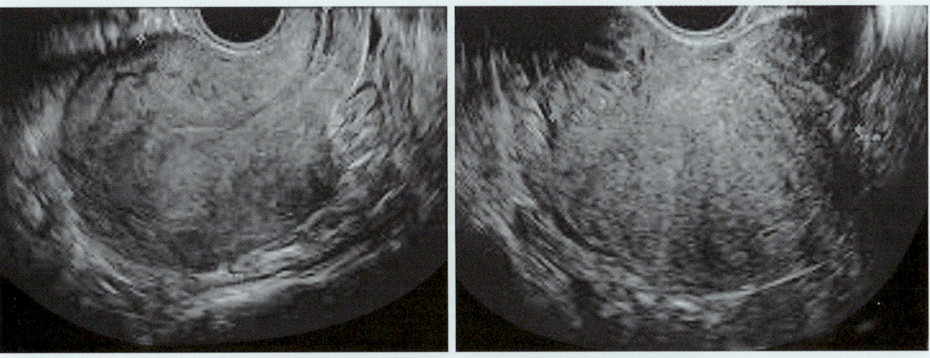

Fig. 1: TVS image of adenomyosis.

Transvaginal two-dimensional ultrasound images of a uterus affected by adenomyosis depicting all Morphological Uterus Sonographic Assessment (MUSA) features of adenomyosis having irregular junctional zone, asymmetrical myometrial thickening, globular uterus, echogenic subendometrial lines and buds; myometrial cysts; and fan-shaped shadowing.

- **Pelvic MRI:**
  - **Indications:** Inconclusive TVUS, differentiation from fibroids, or focal adenomyosis.

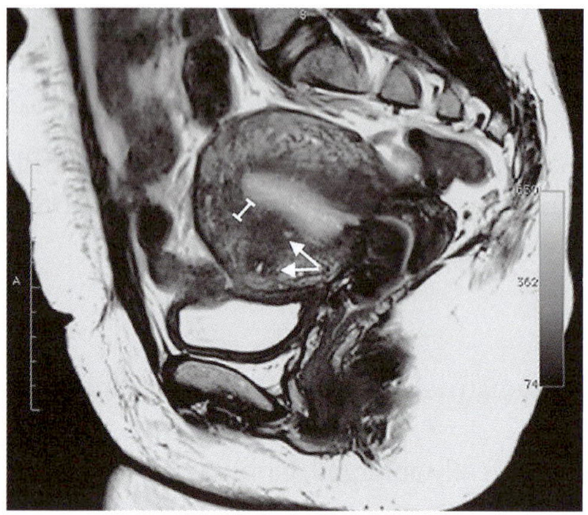

Fig. 2: Uterus with adenomyotic features on Pelvic MRI.

- **Findings:**
  - Junctional zone thickening (>12 mm on T2-weighted images).
  - High-intensity myometrial foci or diffuse adenomyosis.
  - Low-signal-intensity areas (smooth muscle hyperplasia).
- **Sensitivity/Specificity:** 77%/89%.[4]
- **Advantages:** Superior for adenomyoma vs. fibroid differentiation; less operator-dependent.
- **Hysteroscopy:**
  - **Adjunct Role:** Detects endometrial changes (hypervascularization, defects, hemorrhagic cysts).
  - **Limitations:** Not diagnostic alone; used when imaging inconclusive.

- **Histopathology:**

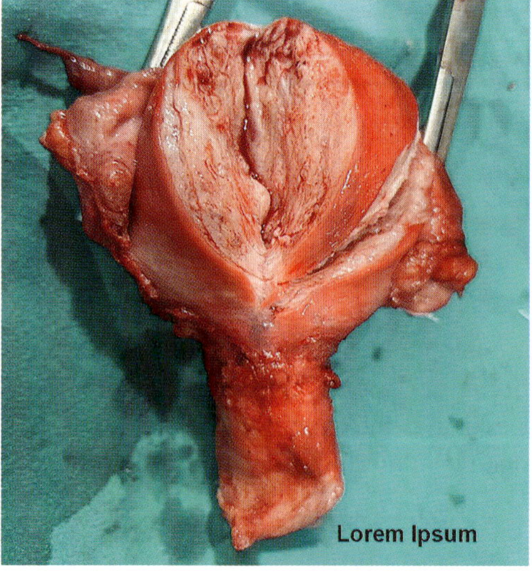

Fig. 3: Adenomyotic features in a specimen of uterus after hysterectomy.

Definitive diagnosis post-hysterectomy via endometrial glands/stroma in myometrium.
- Rarely used due to reliance on non-invasive imaging.

Recent Advances[5]

- Radiomics from T2-weighted MRI enables differentiation of adenomyosis with 85–90% accuracy, serving as a potential biomarker.
- The 2023 FIGO classification integrates imaging-based phenotyping for adenomyosis, aiding personalized management.[6]

Diagnostic Algorithm

- Step 1: Clinical assessment (HMB, dysmenorrhea, globular uterus).
- Step 2: TVUS with MUSA criteria; consider 3D TVUS.
- Step 3: MRI if TVUS inconclusive or focal adenomyosis suspected.
- Step 4: Hysteroscopy or histopathology in complex cases.

Q3. Medical Management of Adenomyosis (2019).

Overview: Medical management of adenomyosis focuses on symptom relief (HMB, dysmenorrhea) and fertility preservation, as no FDA-approved treatments specifically target adenomyosis. Hormonal therapies, adapted from endometriosis protocols, dominate, with nonhormonal options for pain.[7]

Medical Therapies

- **Hormonal Treatments:**
  - **Combined Oral Contraceptives (COCs):**
    - **Mechanism:** Regulate menstrual cycles, reduce endometrial proliferation.
    - **Efficacy:** Decreases HMB by 40–60%, improves dysmenorrhea in 50–70% of patients.
    - **Regimen:** Continuous or cyclic; e.g., ethinyl estradiol/levonorgestrel.
  - **Progestins:**
    - **Options:** Medroxyprogesterone acetate (10–20 mg/day), norethindrone (5 mg/day), dienogest (2 mg/day).
    - **Mechanism:** Induce endometrial atrophy, reduce bleeding.
    - **Efficacy:** Reduces HMB by 60–80%; dienogest particularly effective for pain relief.[8]
  - **Gonadotropin-Releasing Hormone (GnRH) Agonists:**
    - **Options:** Leuprolide (3.75 mg IM monthly), goserelin.
    - **Mechanism:** Induce hypoestrogenic state, shrinking adenomyotic tissue.
    - **Efficacy:** Significant pain reduction (70–90%); limited by menopausal symptoms and bone loss.
    - **Use:** Short-term (3–6 months) with add-back therapy (e.g., low-dose estrogen/progestin).
  - **Levonorgestrel-Releasing Intrauterine System (LNG-IUS):**
    - **Device:** Mirena (52 mg levonorgestrel).
    - **Mechanism:** Local progestin release reduces endometrial growth and vascularity.
    - **Efficacy:** Reduces HMB by 80–90%, pain by 60–70%; effective for 3–5 years.[7]
    - **Advantages:** Fertility-preserving, minimal systemic effects.

- **Nonhormonal Treatments:**
  - **Nonsteroidal Anti-Inflammatory Drugs (NSAIDs):**
    - **Options:** Ibuprofen (400–800 mg 6–8 hourly), mefenamic acid.
    - **Efficacy:** Reduces dysmenorrhea by 30–50%; adjunct to hormonal therapy.
    - **Limitations:** No effect on HMB.
  - **Tranexamic Acid:**
    - **Mechanism:** Antifibrinolytic; reduces menstrual blood loss.
    - **Efficacy:** Decreases HMB by 30–50%; used during menses.

Management Considerations

- **Patient Selection:** LNG-IUS preferred for HMB; GnRH agonists for severe symptoms in perimenopausal women.
- **Fertility:** LNG-IUS and progestins are fertility-sparing; avoid GnRH agonists long-term in women desiring pregnancy.
- **Side Effects:**
  - COCs/Progestins: Irregular bleeding, weight gain.
  - GnRH Agonists: Hot flashes, bone density loss.
  - LNG-IUS: Expulsion risk (5–10%), irregular spotting.

Recent Advances[9]

- GnRH antagonists (e.g., elagolix) show promise for pain relief with fewer hypoestrogenic effects.
- Aromatase inhibitors (e.g., letrozole) are under investigation for adenomyosis, with early trials showing reduced uterine volume.

Algorithm

- Mild Symptoms: NSAIDs + COCs or LNG-IUS.
- Moderate HMB/Pain: LNG-IUS or dienogest.
- Severe Symptoms: GnRH agonists (short-term) or referral for surgical evaluation.

SHORT QUESTIONS AND ANSWERS

Q1. What is Adenomyosis? *(MS, 2015)*

Adenomyosis is a benign condition where endometrial glands and stroma infiltrate the myometrium, causing diffuse or focal lesions. It may involve the inner (junctional zone) or outer myometrium, sometimes contiguous with endometriosis. Symptoms include HMB, dysmenorrhea, and pelvic pain; the uterus is typically globular (10–12 weeks size).[10]

Q2. Morphological Uterus Sonographic Assessment (MUSA) Features of Adenomyosis. *(MS, 2006)*

MUSA features standardize ultrasound diagnosis of adenomyosis:[2]

- **Direct:**
  - Myometrial cysts.
  - Hyperechogenic islands.
  - Echogenic subendometrial lines/buds.

- **Indirect:**
  - Globular uterus.
  - Asymmetrical myometrial thickening.
  - Fan-shaped shadowing.
  - Translesional vascularity.
  - Irregular or interrupted junctional zone.

Q3. Surgical Management of Adenomyosis. *(MS, 2007)*

- **Uterine Artery Embolization (UAE):**
  - **Mechanism:** Reduces blood supply to adenomyotic tissue, causing shrinkage.
  - **Efficacy:** Pain relief in 60–80%, HMB reduction in 50–70%.
  - **Indications:** Symptomatic adenomyosis in women desiring uterine preservation.
- **Adenomyoma Resection:**
  - **Techniques:**
    - **Elliptical:** Wider resection at periphery, narrower near cavity; most common.
    - **Hood/Splice:** For focal lesions.
  - **Procedure:**
    - Intraoperative transvaginal ultrasound mapping to define margins.
    - Laparoscopic resection of adenomyotic plaque, preserving healthy myometrium.
  - **Efficacy:** Improves pain (70–85%), menorrhagia (60–80%), and fertility outcomes.
  - **Indications:** Focal adenomyosis, fertility preservation.
- **Hysterectomy:**
  - **Definitive Treatment:** Total abdominal or laparoscopic hysterectomy.
  - **Efficacy:** Resolves symptoms in >90% of cases.
  - **Indications:** Severe symptoms unresponsive to medical therapy, no desire for fertility.
- **Recent Advances:** Radiomics-guided UAE improves outcomes by targeting focal lesions.[5]

Q4. Differentiation Between Adenomyosis, Fibroid, and Polyp. *(MS, 2006, 2007).*

TABLE 2: Differentiation of adenomyosis, fibroid, and polyp.

Feature	*Adenomyosis*	*Fibroid*	*Polyp*
Definition	Endometrial glands/stroma in myometrium	Benign smooth muscle tumor	Endometrial mucosal growth
Age group	≥45 years (perimenopausal)	30–35 years (reproductive age)	Reproductive/peri-/postmenopausal
Symptoms	HMB, dysmenorrhea, pelvic pain	HMB, pressure symptoms, infertility	Irregular/intermenstrual bleeding
Uterine size	10–12 weeks, symmetrical, globular	Up to 20 weeks, irregular enlargement	Normal size
Examination	Tender uterus (Halban's sign)	Nontender (tender if degenerated/torsed)	Non-tender

Contd...

Contd...

Feature	*Adenomyosis*	*Fibroid*	*Polyp*
Ultrasound	Myometrial cysts, hyperechoic islands, fan-shaped shadowing	Hypoechoic, well-circumscribed, pseudocapsule	Hyperechoic, narrow/ broad base, feeder vessel
Doppler	Translesional vascularity	Peripheral blood vessels	Feeder vessel sign
Investigation of choice	MRI (junctional zone thickening)	Ultrasound-guided fibroid mapping	Hysteroscopy
Management	LNG-IUS, GnRH agonists, hysterectomy	Myomectomy, UAE, hysterectomy	Hysteroscopic polypectomy

REFERENCES

1. Van den Bosch T, Dueholm M, Leone FPG et al. Terms, definitions, and measurements to describe sonographic features of myometrium and uterine masses: MUSA consensus. Ultrasound Obstet Gynecol. 2015;46(3):284-98.
2. Harmsen MJ, Van den Bosch T, de Leeuw RA, et al. (2022). Revised MUSA features of adenomyosis: Delphi consensus. Ultrasound Obstet Gynecol. 2022;60(1):118-31.
3. Bazot M, Daraï E. Role of transvaginal sonography and MRI in adenomyosis diagnosis. Fertil Steril. 2018;109(3):389-97.
4. Dason ES, Maxim M, Sanders A, et al. Guideline No. 437: Diagnosis and management of adenomyosis. J Obstet Gynaecol Can. 2023;45(6):417-29.
5. Burla L, Sartoretti E, Mannil M, et al. MRI-based radiomics for adenomyosis diagnosis. J Clin Med. 2024;13(8):2344.
6. Munro MG. FIGO classification and reporting systems for adenomyosis. J Minim Invasive Gynecol. 2020;27(2):296-308.
7. Schrager S, Yogendran L, Marquez CM, et al. Adenomyosis: Diagnosis and management. Am Fam Physician. 2022;105(1):33-38.
8. Osuga Y, et al. (Dienogest in adenomyosis: A multicenter study. Fertil Steril. 2017;108(6):1039-46.
9. Vannuccini S, et al. (2021). GnRH antagonists and aromatase inhibitors in adenomyosis. Curr Opin Obstet Gynecol. 2021;33(4):297-303.
10. Bluhm M, Dueholm M. Imaging for adenomyosis: Sonographic diagnosis. J Minim Invasive Gynecol. 2020;27(2):267.

Female Genital Tuberculosis

Ruchika Garg

INTRODUCTION

Female Genital Tuberculosis (FGTB) is a significant cause of infertility in developing countries, particularly India, where it accounts for 5–16% of cases.[1] It is typically secondary to pulmonary or extrapulmonary TB, affecting organs like the gastrointestinal tract, spreading via hematogenous or lymphatic routes.[2] FGTB predominantly affects the fallopian tubes (90–100%), endometrium (50–80%), ovaries (20–30%), and cervix (4–15%).[3] Diagnosis is challenging, requiring a high index of suspicion, advanced imaging, and histopathological confirmation. Effective management involves prolonged anti-tubercular therapy (AKT) and fertility counseling.

Epidemiology

- **Global:**
  - **Prevalence:** 5–10% of infertility cases in developing countries; rare in low-TB settings (<1%).[4]
  - **WHO:** TB declared global emergency in 1993; 10 million new cases annually (2023).[5]
- **India:**
  - **Prevalence:** 5–10% of infertility cases; 15–25% in high-risk groups (e.g., urban slums).[6]
  - **2024 Study:** 8% of infertile Indian women had FGTB; 60% had tubal involvement.[7]
  - **TB-HIV co-infection:** 10–15% of TB cases; increases FGTB risk.[8]
- **Risk Factors:** Poverty, malnutrition, HIV, overcrowding, prior pulmonary TB.[9]

TABLE 1: Epidemiology of FGTB.[6,7]

Parameter	*Global*	*India*
Infertility prevalence	5–10%	5–16%
Tubal involvement	90–100%	90–100%
Endometrial involvement	50–80%	50–80%
HIV co-infection	5–10%	10–15%

Pathophysiology

- **Route of Spread:**
  - Hematogenous/lymphatic from pulmonary/extrapulmonary TB (e.g., GI, lymph nodes).[10]
  - Rarely direct spread from adjacent organs (e.g., peritoneum).[11]

- **Organ Involvement**:
  - **Fallopian Tubes**: Bilateral thickening, adhesions, hydrosalpinx; blocks ovum transport.[12]
  - **Endometrium:** Caseation, ulceration; impairs implantation.[13]
  - **Ovaries:** Adhesions, reduced reserve.[14]
  - **Cervix:** Erosions, scarring; rare.[15]
- **Consequences:** Infertility (tubal blockage, endometrial damage), chronic pelvic pain, ectopic pregnancy.[16]

TABLE 2: Organ Involvement in FGTB.[12,13]

Organ	*Involvement*	*Pathology*
Fallopian tubes	90–100%	Adhesions, hydrosalpinx, blockage
Endometrium	50–80%	Caseation, ulceration
Ovaries	20–30%	Adhesions, reduced reserve
Cervix	4–15%	Erosions, scarring

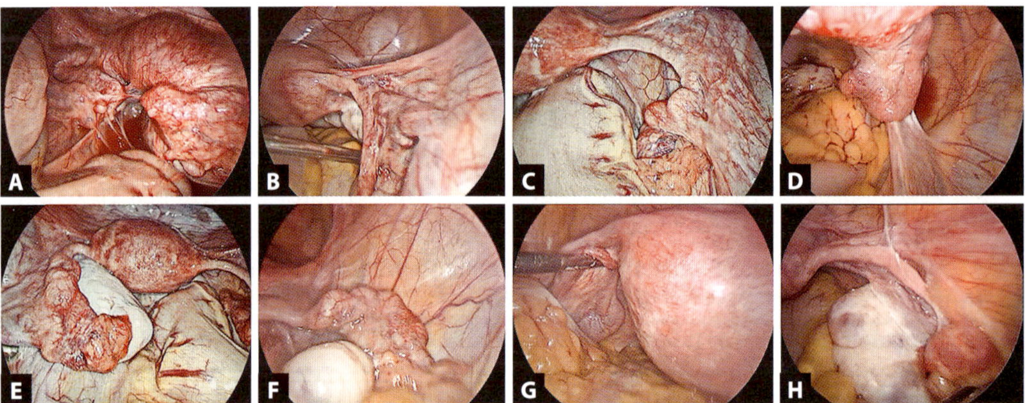

Figs. 1A to H: Laparoscopic images of genital tuberculosis. (A) Bilateral tubo-ovarian masses with adhesions and fluid in pouch of Douglas; (B) Shaggy surface of uterus and tubes; bulbous cornua; (C) Whitish patches on the surface of uterus and pelvic peritoneum and beaded tube; (D) Tubo-ovarian mass; (E, F) Beaded tubes; and (H) Tubal adhesions, distal hydrosalpinx.

4A: Straw-colored fluid inside the abdominal cavity, 4B-F: multiple miliary tubercles over bowel surface (4B), liver (4C), peritoneum (4D), fallopian tubes and hydrosalpinx (4E), pouch of Douglas (4F). *Courtesy*: Pallavi Verma, INHS Asvini, Mumbai.

Clinical Features

- **Infertility:** Primary (60–70%) or secondary; tubal/endometrial damage.[17]
- **Menstrual Irregularities:** Oligomenorrhea, amenorrhea (endometrial involvement).[18]
- **Pelvic Pain:** Chronic, dull; worse with menstruation.[19]
- **General Symptoms:** Fever, weight loss, night sweats (systemic TB).[20]
- **HIV Co-infection:** More severe symptoms, rapid progression.[21]

TABLE 3: Clinical features of FGTB.[17,19]

Symptom	*Prevalence*	*Description*
Infertility	60–70%	Primary/secondary; tubal blockage
Pelvic pain	40–50%	Chronic, dull
Oligomenorrhea	20–30%	Endometrial involvement
Systemic (fever, etc.)	10–20%	Active pulmonary/extrapulmonary TB

Diagnosis

- **Clinical Suspicion:** Infertility, pelvic pain, history of TB exposure, or HIV.[22]
- **Investigations:**
  - **Hysteroscopy/Laparoscopy:** Visualizes adhesions, tubal blockage; biopsy for histopathology.[23]
  - **Histopathology:** Caseating granulomas in endometrial/tubal tissue.[24]
  - **TB PCR:** High sensitivity (80–90%) for endometrial samples.[25]
  - **AFB Culture:** Gold standard; low sensitivity (30–40%).[26]
  - **Imaging:**
    - Ultrasound: Hydrosalpinx, endometrial thinning.[27]
    - Hysterosalpingography (HSG): Beaded tubes, uterine synechiae.[28]
  - **Mantoux Test/IGRA:** Screens for latent TB; nonspecific.[29]
- **Challenges:** Its diagnosis is notoriously difficult due to its paucibacillary nature, vague clinical presentation, and the limitations of available diagnostic tools.
- **Key Reasons for Diagnostic Difficulty:**
  - **Insidious and Nonspecific Clinical Presentation:**
    - Patients are often asymptomatic or present with nonspecific symptoms like chronic pelvic pain, menstrual irregularities (oligo/amenorrhea), or infertility.
    - Clinical signs can mimic other pathologies like pelvic inflammatory disease (PID), endometriosis, or ovarian cancer.
    - The "classic" symptoms of TB (fever, night sweats, weight loss) are frequently absent.
- **Paucibacillary Nature and Anatomical Inaccessibility:**
  - FGTB is primarily a latent infection with very few actively replicating bacilli in the genital tract.
  - The disease often affects the endometrium and fallopian tubes, making the collection of adequate tissue samples challenging without invasive procedures like hysteroscopy or laparoscopy.
  - The bacilli are shed intermittently in the endometrium, leading to false-negative results if sampling is mistimed.
- **Limitations of Diagnostic Modalities:**
  - **AFB Smear/Culture:** Endometrial tissue or menstrual blood has a very low yield for Acid-Fast Bacilli (AFB) smear (<5%) and even for culture on Löwenstein-Jensen (LJ) medium (sensitivity 50–60%). Culture, the gold standard, takes 6–8 weeks.

- **Nucleic Acid Amplification Tests (NAATs like PCR):** While rapid and specific, PCR can be *too sensitive*, detecting nonviable bacilli from an old, healed infection, leading to false positives. Its sensitivity on clinical samples remains variable (50–80%).
- **Histopathology:** Finding a definitive caseating granuloma on endometrial biopsy is diagnostic, but its sensitivity is low (25–50%) due to the patchy involvement of the endometrium. A single biopsy can easily miss the affected tissue.
- **Imaging (USG/HSG):** Hysterosalpingography (HSG) may show classic signs like beaded tubes, rigid pipe-stem tubes, or tubal blockages, but these are not specific for TB and can be seen in other chronic infections.

▪ **Lack of a Single, Gold-Standard Outpatient Test:**
- There is no simple, highly sensitive, and specific noninvasive test (like a blood test) for FGTB.
- The definitive diagnosis often requires a **"Composite Reference Standard"**—combining clinical suspicion, laparoscopy findings (e.g., tubercles, adhesions), histology, culture, and PCR. The need for this multimodal approach itself underscores the difficulty.

Diagnosing FGTB requires a high index of suspicion, particularly in a patient with unexplained infertility from a TB-endemic region. No single test is infallible. A combination of clinical assessment, imaging, histopathology, and microbiological/molecular tests is essential.

- Low bacterial load in genital tissues; negative cultures common.[30]
- Overlap with endometriosis, pelvic inflammatory disease (PID).[31]

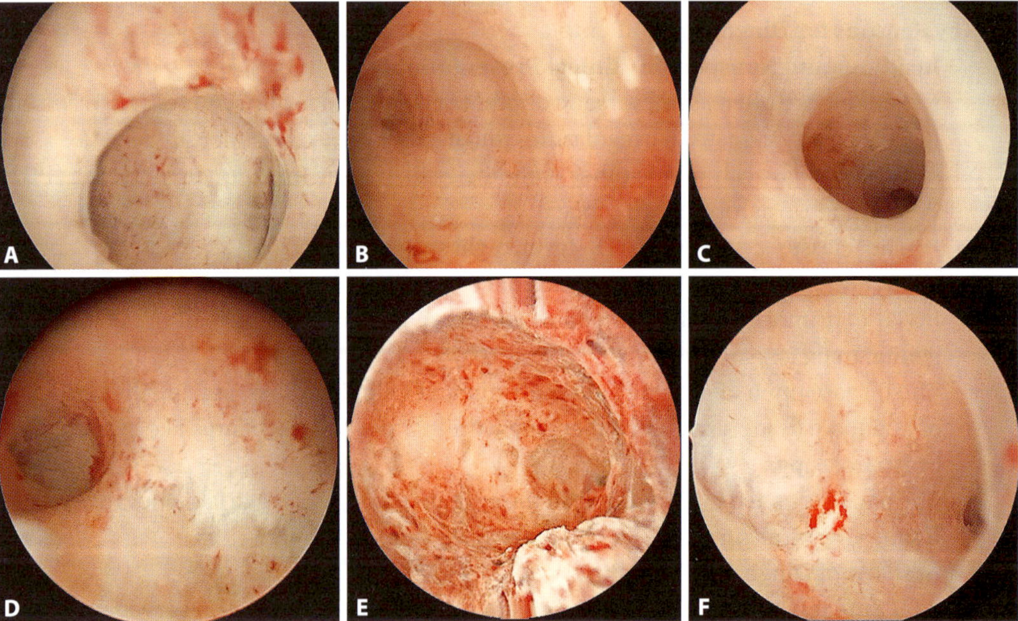

Figs. 2A to F: Hysteroscopic images of genital tuberculosis: (A) Pale endometrium with fundal adhesions; (B) Pale endometrium with caseous nodules; (C) and (D): Deep-seated ostia with fundal and periosteal adhesions; (E) Extensive endometrial scarring; (F) Pale endometrium with caseous nodules.

TABLE 4: Diagnostic Modalities for FGTB.[25,26]

Method	*Sensitivity*	*Specificity*	*Role*
TB PCR	80–90%	90%	Rapid, high sensitivity
AFB Culture	30–40%	95%	Gold standard, low yield
Histopathology	50–60%	90%	Caseating granulomas
Laparoscopy	70–80%	80%	Visualizes lesions, biopsy

Management

- **Antitubercular Therapy (AKT):**
  - **Category I (New Cases):**
    - **Intensive Phase (2 months)**: Daily rifampicin (R), isoniazid (H), pyrazinamide (Z), ethambutol (E).[32]
    - **Continuation Phase (4 months)**: Daily R, H.[33]
    - **Dosing (WHO 2020):**
      - Weight <45 kg: HRZE 300/450/1250/800 mg.
      - Weight >45 kg: HRZE 300/600/1750/1200 mg.[34]
    - **DOTS**: Thrice-weekly HRZE (2 months), HR (4 months); ensures 85% cure rate.[35]
  - **Category II (Relapse/Failure):**
    - Intensive Phase (3 months): Streptomycin (IM) + HRZE thrice weekly.
    - Continuation Phase (5 months): HRE thrice weekly.[36]
  - **MDR-TB:**
    - **Intensive Phase (6–9 months):** Kanamycin, levofloxacin, ethionamide, cycloserine, Z, E.
    - **Continuation Phase (18 months):** Levofloxacin, ethionamide, cycloserine, E.[37]
    - **2024 WHO Update:** Injection-free regimens (bedaquiline, delamanid) for MDR-TB.[38]
  - **Non-DOTS:** Daily HRZE (2 months), HR (4 months); less preferred due to adherence issues.[39]
  - **Monitoring:**
    - Monthly clinical review; no routine liver function tests unless hepatic symptoms.[40]
    - Pyridoxine for isoniazid-induced neuropathy.[41]
  - **Adverse Effects:**
    - Isoniazid: Peripheral neuropathy, hepatitis.
    - Rifampicin: Hepatitis, skin reactions.
    - Ethambutol: Optic neuritis.[42]

TABLE 5: AKT Regimens for FGTB.[34,37]

Category	*Phase*	*Drugs*	*Duration*
Category I	Intensive (2 months)	HRZE (daily/thrice weekly)	2 months
	Continuation (4 months)	HR (daily/thrice weekly)	4 months
Category II	Intensive (3 months)	SRHZE (thrice weekly)	3 months
	Continuation (5 months)	HRE (thrice weekly)	5 months
MDR-TB	Intensive (6–9 months)	Kanamycin, levofloxacin, ethionamide	6–9 months
	Continuation (18 months)	Levofloxacin, ethionamide, cycloserine	18 months

FGTB in HIV-Positive Women

- **Epidemiology:** 10–15% of Indian TB cases; higher FGTB risk.[43]
- **Management:**
  - AKT as per Category I/II; rifampicin interacts with antiretrovirals (ARVs).[44]
  - **Options:**
    - Defer ARV until TB treatment completion.
    - Use efavirenz-based ARV with rifampicin.[45]
    - Switch to nonrifampicin AKT in continuation phase.[46]
- **Challenges:** Drug interactions, immune reconstitution syndrome.[47]

Fertility Outcomes

- **Impact:**
  - Tubal blockage: 70–80% infertility cases.[48]
  - Endometrial damage: Poor implantation.[49]
- **Management:**
  - **Post-AKT:** In vitro fertilization (IVF) for tubal factor infertility; success rate 20–30%.[50]
  - **2024 Study:** 25% pregnancy rate in FGTB patients post-AKT with IVF.[51]
- **Counseling:** Discuss poor prognosis, ART options, adoption.[52]

WHO/RNTCP Guidelines

- **WHO (2020):**[53]
  - **Diagnosis:** High suspicion; use TB-PCR, histopathology for extrapulmonary TB.
  - **Treatment:** 6-month DOTS (2 HRZE/4 HR); injection-free MDR regimens.
  - **Monitoring:** Adherence via DOTS; manage side effects promptly.
- **RNTCP (2023):**[54]
  - **Coverage:** 100% geographical; 71% case detection, 87% treatment success.
  - **Strategy:** DOTS with fixed-dose combinations (FDCs); 4-drug FDC (HRZE 75/150/400/275 mg).
  - **MDR-TB:** Bedaquiline-based regimens; 18–24 months.[55,56]

Indian Context

- **Burden:** 5–16% of infertility.
- **Challenges:**
  - Diagnostic delay (2–3 years) due to low suspicion, limited PCR access.[57]
  - High MDR-TB prevalence (3–5% of cases).[58]
  - Cost of IVF (~₹2–3 lakh/cycle) limits fertility treatment.[59]
- **Strategies**:
  - Free DOTS via RNTCP; ASHA-led TB screening.[60]
  - **2024 Study:** Only 50% of FGTB patients complete AKT due to stigma.[61]

Newer anti-tubercular therapy in 2025 for the management of multidrug-resistant and rifampicin-resistant tuberculosis, bedaquiline, delamanid and pretomanid. Bedaquiline, a diarylquinoline that inhibits mycobacterial ATP synthase, and the nitroimidazoles delamanid and pretomanid, which disrupt mycolic acid synthesis and respiratory processes, are now core components of short, all-oral 6–9 month regimens for MDR/RR/XDR-TB, replacing older, toxic injectable-based protocols. These drugs are commonly combined with repurposed agents such as linezolid, clofazimine and later-generation fluoroquinolones in standardized regimens like BPaL and BPaLM, achieving high cure rates and significantly reduced treatment duration while maintaining acceptable safety with careful monitoring for QT prolongation and myelosuppression. Current research is focused on next-generation diarylquinolines and oxazolidinones to improve sterilizing activity, shorten therapy further, and mitigate cardiac and mitochondrial toxicity, and multiple phase II–III trials are under way.

REFERENCES

1. Sharma JB, et al. FGTB review. J Obstet Gynaecol India. 2016;66(Suppl 1):S337-43.
2. Gupta N, et al. FGTB pathophysiology. Fertil Steril. 2017;108(3):e123-9.
3. Mondal SK, et al. FGTB organ involvement. Indian J Pathol Microbiol. 2018;61(4):521-6.
4. WHO. Global TB Report 2023. Geneva: WHO; 2023.
5. Dye C, et al. TB epidemiology. Lancet. 2016;367(9514):938-40.
6. Malhotra N, et al. FGTB infertility India. J Hum Reprod Sci. 2019;12(3):234-40.
7. Patel S, et al. FGTB prevalence 2024. Fertil Steril. 2024;121(2):345-51.
8. Gupta A, et al. TB-HIV co-infection India. Indian J Med Res. 2017;145(6):723-9.
9. Narula M, et al. TB risk factors. J Assoc Physicians India. 2016;64(8):34-40.
10. Kumar P, et al. FGTB spread. J Clin Diagn Res. 2018;12(9):QC01-5.
11. Sharma SK, et al. Extrapulmonary TB. Indian J Med Res. 2017;145(3):292-304.
12. Banerjee S, et al. Tubal pathology FGTB. J Minim Invasive Gynecol. 2016;23(6):873-80.
13. Jindal UN, et al. Endometrial TB. Fertil Steril. 2016;106(3):e234-40.
14. Gupta R, et al. Ovarian involvement FGTB. Indian J Radiol Imaging. 2018;28(2):143-8.
15. Mondal SK, et al. Cervical TB. J Cytol. 2017;34(2):111-4.
16. Kulshrestha V, et al. FGTB complications. J Obstet Gynaecol India. 2017;67(5):321-7.
17. Shahdad S, et al. FGTB infertility. Int J Reprod Contracept Obstet Gynecol. 2016;5(8):2563-8.
18. Tripathy SN, et al. Menstrual changes FGTB. J Indian Med Assoc. 2017;115(4):45-9.
19. Sharma JB, et al. Pelvic pain FGTB. Indian J Tuberc. 2016;63(2):115-20.
20. Gupta VK, et al. Systemic symptoms TB. J Assoc Physicians India. 2018;66(6):56-61.
21. Pawlowski A, et al. TB-HIV clinical features. Clin Infect Dis. 2016;54(9):1306-13.
22. Muneer A, et al. FGTB suspicion. J Clin Diagn Res. 2017;11(9):QC06-10.
23. Baxi A, et al. Hysteroscopy in FGTB. J Minim Invasive Gynecol. 2016;23(5):673-9.
24. Thangappah RB, et al. Histopathology FGTB. Indian J Pathol Microbiol. 2017;60(3):321-6.
25. Bhanothu V, et al. TB PCR in FGTB. J Med Microbiol. 2016;65(8):819-27.
26. Kashyap B, et al. AFB culture sensitivity. Indian J Med Microbiol. 2017;35(2):234-9.
27. Gupta N, et al. Ultrasound in FGTB. Indian J Radiol Imaging. 2016;26(4):456-62.
28. Sharma JB, et al. HSG in FGTB. Fertil Steril. 2018;110(4):e234-41.
29. Menzies D, et al. IGRA in TB. N Engl J Med. 2016;364(15):1441-8.
30. Arora VK, et al. FGTB diagnostic challenges. Indian J Tuberc. 2017;64(3):165-70.
31. Sharma JB, et al. FGTB vs. endometriosis. J Obstet Gynaecol India. 2016;66(4):234-40.
32. WHO. TB treatment guidelines 2020. Geneva: WHO; 2020.
33. Nahid P, et al. ATS TB guidelines. Clin Infect Dis. 2016;63(7):e147-95.
34. WHO. FDC dosing 2020. Geneva: WHO; 2020.
35. RNTCP. DOTS strategy India. New Delhi: MoHFW; 2016.
36. Jindal SK, et al. Category II TB. Indian J Chest Dis Allied Sci. 2017;59(2):67-73.
37. WHO. MDR-TB guidelines 2019. Geneva: WHO; 2019.

38. WHO. Rapid communication MDR-TB 2024. Geneva: WHO; 2024.
39. Moonan PK, et al. Non-DOTS TB. Int J Tuberc Lung Dis. 2016;15(9):1164-70.
40. Ramachandran R, et al. AKT monitoring. Indian J Tuberc. 2017;64(4):234-9.
41. Snider DE, et al. Pyridoxine in TB. Am Rev Respir Dis. 2016;122(2):332-4.
42. Dorman SE, et al. AKT side effects. Clin Infect Dis. 2016;50(5):708-14.
43. Gupta A, et al. TB-HIV India. Indian J Med Res. 2017;145(6):723-9.
44. Maartens G, et al. TB-HIV drug interactions. N Engl J Med. 2016;370(24):2340-8.
45. Manosuthi W, et al. Efavirenz in TB-HIV. Clin Infect Dis. 2016;50(9):1267-74.
46. Swaminathan S, et al. TB-HIV management India. Indian J Med Res. 2017;135(6):785-91.
47. Meintjes G, et al. IRIS in TB-HIV. Lancet Infect Dis. 2016;10(7):489-98.
48. Malik S, et al. Tubal infertility FGTB. J Hum Reprod Sci. 2016;9(4):234-9.
49. Ghosh K, et al. Endometrial damage FGTB. Fertil Steril. 2017;108(3):e234-40.
50. Jindal UN, et al. IVF in FGTB. J Assist Reprod Genet. 2016;33(9):1175-81.
51. Sharma A, et al. IVF outcomes FGTB 2024. Fertil Steril. 2024;121(4):456-62.
52. Ethics Committee, ISAR. FGTB counseling. J Hum Reprod Sci. 2017;10(3):234-40.
53. WHO. Extrapulmonary TB guidelines 2020. Geneva: WHO; 2020.
54. RNTCP. Annual report 2023. New Delhi: MoHFW; 2023.
55. Sachdeva KS, et al. MDR-TB India. Indian J Med Res. 2017;145(6):712-8.
56. MoHFW. India TB report 2023. New Delhi: MoHFW; 2023.
57. Rao M, et al. FGTB diagnostic delays. Indian J Med Res. 2019;150(6):543-50.
58. Gupta VK, et al. MDR-TB prevalence India. J Assoc Physicians India. 2018;66(6):56-61.
59. Malhotra N, et al. IVF costs India. Fertil Steril. 2018;110(4):e234-41.
60. MoHFW. ASHA TB program. New Delhi: 2023.
61. Patel N, et al. FGTB stigma India. J Obstet Gynaecol India. 2024;74(1):89-95.

Vaginal Discharge

Ruchika Garg, Shaifali Singh

INTRODUCTION

Vulvovaginitis is a commonly encountered problem in practice. It usually presents with irritation and discharge.

Candidiasis and bacterial vaginosis are the most common causes.

Other causes are *Trichomonas vaginalis* and herpes. Other STIs like chlamydia and gonorrhea present with vaginal discharge.

Noninfective causes include lichen simplex, contact dermatitis, seborrheic dermatitis, and eczema.

In prepubertal girls, threadworm, group A streptococci, and staphylococci may be the cause.

PRURITUS VULVAE

The most common causes of pruritus vulvae are:

- Vulvovaginal candidiasis
- *Dermatoses*:
    - Lichen sclerosis
    - Lichen planus
    - Psoriasis
    - Lichen simplex/vulval eczema
- VIN suspected in chronic cases (*see chapter on Vulval Lesions*)
- Paget's disease
- Atrophy/estrogen deficiency (*given below*)
- Vulvodynia
- *Infections: T. vaginalis* (*given below*), molluscum contagiosum, herpes
- Scabies
- *Worm infestation:* Threadworm, pinworm
- Allergy, tight clothes, contact dermatitis
- *Systemic causes:* Diabetes mellitus, drug allergy

Pruritus vulvae may be acute or chronic.

RECURRENT VULVOVAGINITIS

It will include a brief difference between leukorrhea with no irritation versus vulvovaginitis with irritation. Infective causes of recurrent vulvovaginitis will include candidiasis, herpes simplex, and *Trichomonas* vaginitis. STIs like chlamydia and gonorrhea can also cause recurrent infections with vaginal discharge but this can be prevented by safe sexual practices. DD of bacterial vaginosis with offensive vaginal discharge but no inflammation.

Noninfective causes (dermatoses) mentioned above can be listed.

General advice for all cases: Avoid irritant soaps, use emollients and moisturizers. Wear breathable undergarments.

LEUKORRHEA

Vaginal discharge to some extent is normal and beneficial for women of reproductive age. **Hormonal fluctuations** induce changes in the quantity and type of cervical mucus during the menstrual cycle. **Increase in estrogen levels prior to ovulation results in change in cervical mucus** from nonfertile (thick and sticky) to fertile (thin and slippery).

Normal vaginal flora is dominated by *Lactobacillus* species. There is a predominance of typical gram-positive rods known as *Doderlein's bacilli* observed on microscopy. There are over 20 species of lactobacilli in premenopausal women. Lactobacilli protect the vaginal ecosystem through production of antimicrobial molecules. Lactic acid maintains the pH between 3.5 and 4.5. Hydrogen peroxide inhibits the growth of *Gardnerella vaginalis, Bacteroides,* and *Mobiluncus* which cause dysbiosis. It has been found that a small amount of *Bifidobacterium, Candida, Corynebacterium, Enterococcus, Escherichia, Staphylococcus,* and *Streptococcus* also inhabit the genital tract.

Leukorrhea occurs **before menarche**. A **clear white vaginal discharge** is noted. It occurs because of **desquamated epithelial cells** and **mucous** from estrogenized mucosa. It can begin before thelarche. Unopposed estrogen causes profuse secretions that decrease with concomitant progesterone. As puberty progresses the vaginal pH decreases. Therefore, before puberty infections are caused by gram-positive cocci and gram-negative rods that cause vulvovaginitis but after puberty yeast colonizes. Leukorrhea is **not associated with irritation**. The discharge contains abundant epithelial cells.

CAUSES OF PHYSIOLOGICAL VAGINAL DISCHARGE

- Physiological excess estrogen
- Cervical causes
- Vaginal causes

Physiological Excess

Normally secretion is increased in conditions with increased estrogen levels such as:

- *Puberty:* Elevated endogenous estrogen levels cause the **endocervical epithelium to notably overgrow**, potentially encroaching on the ectocervix and resulting in **cervical ectopy**.
- *During the menstrual cycle:* The **peak surge in estrogen around ovulation** leads to an increase in the **cervical glands' secretory activity**.
- During pregnancy, **increased vascularity and elevated estrogen** cause an increase in cervical gland production and vaginal transudate.
- Bartholin's glands are responsible for copious secretions during **sexual excitation**.

Cervical Causes

- *Noninfective:* Excessive cervical secretion is caused by cervical lesions such as **cervical ectopy**, **mucous polyps**, and ectropion (exposed cervical glands to the vagina).
- **Infective causes:** Acute and chronic cervicitis

Vaginal Causes

- *Noninfective:* Increased vaginal transudate can occur in conditions associated with increased pelvic congestion like **COC use**, **vaginal adenosis** (benign condition where glandular epithelium is present in the vagina, the squamous epithelium fails to replace the columnar epithelium during embryogenesis, it may be associated with exposure to DES), **uterine prolapse, acquired retroverted uterus**, and **chronic pelvic inflammation**. **Ill health** may also cause excessive discharge due to excess exfoliation of the superficial cells.
- **Infective:** Vaginitis

	Physiological causes	*Pathological causes*
Cervical causes	• Cervical ectropion under influence of estrogen • Change in cervical mucous at ovulation • Increased cervical vascularity in pregnancy	Mucous polyp, infection cervicitis
Vaginal causes	COC	Infective vaginitis, prolapse, retroverted uterus, vaginal adenosis with a classic red grape-like mucosa of vaginal fornices (it does not stain with iodine solution)
Bartholin's glands	Increased secretion during sexual excitation	

MANAGEMENT

History:

- Duration and amount of discharge and its association with menstrual cycle
- History of contraception use
- History of vaginal itching
- Associated dysuria, dyspareunia, and pelvic pain
- High-risk sexual behavior and previous history of excessive vaginal discharge

Examination:

- **Abdominal examination:** For presence of tenderness or pelvic mass
- **Vulva inspection:** For signs of vulvitis, ulcers, discharge, or other lesions; color, consistency, and pH of discharge
- **Speculum examination:** For the **color, amount, and consistency of discharge** and to examine cervix and vaginal walls; **mucopus, or mucopurulent secretions** in the endocervical canal, and symptoms of inflammation, such as **edema or friability** must

be checked during the examination. Mucopus or **cervical inflammation** may be a sign of cervicitis.

- **Bimanual pelvic examination** is done to detect presence of **tenderness or mass** in the adnexal and/or uterine region, as well as **cervical motion tenderness**.

Investigations:

- **Pap smear** should be taken before per vaginal examination.
- Microscopic examination of vaginal discharge: Also known as a **"vaginal smear"** or a **"wet mount"**—can be examined for indications of infection; the specimen is processed on a glass slide and evaluated under a **microscope to detect infections such as T. vaginalis**, associated **bacteria, leukocytes, and clue cells**.
- KOH test and **whiff test**
- Vaginal discharge for **Gram staining**
- **Urine** for routine microscopy and culture sensitivity
- HIV serology, VDRL, HBsAg

Table 1 provides the period, associated symptom, and possible diagnosis of abnormal vaginal discharge.

TABLE 1: Abnormal vaginal discharge.

Period	*Associated symptom*	*Possible diagnosis*
Early neonatal period	–	Leukorrhea
Premenarchal period	–	Leukorrhea
	Offensive	Foreign body
	Vulval itching	Threadworm
Reproductive period		
Nonpregnant (related to menstrual cycle)	–	Leukorrhea
COC users	–	Leukorrhea
	Pruritus	Moniliasis
Any period		
	–	Ill health
	Pruritus	Infective vaginitis
	Offensive	Foreign body, neoplasm
During antibiotic therapy	Pruritus	Moniliasis
Diabetes mellitus	Pruritus	Moniliasis
Pregnancy	–	Leukorrhea
	Pruritus	Vaginitis (moniliasis)
Postmenopausal	–	Senile vaginitis
	Pruritus/diabetes mellitus	Moniliasis
	Offensive	• Pyometra • Neoplasm

General Management

- General improvement of health
- Maintenance of **local hygiene**
- Surgical treatment like **electrocautery, cryosurgery, or trachelorrhaphy** for cervical lesions
- Pelvic lesions leading to vaginal leukorrhea require appropriate therapy.
- If symptoms are excessive, **hormonal pills may have to be stopped** temporarily.
- Treatment for **determined infection**

COMMON CAUSES OF VAGINITIS

- Gonococcal
- Chlamydia
- Trichomoniasis
- *Candida*
- Bacterial vaginosis

Gonococcal Vaginitis

Causative organism: *Neisseria gonorrhoeae* (gram-negative *Diplococcus*)

Primary sites of infection: Endocervix (cervicitis), **urethra** (urethritis), Bartholin's glands (bartholinitis) and Skene's glands; other sites of infection are **oropharynx, anorectal region,** and **conjunctiva**.

Incubation period: 3–7 days

The principal site of gonococcal invasion is the **columnar and transitional epithelium of genitourinary tract**.

Vaginitis is not possible in adults because squamous epithelium is resistant to gonococcal invasion but can cause vulvovaginitis in childhood.

Clinical Features

Local symptoms: Dysuria (25%) is the most common urinary symptom. 50% of women have **vaginal discharge** that is excessively uncomfortable. **Mucopurulent urethral discharge** is present. **Swelling over the labia** and intense unilateral pain are symptoms of Bartholin's gland involvement. There could also be discomfort in the rectum, pain, and discharge. There may also be additional symptoms like **intermenstrual bleeding** and pharyngeal infection. 25% patients have abdominal pain generally those with coinfection with chlamydia.

Local signs: Labia could be **swollen** and irritated. There is vaginal discharge that is **mucopurulent**. Purulent exudate leaks out of the congested Bartholin's duct openings and the **external urethral meatus** when pressure is exerted. A **Bartholin's abscess** may form. Concomitant proctitis may occur.

On per speculum examination: Congested ectocervix with **elevated mucopurulent cervical** secretions

Local spread: Gonococcal infection may ascend up and cause **acute PID** in 15% of untreated cases. Infection spreads along the spermatozoa and involve **upper genital organs causing endometritis and salpingitis**.

Distant/metastatic: There may be signs of **septicemia** and **perihepatitis**. Perihepatitis is caused by an infection that spreads to the liver capsule. 10–15% of cases result in **adhesions** to the abdominal wall. Hematogenous spread can cause **arthritis, tenosynovitis, and skin lesions**.

Complications

- Acute PID
- Chronic PID—if not treated adequately
- Chronic pelvic pain
- Dyspareunia
- Infertility
- Ectopic pregnancy
- Tubo-ovarian mass
- Bartholin's gland abscess

Diagnosis

- **Gram staining and culture** of **discharge** often shows gram-negative diplococci within polymorphonuclear leukocytes.
- **Nucleic acid amplification testing (NAAT)** can be performed in **urine or endocervical discharge**. It is very sensitive (>95%). **Vulvovaginal swabs** may be used but **first void sample** should be tested preferably.

Treatment

- Injection ceftriaxone 1 g intramuscularly as a single dose is recommended.
- Dual therapies may be given for treatment failure.
- Cefixime 400 mg with azithromycin 2 g may be used if intramuscular dose is refused.
- Gentamicin intramuscular and azithromycin 2 g.
- Azithromycin monotherapy is not recommended due to macrolide resistance.

In Case of Disseminated Gonorrhea

Investigate sexual partners with contact within 2 weeks if symptomatic. Treat the male partner.

Check for syphilis and chlamydial infection.

Surgical intervention such as cyst removal and abscess drainage in case of Bartholin's abscess is done.

Ceftriaxone 1 g IM/IV daily × 7 days minimum (or until 24-48 hours afebrile), transitioning to oral if susceptible.

Appropriate treatment for gonococcal infections and careful monitoring until the patient has been declared cured are the best ways to prevent recurrences. Avoid sexual contact till treated. Treat the sexual partner concurrently. Advise the women to refrain from having multiple sexual partners and to use condoms.

Follow-up and test of cure is needed to detect failed treatment, failed compliance, and to assess for side effects.

Chlamydial Vaginitis

Causative organism: *Chlamydia trachomatis* (obligatory intracellular gram-negative bacteria)

Serotype:

- D-K causes vaginal discharge (lower genital tract infection) and PID.
- L1, L2, and L3 cause lymphogranuloma venereum.

Incubation period: 6–14 days, can be up to 21 days

It affects young adults. Patients with more than one partner are high risk for chlamydia. Partner concordance is 75%. 50% infections may resolve spontaneously.

Sites of infection: Urethra, Bartholin's glands, and cervix; it can also cause throat infection and conjunctivitis.

Chlamydia affects **columnar and transitional epithelium of the genitourinary tract**. Lesion is limited superficially with no deeper penetration. It may ascend upward like to produce acute **PID**. In 20–40% women it is associated with gonococcal infection.

Clinical Features

Chlamydial infection is usually **asymptomatic and nonspecific**. Presenting symptoms are **vaginal discharge, dysuria, dyspareunia, postcoital bleeding, and intermenstrual bleeding**. It may also cause **lower abdominal pain**.

Local examination findings include **mucopurulent cervical edema and discharge**. Cervix may **bleed** on touch.

On bimanual examination, there may be **pelvic tenderness and lower abdominal tenderness**.

Complications

- **Urethritis** and **bartholinitis:** Manifested by dysuria and purulent vaginal discharge
- **Endometritis, salpingitis, and PID:** Mostly asymptomatic; scarring of fallopian tubes result in **infertility, chronic pelvic pain, and ectopic pregnancy**.
- **SARA (sexually acquired reactive arthritis) in <1% cases**
- **Perihepatitis (Fitz-Hugh-Curtis syndrome):** More common in chlamydia than *Gonococcus*.

Hence early diagnosis and treatment is essential to prevent complications.

Diagnosis

In females, the **vulvovaginal swab is most sensitive. Urethral and rectal swabs** may be taken. Endocervical swabs less sensitive.

Chlamydial **NAAT** *and detection by* **PCR**: Most sensitive and specific test (95%); **first void sample of urine** most effective and specific

Chlamydia antigen can be detected from endocervical samples (lipopolysaccharide) via ELISA technique. Less sensitivity and specificity compared to NAAT

Chlamydia can be demonstrated in tissue culture (McCoy cell monolayers), is 100% specific but expensive, technically difficult, and takes 3–7 days to obtain result.

Test for LGV serotypes in patients with proctitis.

Treatment

- *Doxycycline:* 100 mg BID for 7 days, or
- *Azithromycin:* 1 g orally OD; however, this is avoided due to macrolide resistance.
- *Ofloxacin:* 200 mg orally BID for 7 days or
- *Erythromycin:* 500 mg orally BID for 10–14 days

Sexual partner should also be treated with same drug regimen.

Chlamydia reinfection may occur after 2–5 months and must be distinguished from a treatment failure. Repeat test is recommended as per UK National Guideline after 3 months in patients below 25 years of age as chlamydia is the common STI in UK. Recurrent chlamydia infections are associated with higher chances of PID and infertility.

Patient is advised to avoid sexual intercourse even with condom till treated.

In pregnancy with chlamydia, doxycycline and ofloxacin are contraindicated. The following options may be used:

- Azithromycin 1 g single dose, or
- Erythromycin 500 mg QDS for 7 days
- Amoxicillin 500 mg TDS for 7 days

A test of cure is recommended after 3 weeks.

Chlamydia may be transmitted to the neonate throught the genital tract and can cause ophthalmia neonatorum which presents after first 5–12 days of life. It can also cause *Chlamydia pneumoniae* up to 1–3 months of life. NAAT test is ideally done. It is treated with oral erythromycin or azithromycin.

Trichomonal Vaginitis

Causative organism is flagellated protozoan parasite, *T. vaginalis.*

Incubation period: 3–28 days, with an average of 7 days

Site of infection: In females 90% cases urethra is infected, along with paraurethral glands and vagina. In males, urethra, subprepuce, and penis are the sites affected.

It is the **most common cause pruritus vulvae**. It is a disease of **reproductive age-group**; however, **young girls and postmenopausal women** may be infected.

Modes of transmission: Most common mode of transmission is **sexual**, but women can become infected by **poor hygiene** and use of contaminated towels or clothes. Infection is favored by a **decreased immunity** and **raised pH during menstruation (pH 5–6)**. Women can also be infected with trichomoniasis during **pregnancy** and can be associated with gonococcal infection. Men harbor *T. vaginalis* in their urethra and prostate.

Clinical Features (Fig. 1)

- *Symptoms*: **20% (10–50%) of infected the women are asymptomatic.**

- *Typical discharge:* **Profuse, thin, frothy, slightly green-yellow** in color **vaginal discharge with foul smell and vulval itching** may be presenting features. Vulval ulcers and lower abdominal discomfort may be present.
- Males may present with **urethral discharge**.
  Itching or burning in vagina irritating
  Urinary complaints like increase in **frequency and dysuria** may be present.
  Abdominal pain, low backache, and dyspareunia are also associated with trichomonal vaginitis infection.

Usually, asymptomatic in women, but features of urethritis; and in males urethritis, balanoposthitis, epididymitis, and prostatitis may be present.

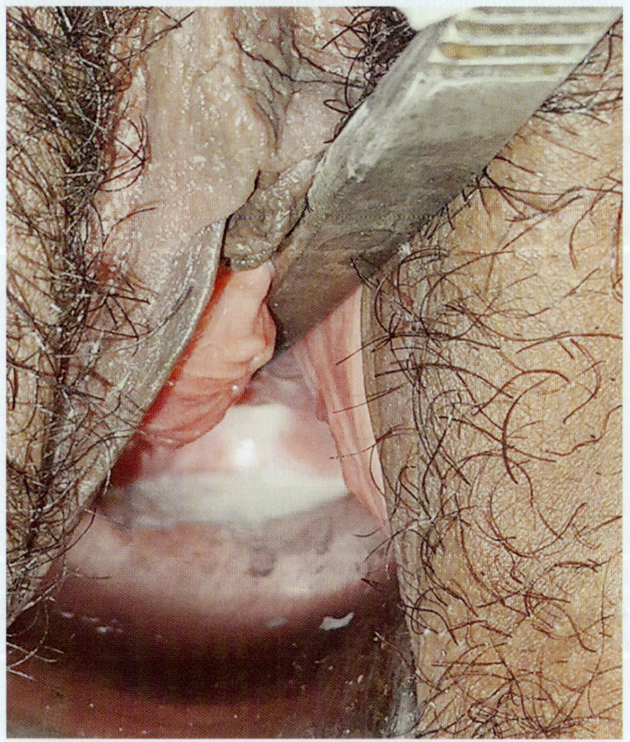

Fig. 1: Discharge of trichomoniasis.

Signs

Per speculum examination: **Vagina is inflammed**, tender, and angry-looking. Multiple, small, punctate, **strawberry spots** on vaginal vault and portio vaginalis of cervix (strawberry cervix/vagina), along with **yellow-green frothy discharge** are diagnostic of trichomoniasis. The characteristic frothy discharge is diagnostic but presence of secondary infection may change and mask the primary findings.

5–15% may have no significant signs.

Specimen

- Swab taken from the posterior fornix
- Urine sample may be taken.

Diagnosis: For **wet film** vaginal discharge is mixed with saline and taken on a slide with a cover slip and examined under microscope. When stained with Gram stain and Leishman stain, *Trichomonas* is in continuous motion which distinguishes it from pus cells may be seen in 10 minutes. *Trichomonas* is also associated with a mixed group of secondary infecting organisms like *Escherichia coli* and pathogenic cocci.

Acridine orange may stain dead *Trichomonas*.

Culture: 98% sensitivity

Other sensitive tests for diagnosing trichomoniasis are PCR and antigen testing.

Pap smear: Grayish, blue, pear-shaped structure without flagella is found to be attached to glycogen-rich superficial squamous cells.

More sensitive tests like **PCR and NAAT** are also available.

Test for **other sexually transmitted diseases** like HIV, syphilis, gonorrhea, chlamydia, etc.

Treatment

- **Metronidazole 500 mg oral BID** for 7 days or **2 g single dose**
- Tinidazole 2 g single dose to both partners can also be prescribed.

Abstinence or use of barrier methods is advised during course of treatment. Treat both partners together irrespective of result of investigation. Effectiveness of metronidazole is 85% effective and is best taken after meal to avoid nausea and vomiting.

Metronidazole 2 g for 1 day can also be given for better patient compliance, multidose treatment is more effective than single dose treatment.

If metronidazole causes vomiting, alternative drugs can be used.

Alcohol is avoided as it can cause disulfiram-like reaction with metronidazole.

- Tinidazole 500 mg BID for 7 days or
- Secnidazole 1,000 mg OD for 2 days

In pregnancy, metronidazole is avoided in the first trimester. Treatment should be started in the second trimester. However, high-dose treatment should be avoided. *Trichomonas* infection can cause preterm labor, low birth weight, and postpartum sepsis.

Retesting for trichomoniasis is recommended for all women 3 months after completion of treatment or whenever women present to OPD because of high risk of reinfection.

For recurrent Trichomonas vaginitis, repeat the course metronidazole 500 BD for 7 days or high-dose metronidazole 800 mg TDS for 7 days' treatment may be given; if the cause of relapse is noncompliance.

Treatment options for **resistant recurrent infection**: High-dose **oral plus vaginal tinidazole** (2 g daily orally and 500 mg vaginally twice daily for 14 days) or **high dose oral tinidazole plus vaginal paromomycin** for 14 days

For detection of reinfection or persistence of infection, culture is preferred over NAAT. Repeat NAAT can only be conducted 3 weeks after completion of treatment, as it can detect clinically irrelevant residual nucleic acid.

Candidiasis/Moniliasis

Candidiasis is a fungal infection caused by *Candida* or Monilia.

Organism: Candida albicans species, which is mostly responsible for human infection is gram-positive yeast

It is a commensal which grows on moist skin, respiratory, GI mucosa, and female genital tract.

25% women harbor *Candida* in vagina. 75% of all women at least once in their lifetime develop vulvovaginal candidiasis.

It may be acute candidiasis or recurrent candidiasis where at least 4 episodes occur in 12 months. 6% have recurrent candidiasis.

Risk factors for candidiasis are:

- HIV
- Pregnancy
- Steroid therapy
- Long-term antibiotic usage
- Hormonal birth control
- Diabetes mellitus
- Obesity
- Poor personal hygiene
- Anemia

Clinical features

Pruritus vulva, vaginal irritation, redness, swelling, presence of flaky and **thick curdy discharge which is nonoffensive** and **painful urination**.

Speculum examination: Vulval **edema, fissures, excoriation**, vaginal congestion, and thick curdy white discharge; vulva and perineum may show **rash with satellite lesions**.

Diagnosis: Diagnosis is made if women present with **typical clinical features** along with identification of *Candida* in either **wet preparation or culture**. **High vaginal swab** may be **Gram stained** to see *C. albicans* blastospores, pseudohyphae, and neutrophils. Absence of neutrophils shows no inflammation which indicates colonization only. 10% KOH solution dissolves all other cellular debris present in vaginal secretion leaving the budding yeast, hyphae or pseudohyphae, and mycelia or spores of *Candida*.

Culture is indicated if wet mount is negative in **symptomatic women**, but treatment should not be started in asymptomatic, culture-positive women as it cannot differentiate between colonization and infection. On culture on Sabouraud's agar colonies appears as black rounded with diameter of 1–2 mm colonies and yeast-like odor. Empirical treatment should be given if culture is not possible. Culture is necessary to confirm at least one of the four episodes of recurrent candidiasis in a year.

Candida can be identified by **Gram staining** of vaginal discharge or presence of **thick red stained hyphae and dark red spores on pap smear**.

Treatment

- **Avoid irritant soaps** and use emollients and moisturizers. Wear breathable undergarments.
- Treat **diabetes mellitus**, treat **anemia**.
- Vaginal application of antifungal creams or pessaries such as clotrimazole, miconazole, tioconazole, butoconazole, and terconazole used for 3–7 days is proved to be very effective.
- **Fluconazole 150 mg orally** single dose is effective.
- **Clotrimazole 500 mg single day** is also effective.

Sexual intercourse can continue. However, **topical antifungals may weaken latex condoms** and diaphragms.

For recurrent infection:

- Fluconazole orally 150 mg every 72 hours for 3 doses and then weekly for 6 months
- Alternatively use imidazole topical 7–14 days and then clotrimazole pessary once a week for 6 months may be used.

Non-albicans vulvovaginal candidiasis (NAC):

- Nystatin 100,000 units twice daily for 14 days is very effective in NAC vaginitis.
- Boric acid suppositories 600 mg vaginally once or twice daily for 2 weeks
- Other treatment options are 17% flucytosine vaginally for 2 weeks, high-dose fluconazole, amphotericin B, and oral posaconazole.

Supportive care like probiotics are also potentially helpful in prevention of reinfection.

Bacterial Vaginosis

Bacterial vaginosis is a vaginal dysbiosis. It is caused by lactic acid-producing *Lactobacillus* species which are **replaced by anaerobic organism such as G. vaginalis, Bacteroides species, Peptococcus species, Mobiluncus, and Mycoplasma**. There is marked decrease in number of lactobacilli in these women.

Clinical Features

- Homogeneous malodorous **(fishy)** creamy (milk-like) **vaginal discharge** which is **adherent** to the vaginal wall and vestibule is pathognomonic of bacterial vaginosis. **pH of vaginal fluid is >4.5**. The term vaginosis is preferred over vaginitis, as there is **no vaginal inflammation**.
- It is the **most common** cause of pathological vaginal discharge worldwide. Although, most of the women are asymptomatic (50%).
- Prevalence is high in women following **high-risk** sexual behavior and in copper-containing **IUD users**. Other risks include **smoking and douching**. Its prevalence not increases in women using hormonal contraceptives. There is increased risk in patients who undergo termination of pregnancy.
- Bacterial vaginosis is not an STI. These women should be screened for other STIs like HIV, gonococcal vaginitis, chlamydial vaginitis, and syphilis.
- Male partners are mostly asymptomatic.

Complications
- Abortion
- Recurrent infection can lead to pelvic inflammatory disease
- Second trimester miscarriage
- Preterm birth
- Preterm premature rupture of membrane
- Chorioamnionitis
- Endometritis
- Vaginal cuff cellulitis following hysterectomy

Diagnosis: **Amsel's** diagnostic criteria are (at least **three of the four** findings are diagnostic of bacterial vaginosis):
1. Homogeneous vaginal discharge
2. Vaginal **pH >4.5** (litmus paper test)
3. **Positive whiff test**
4. Presence of clue cells on wet mount (>20% of cells)

Gram-stained vaginal smear: Presence of more anaerobic vaginosis causing bacteria, with few or absent lactobacilli.

Whiff test: It is considered positive if fishy (amine) odor is detected on adding 10% KOH solution with a drop of vaginal discharge.

Clue cells: A smear of vaginal discharge is prepared with drops of normal saline and is observed under a microscope. If the **vaginal epithelial cells are heavily stippled with coccobacilli** and their **cell borders are obscured**, these cells are known as clue cells (>20% is diagnostic of BV).

Mere isolation of *Gardnerella* is not diagnostic. But a high concentration of *Gardnerella* confirms the diagnosis.

See PID chapter for Hay Ison's criteria.

Differential diagnosis of vaginal discharge is given in **Table 2.**

Treatment

General measures avoid antiseptics, shower gels, and shampoo in bath tub. Avoid douche.
- Metronidazole 500 mg oral BID for 7 days or 2 g stat
- Metronidazole (0.75%) topical gel 5 g (full applicator) daily for 5 days
- Clindamycin 2% cream 5 g (full applicator) HS for 7 days

Alternatively, oral preparations can be given:
- Oral clindamycin can be use in 300 mg BID for 7 days
- Secnidazole 2 g oral granules single dose
- Tinidazole 2 g orally daily for 2 days
- Tinidazole 1 g orally daily for 5 days

Sexual partner of infected women should be treated simultaneously.

TABLE 2: Differential diagnosis of vaginal discharge.

Characteristic	*Trichomoniasis*	*Candidiasis*	*Bacterial vaginosis*	*Chlamydia*	*Normal vaginal discharge*
Color	Greenish yellow	Curdy white	Gray-white	Mucopurulent	White
Consistency	Thin, frothy	Thick	Thin	Thick	Thin
Whiff test	Negative	Negative	Positive (fishy amine)	Negative	Negative
pH	≥5	≤4.5	≥5	≤4.5	≤4.5
Pruritus	+++	++	Nonirritating	–	–
Diagnosis (wet mount M/C)	Motile trichomonas	Hyphae or spores	Clue cells ≥ 20%	Chlamydia NAAT	–
Treatment	Metronidazole	Fluconazole	Metronidazole	Azithromycin	–

Q1. Senile Vaginitis MUHS, 2020. *(10 marks)*

This is a different entity which is associated with the genitourinary syndrome of menopause. It is also called atrophic vaginitis.

Cause: Inflammation is due to thinning of the vaginal epithelium due to estrogen deficiency.

Symptoms: Vaginal dryness, itchiness, and burning micturition; it is associated with symptoms of painful intercourse. It may present with soreness and bleeding after intercourse. There is increased susceptibility to infection.

Sign: Dryness is a sign.

Complications

- Urinary tract infection
- Aerobic vaginitis is a dysbiosis that may occur in patients with atrophic vagina. It occurs due to desquamation with decrease in lactobacilli; increase in *E. coli*, enterococci, staphylococci, and streptococci. It is associated with foul-smelling discharge and redness and edema of the vagina with an increased PH.

Treatment

- Lubrication for sexual intercourse
- Low-dose local estrogen cream or genitourinary symptoms

Syndromic Management Approach (Table 3)

Five steps of syndromic management:

1. History and examination
2. Diagnosis and treatment using flowcharts
3. Education and counseling regarding safe sex practices
4. Partner treatment
5. Record keeping and reporting

It classifies STI/RTI into easily identifiable **syndromes** which are a **combination of the symptoms and signs** as observed by healthcare provider. **Recommended treatment is effective for all** the diseases that **could cause the particular syndrome**.

Syndromic approach is comprehensive, i.e., it includes **patients treatment, education,** and **counseling**.

Drugs are provided in syndromes base color coded kits, numbered from 1 to 7.

Advantages of syndromic approach:
- Standardized and **prompt**
- **Cost-effective** and easy to integrate
- Patient is diagnosed and treated in a **single visit**
- Problem-oriented—**all possible STIs** are treated at once
- Highly effective for syndromes like **urethral discharge and genital ulcer disease**, also satisfactory for lower **abdominal pain**
- **Avoids** use of **laboratory tests**
- Widely practiced worldwide
- Easy to learn and practice
- Can be used by providers at all levels
- Provides adequate time for counseling

Limitations
- It does **not** detect asymptomatic patients.
- **Over-treatment** of patients with single infection
- Financial cost of over-treatment and side effects
- Increase potential for creation of **antibiotic resistance**, especially if full course is not completed
- Some cases of vaginal discharge may remain unresponsive.

TABLE 3: Syndromic case management protocol.

Kit No.	*Syndrome*	*Color*	*Drugs*
Kit 1	• Urethral discharge • Cervical discharge • Anorectal discharge • Painful scrotal swelling • Presumptive treatment	Gray	Tab. Azithromycin 1 g and Tab. Cefixime 400 mg single dose
Kit 2	Vaginal discharge	Green	Tab. Secnidazole 2 g and Tab. Fluconazole 150 mg single dose
Kit 3	Non-herpetic genital ulcer	White	Inj. Benzathine penicillin 2.4 MU stat and Tab. Azithromycin 1 g single dose
Kit 4	Non-herpetic genital ulcer (allergic to penicillin)	Blue	Tab. Doxycycline 100 mg twice daily for 15 days and Tab. Azithromycin 1 g single dose
Kit 5	Herpetic genital ulcer	Red	Tab. Acyclovir 400 mg thrice daily for 7 days
Kit 6	Lower abdominal pain	Yellow	Tab. Cefixime 400 mg 14 days and Tab. Metronidazole 400 mg twice daily and Cap. Doxycycline 100 mg twice daily for 14 days
Kit 7	Inguinal bubo	Black	Tab. Doxycycline 100 mg twice daily for 21 days and Tab. Azithromycin 1 g single dose

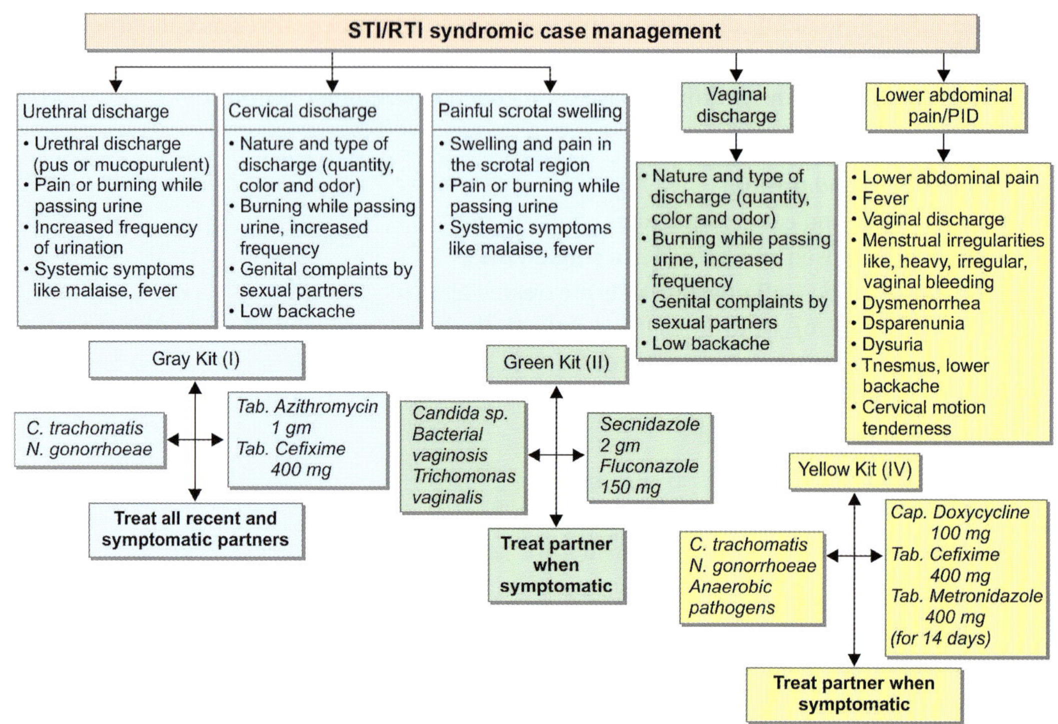

MULTIPLE CHOICE QUESTIONS

Q1. Which worm infestation is common in young girls and can cause vaginal itching and discharge?

a. Threadworm
b. Pinworm
c. Both A and B
d. None of the above

Ans. c. Both A and B

Q2. Which type of vaginitis is common in patients of diabetes mellitus and with use of antibiotics?

a. Candidiasis
b. Trichomoniasis
c. Bacterial vaginosis
d. Gonococcal

Ans. a. Candidiasis

Q3. Complications associated with bacterial vaginosis in pregnancy are:

a. Second trimester miscarriage
b. Preterm birth and PROM
c. Postpartum endometritis
d. All of the above

Ans. d. All of the above

Q4. Amsel's diagnostic criteria for bacterial vaginosis includes:

a. Curdy vaginal discharge
b. Vaginal pH <4.5 (litmus paper test)
c. Positive whiff test
d. Clue cells (>50% of cells)

Ans. c. Positive whiff test

Q5. What is whiff test? Fishy odor when a drop of vaginal discharge is mixed with______

a. 5% potassium hydroxide solution
b. 10 % sodium hydroxide solution
c. 5% sodium hydroxide solution
d. 10 % potassium hydroxide solution

Ans. d. 10 % potassium hydroxide solution

Q6. Name the syndrome for which kit 6 is used:

a. Vaginal discharge
b. Urethral discharge
c. Lower abdominal pain
d. Inguinal bubo

Ans. c. Lower abdominal pain

Q7. Which hormone is responsible for secretary activity in genital tract?

a. Progesterone
b. Estrogen
c. Both of the above
d. None of the above

Ans. b. Estrogen

Q8. What is the average vaginal pH in reproductive age?

a. 5.5
b. 7
c. 6.5
d. 4.5

Ans. d. 4.5

Q9. Drug of choice for bacterial vaginosis is:

a. Metronidazole
b. Erythromycin
c. Tetracycline
d. Nystatin

Ans. a. Metronidazole

SUGGESTED READING

1. Frackelton R, Jones K, Hamer B, et al. Managing contacts of chlamydia: should clinics implement a test and wait process? Int J STD AIDS. 2021;32(1):38-44.
2. Kissinger PJ, Gaydos CA, Seña AC, et al. Diagnosis and Management of Trichomonas vaginalis: Summary of Evidence Reviewed for the 2021 Centers for Disease Control and Prevention Sexually Transmitted Infections Treatment Guidelines. Clin Infect Dis. 2022;74(Suppl_2):S152-S161.

Chronic Pelvic Pain

Ruchika Garg, Shaifali Singh

PART 1: CHRONIC PELVIC PAIN

DEFINITION

Chronic pelvic pain (CPP) is defined as pelvic pain persisting in the same location for **>6 months**, causing **functional disability** or requiring **treatment**. It is localized to the **pelvis**, **anterior abdominal wall below the umbilicus**, or **lower back**.

ETIOPATHOGENESIS OF CHRONIC PELVIC PAIN

Chronic pelvic pain arises from complex interactions between gynecological, gastrointestinal, urological, neurological, musculoskeletal, and psychological factors. Its pathogenesis involves **central sensitization** and **neural plasticity**, leading to persistent pain even after peripheral pathology resolves **(Table 1)**.

TABLE 1: Etiopathogenesis of CPP.

System	*Causes*	*Pathogenesis*
Reproductive	• *Cyclic:* Mittelschmerz, dysmenorrhea, premenstrual syndrome, pelvic congestion syndrome, endometriosis, adenomyosis, ovarian remnant syndrome, uterine fibroids, IUDs • *Acyclic:* Endometriosis, pelvic inflammatory disease (PID), tubo-ovarian abscess, retroverted uterus, prolapse, ovarian cysts, pelvic adhesions, pelvic varicosities, psychosomatic causes	• *Endometriosis:* Prostaglandin/cytokine production (PGE, PGF2α) from petechial lesions; nerve supply in implants causes peripheral/central sensitization • Deep infiltrating endometriosis (rectovaginal, bowel, ureters, bladder) strongly correlates with pain (dyspareunia, dyschezia) • *Adhesions:* Variable pain correlation; these may trap nerves or distort anatomy • *Central sensitization:* Silent nociceptive C-fibers activate, flooding dorsal horn with noxious stimuli, leading to spontaneous neuronal activity, enlarged receptive fields, and lowered firing thresholds
Gastrointestinal	• IBS, inflammatory bowel disease (Crohn's, ulcerative colitis), appendicitis, hernia, intestinal neoplasms	• *IBS:* Visceral hypersensitivity from decreased descending inhibition; central sensitization amplifies pain • Shared innervation (T10–L1) with reproductive organs complicates differentiation

System	*Causes*	*Pathogenesis*
Urological	• Interstitial cystitis (IC)/painful bladder syndrome (PBS), recurrent cystourethritis, sensory urgency, renal stones, bladder tumors, ureteral obstruction	• *IC/PBS:* Defective glycosaminoglycan (GAG) layer allows urine irritants to reach subepithelial nerves; increased mast cell activity, substance P, and nerve growth factor; autoimmune mechanisms; central sensitization causes phantom pain post-cystectomy
Neurological/ musculoskeletal	• Nerve entrapment (iliohypogastric, ilioinguinal, pudendal), myofascial pain syndrome (MPS), pelvic floor dysfunction	• *Nerve entrapment:* Postsurgical (e.g., Pfannenstiel, laparoscopy), trauma, or muscle contraction traps nerves (T12–L2) • *MPS*: Trigger points in skeletal muscle/fascia from intra-abdominal pathology, trauma, or viscerosomatic reflexes • *Central sensitization:* Allodynia, hyperalgesia, and widened receptive fields amplify pain
Psychological	• Anxiety, depression, past trauma (e.g., sexual abuse), stress	• Altered brain networks (reward, motivation, and pain modulation) increase pain vulnerability • Early trauma, conditioning, and fear perpetuate chronicity via CNS changes
Systemic	• Fibromyalgia, abdominal migraine, acute intermittent porphyria, SLE, lymphoma, neurofibromatosis	• Systemic inflammation or neurological dysfunction contributes to pain amplification

KEY PATHOGENIC MECHANISMS

- *Central sensitization:* Persistent noxious input leads to dorsal horn neuronal changes (spontaneous activity, enlarged receptive fields, and lowered firing thresholds), causing allodynia, hyperalgesia, and widened pain fields.
- *Neural plasticity:* Maladaptive CNS changes maintain pain despite resolution of peripheral pathology.
- *Visceral hypersensitivity:* Silent nociceptive C-fibers activate, flooding spinal cord with stimuli, amplifying pain perception.
- *Psychological factors:* Anxiety, depression, and trauma modulate sensory/affective pain components via altered brain pathways.
- *Comorbidities:* Endometriosis, interstitial cystitis (IC), irritable bowel syndrome (IBS), and fibromyalgia often coexist, requiring concurrent treatment.

CLINICAL IMPLICATIONS

- Pain severity may not correlate with pathology (e.g., mild endometriosis causing severe pain).
- Multidisciplinary evaluation is essential due to overlapping etiologies.
- **RCOG (2022):** It emphasizes assessing psychological comorbidities to tailor treatment.

PART 2: EVALUATION AND MANAGEMENT OF CHRONIC PELVIC PAIN IN A 38-YEAR-OLD PATIENT

A 38-year-old woman presents with CPP for 1 year. The following outlines a structured approach to **evaluation** and **management**, emphasizing a multidisciplinary and patient-centered strategy.

EVALUATION

History-Taking

- ***Pain characteristics:***
  - Onset, site, character (cramping, stabbing, dull), duration, aggravating/relieving factors (e.g., posture, menses, coitus), and radiation
  - Use verbal/visual analog scale (0–10) to quantify pain.
- ***Gynecological history:*** Dysmenorrhea, dyspareunia, abnormal vaginal discharge, heavy menstrual bleeding, infertility, and prolapse symptoms
- ***Gastrointestinal history:*** Constipation, diarrhea, bloating, bloody stools, and relation to defecation
- ***Urological history:*** Urgency, frequency, dysuria, hematuria, suprapubic pain, and postvoid fullness
- ***Psychological/other history:*** Anxiety, depression, past trauma, antidepressant use, and chronic diseases (e.g., spondylitis, disc prolapse)

Physical Examination

- ***General/abdominal:***
  - Inspect for scars, hernias; palpate for tenderness, masses.
  - **Carnett test**: It differentiates abdominal wall pain (increased with muscle tensing) from visceral pain (decreased).
- ***Pelvic examination:***
  - Speculum: It assesses cervical/vaginal discharge.
  - Bimanual/rectovaginal: It detects masses, prolapse, and tenderness (e.g., uterosacral ligaments in endometriosis).
- ***Musculoskeletal/neurological:***
  - It assesses pelvic floor, lower back, trigger points, and nerve entrapment (iliohypogastric/ilioinguinal).

Investigations

- ***Gynecological:***
  - Ultrasound (pelvis/abdomen) for fibroids, cysts, adenomyosis
  - MRI/CT if complex pathology (e.g., endometriosis, PAS) suspected
  - Hysteroscopy/endometrial biopsy for intrauterine pathology
  - Laparoscopy: Diagnostic/therapeutic for endometriosis/adhesions (see SAQ 1)
- ***Gastrointestinal:*** Stool analysis, ultrasound, colonoscopy/sigmoidoscopy (consult gastroenterologist)
- ***Urological:*** Urine microscopy, culture, ultrasound (pre/postvoid volume), CT urography, cystoscopy if indicated

- ***Neurological/musculoskeletal:*** Refer to neurologist/orthopedist for nerve entrapment or MPS evaluation.

Diagnostic approach for CPP is given in **Table 2**.

TABLE 2: Diagnostic approach for CPP.

System	*Key history*	*Examination*	*Investigations*
Gynecological	Dysmenorrhea, dyspareunia, abnormal bleeding	Bimanual, speculum, rectovaginal	Ultrasound, MRI/CT, laparoscopy, hysteroscopy
Gastrointestinal	Constipation, diarrhea, bloating, bloody stools	Abdominal palpation, rectal exam	Stool analysis, colonoscopy, ultrasound
Urological	Urgency, frequency, dysuria, hematuria	Suprapubic/pelvic floor tenderness	Urine analysis, ultrasound, cystoscopy
Neurological/musculoskeletal	Trigger points, nerve pain, posture-related pain	Carnett test, pelvic floor assessment	Neurological/orthopedic referral

MANAGEMENT

General Principles

- Multidisciplinary approach involving gynecology, gastroenterology, urology, psychology, and physical therapy
- *Goals:* Pain relief, functional restoration, addressing psychological comorbidities
- Use pain diary (2 menstrual cycles) to track pain (0–10), mood, and triggers (stress, food, and activity).

Management modalities for CPP are given in **Table 3**.

TABLE 3: Management modalities for CPP.

Modality	*Details*	*Indications*
Psychotherapy	Cognitive behavioral therapy (CBT), mindfulness, stress management, hypnosis	Depression, anxiety, past trauma, sexual difficulties
Pharmacotherapy	• *NSAIDs/hormonal therapy:* Suppress ovulation (dysmenorrhea, luteal pain) • *Tricyclic antidepressants (e.g., amitriptyline), gabapentin, and pregabalin:* Neuropathic pain, central sensitization • *Local anesthetics:* Ilioinguinal/pudendal blocks, trigger point injections • *Antispasmodics (dicyclomine, hyoscyamine):* IBS • *Opioids:* Last resort, with narcotic contract	Dysmenorrhea, endometriosis, neuropathic pain, IBS
Physical therapy	Pelvic floor therapy, posture correction, trigger point release	Myofascial pain, pelvic floor dysfunction, fibromyalgia
Laparoscopy	Diagnostic (endometriosis, adhesions); therapeutic (adhesiolysis, cauterization)	Refractory cyclic/noncyclic pain (see SAQ 1)
Hysterectomy	Vaginal/laparoscopic for completed families with adenomyosis, severe endometriosis	Refractory pain without correctable pathology (ACOG criteria)

Specific Considerations

- ***Endometriosis:*** Hormonal therapy (e.g., progestins, GnRH agonists) or laparoscopy; pain may persist due to central sensitization.
- ***IBS/IC:*** Combine medical (antispasmodics, amitriptyline) and behavioral therapy (see SAQs 3, 4).
- ***ACOG (2024):*** Hysterectomy is indicated only for women with CPP > 6 months without correctable pathology, after discussing risks/benefits (PREPARE mnemonic: Procedure, Reason, Expectation, Probability, Alternatives, Risks, Expense).
- ***NICE (2024):*** Regular follow-up to monitor pain and adjust treatment.

SHORT QUESTIONS AND ANSWERS

Q1. Role of Laparoscopy in Chronic Pelvic Pain.

- ***Definition:*** CPP is pelvic pain >6 months causing disability or requiring treatment, encompassing gynecological, gastrointestinal, urological, and musculoskeletal causes.
- ***Role of laparoscopy:***
- **Diagnostic:** Detects endometriosis, adhesions, small inflammatory masses; peritoneal biopsies confirm pathology (RCOG 2012)
- **Therapeutic:** Adhesiolysis, cauterization of endometriotic lesions
- **Indications:** Refractory cyclic/noncyclic pain after excluding non-gynecological causes; trial of hormonal therapy (3–6 cycles) for cyclic pain
- **Limitations:**
  - *Risks:* Death (1/10,000), visceral injury (2.4/1,000)
  - Adenomyosis, some endometriosis, and IBS not visible
  - Poor correlation between macroscopic findings and pain severity
- **Techniques:** Conscious pain mapping, presacral neurectomy, or laparoscopic uterosacral nerve ablation (LUNA); LUNA not superior to laparoscopy alone
- **RCOG (2012):** Reserve for high suspicion of adhesions/endometriosis or fertility concerns; discuss risks/benefits.

Q2. Residual Ovarian Disease (Trapped Ovarian Syndrome) and Remnant Ovarian Syndrome

- ***Residual ovarian disease (trapped ovarian syndrome):***
  - **Definition:** Pain from conserved ovaries post-hysterectomy, becoming cystic, enlarged, or trapped in adhesions; rarely neoplastic
  - **Symptoms:** Cyclic pain (ovulation), CPP, deep dyspareunia, acute pain, or adnexal mass
  - **Investigations:** Ultrasound, MRI, CT (if malignancy suspected)
  - **Management:**
    - Medical: Progestins, combined oral contraceptives, GnRH analogs
    - Surgical: Laparoscopic/laparotomic oophorectomy (challenging due to adhesions; risk of ureter/bowel injury)
    - Malignancy: Staging laparotomy, chemotherapy

- ***Remnant ovarian syndrome:***
  - **Definition:** Pain from ovarian tissue left post-hysterectomy, often due to adhesions (endometriosis, PID)
  - **Symptoms:** Lateralizing CPP, cyclic with ovulation/luteal phase, sharp/stabbing, dyspareunia, constipation, flank pain; tender pelvic mass
  - **Investigations:** Ultrasound, MRI; clomiphene citrate (100 mg, 7–10 days) to enhance ovarian tissue visibility; premenopausal FSH levels
  - **Management:**
    - Medical: Progestins, oral contraceptives, GnRH analogs
    - Surgical: Laparoscopy/laparotomy (adhesion-related risks)
    - Clomiphene presurgery to aid visualization

Q3. Irritable Bowel Syndrome

- ***Definition:*** Chronic abdominal/pelvic pain with altered bowel habits (constipation, diarrhea, or alternating)
- ***Symptoms:*** Pain (exacerbated by eating, stress, menses), bloating, flatulence; relieved post-defecation
- ***Diagnosis:*** Rome IV criteria (pain >6 months, ≥1/week in last 3 months, with ≥2 of: related to defecation, altered stool frequency/form)
- ***Signs***: Tender sigmoid colon, rectal discomfort, hard feces
- ***Investigations:*** CBC, thyroid profile, stool analysis, sigmoidoscopy/colonoscopy (if refractory or older patients)
- ***Management:***
  - Reassurance, lifestyle changes (avoid lactose, fructose, alcohol)
  - Antispasmodics (dicyclomine, hyoscyamine), laxatives, tricyclic antidepressants (low-dose for pain), SSRIs/SNRIs for depression

Q4. Interstitial Cystitis/Painful Bladder Syndrome

- ***Definition:*** Suprapubic pain with bladder filling, plus frequency, urgency, nocturia, without infection/pathology; IC includes cystoscopic/histologic findings
- ***Etiology:*** Defective GAG layer, mast cell activity, substance P, nerve growth factor, autoimmune mechanisms, central sensitization
- ***Symptoms:*** Suprapubic/pelvic/vaginal pain, frequency, urgency, nocturia, occasional hematuria; pain relieved by voiding
- ***Signs:*** Suprapubic/anterior vaginal wall tenderness, microhematuria
- ***Diagnosis:*** Exclusion-based; cystoscopy (glomerulations) not mandatory
- ***Management:***
  - Behavioral: Bladder training, stress management, and dietary restrictions
  - Pharmacotherapy: Amitriptyline (10–150 mg/day), pentosan polysulfate (FDA-approved), urinary alkalinizers
  - Intravesical: Lidocaine, heparin, DMSO (FDA-approved), botulinum toxin (investigational)
  - Sacral neuromodulation for refractory cases

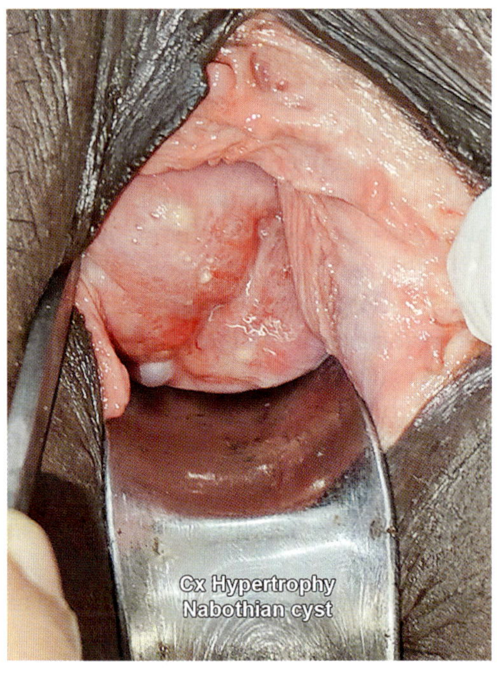

SUGGESTED READING

1. American College of Obstetricians & Gynecologists. Chronic Pelvic Pain. ACOG Practice Bulletin, Number 218. Obstet Gynecol. 2020;135(3):e98-e109.
2. Costantine MM. Physiologic and pharmacokinetic changes in pregnancy. Front Pharmacol. 2014;5:65.
3. Holmgren G, Sjöholm L, Stark M. The Misgav Ladach method for cesarean section: Method description. Acta Obstet Gynecol Scand. 1999;78(7):615-21.
4. Howard FM. Chronic pelvic pain. Obstet Gynecol. 2003;101(3):594-611.
5. National Institute for Health and Care Excellence. (2021). Chronic pain (primary and secondary) in over 16s: assessment of all chronic pain and management of chronic primary pain. NICE guideline: NG193. [online] Available from https://www.nice.org.uk/guidance/ng193 [Last accessed December 2025].
6. Royal College of Obstetricians & Gynaecologists. (2012). The Initial Management of Chronic Pelvic Pain (Green-top Guideline No. 41). [online] Available from https://www.rcog.org.uk/guidance/browse-all-guidance/green-top-guidelines/the-initial-management-of-chronic-pelvic-pain-green-top-guideline-no-41/ [Last accessed December 2025].
7. Sanghavi M, Rutherford JD. Cardiovascular physiology of pregnancy. Circulation. 2014;130:1003-8.

Pelvic Inflammatory Disease

Ruchika Garg

INTRODUCTION

Pelvic inflammatory disease (PID) is an acute or chronic infection of the upper genital tract in women, involving the uterus, fallopian tubes, ovaries, and/or adjacent pelvic structures. It ranges from mild-to-moderate [no tubo-ovarian abscess (TOA)] to severe (systemic symptoms or TOA). PID is a major cause of infertility, ectopic pregnancy, and chronic pelvic pain, with significant reproductive health implications.

EPIDEMIOLOGY

- ***Global:***
  - Incidence: 2–8% among reproductive-age women
  - Complications: 15–20% develop infertility, ectopic pregnancy, or chronic pain
- ***India:***
  - Prevalence: 23–43% (NFHS-2, 1998–99)
  - Common causes: Postabortion, puerperal sepsis, IUD insertions
  - Silent PID: Significant contributor to tubal infertility; often undiagnosed
- ***Trends:*** High burden in young, sexually active women; genital tuberculosis (TB) prevalent in India

ETIOLOGY

- ***Microorganisms:***
  - **Sexually transmitted:**
    - *Chlamydia trachomatis*
    - *Neisseria gonorrhoeae*
    - *Mycoplasma genitalium*
  - **Polymicrobial:**
    - Anaerobes (*Bacteroides fragilis, Gardnerella vaginalis*)
    - Enteric gram-negative rods (*Escherichia coli*)
    - Group B streptococci
  - **Nonsexually transmitted:** Genital TB (India-specific

- ***Risk factors:***
    - Multiple sexual partners, unprotected intercourse, recent IUD insertion, douching, bacterial vaginosis (BV)
    - Hormonal changes during ovulation/menstruation reduce cervical mucus barrier

PATHOGENESIS

- ***Routes of spread:***
- **Ascending:** Most common; vaginal/cervical infection ascends to upper genital tract.
- **Hematogenous:** Rare; seen in TB
- **Local spread:** From adjacent structures (e.g., appendicitis)

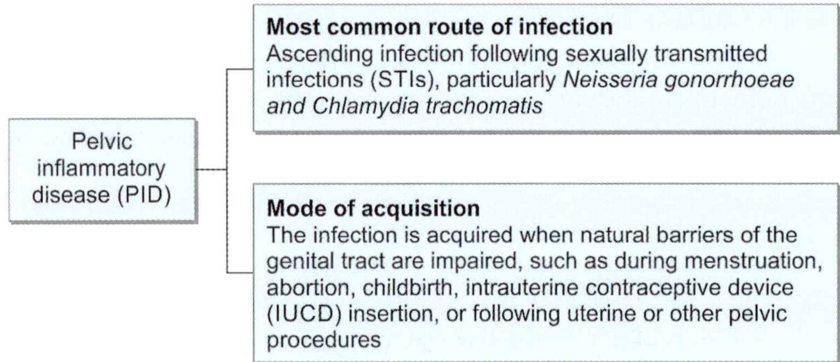

- ***Process:***
    - Cervical infection (often asymptomatic) leads to endometritis, salpingitis, or parametritis.
    - Spread to pelvic cavity causes peritonitis or perihepatitis (Fitz-Hugh-Curtis syndrome).
    - Tubal damage results in adhesions, hydrosalpinx, or TOA.
- ***Antibiotic disruption:*** It alters vaginal flora, promoting overgrowth of nonpathogenic organisms.

CLINICAL FEATURES

- ***Presentation:*** Acute or chronic; varies by organism
- ***Symptoms:***
    - Lower abdominal pain (hallmark)
    - Dyspareunia, abnormal vaginal discharge (purulent, foul-smelling)
    - Menorrhagia, dysmenorrhea, irregular bleeding
    - Dysuria, fever, nausea, vomiting, bloating
    - Severe cases: High fever, tachycardia, right upper quadrant pain (perihepatitis)
- ***Signs:***
    - Cervical motion tenderness, uterine/adnexal tenderness
    - Friable cervix, cervical discharge, pelvic mass (TOA)

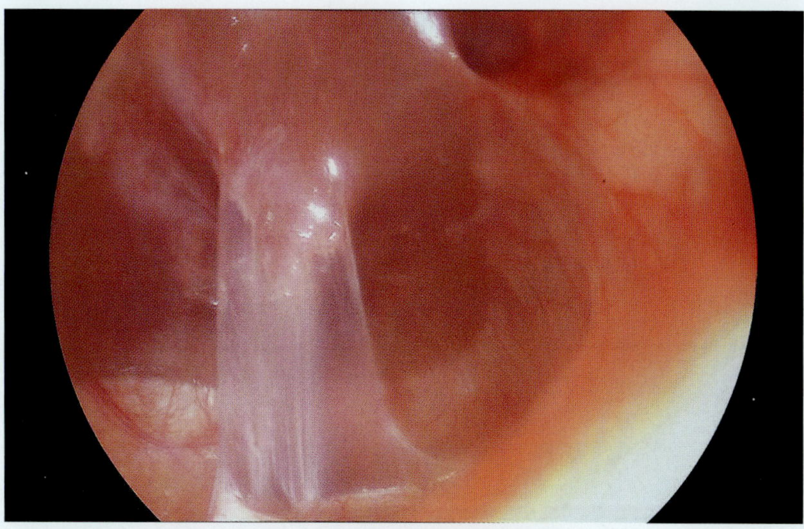

Fig. 1: Violin string appearance, adhesions in PID.

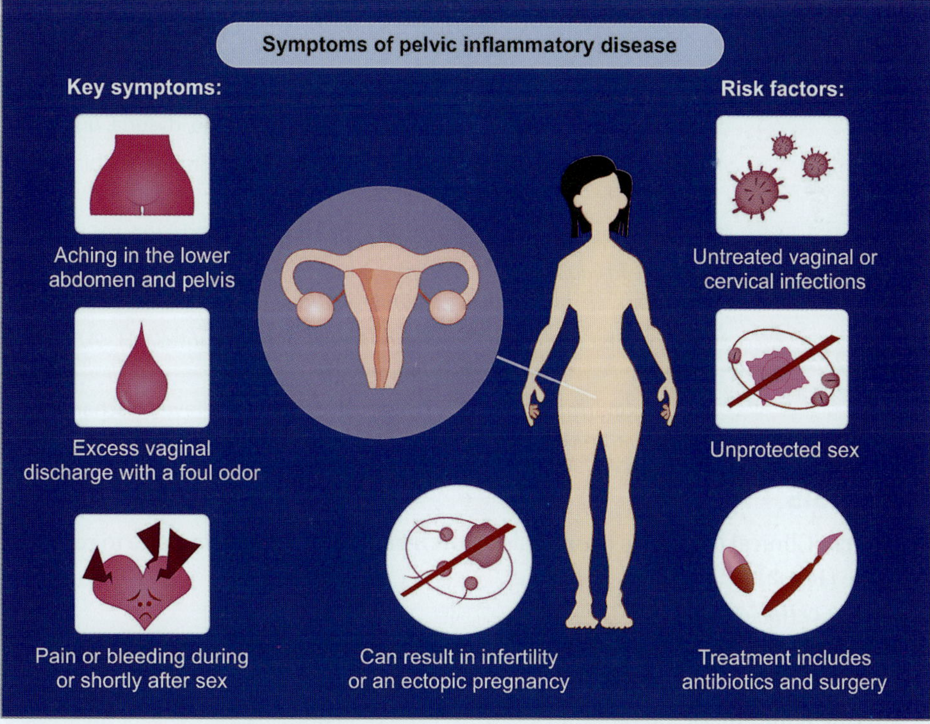

Fig. 2: Symptoms and risk factors of PID.

- **Silent PID:** Minimal/no symptoms; diagnosed during infertility workup

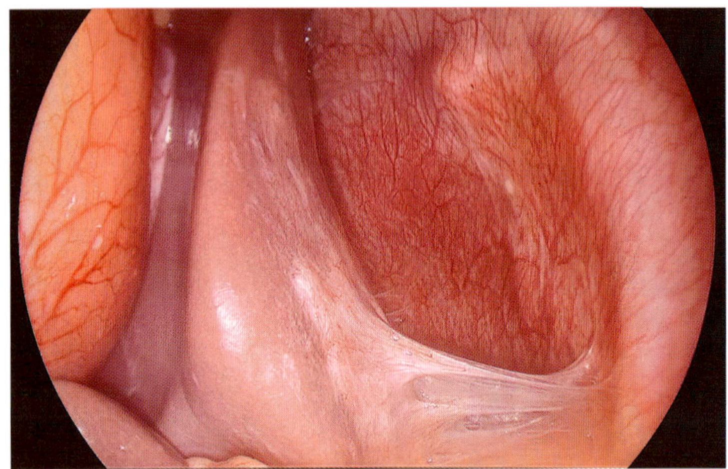

Fig. 3: Perihepatic adhesions Fitz–Hugh–Curtis syndrome.

Table 1 provides clinical features of common STIs/RTIs.

TABLE 1: Clinical features of common STIs/RTIs.

Infection	*Pathogen*	*Features*
Gonorrhea	*Neisseria gonorrhoeae*	Mucopurulent discharge, dysuria, urethritis
Chlamydia	Chlamydia trachomatis	Silent PID, purulent discharge, friable "beefy" cervix
Trichomoniasis	Trichomonas vaginalis	Frothy, foul-smelling discharge, pH >5, itching
Bacterial vaginosis	*Gardnerella vaginalis*, anaerobes	Fishy odor, gray discharge, pH >4.5, no inflammation
Candidiasis	Candida albicans	Curd-like discharge, pruritus, pH <4.5, no foul smell
PID	Mixed (gonorrhea, chlamydia, anaerobes)	Lower abdominal pain, fever, discharge, cervical/adnexal tenderness, mass

DIAGNOSIS

- ***Approach:*** Clinical diagnosis of exclusion; low threshold for suspicion due to reproductive sequelae **(Fig. 2)**
- ***Minimum criteria (CDC, 2021):***
  - Pelvic/lower abdominal pain with no other cause, plus one of:
  - Cervical motion tenderness
  - Uterine tenderness
  - Adnexal tenderness
- ***Additional criteria:***
  - Fever (>38.3°C)

- Mucopurulent cervical discharge, cervical friability
- Elevated ESR/CRP
- Saline microscopy: Abundant WBCs in vaginal secretions
- Nucleic acid amplification test (NAAT): *N. gonorrhoeae, C. trachomatis*

- ***Supportive tests:***
  - Chlamydia antibodies (IgG/IgM), syphilis/HIV/UTI screening
  - Imaging: USG/MRI (TOA, hydrosalpinx, pelvic congestion)
  - Endometrial biopsy: Histologic endometritis (rare)
  - Laparoscopy: Gold standard but invasive **(Figs. 1 and 3)**
- ***Differential diagnosis***: Differential diagnosis includes ectopic pregnancy, appendicitis, ovarian torsion, and endometriosis.

Clinical diagnosis of PID is given in **Flowchart 1**.

Flowchart 1: Clinical diagnosis of PID.

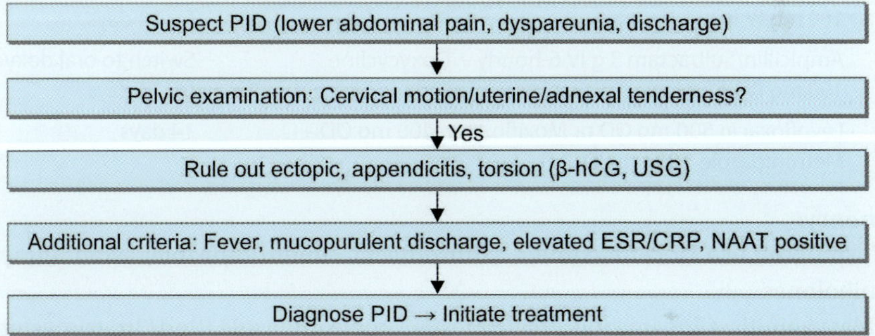

TREATMENT

- ***Approaches:***
  - **Presumptive:** Empirical therapy for at-risk women with minimum criteria
  - **Etiological:** Laboratory-based; delays treatment, risk of loss to follow-up
  - **Syndromic:** WHO-developed; immediate treatment in resource-limited settings

Comparison of diagnostic approaches is given in **Table 2**.

TABLE 2: Comparison of diagnostic approaches.

Aspect	*Etiological*	*Syndromic*
Accuracy	High (laboratory-based)	Lower (overtreatment risk)
Treatment delay	Yes (await results)	No (immediate)
Cost	High (laboratory tests)	Low (no laboratory tests needed)
Follow-up	Risk of loss	Minimal loss
Asymptomatic cases	Detected	Missed

- ***Rationale:*** Broad-spectrum antibiotics covering *N. gonorrhoeae, C. trachomatis*, anaerobes, and BV-associated organisms

Table 3 provides treatment protocols (CDC/NACO, 2021).

TABLE 3: Treatment protocols (CDC/NACO, 2021).

Regimen	*Drugs*	*Duration*
Outpatient (mild/moderate PID)		
I	Ceftriaxone 500 mg IM single dose + Doxycycline 100 mg BD ± Metronidazole 500 mg BD	14 days (Doxycycline ± Metronidazole)
II	Cefoxitin 2 g IM single dose + Doxycycline 100 mg BD ± Metronidazole 500 mg BD	14 days (Doxycycline ± Metronidazole)
III	Ceftriaxone 500 mg IM single dose + Azithromycin 1 g weekly	2 weeks
Inpatient (severe PID/TOA)		
I	Clindamycin 900 mg IV 8-hourly + Gentamicin 2 mg/kg loading, then 1.5 mg/kg 8-hourly	Switch to oral Clindamycin/ Doxycycline for 14 days
II	Cefotetan 2 g IV BD or Cefoxitin 2 g IV 6-hourly + Doxycycline 100 mg IV BD	Switch to oral doxycycline for 14 days
III	Ampicillin/Sulbactam 3 g IV 6-hourly + Doxycycline 100 mg IV BD	Switch to oral doxycycline for 14 days
IV	Levofloxacin 500 mg OD or Moxifloxacin 400 mg OD + Metronidazole 500 mg BD	14 days

- ***Pregnancy:***
  - Hospitalize; use IV cefotaxime + azithromycin + metronidazole; avoid tetracyclines/ quinolones
  - Treat vaginitis: Clotrimazole (1st trimester), metronidazole (2nd/3rd trimester)
- ***IUD users:*** No routine removal; remove if no improvement in 48–72 hours
- ***TOA:***
  - Medical therapy (as above); surgical drainage (laparoscopy/laparotomy) or USG-guided aspiration if no response
  - 10–15% risk of rupture; monitor for sepsis

Drug pharmacokinetics and side effects are given in **Table 4**.

TABLE 4: Drug pharmacokinetics and side effects.

Drug	*Spectrum*	*Pharmacokinetics*	*Side effects*	*Contraindications*
Ceftriaxone	Gonorrhea, gram-negative	IM/IV, *t½* 8.5 h, biliary/ renal excretion	GI upset, rash, leukopenia	Penicillin/cephalosporin allergy
Azithromycin	Chlamydia, gram-positive	Oral, *t½* 68 h, biliary excretion	Arrhythmias, hepatotoxicity	Renal failure (GFR <10 mL/min)
Metronidazole	Anaerobes, protozoa	Oral, >90% bioavailability, liver metabolism	Metallic taste, neuropathy, nausea	1st trimester pregnancy, disulfiram use
Doxycycline	Chlamydia, gram-positive/negative	Oral, 95% bioavailability, biliary/renal	Photosensitivity, GI upset	Pregnancy, children <8 years
Levofloxacin	Gram-positive/ negative, anaerobes	Oral, renal excretion	Tendonitis, CNS effects, QT prolongation	Pregnancy, epilepsy, Marfan's syndrome

COMPLICATIONS

- ***Reproductive:***
  - Infertility: 12% after 1 episode, 25% after 2, >50% after 3
  - Ectopic pregnancy: Sevenfold risk
  - Chronic pelvic pain: 18–30% of cases
- ***Pregnancy-related:*** Preterm labor, stillbirth, miscarriage
- ***Systemic:*** Sepsis, perihepatitis, neurological/cardiovascular issues

PREVENTION

- ***Primary:***
  - Safe sex (condoms), partner education, STI screening
  - HPV/hepatitis B vaccination
- ***Secondary:***
  - Early treatment, contact tracing, partner treatment
  - Avoid douching; regular STI testing in high-risk groups
- ***National strategies (NACO):***
  - STI control programs, prepackaged STI kits, youth education
  - Opportunistic screening during abortion/pregnancy care

GUIDELINES

- ***CDC (2021):***
  - Low diagnostic threshold; empirical treatment for minimum criteria
  - Outpatient therapy for mild/moderate PID; inpatient for severe/TOA/pregnancy
  - Partner treatment for last 60 days; retest chlamydia/gonorrhea at 3 months.
- ***NACO (2020):***
  - Syndromic approach for resource-limited settings; prepackaged kits
  - Emphasize contact tracing, safe sex counseling
- ***WHO (2021):***
  - Syndromic management for STIs; broad-spectrum antibiotics for PID
  - Integrate STI prevention into family planning services.

INDIAN CONTEXT

- ***Burden:*** 23–43% prevalence; TB and postabortion sepsis significant
- ***Challenges:***
  - Silent PID delays diagnosis; limited laboratory access in rural areas
  - Stigma reduces STI reporting; high unprotected sex among youth
- ***Strategies:***

  NACO's STI kits in primary health centers

  ASHA workers for education and contact tracing
- ***2022 study:*** Only 40% of PID cases in rural India treated per guidelines; 20% had silent PID.

CLINICAL CASE SCENARIO

Case: A 28-year-old woman presents with lower abdominal pain, dyspareunia, and purulent vaginal discharge for 5 days. Pelvic examination reveals cervical motion tenderness and adnexal tenderness. Patient has no fever; β-hCG negative.

Management

- **Diagnosis:** Mild PID (clinical criteria met; rule out ectopic)
- **Counseling:** Explain PID sequelae, safe sex, partner treatment.
- **Treatment:** Ceftriaxone 250 mg IM single dose + Doxycycline 100 mg BD + Metronidazole 500 mg BD for 14 days
- **Testing:** NAAT for gonorrhea/chlamydia, HIV/syphilis screen
- **Follow-up:** Review in 48–72 hours; ensure partner treatment.
- **Outcome:** Symptoms resolve; NAAT positive for chlamydia; retest at 3 months.

Examination tip: Highlight low diagnostic threshold, syndromic approach, and partner management.

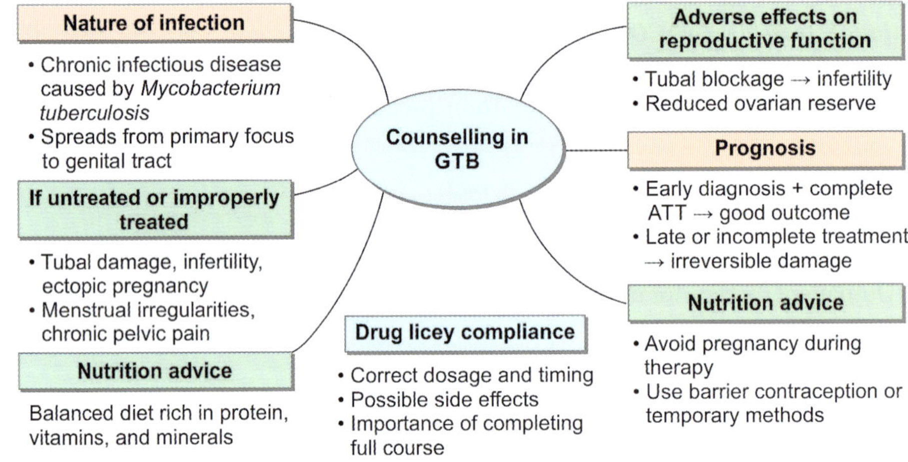

KEY POINTS

- ***Prevalence in India:*** 23–43%; high silent PID burden
- ***Etiology:*** Polymicrobial; chlamydia, gonorrhea, anaerobes, TB (India-specific)
- ***Diagnosis:*** Clinical; cervical motion tenderness + supportive tests (NAAT, USG)
- ***Treatment:*** Broad-spectrum antibiotics; outpatient for mild, inpatient for severe
- ***Complications:*** Infertility (12–50%), ectopic pregnancy (7× risk), chronic pain
- ***Prevention:*** Safe sex, STI screening, NACO's syndromic kits

Box 1 lists the important examination points.

BOX 1: Important examination points.

- ***Minimum criteria:*** Cervical motion/uterine/adnexal tenderness
- ***Syndromic approach:*** Immediate treatment, high cure rates, misses asymptomatic cases
- ***Partner treatment:*** Essential for last 60 days' contacts
- ***TOA:*** Medical therapy first; surgical drainage if no response

SUGGESTED READING

1. Arora R, et al. STI screening in family planning. Indian J Med Res. 2020;152(4):S89-96.
2. Brunham RC, Gottlieb SL, Paavonen J. Pelvic inflammatory disease. N Engl J Med. 2015;372(21):2039-48.
3. Burney RO, et al. Differential diagnosis of PID. Fertil Steril. 2018;110(4):674-81.
4. CDC. PID diagnosis criteria. MMWR. 2021;70(4):1-36.
5. CDC. PID treatment guidelines 2021. MMWR. 2021;70(4):87-94.
6. CDC. STI treatment guidelines 2021. MMWR.
7. Cohen CR, et al. PID and pregnancy outcomes. Lancet Infect Dis. 2019;19(2):e54-60.
8. Dayal S, Singh A, Chaturvedi V, et al. Pattern of pelvic inflammatory disease in women who attended the tertiary care hospital among the rural population of North India. Muller J Med Sci Res. 2016;7:100-4.
9. Duff P. PID in pregnancy. Am J Perinatol. 2017;34(5):452-9.
10. Eschenbach DA. IUD and PID risk. Contraception. 2019;100(4):262-8.
11. Fitz-Hugh-Curtis Syndrome. Am J Obstet Gynecol. 2020;222(6):S896-902.
12. Flagyl (Metronidazole) [package insert]. New York: Pfizer; 2022.
13. Garrett NJ, et al. Syndromic vs. etiological STI management. Lancet Infect Dis. 2018;18(8):e242-50.
14. Golden MR, et al. Partner management in STI. Clin Infect Dis. 2019;64(Suppl 3):S138-44.
15. Granberg S, et al. TOA rupture risk. Ultrasound Obstet Gynecol. 2018;51(6):755-61.
16. Gravett MG, et al. STI treatment in pregnancy. Obstet Gynecol. 2018;132(2):e113-24.
17. Haggerty CL, Totten PA, Tang G, et al. Identification of novel microbes associated with pelvic inflammatory disease and infertility. Sex Transm Infect. 2016;92(6):441-6.
18. Hillier SL, et al. Cervical mucus barrier in PID. J Infect Dis. 2018;217(5):S45-50.
19. Hillis SD, et al. Ectopic pregnancy risk post-PID. Am J Obstet Gynecol. 1997;177(3):529-36.
20. International Institute of Population Sciences. National Family Health Survey 1998–99. Mumbai: IIPS; 2000.
21. Jejeebhoy SJ, et al. Unprotected sex among Indian youth. Reprod Health Matters. 2017;25(1):45-62.
22. Kreisel K, et al. Severe PID manifestations. Sex Transm Dis. 2021;48(4):256-62.
23. Lexicomp. Cephalosporin pharmacokinetics. Wolters Kluwer; 2023.
24. Low N, et al. Douching and STI risk. Sex Transm Dis. 2016;43(4):215–21.
25. Marrazzo JM, et al. STI prevention strategies. Clin Infect Dis. 2020;70(7):S132-8.
26. Meyer T. NAAT in STI diagnosis. Clin Microbiol Infect. 2016;22(8):S36-42.
27. Ministry of Health and Family Welfare. ASHA program for STI education. New Delhi: 2020.
28. Mitchell C, et al. PID microbiology. Clin Infect Dis. 2020;70(5):879-85.
29. Mol BW, et al. Laparoscopy in PID. Hum Reprod Update. 2017;23(4):458-66.
30. National AIDS Control Organisation. STI management guidelines 2020. New Delhi: Ministry of Health and Family Welfare.
31. National AIDS Control Organisation. STI treatment protocols. New Delhi: Ministry of Health and Family Welfare; 2020.
32. National AIDS Control Organisation. STI/RTI clinical features. New Delhi: Ministry of Health and Family Welfare; 2020.
33. National AIDS Control Organisation. Training of Medical Officers to deliver STI/RTI Services. New Delhi: Ministry of Health and Family Welfare; 2020.
34. National AIDS Control OrganisationNACO. STI control program. New Delhi: Ministry of Health and Family Welfare; 2021.
35. Ness RB, et al. Chronic pelvic pain after PID. Obstet Gynecol. 2002;99(5):801-7.
36. Ness RB, Hillier SL, Kip KE, et al. Bacterial vaginosis and risk of pelvic inflammatory disease. Obstet Gynecol. 2004;104(4):761-9.
37. Paavonen J, et al. PID mechanisms. Lancet Infect Dis. 2019;19(7):e232-43.

38. Patel V, et al. Silent PID in rural India. BMC Womens Health. 2019;19(1):102.
39. Peipert JF, et al. Antibiotic disruption in PID. Obstet Gynecol. 2018;131(4):701-7.
40. Revzin MV, et al. Imaging in PID. Radiol Clin North Am. 2019;57(6):1109-24.
41. Rosen M, et al. TOA management. Obstet Gynecol Surv. 2020;75(3):184-92.
42. Ross J, et al. PID clinical features. BMJ. 2017;356:j1043.
43. Savaris RF, et al. PID diagnostic flowchart. Am J Obstet Gynecol. 2020;222(5):S879-85.
44. Sharma JB, et al. Genital TB in India. Indian J Med Res. 2018;148(Suppl):S10-9.
45. Sharma JB, et al. PID burden in India. J Midlife Health. 2021;12(2):78-85.
46. Simms I, et al. Systemic STI complications. Sex Transm Infect. 2017;93(3):201-6.
47. Singh A, et al. PID treatment gaps in rural India. Indian J Obstet Gynecol. 2022;10(3):167-73.
48. Soper DE. PID diagnosis and management. Obstet Gynecol Clin North Am. 2019;46(2):233-46.
49. Sweet RL. PID pathogenesis. Am J Obstet Gynecol. 2017;216(3):S97-103.
50. Walker CK, et al. PID antibiotic rationale. Clin Infect Dis. 2019;68(6):S60-6.
51. Weström L, Joesoef R, Reynolds G, et al. Pelvic inflammatory disease and fertility. A cohort study of 1,844 women with laparoscopically verified disease and 657 control women with normal laparoscopic results. Sex Transm Dis. 1992;19(4):185-92.
52. Westrom L. PID sequelae. Sex Transm Dis. 1994;21(2 Suppl):S24-8.
53. WHO. HPV and hepatitis B vaccination. Geneva: WHO; 2021.
54. Wiesenfeld HC, et al. BV and PID. Clin Infect Dis. 2017;64(6):S111-5.
55. Wiesenfeld HC. PID physical findings. Clin Obstet Gynecol. 2019;62(1):49-57.
56. Wølner-Hanssen P. Silent PID. Lancet. 2018;391(10129):1406-7.
57. Workowski KA, Bachmann LH, Chan PA, et al. Sexually Transmitted Infections Treatment Guidelines, 2021. MMWR Recomm Rep. 2021;70(4):1-187.
58. World Health Organization. STI management 2021. Geneva: WHO; 2021.
59. World Health Organization. STI syndromic approach. Geneva: WHO; 1991.
60. World Health Organization. Syndromic management of STIs. Geneva: WHO; 2021.

Pelvic Congestion Syndrome

Ruchika Garg

Pelvic congestion syndrome (PCS) is a recognized cause of chronic pelvic pain (CPP) in women, characterized by dilated pelvic veins, often linked to ovarian vein incompetence or venous stasis. Its relevance in postgraduate gynecology theory exams, such as MS/DNB Gynecology in India, depends on its clinical significance, diagnostic challenges, and evolving management strategies.

- **Indian Context:**
  - PCS is underdiagnosed in India due to limited access to advanced imaging (e.g., MR venography) and low awareness among clinicians.[6]

OVERVIEW OF PELVIC CONGESTION SYNDROME

- **Definition:** PCS is a condition of chronic pelvic pain (>6 months) due to pelvic venous dilatation, often involving ovarian or internal iliac veins, leading to venous stasis and pain.[8]
- **Epidemiology:**
  - **Global:** Prevalence 12–33% among women with CPP; 10–20% of gynecological consultations.[9]
  - **India:** Estimated 15–25% of CPP cases; underreported due to diagnostic delays (average 4 years).[10]
  - **2024 Study:** 18% of Indian women with CPP had PCS on Doppler ultrasound.[11]
- **Risk Factors:** Multiparity, postpregnancy hormonal changes, prolonged standing, estrogen-mediated vein wall weakening.[12]

TABLE 1: Epidemiology of PCS.[9,11]

Parameter	*Global*	*India*
Prevalence in CPP	12–33%	15–25%
Gynecological visits	10–20%	10–15%
Diagnostic delay	2–4 years	3–5 years

Pathophysiology (Fig. 1)

- **Mechanism:**
  - Ovarian vein engorgement stretches intima, distorting endothelium, releasing vasoactive substances (e.g., nitric oxide), and causing inflammation and pain.[13]
  - Venous stasis due to incompetent valves or anatomical anomalies (e.g., nutcracker syndrome).

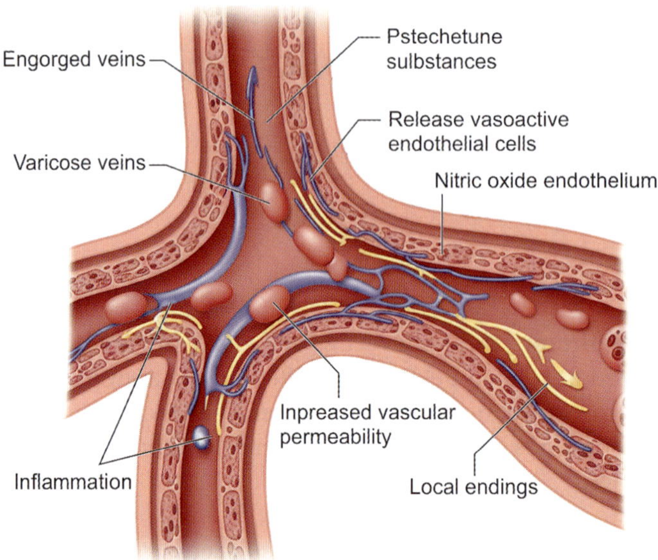

Fig. 1: Pathophysiology of PCS.

- **Hormonal Role:** Estrogen weakens vein walls, exacerbated post pregnancy.[15]
- **Symptoms:**
  - Dull, aching pelvic pain (unilateral/bilateral), worse on standing, post-intercourse, or end of day; relieved by lying down.[16]
  - Associated: Low back pain, leg aches, vulvar varicosities, dysmenorrhea, dyspareunia.[17]
  - Psychological: Anxiety, depression due to chronic pain.[18]

TABLE 2: Clinical features of PCS.[16,17]

Symptom	*Description*	*Prevalence*
Pelvic pain	Dull ache, worse standing/postcoitus	90%
Low back pain	Radiating to lower back	60%
Vulvar varicosities	Visible veins in vulva/thighs	30%
Dyspareunia	Pain during/after intercourse	50%

Diagnosis

- **Clinical Criteria:**
  - CPP >6 months, tender ovaries on pelvic exam, symptoms worse on standing.[19]
- **Imaging:**
  - **Transvaginal Ultrasound (TVUS):** First-line; detects ovarian vein diameter >5–8 mm, low flow velocity, or pelvic varicosities.[20]
  - **Doppler Ultrasound:** Identifies reverse flow during Valsalva.[21]
  - **MR Venography/CT:** Noninvasive; confirms varicosities if TVUS inconclusive.[22]
  - **Venography:** Gold standard; shows vein diameter >5–10 mm, reflux.[23]
  - **Laparoscopy:** Rules out other causes (e.g., endometriosis); not diagnostic for PCS due to vein compression by pneumoperitoneum.[24]

- **Challenges:**
  - Overlap with endometriosis symptoms (e.g., dyspareunia, dysmenorrhea).[25]
  - Imaging alone nondiagnostic; clinical correlation essential.[26]

TABLE 3: Diagnostic modalities for PCS.[20,23]

Modality	*Role*	*Sensitivity*	*Specificity*
TVUS	First-line; detects varicosities	80%	60%
Doppler	Identifies reflux	85%	70%
MR Venography	Confirms varicosities	90%	80%
Venography	Gold standard; diagnostic/therapeutic	95%	90%

Management

- **Medical Therapy:**
  - **NSAIDs:** First-line for pain relief; 60–70% efficacy for mild symptoms.[27]
  - **Medroxyprogesterone Acetate (MPA):** High-dose (30 mg/day) suppresses ovarian function, reduces venous dilatation; 50% pain relief.[28]
  - **GnRH Agonists:** Induce hypoestrogenic state; effective for severe pain but limited by side effects (e.g., osteoporosis).[29]
  - **Dihydroergotamine (IV):** Rarely used; vasoconstrictive effect.[30]
- **Interventional Therapy:**
  - **Embolization/Sclerotherapy:** Transcatheter ovarian vein embolization (coils, sclerosing agents); 80% pain reduction, minimally invasive.[31]
  - **2024 Study:** Embolization improved QOL in 75% of PCS patients at 12 months.[32]
- **Surgical Options:**
  - Laparoscopic ovarian vein ligation: Anecdotal; high morbidity, less effective.[33]
  - Hysterectomy: Residual pain in 33%, 20% recurrence; not preferred.[34]
- **Lifestyle:** Compression stockings, weight management, avoid prolonged standing.[35]

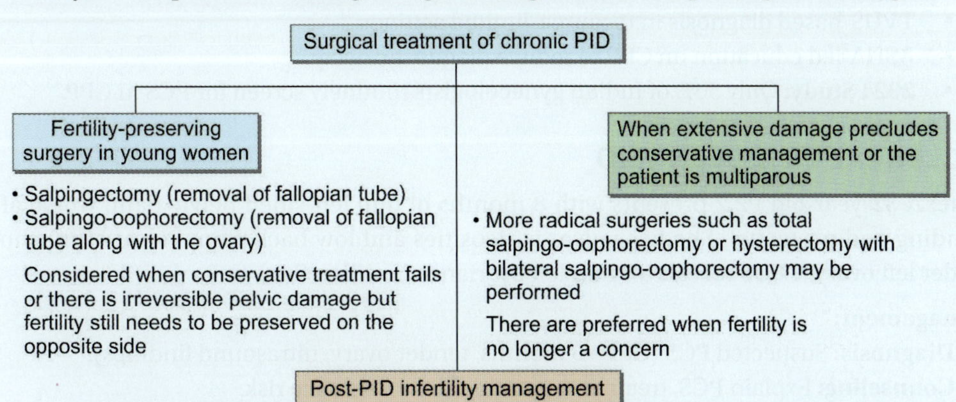

TABLE 4: Treatment options for PCS.[27,31]

Therapy	*Mechanism*	*Efficacy*	*Side Effects*
NSAIDs	Pain relief	60–70%	GI upset, renal risk
MPA	Suppresses ovarian function	50%	Weight gain, mood changes
GnRH Agonists	Hypoestrogenic state	60%	Osteoporosis, hot flashes
Embolization	Blocks varicose veins	80%	Infection, coil migration

RCOG/NICE Guidelines

- **RCOG (2017):**[36]
  - **Diagnosis:** TVUS first-line; venography if intervention planned.
  - **Management:** NSAIDs, hormonal therapy (MPA, GnRH agonists); embolization for refractory cases.
  - **Counseling:** Discuss recurrence risk, psychological impact.
- **NICE (2017, updated 2023):**[37]
  - **Diagnosis:** CPP >6 months; rule out endometriosis, PID via ultrasound/lap.
- **Treatment:**
  - First-line: NSAIDs, progestins.
  - Second-line: Embolization if imaging confirms varicosities.
  - Multidisciplinary approach for CPP management.
- **Research:** Limited high-quality evidence for PCS treatments; embolization studies ongoing.

Indian Context

- **Burden:** 15–25% of CPP cases; diagnostic delay due to low awareness.[38]
- **Challenges:**
  - Limited access to MR venography, embolization in rural areas.[39]
  - High cost of interventional radiology (~₹50,000–1,00,000).[40]
- **Strategies:**
  - TVUS-based diagnosis in resource-limited settings.[41]
  - ASHA-led education on CPP to reduce diagnostic delay.[42]
  - **2024 Study:** Only 30% of Indian gynecologists routinely screen for PCS in CPP.[43]

CLINICAL CASE SCENARIO

Case: A 32-year-old P2,2 presents with 8 months of dull left-sided pelvic pain, worse after standing and postcoital. She has vulvar varicosities and low back pain. Pelvic exam shows tender left ovary. TVUS reveals a 7 mm left ovarian vein with reflux.

Management:

- **Diagnosis:** Suspected PCS (CPP >6 months, tender ovary, ultrasound findings).
- **Counseling:** Explain PCS, treatment options, and recurrence risk.
- **Treatment:**
  - Start with NSAIDs (e.g., ibuprofen 800 mg TDS) for 4 weeks.

    Trial medroxyprogesterone acetate 30 mg/day for 3 months. **Daflon**®, an oral phlebotropic drug, consisting of 90% micronized diosmine and 10% flavonoids expressed as hesperidine improves venous tone and lymphatic drainage and reduces capillary permeability by protecting the microcirculation from inflammatory process.[27]

Mechanism of action: By inhibiting endothelial activation, micronized purified flavonoid fraction (MPFF) (Daflon 500 mg), an edema-protective agent.

It blocks the action of prostaglandins and thromboxane A2 which further prevents the inflammatory cascade resulting from the leukocyte–endothelium interaction. This subsequently delays the appearance of reflux and inhibits the initiation of the vicious circle ending in enhanced venous pressure. Rheological disturbances also play a major role in the appearance of these disorders. Furthermore, venous hypertension provokes leakage from the vessels and capillaries exhibiting increased permeability, leading to increases in hydrostatic load, and overloading of the lymphatic network, which subsequently results fluid exudation causing edema.[28]

Venoactive drugs, containing the bioflavonoids diosmin and hesperidin, play a key role in the medical therapy of PCS. Previous studies have shown that by improving venous tone, MPFF may restore pelvic circulation and provide relief from the symptoms of chronic pelvic pain and a feeling of heaviness in the pelvic area.[29]

Side effects are possibly safe for most people when used for short term. However, it can cause some side effects such as gastritis, diarrhea, dizziness, headache, skin redness and hives, muscle pains, and altered heart rate.

- Contraindicated in bleeding disorders, its safety during pregnancy and breast feeding is not known.
- Refer to interventional radiology for venography/embolization if there is no improvement.

- **Follow-Up:** Reassess pain at 3 months; repeat TVUS if symptoms persist.
- **Outcome:** Pain reduced by 50% with MPA; embolization planned for residual symptoms.
  - **Exam Tip:** Emphasize TVUS as first-line, venography as gold standard, and embolization as effective for severe cases. Differentiate PCS from endometriosis.
  - **LAQ**: "Discuss the etiology, diagnosis, and management of chronic pelvic pain in women, including the role of pelvic congestion syndrome."
  - "Write a note on pelvic congestion syndrome: diagnosis and treatment."
  - **MCQ:** "Which imaging modality is the gold standard for diagnosing PCS?" (Answer: Venography) **(Fig. 2)**.[5]

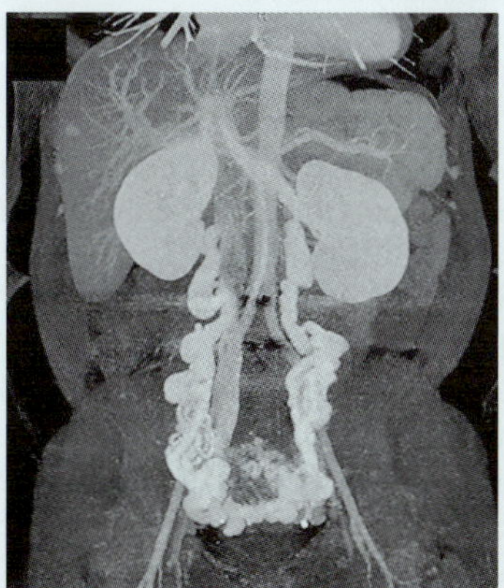

Fig. 2: Pelvic venogram in a patient of pelvic congestion syndrome.

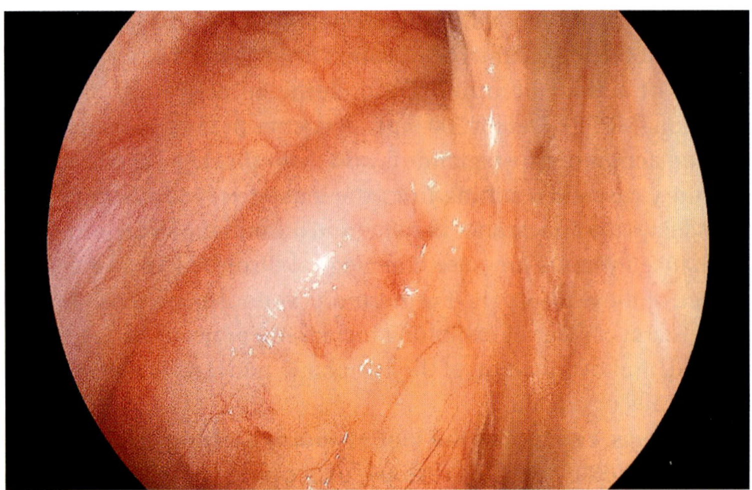

Sharma's Parachute Sign ascending colon being completely attached to the anterior abdominal wall, with its mesocolon resembling an open parachute in genital tuberculosis.

KEY POINTS

- **Exam Relevance:** PCS is occasionally asked as part of Chronic Pelvic pain differential Diagnosis in MS/DNB exams.
- **Prevalence in India:** 15–25% of CPP; underdiagnosed due to limited imaging access.
- **Diagnosis:** TVUS first-line; venography gold standard; clinical correlation essential.
- **Management:**
  - **NSAIDs, MPA** first-line; **embolization** for refractory cases.
  - Limited evidence for GnRH agonists, surgical ligation.
  - **Challenges**: High cost, diagnostic delays in India.

BOX 1: Important points to remember.

- **Key Symptom:** Dull pelvic pain, worse standing/post-coitus, relieved lying down
- **TVUS:** First-line; ovarian vein >5 mm, reflux diagnostic
- **Embolization:** 80% pain relief; minimally invasive

REFERENCES

1. Bendek B, Afuape N, Banks E, et al. PCS review. Curr Opin Obstet Gynecol. 2020;32(4):237-42.
2. Khan KS, et al. CPP in gynecology. Acta Obstet Gynecol Scand. 2016;91(5):525-8.
3. DNB Gynecology Question Bank. New Delhi: 2021.
4. Champaneria R, et al. PCS prevalence. BJOG. 2016;123(3):373-81.
5. Park SJ, Lim JW, Ko YT, et al. PCS ultrasound diagnosis. AJR Am J Roentgenol. 2016;182(3):683-8.
6. Gupta VK, et al. PCS in India. J Indian Med Assoc. 2018;116(5):34-40.
7. Sharma A, et al. CPP differentials India. J Obstet Gynaecol India. 2023;73(2):123-9.
8. Meissner MH, et al. PCS pathophysiology. J Vasc Surg. 2017;65(2):e25-e31.
9. Clark MR, et al. PCS update. Semin Intervent Radiol. 2023;40(4):362-71.
10. Rao S, et al. CPP burden India. Indian J Med Res. 2019;150(6):567-73.

11. Patel N, et al. PCS ultrasound India. Fertil Steril. 2024;121(3):456-62.
12. Gavrilov S, et al. PCS risk factors. Diagnostics. 2022;12(1):145.
13. Beard RW, et al. PCS pathophysiology. Lancet. 2016;2:946-9.
14. Rastogi N, et al. PCS and nutcracker syndrome. Ann Vasc Surg. 2017;26(5):732.e7-11.
15. Stones RW, et al. PCS hormonal factors. Clin Obstet Gynecol. 2017;46(4):831-6.
16. Bendek B, et al. PCS symptoms. Curr Opin Obstet Gynecol. 2020;32(4):237-42.
17. Bartl T, et al. PCS case report. BMC Womens Health. 2021;21(1):181.
18. Kavallieros K, et al. PCS psychological impact. J Vasc Surg Venous Lymphat Disord. 2022;10(4):789-95.
19. Merck Manual. PCS diagnosis. 2023.
20. Labropoulos N, et al. PCS ultrasound protocol. J Vasc Surg. 2018;67(3):e45-e50.
21. Gavrilov S, et al. Doppler in PCS. Diagnostics. 2022;12(1):145.
22. Kim HS, et al. PCS imaging. J Vasc Interv Radiol. 2016;17(2):289-97.
23. Venbrux AC, et al. PCS venography. J Vasc Interv Radiol. 2017;18(6):735-42.
24. Phillips D, et al. PCS laparoscopy limitations. Gynecol Surg. 2016;13(4):245-51.
25. Robinson JC, et al. CPP differentials. Curr Opin Obstet Gynecol. 2017;5:740-3.
26. Steenbeek MP, et al. PCS imaging review. Acta Obstet Gynecol Scand. 2018;97(8):1016-24.
27. Brown CL, et al. PCS medical therapy. J Pain Res. 2017;10:147-53.
28. Farquhar CM, et al. MPA in PCS. Fertil Steril. 2016;106(3):e234-40.
29. Soysal ME, et al. GnRH agonists PCS. Hum Reprod. 2017;32(8):1583-90.
30. Reginald PW, et al. Dihydroergotamine PCS. Br J Obstet Gynaecol. 2016;93(3):270-5.
31. Kim HS, et al. PCS embolization outcomes. J Vasc Interv Radiol. 2016;17(2):289-97.
32. Kumar A, et al. PCS embolization India. J Interv Radiol. 2024;30(2):123-30.
33. Gargiulo T, et al. PCS surgical ligation. Fertil Steril. 2017;108(3):e123-9.
34. Chung MH, et al. PCS hysterectomy outcomes. J Minim Invasive Gynecol. 2016;23(6):873-80.
35. Smith PC, et al. PCS lifestyle management. Phlebology. 2017;32(5):297-304.
36. RCOG. CPP management. Green-top Guideline No. 41. London: RCOG; 2017.
37. NICE. CPP: diagnosis and management. London: NICE; 2023.
38. Mishra VV, et al. CPP India. J Hum Reprod Sci. 2017;10(4):243-50.
39. Malhotra N, et al. PCS access India. Fertil Steril. 2018;110(4):e234-41.
40. Gupta S, et al. PCS cost India. J Obstet Gynaecol India. 2023;73(1):89-95.
41. Rao M, et al. TVUS in CPP. Indian J Med Res. 2019;150(6):543-50.
42. MoHFW. ASHA CPP program. New Delhi: 2023.
43. Sharma P, et al. PCS screening India. J Obstet Gynaecol India. 2024;74(1):123-9.

Thin Endometrium

Ruchika Garg, Neelansha Varshney

INVESTIGATIONAL THERAPIES

Thin endometrium, defined as endometrial thickness (EMT) <7 mm, is a significant challenge in assisted reproductive technology (ART), reducing implantation and pregnancy rates due to impaired endometrial receptivity.[1] Despite advances in ultrasound markers like EMT, blood flow, and uterine volume, their specificity for predicting receptivity remains low. A triple-line endometrial pattern on the day of human chorionic gonadotropin (hCG) trigger is associated with successful implantation, with a minimum EMT of 6 mm generally required, though pregnancies have occurred at 4 mm.[2] This chapter provides an examination-focused overview for MS/DNB gynecology students, integrating updated prevalence, RCOG/NICE guidelines, Indian context, and a clinical case scenario.

EPIDEMIOLOGY

- *Global:*
  - Prevalence: 2.4–10% in ART cycles; higher in women with recurrent implantation failure (RIF)[3]
  - Impact: Pregnancy rates drop to <20% with EMT <7 mm versus 40–50% with EMT ≥8 mm[4]
- *India:*
  - Prevalence: 5–15% in ART patients; linked to clomiphene citrate (CC) use, intrauterine adhesions[5]
  - 2024 Study: 8% of Indian ART patients had EMT <7 mm; 60% had reduced pregnancy rates.[6]
- *Risk factors:* Age >35, obesity, smoking, prior uterine surgery, prolonged progesterone/oral contraceptive use[7]

PATHOPHYSIOLOGY

- *Mechanisms of thin endometrium:*
  - Intrauterine adhesions (Asherman syndrome): Postsurgical scarring reduces endometrial proliferation.[8]
  - CC: Antiestrogenic effects impair endometrial growth.
  - Prolonged progesterone/contraceptives: These suppress endometrial proliferation.
  - Infections: Chronic endometritis disrupts endometrial receptivity.[9]
  - Impaired blood flow: Reduced uterine artery perfusion limits endometrial development.[10]

- *Endometrial receptivity:*
  - Requires adequate EMT (≥7 mm), triple-line pattern, and optimal vascularity[11]
  - Thin endometrium lacks sufficient glandular and stromal development, impairing embryo implantation.[12]

Causes of thin endometrium are given in **Table 1**.

TABLE 1: Causes of thin endometrium.[8,10,13]

Cause	*Mechanism*	*Impact*
Intrauterine adhesions	Scarring postsurgery	Reduced endometrial proliferation
Clomiphene citrate	Antiestrogenic effect	Impaired endometrial growth
Prolonged progesterone/OCPs	Suppression of endometrial proliferation	Thin, nonreceptive endometrium
Chronic endometritis	Inflammation	Disrupted receptivity
Poor uterine blood flow	Reduced perfusion	Limited endometrial development

Measurement of EMT: It is shown in **Figure 1**.

- *Technique:*
  - Transvaginal ultrasound (TVUS): Preferred over transabdominal due to higher resolution[14]
  - Sagittal plane: Measure thickest echogenic area from stratum basalis to stratum basalis, excluding myometrial lucency.[15]
  - Timing: Day of hCG trigger or midluteal phase in frozen embryo transfer (FET) cycles[16]
  - Bladder: Empty to avoid distortion[17]
- *Cutoffs:*
  - Minimum: 6 mm for implantation; pregnancies reported at 4 mm[18]
  - Optimal: 7–10 mm; most ART centers use ≥8 mm as threshold.[19]
- *Triple-line pattern:* Hypoechoic central line with hyperechoic outer layers; indicates receptivity[20]

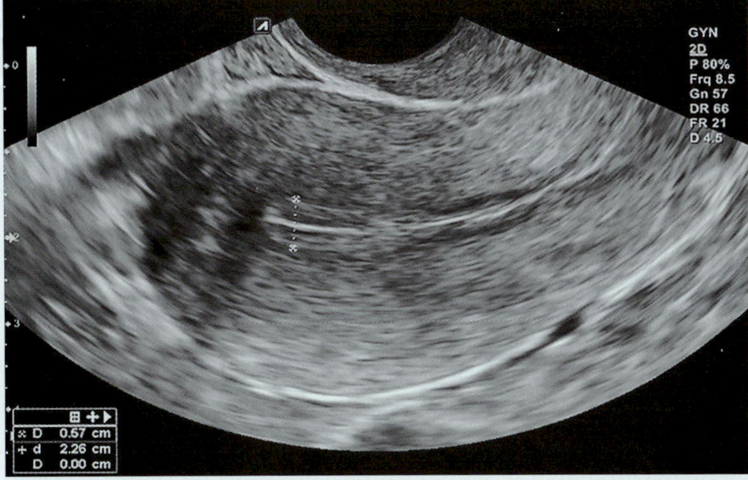

Fig. 1: EMT measurement.[15]

- Sagittal TVUS showing double-layer EMT from basalis to basalis, measured 1 cm from fundal tip.

DIAGNOSIS

- *Ultrasound markers:*
  - EMT: <7 mm on hCG trigger day or FET preparation indicates thin endometrium[21]
  - Endometrial pattern: Triple-line preferred; homogenous or hyperechoic patterns less favorable[22]
  - Blood flow: Doppler assessment of uterine artery pulsatility index (PI); low specificity[23]
- *Hysteroscopy:* Detects adhesions, polyps, or endometritis in refractory cases[24]
- *Endometrial biopsy:* Assesses receptivity markers (e.g., integrin expression) in research settings.[25]

  Flowchart 1 provides evaluation of thin endometrium.

Flowchart 1: Evaluation of thin endometrium.[26]

TVUS: EMT <7 mm on hCG trigger/FET preparation

↓

Assess endometrial pattern (triple-line?) and blood flow

↓

History: CC use, prior surgery, progesterone/OCP exposure

↓

Hysteroscopy if adhesions/endometritis suspected

↓

Initiate cause-specific treatment

TREATMENT MODALITIES

- *Goal:* Increase EMT to ≥7 mm, enhance receptivity, and improve implantation rates.[27]
- *Approaches:* Cause-specific; multifactorial cases require combined therapies.[28]

Low-dose aspirin:

- *Mechanism:* Reduces uterine artery impedance, improves blood flow[29]
- *Dose:* 75 mg/day from cycle day 1 to embryo transfer[30]
- *Evidence:*
  - Small RCT ($n = 28$): No significant improvement in EMT, pregnancy, or live birth rates in women with EMT < 8 mm[31]
  - Cochrane Review (2019): No substantial benefit for EMT or pregnancy outcomes[32]
- *Side effects:* GI upset, bleeding risk[33]

Luteal estradiol:

- *Mechanism:* Promotes endometrial proliferation, reduces oxygen tension for implantation[34]
- *Forms:*
  - Oral: Micronized estradiol, estradiol valerate (2–6 mg/day)[35]
  - Vaginal: Higher endometrial estradiol levels; preferred for refractory cases[36]

REFERENCES

1. Burney RO, Giudice LC. Pathogenesis and pathophysiology of endometriosis. Fertil Steril. 2012;98(3):511-9.
2. Giudice LC, Kao L. Endometriosis. Lancet. 2004;364:1789-99.
3. Ilangavan K, Kalu E. High prevalence of endometriosis in infertile women with normal ovulation and normospermic partners. Fertil Steril. 2010;93:e10.
4. Guo SW, Wang Y. The prevalence of endometriosis in women with chronic pelvic pain. Gynecol Obstet Invest. 2006;62:121-30.
5. Rocha AL, Reis FM, Petraglia F. New trends for the medical treatment of endometriosis. Expert Opin Investig Drugs. 2012;21(7):905-19.
6. Bedaiwy MA, Alfaraj S, Yong P, et al. New developments in the medical treatment of endometriosis. Fertil Steril. 2017;107(3):555-65.
7. Shakiba K, Bena JF, McGill KM, et al. Surgical treatment of endometriosis: a 7-year follow-up on the requirement for further surgery. Obstet Gynecol. 2008;111(6):1285-92.
8. Allen C, Hopewell S, Prentice A, et al. Nonsteroidal anti-inflammatory drugs for pain in women with endometriosis. Cochrane Database Syst Rev. 2009;2:CD004753.
9. Jensen JT, Schlaff W, Gordon K. Use of combined hormonal contraceptives for the treatment of endometriosis-related pain: a systematic review of the evidence. Fertil Steril. 2018; 110(1):137-152.e1.
10. Razzi S, Luisi S, Ferretti C, et al. Use of a progestogen only preparation containing desogestrel in the treatment of recurrent pelvic pain after conservative surgery for endometriosis. Eur J Obstet Gynecol Reprod Biol. 2007;135:188-90.
11. Olive DL. Medical therapy of endometriosis. Semin Reprod Med. 2003;21:209-22.
12. Aznaurova YB, Zhumataev MB, Roberts TK, et al. Molecular aspects of development and regulation of endometriosis. Reprod Biol Endocrinol. 2014;12:50.
13. Harada T, Momoeda M, Taketani Y, et al. Low-dose oral contraceptive pill for dysmenorrhea associated with endometriosis: a placebo-controlled, double-blind, randomized trial. Fertil Steril. 2008;90:1583-8.
14. Menakaya U, Infante F, Condous G. Consensus on current management of endometriosis. Hum Reprod. 2013;28:3162-3.
15. Casper RF. Progestin-only pills may be a better first-line treatment for endometriosis than combined estrogen-progestin contraceptive pills. Fertil Steril. 2017;107:533-6.
16. Ferrero S, Barra F, Leone Roberti Maggiore U. Current and Emerging Therapeutics for the Management of Endometriosis. Drugs. 2018;78(10):995-1012.
17. Practice Committee of the American Society for Reproductive Medicine. Treatment of pelvic pain associated with endometriosis: a committee opinion. Fertil Steril. 2014;101(4):927-35.
18. Harrison RF, Barry-Kinsella C. Efficacy of medroxyprogesterone treatment in infertile women with endometriosis: a prospective, randomized, placebo-controlled study. Fertil Steril. 2000;74(1):24-30.
19. Vercellini P, Pietropaolo G, De Giorgi O, et al. Treatment of symptomatic rectovaginal endometriosis with an estrogen-progestogen combination versus low-dose norethindrone acetate. Fertil Steril. 2005;84(5):1375-87.
20. Buggio L, Somigliana E, Barbara G, et al. Oral and depot progestin therapy for endometriosis: towards a personalized medicine. Expert Opin Pharmacother. 2017;18(15):1569-81.
21. Harada T, Taniguchi F. Dienogest: a new therapeutic agent for the treatment of endometriosis. Women Health (Lond). 2010;6(1):27-35.
22. Schindler AE. Dienogest in long-term treatment of endometriosis. Int J Womens Health. 2011;3:175-84.

23. Bizzarri N, Remorgida V, Leone Roberti Maggiore, et al. Dienogest in the treatment of endometriosis. Expert Opin Pharmacother. 2014;15:1889-902.
24. Momoeda M, Taketani Y, Terakawa N, et al. A randomized, double-blind, multicenter, parallel, dose-response study of dienogest in patients with endometriosis. Jpn Pharmacol Ther. 2007;35:769-83.
25. Strowitzki T, Faustmann T, Gerlinger C, et al. Dienogest in the treatment of endometriosis-associated pelvic pain: a 12-week, randomized, double-blind, placebo-controlled study. Eur J Obstet Gynecol Reprod Biol. 2010;151:193-8.
26. Strowitzki T, Marr J, Gerlinger C, et al. Dienogest is as effective as leuprolide acetate in treating the painful symptoms of endometriosis: a 24-week, randomized, multicentre, open-label trial. Hum Reprod. 2010;25(3):633-41.
27. Petraglia F, Hornung D, Seitz C, et al. Reduced pelvic pain in women with endometriosis: efficacy of long-term dienogest treatment. Arch Gynecol Obstet. 2012;285(1):167-73.
28. Harada M, Osuga Y, Izumi G, et al. Dienogest, a new conservative strategy for extragenital endometriosis: a pilot study. Gynecol Endocrinol. 2011;27(9):717-20.
29. Yamanaka A, Hada T, Matsumoto T, et al. Effect of dienogest on pain and ovarian endometrioma occurrence after laparoscopic resection of uterosacral ligaments with deep infiltrating endometriosis. Eur J Obstet Gynecol Reprod Biol. 2017;216:51-5.
30. Angioni S, Nappi L, Pontis A, et al. Dienogest. A possible conservative approach in bladder endometriosis. Results of a pilot study. Gynecol Endocrinol. 2015;31(5):406-8.
31. Morotti M, Sozzi F, Remorgida V, et al. Dienogest in women with persistent endometriosis-related pelvic pain during norethisterone acetate treatment. Eur J Obstet Gynecol Reprod Biol. 2014;183:188-92.
32. Leone Roberti Maggiore U, Remorgida V, Scala C, et al. Desogestrel-only contraceptive pill versus sequential contraceptive vaginal ring in the treatment of rectovaginal endometriosis infiltrating the rectum: a prospective open-label comparative study. Acta Obstet Gynecol Scand. 2014;93:239-47.
33. Lan S, Ling L, Jianhong Z, et al. Analysis of the levonorgestrel-releasing intrauterine system in women with endometriosis. J Int Med Res. 2013;41(3):548-58.
34. Vercellini P, Frontino G, De Giorgi O, et al. Comparison of a levonorgestrel-releasing intrauterine device versus expectant management after conservative surgery for symptomatic endometriosis: a pilot study. Fertil Steril. 2003;80:305-9.
35. Gomes MK, Rosa-e-Silva JC, Garcia SB, et al. Effects of the levonorgestrel-releasing intrauterine system on cell proliferation, Fas expression and steroid receptors in endometriosis lesions and normal endometrium. Hum Reprod. 2009;24:2736-45.
36. Lockhat FB, Emembolu JO, Konje JC. The evaluation of the effectiveness of an intrauterine-administered progestogen (levonorgestrel) in the symptomatic treatment of endometriosis and in the staging of the disease. Hum Reprod. 2004;19:179-84.

Imaging in Gynecology

Sharmeen Vazifdar, Gaurav Desai

INTRODUCTION

In routine gynecology practice, imaging methods are used to confirm or exclude a diagnosis that is suspected on medical history taking and detailed clinical examination. The first-choice imaging technique in the management of most gynecological conditions is ultrasonography, while other imaging methods have been used as second step to evaluate patients in case of diagnostic dilemmas.[1-3]

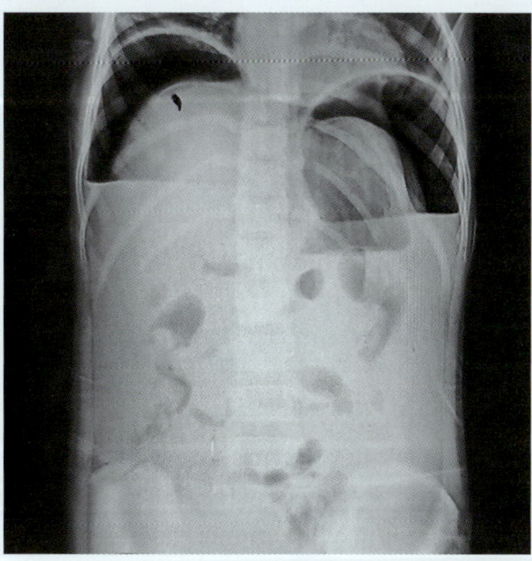

X-ray showing gas under diaphragm perforation.

KEY QUESTIONS

1. What are the various imaging modalities used to investigate a gynecology case?
2. What is the role of ultrasonography in gynecology?
3. What are the key differences between transabdominal and transvaginal sonography?
4. What are the advantages of transvaginal sonography over transabdominal?
5. What are the advantages of CT scan?
6. What are the applications of MRI in gynecology?
7. Where are plain X-rays used in gynecology cases?
8. What is the role of HSG in gynecology?
9. What are the principles of PET scan?

IMAGING MODALITIES

The various imaging modalities in gynecology are:
1. Ultrasonography
2. Computed Tomography (CT) Scan
3. Magnetic Resonance Imaging (MRI)
4. Conventional radiology: X-rays, Hysterosalpingography (HSG)
5. Positron Emission Tomography (PET) Scan

ULTRASONOGRAPHY

INTRODUCTION

The first choice for screening is ultrasonography. In ultrasonography, the sound waves travel through soft tissues and fluid and then bounce back from dense surfaces to create an ultrasound image. It is a noninvasive imaging technique.

Indications

Gynecological ultrasonography can be used in the diagnosis of:
- Pelvic pain.
- Dysmenorrhea (painful menses).
- Menorrhagia (excessive menstrual bleeding).
- Metrorrhagia (irregular uterine bleeding).
- Menometrorrhagia (excessive bleeding irregularly).
- Evaluation and/or monitoring of infertile patients.
- Delayed menses or precocious puberty.
- Postmenopausal bleeding.
- Abnormal pelvic examination.
- Evaluation of congenital anomalies.
- Excessive bleeding, pain, or fever after pelvic surgery or delivery.
- Localization of intrauterine contraceptive device.
- Screening for malignancy in patients with an increased risk
- In the diagnostic workup of pelvic masses suspected on the basis of history and pelvic clinical examination
- In the differential diagnosis of other acute abdominopelvic diseases (appendicitis, diverticulitis, inflammatory bowel diseases)
- In the peri- and postmenopausal diagnostic evaluation of women with atypical uterine bleeding

Ultrasonography can be by two routes: (A) transabdominal and (B) transvaginal.

A. Transabdominal Sonography

In transabdominal sonography, the sonography probe is placed on the abdomen, and the distended bladder underneath is used to bounce off the sound waves and view the pelvic structures. Therefore, for a pelvic sonogram performed transabdominally the patient's urinary bladder should be distended adequately to displace the small bowel and its contained gas from the field of view. However, the visualization is limited by attenuation from the body wall and the distance of the transducer from the area of interest.

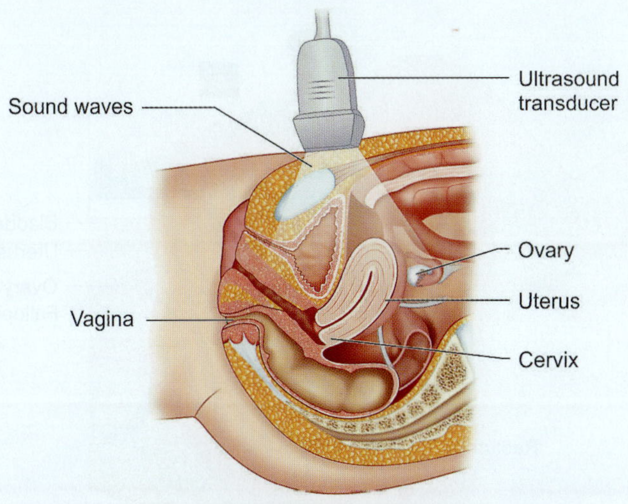

Transabdominal sonography.

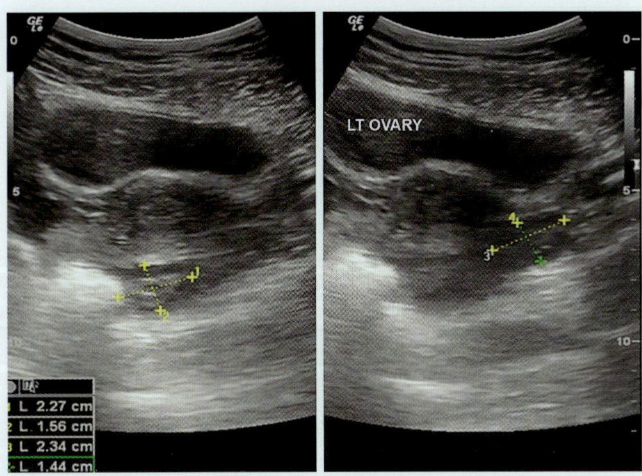

Sagittal and transverse views of the pelvis.

Left image is the sagittal view of the pelvis. Bladder is the dark area. Uterus is the area to the right as marked with the arrow. The bright line in the uterus is the endometrium. The cervix is posteriorly and vagina is to the right side. When the transducer probe is rotated 90° counter-clockwise, you see the orientation to the right.

B. Transvaginal Ultrasonography

In the transvaginal sonography, a transducer is inserted into the vagina. Sagittal, coronal, and oblique images of the pelvic viscera may be obtained. Transvaginal scanning is now the examination technique of choice. However, certain conditions do not allow transvaginal sonography: The integrity of the hymen, women's refusal to undergo an imaging technique that they consider invasive.

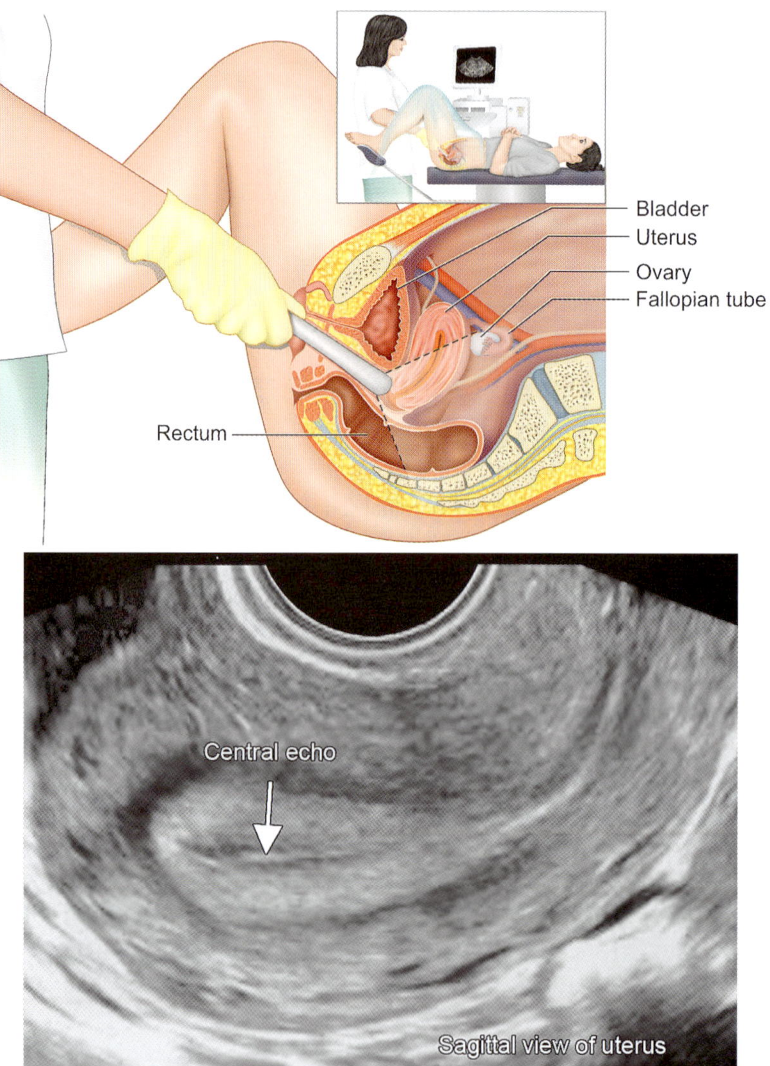

Advantages of transvaginal ultrasonography over transabdominal ultrasonography.

Transvaginal ultrasonography has several advantages over transabdominal ultrasonography:

1. In transvaginal ultrasonography, the transducer is placed closer to the scanning target, therefore giving better resolution.
2. A full or partially full bladder is needed in transabdominal ultrasonography whereas in transvaginal ultrasonography a full urinary bladder is not needed, resulting in a procedure that is more acceptable to patients.

3. The quality of images of transvaginal ultrasonography has been found to be better than transabdominal ultrasonography in most instances, although the depth of penetration is comparatively limited.
4. The transvaginal approach has superior tissue characterization of the uterus and ovaries.

Abdominal scan	*Vaginal scan*
• Low frequency • Abdominal transducer C1-5 (1–5 MHz) • Poor resolution • Good overview • Scan the abdomen • Full bladder	• High frequency • Vaginal transducer R1C5 (5–9 MHz) • Superb resolution • Poor overview • Abdomen not seen • Empty bladder

Sequence for visualizing and checking pelvic organs during ultrasonographic evaluation: First check the bladder—walls, distension. Then uterus for position, dimensions, myometrium, endometrium cervix, and volume, followed by both ovaries and adnexa for ovarian dimension, morphology, and then cul-de-sac for fluid.

COMPUTED TOMOGRAPHY (CT) SCAN

INTRODUCTION

Computed tomography (CT) Scan came into clinical practice in the early 1970s. It was the first imaging modality that could achieve a view of anatomy in multiple "slices". CT combines X-ray images taken from different angles around the body and uses computer processing to create cross sectional images of the bones, blood vessels, and soft tissues inside the body. CT provides more detailed information than plain X-rays. It has excellent spatial resolution and allows better interpretation of images

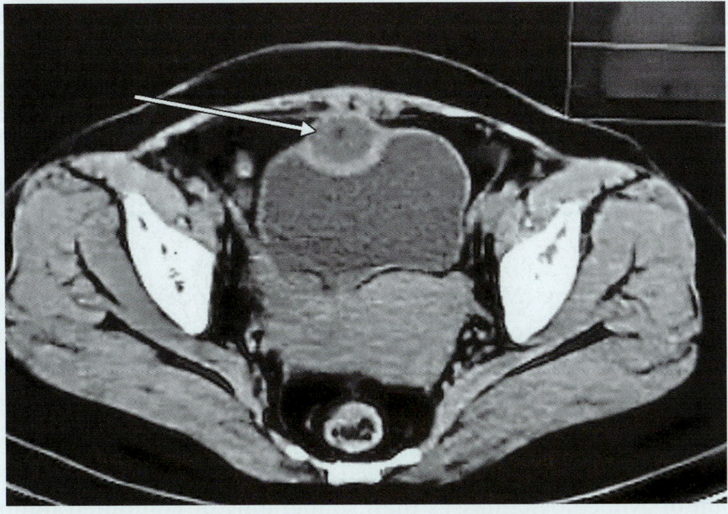

CT scan of female pelvis axial view.

The optional, yet common use of IV contrast helps with differentiation of tissues such as blood vessels, lymph nodes, and the presence of tumors.

ADVANTAGES OF CT

CT plays an important role when the results of ultrasonography are inconclusive or unclear. CT scan helps to evaluate pelvic mass, particularly in staging of malignant conditions. Large masses are best evaluated due to the larger field of view and to better characterize and delineate advanced pelvic diseases such as PID; to aid in the preoperative staging of ovarian, uterine, and cervical malignancies; to assess treatment response of gynecologic malignancies; and to assess for tumor recurrence. CT is the best modality to evaluate postoperative complications such as abscesses, fistulas, hematomas, ureteral injuries, and retroperitoneal complications. CT-guided biopsies and procedure to drain pelvic fluid collections can also be done. Women frequently have CT imaging performed as a first step in the evaluation of pelvic or abdominal pain.

DISADVANTAGES OF CT

The major disadvantage of CT is the exposure to ionizing radiation. Radiation exposure should be weighed against the benefits when a decision is being made to order this imaging technique. The radiation level of CT is between 5 and 10 mSv as compared to which relative level of radiation exposure in ultrasonography and MRI is zero. If abdominal or pelvic CT is done with and without contrast, the exposure can be in the range of greater than 10 mSv, which is considered as being high exposure.

CONTRAINDICATIONS

- Pregnancy: CT should be used with extreme caution for diagnostic purposes in pregnancy, especially in the first trimester
- Related to contrast: In patients who are either allergic to contrast, those with renal compromise, those who are at high risk for acute radio contrast nephrotoxicity, and those in renal failure.[4]

MAGNETIC RESONANCE IMAGING (MRI)

INTRODUCTION

Magnetic resonance imaging (MRI) is one of the great modern advances in the field of imaging and has vast clinical applications in medical science. In MRI, radiofrequency pulses are directed at living body tissue/organ in magnetic field; the tissue emits back (reflected) the modulated radiofrequency signals which are used to construct the image of emitting tissue or organ. It also provides cross-sectional images of the body and gives good soft-tissue detail of pelvic organs. MRI is highly advanced. It has greater accuracy and specificity for characterization of gynecologic masses than sonography or computed tomography (CT). However, due to its cost, it should generally be performed after pelvic sonography. It is superior to USG and CT but is expensive.

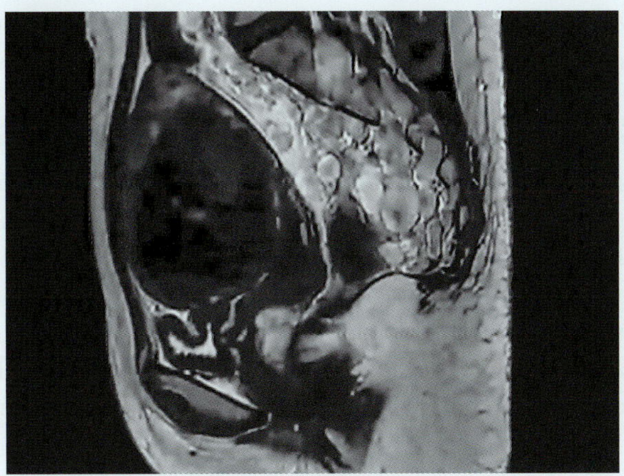

Normal female pelvis T2 sagittal view.

APPLICATION OF MRI IN GYNECOLOGY

The use of MRI in gynecology was first found in 1983. Due to natural contrast provided by pelvic fat, urine in the bladder and gas in the bowel, the pelvis is particularly well suited to MRI. There is less movement induced blurring than in the upper abdomen and chest. It has the advantage of not using ionizing radiation, allows multiplanar imaging, and is suitable for imaging in pregnancy and in the childbearing years. Recently, there have been improvements in hardware and software design, thus giving even better resolution of images along with shorter examination times. It is indicated when USG diagnosis is inadequate or for staging of carcinoma.

INDICATIONS

MRI is used to:

- Study normal uterus and adnexa—with the aim to have clear image of myometrium, endometrium, ovary, and follicles within the ovary.
- Myoma—to differentiate myoma from adenomyoma. Localization of myoma—subserous/intramural or submucous.
- Accurate diagnosis adenomyosis
- Diagnose congenital uterovaginal anomalies—bicornuate septate, subseptate, unicornuate, didelphys, rudimentary horn and vaginal atresia and associated renal anomalies.
- Gynecological cancers

    Staging of gynecologic malignancy is based on the International Federation of Gynecology and Obstetrics (FIGO) system, and cross-sectional imaging is helpful in preoperative planning

- Cervical cancer—extent of parametrial and pelvic organs, pelvic lymph nodes, endocervical.
- Endometrial cancer—myometrial invasion, downward extension to cervix
- Ovarian cancer—malignant versus benign mass, ascites, retroperitoneal node >1 cm, bowel bladder anorectal parietal peritoneum, liver or omental metastasis
- Pregnancy complicated by genital cancer

- More recently, MRI has been used to image the pelvic floor for assessing the degree of prolapse, the compartments involved and, postoperatively, the results of surgery.

ADVANTAGES OF MRI OVER OTHER TYPES OF IMAGING TECHNIQUES

MRI has several advantages over computed tomography (CT) and ultrasonography.

- It is noninvasive. The imaging components include a large static magnetic field and an electromagnetic field produced by radiofrequency (RF) waves.
- It is capable of multiplanar imaging.
- MRI has good tissue-differentiating capabilities,
- MRI is its intrinsically sensitive to flowing blood. As with Doppler ultrasonography, flow direction and speed may be determined. It is possible to assess both arterial and venous abnormalities by MRI.
- It is the most sensitive for diagnosis of adenomyosis.
- It can accurately diagnose congenital malformation of the genitourinary tract; retroperitoneal node >1 cm can be identified; deposits on bowel, bladder, and liver can be identified in cases of cancers.
- It can assess infiltration of myometrial cervical wall, adjoining organs, and parametrium, thus helping in preoperative staging of genital carcinomas.
- It is safe in pregnancy—useful in diagnosing obstetric conditions as well as differentiation of tumors (benign/malignant) complicating pregnancy.
- MRI is superior to CT in diagnosing lymph gland metastasis in any pelvic malignancy. It can also be used to evaluate origin and nature of any pelvic mass like tubo-ovarian mass or abscess, endometrioma, and ovarian tumor.

TABLE 1: Utility of MRI in gynecology compared with Ultrasonography and CT.

	MRI	*Ultrasonography*	*CT*
Normal pelvic anatomy	+++	+++	+++
Leiomyomas	+++	++	++
Adenomyosis	++	–	?
Endometrial cancer	++	–	+
Myometrial invasion	+++	–	+/–
Cervical cancer	+++	–	++
Vaginal cancer	++	–	+
Simple/functional	++	+++	+
Hemorrhagic	++	+	+
Dermoid	+++	++	+
Endometrioma	+	–	–
Ovarian cancer	+/–	+/–	+
Müllerian anomalies	++	++	?
Tumor involvement of	+/–	–	+/–
Pelvic thrombophlebitis	++	+	+

IMAGING ON MRI

T1- and T2-weighted images are obtained by varying the time of application of radiofrequency pulses and sampling the emitted signals. Various tissues appear with varying intensity and brightness in T1 and T2 images. Depending on their molecular morphology, different tissues emit different radiofrequency signals and hence different intensity and brightness. Paramagnetic contrast agents like Gadolinium-DTPA are used for better demarcation of adjoining tissue.

The appearance of an image changes markedly depending on the emphasis of T1 or T2 relaxation times. For example, on a T1-weighted image, fat appears bright (white), whereas fluid appears dark. On a more T2-weighted image, fat appears gray, whereas fluid appears bright (white). Most but not all pathology, because of its increased water content, mimics fluid; that is, it is dark on T1-weighted images and bright on T2-weighted images.

TABLE 2: Magnetic resonance signal intensity of tissue.

Tissue	*T1-Weighted images*	*T2-Weighted images*
Fat	Increased	Slightly increased
Blood	Variably increased or decreased	Variably increased or decreased
Pus	Slightly decreased	Increased
Inflammation	Decreased	Increased
Edema	Decreased	Increased
Serous fluid	Decreased	Increased

SAFETY OF MRI

No ill effects have been demonstrated with exposure levels currently used in imaging.

It can be safely used for imaging when indicated in pregnancy.

CONTRAINDICATIONS

A potential risk during MRI is injury from flying metal objects that are drawn to the magnet. Accordingly, patients entering the MRI unit should be wearing no metallic objects (e.g., hairpins, pens).

MRI in patients with cardiac pacemakers is contraindicated due to the effects of magnetic field on the device.

MRI in patients with surgical ferrous intracranial aneurysm clips and embedded shrapnel are also contraindicated.

Finally, one significant concern is claustrophobia, because patients lie on a sliding bed that is then placed within the magnet, which is approximately 52 cm in diameter and 6 feet long. Approximately 1–5% of patients are mildly uncomfortable. Appropriate patient support or medication may be necessary to complete the requested study.[5]

CONVENTIONAL RADIOLOGY

INTRODUCTION

Conventional radiology involves the use of X-rays. X-rays are a form of electromagnetic radiation.

A. X-RAYS

In gynecology, the following radiological examinations are used:

- Chest X-ray is needed to exclude secondary metastasis in malignant conditions of the pelvis and for pleural effusion in Meig's and pseudo-Meig's syndrome.
- Plain X-ray abdomen is used to locate lost intrauterine devices (IUDs).
- Chest X-ray is required in preoperative evaluation of patients.

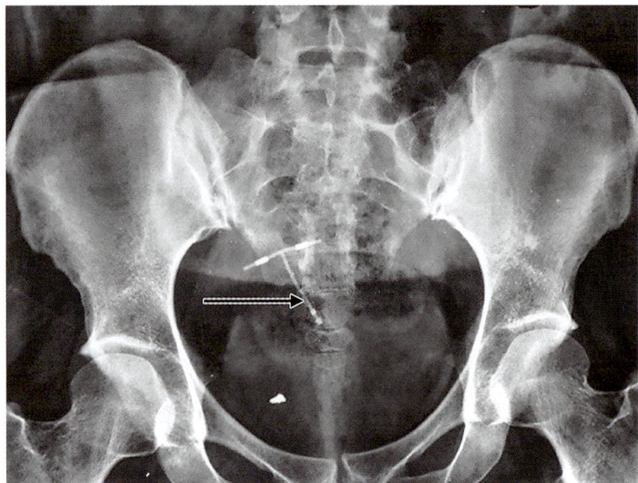

X-ray image of displaced Intrauterine Contraceptive Device (IUCD).

B. HYSTEROSALPINGOGRAPHY (HSG)

Introduction

It is a procedure in which radiopaque dye (iodine dye) is introduced from the vagina into the uterine cavity. This dye then travels through the fallopian tube and comes out through the fimbrial end of the tubes, spilling into the peritoneal cavity. Hysterosalpingography (HSG) has been the first line of investigation anatomy and contour of uterine cavity along with fallopian tube and its patency. It can be used to detect the uterine malformation, synechiae, fibroids, distorted uterine cavity, and patency of the fallopian tube.

Indications

- To check tubal patency while investigating for infertility.
- To check for tubal abnormality—tubal polyps, tubal malignancy, hydrosalpinx salpingitis isthmica nodosa (SIN) , tubal spasm: can be physiological, salpingectomy

- To detect uterine abnormality—uterine congenital anomalies, Submucosal uterine fibroids, uterine malignancy, adenomyosis, intrauterine adhesions, uterine (endometrial) polyps.
- For diagnosis of uterine synechiae
- Lost intrauterine contraceptive device (IUCD)

Procedure

Written informed consent is obtained and then HSG is performed under aseptic conditions. The patient is placed in supine position on the radiology table and cervix is visualized. Then the patient is placed where the X-ray is to be taken and disinfection of the perineum and vagina is to be done; then a sterile Cusco speculum is inserted into the vagina. The cervix is held with a tenaculum. Then, a Leech-Wilkinson cannula is placed in the cervical canal and through it 10–15 cc of iohexol is injected into the uterus to visualize the cervical canal, uterine cavity, and fallopian tubes. Three to six images are taken of the patients, the first of which is after the complete injection of the contrast agent; the time taken to complete the procedure with contrast agent injection is 3-30 minutes.

Timing: Day 7–9 of the menstrual cycle

HSG can is performed in the first 10 days after the last menstrual cycle (between the 4th and 13th days of the menstrual cycle). In this way, the possibility of unintentional irradiation of the developing fetus in an undetected early pregnancy and the possibility of ectopic pregnancy are prevented.

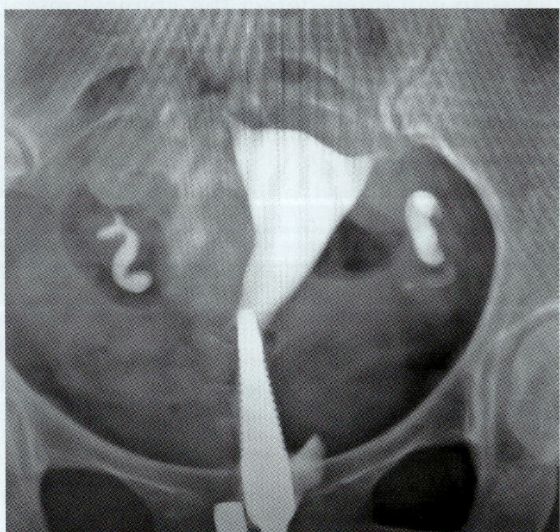

Contraindications

- The primary contraindication is pregnancy. Therefore, timing is after menstruation. In addition, a beta-HCG test is ordered to confirm the absence of pregnancy.
- Active pelvic infection is a contraindication since there is a high-risk factor for infection following this procedure.
- Recent surgery on the tubes or the uterus is also a contraindication due to the likelihood of uterine perforation or tubal rupture, or due to the weakness of the healing tissues.

- Hypersensitivity to contrast agents is obviously a contraindication to its use in this procedure.
- Active bleeding from the vagina and suspected malignancy are also contraindications to its performance.

PET SCAN

INTRODUCTION

Positron emission tomography (PET) scanning is an imaging technique which utilizes radiotracers for measuring various metabolic processes in the body. Various changes in metabolism, blood flow, and regional chemical composition can be analyzed by it. The PET images are typically combined with CT or MRI and are called PET-CT or PET-MRI scans. It has primary use in the field of oncology.

INDICATIONS

PET presently has the highest sensitivity among all the imaging modalities in identifying malignant cells (10^8–10^9 cells). The specificity is higher than routine conventional imaging like CT and MRI.

TRACER IN PET

In PET scan, a radioactive drug called a tracer is used, which shows both typical and atypical metabolic activity. A PET scan can often detect the atypical metabolism of the tracer in diseases before the disease shows up on other imaging tests, such as CT and MRI. The tracer is most often injected into a vein in the arm. After that, the tracer then collects into areas of the body that have significantly higher levels of metabolic activity or biochemical activity. This is what often pinpoints the exact location of the disease.

Radiotracers can be injected, swallowed, or inhaled depending upon the site of the body which is to be examined. The tracer then gets trapped in different tissues of the body depending upon the affinity. Areas of higher activity will show higher uptake and brighter spots on images. A computer then uses this data to form a 3D image of the tracer that is in the body. Various tracers are utilized depending on the targets. A contrast may be administered intravenously or orally if a PET-CT is to be done. Tracer used commonly is called fluorine-18 (18F) fluorodeoxyglucose (FDG), also known as [18F] FDG PET. 18F-FDG, being a glucose analog, gets taken up by the cells instead of regular glucose for metabolism. Glucose gets phosphorylated by hexokinases. The values of the mitochondrial form of this enzyme are raised in cancers that are rapidly growing. In areas of cancer, the metabolic activity is increased; hence, the glucose uptake is also increased. So, this 18F-FDG also gets picked up significantly in these areas, and then this shows up as a bright spot on the PET scan. In a similar manner, this helps in detection of metastasis also.

PET-CT ROLE IN ONCOLOGY

PET scan is excellent for staging of the disease—good in identifying nodal and distant metastasis. It is the best modality to identify response to chemotherapy or radiotherapy. It is helpful in evaluation of disease recurrence.

COMPLICATIONS

PET-CT has complications involved with contrast administration, including possible anaphylaxis, contrast-induced nephropathy, etc. Generally, the radiotracers used do not cause any significant side effects.

CONTRAINDICATIONS

- *Pregnancy:* PET-CT involves radioactive material, and exposure to radiation in the dose of 14 mSv. Therefore, it is contraindicated in pregnant ladies as radioactivity can affect the fetus.
- *Breastfeeding:* A breastfeeding woman should limit close contact with infants or pregnant women for up to 12 hours. Breast milk may be discarded until 12 hours and after about 24 hours, it is considered safe to breastfeed again.

REFERENCES

1. Froyman W, Timmerman D. Role of imaging in gynaecology. In: Dewhurst's Textbook of Obstetrics & Gynaecology. Blackwell Publishing; 2018. pp. 499-518.
2. Busse RM. Imaging modalities in gynecology. Donald School J Ultrasound Obstet Gynecol. 2010;4(1):1-2.
3. Taylor H, Moore C. Imaging in gynaecology. Curr Obstet Gynaecol. 2006;16(3):154-60.
4. Busse RM. Imaging modalities in gynecology. Donald School J Ultrasound Obstet Gynecol. 2010;4(1):1-2.
5. Kay H, Spritzer C. Glob. libr. women's med. (ISSN: 1756-2228) 2008; DOI 10.3843/GLOWM.10067 FIGO guidelines.

SECTION 6

Menopause

CHAPTER 48

Menopause

Ruchika Garg

BACKGROUND

Menopause is a phenomenon that occurs universally and with increased life expectancy, many females in most parts of the world tend to spend almost 1/3rd of their lifetime beyond 50 years of age. The world's elderly population will be more than double from 1998 to 2025, rising from 264 million in 2009 to 416 million in 2050.[1] In 1990, it was estimated that there were almost 500 million women aged 50 years or over worldwide and this number is expected to increase to 1.2 billion by 2030. By that time, 76% will be living in developing countries. About 50 million women worldwide reach menopause each year.[2] The term menopause relates to permanent cessation of menses that marks the end of a woman's reproductive years due to loss of ovarian follicular activity and is a retrospective diagnosis. The event is said to have occurred after 12 consecutive months of amenorrhea for which no physiological or pathological cause has been ascertained. The term climacteric or perimenopausal phase has been replaced by menopausal transition and begins 4–7 years preceding menopause during which the endocrinological, biological, and clinical features of declining ovarian activity appears.

The average or median age of menopause globally is between 50 and 52 years[3] and in India it is approximately 47 years of age.[4] Various demographic (race, ethnicity, education, employment), menstrual and reproductive history (parity and OCP use), familial, genetic and lifestyle (e.g. smoking, weight, physical activity and diet) are important determinants of the age at which menopause is attained.[4] Age at natural menopause may be a surrogate marker of overall health and general well-being as late age of menopause (52 years and beyond) has been associated with:

- Improved overall survival and life expectancy along with decrease in overall mortality.[5,6]
- Decreased risk of cardiovascular diseases (ischemic heart diseases), stroke, atherosclerosis.[7-11]
- Decreased risk of osteoporosis and fractures.[12,13]
- Slight increased risk of endometrial, breast, and ovarian cancers.[14,15]

Lifestyle interventions for management of postmenopausal osteoporosis

Calcium and vitamin D intake

1,200 mg/day calcium
800–1,000 IU/day vitamin D
Reduce fracture risk by 10–15%

Weight-bearing exercise

30 min, 5 days/week improves BMD by 1–2%

Fall prevention

E.g., balance training reduces fracture incidence by 20%

Smoking cessation and alcohol moderation

Milk products green vegetables

Swimming

Although menopause is a ubiquitous event occurring in all women, the timing of onset and duration of menopausal transition and the attainment of final menstrual period are unique to every female.

Premature menopause, also known as premature ovarian insufficiency, refers to cessation of menses before 40 years of age and it has been observed that the incidence of POI, i.e., 1%, has been on a rising trend.[4] Surgical menopause is the term which is used in females when they have undergone hysterectomy with or without bilateral oophorectomy before the attainment of natural menopause. Females who have undergone hysterectomy before the age of 45 years for benign and malignant conditions are at an increased risk of mortality, especially from ischemic heart disease if not treated with HRT.[16]

CLASSIFICATION AND STAGING OF MENOPAUSAL TRANSITION AND MENOPAUSE

There were many classification systems, but the most accepted is the Stages of Reproductive Aging Workshop (STRAW) classification which was proposed in 2001 after extensive and thorough research. STRAW describes the various stages of reproductive life in females as well as it brings uniformity in nomenclature and the characteristic transformation at every stage across the studies conducted.[17] It was revised in 2010 and was renamed as Re STRAW +10 which was upgraded to incorporate the biochemical or hormonal changes along with ultrasound findings throughout the reproductive aging.

The STRAW proposed a system that divides female reproductive aging into five stages before the final menstrual period, and two afterward. Each of these stages is divided into substages on the basis of menstrual cycle pattern and investigations [serum levels of follicle-stimulating hormone (FSH), anti-Mullerian hormone (AMH), and ultrasound-based ovarian antral follicle count (AFC)].

TABLE 1: Phases of female reproductive life span.

Reproductive period			*Menopausal transition*		*Final menstrual period*	*Post menopausal*	
Early	Peak	Late	Early	Late	FMP	Early	Late
–5	–4	–3a, b	–2	–1	0	+1a,b,c	+2

- Three stages [early (–5), peak (–4), and late (–3) reproductive] describe the years before the perimenopause. Stage –3 is characterized by regular cycles but elevated levels of follicle-stimulating hormone (FSH) in the follicular phase. Stage –3 has been subdivided into substages –3b and –3a. In substage –3b, the menstrual cycle remains unchanged along with normal serum levels of FSH in early follicular phases but AFC and AMH tend to become low. The only difference between substages –3b and –3a is that in –3a early follicular phase FSH level increases leading to shorter menstrual cycles.
- Stage –2 (early menopause transition) is characterized by variable cycle length.
- Stage –1 (late menopause transition) is characterized by two or more stopped cycles and 60 or more days of amenorrhea.
- Stage + 1 is the first 5 years after the final menstrual period.
- Stage + 2 is the late post menopause.

HORMONAL AND MENSTRUAL CHANGES ACROSS THE MENOPAUSAL TRANSITION

- **Ovarian Changes:** The size of ovary in postmenopausal females is 10 cm3 compared to 20 cm3.in reproductive age females. The functional unit of ovary is the ovarian follicle and approximately 30 follicles are recruited in each menstrual cycle out of which 1 becomes a dominant follicle surrounded by granulosa cells along with theca cells. All the follicles develop from the population of primordial follicles which are maximum during the intrauterine life (6 million), 1-2 million at birth, and 500,000 at puberty. There is substantial acceleration/exponential loss of follicles when the female reaches beyond 40 years of age. By the time, menopause is attained only 1,000 follicles remain which are atretic and of substandard quality and also they become less responsive to gonadotrophins as compared to the reproductive age period.
- **Hormonal Changes:** The endocrinology of menopause can be summarized as a sequence of events that results in replacement of the cyclical secretory pattern of gonadotropins (FSH, LH) and gonadal steroids (estrogen, progesterone) and peptides (inhibin) by a monophasic pattern of increased levels of gonadotropins along with decreased levels of estrogen, progesterone, and inhibins. Secretion of androgens, particularly testosterone, is not affected by the event of menopause.
  - Follicle Stimulating Hormone (FSH):[7] As the ovarian function declines, the pituitary gland increases FSH release in an attempt to stimulate the ovaries to produce more estrogen. Monotropic rise in FSH (>40 IU/L) is the hallmark of MT and is often used

as a diagnostic marker for menopause. It is more indicative of egg quantity rather than quality, especially during the early transition. Significant changes in central neural processes that produce LH surge in mid-reproductive life also become dysfunctional leading to an irregular cycle (skipping of menstrual cycles or intermenstrual interval >7 days) during early transition. FSH increases are more sustained over time during the late menopausal transition when there is amenorrhea for more than 3 months and the rise is most remarkable in the years preceding FMP.

- Gonadal Steroids:[8-10] The two gonadal steroids involved in physiology of menopause are estrogen and progesterone out of which estrogen levels fluctuate and more closely resemble the various stages of menopausal transition as well as post menopause. The four major naturally occurring estrogens are esterone (E1), estradiol (E2), estriol (E3), and estetrol (E4). Estradiol is the predominant estrogen during reproductive years both in terms of absolute serum levels and in terms of estrogenic activity. During menopause, estrone is the predominant circulating estrogen and has the weakest estrogenic activity. In early menopausal transition, estradiol levels are initially elevated in the early follicular phase as a result of accelerated folliculogenesis and shortening of the follicular phase. There occurs a rapid decline beginning 2 years before the FMP followed by reaching a plateau level 2 years thereafter; therefore, it is the last biomarker from MT to FMP. Progesterone levels do not show marked fluctuations during menopausal transition but eventually become undetectable during menopause; therefore, progesterone cannot be used as a marker. The hormonal changes during menopause can lead to various physical and emotional symptoms.
- Inhibin:[18] Inhibin B is the product of granulosa cells of the cohort of follicles and in a normal ovarian cycle its level is highest in the early follicular phase followed by peak in midcycle and declines thereafter. It represents the overall quality of the follicle along with its numbers. Inhibin B becomes undetectable in the preceding 4–5 years before complete cessation which is consistent with a decrease in both the size of primordial follicle pool and the cohort of follicles recruited from that pool in each menstrual cycle. The fall in Inhibin B parallels the rise in FSH which supports the evidence that inhibin B plays an important role in negative feedback regulation of FSH secretion.

  Inhibin A is the product of the dominant follicle as well as also produced by corpus Luteum; therefore its levels are highest during mid-cycle and also detected during luteal phase. The Inhibin levels eventually vanish after the attainment of menopause. The measurement of inhibin B is more important than inhibin A as it is one of the earliest harbingers of menopausal transition.
- Anti-mullerian Hormone (AMH)/MIS: AMH is produced by primary, secondary, and early antral follicles and more closely correlate with the follicle cohort, and therefore its concentration declines throughout the reproductive life with minimal intercycle variations and constitute the earliest and the most efficient way to predict the women's progress toward menopause. It can be hoped in near future that AMH becomes a menopause test with the development of a comprehensive sensitive assay.

- Testosterone and DHEA-S:[19] Both testosterone and DHEA metabolites show age-related decline as ovarian androgen production decreases, but there has been an increase in adrenal-derived androgens during the MT in majority of females. Due to falling estrogen levels, there is a decline in SHBG leading to rise in free testosterone besides being contributed by adrenals in postmenopausal females. The complimentary contributions of DHEA metabolites to total androgenicity should not be ignored but DHEAS levels across the MT are still under research and no conclusions can be made.

MENSTRUAL CHANGES[20]

During the menopausal transition, the pattern of menstrual bleeding changes with respect to regularity, timing, and nature, i.e., cycles may become irregular in length and flow along with periods of heavier or lighter bleeding and missed periods. Eventually, menstruation stops completely, and menopause is confirmed when a woman has not had a menstrual period for 12 consecutive months. The nature and timing of bleeding vary within an individual and also among different women.

- During the STRAW stage –2, i.e., early menopausal transition, there is an increase in the irregularity of the cycles which is defined as recurrence of 7-day difference in cycle length over a period of 10 consecutive cycles. The duration of the follicular phase is the major determinant of cycle length.
- Menstrual cycles become increasingly irregular due to short/inadequate luteal phase or anovulation. Insufficient FSH responsiveness results in decreased luteal phase estrogen and progesterone secretion leading to lack of corpus luteum which results in only estrogen secretion (hyperestrogenic states) without progesterone secretion eventually resulting in profuse bleeding.
- During late menopausal transition, STRAW stage –1 is characterized by amenorrhea lasting for 3 months due to increased chances of anovulation during this period.
- Early postmenopause STRAW stage +1a, b, c includes post 1 year beyond FMP and early post menopause which spans a total of 5–8 years.

SYMPTOMS[21]

SWAN (a study of women's health across the nation, multicentric, multiethnic longitudinal study across 7 clinical sites with 3,302 females enrolled between 42 and 52 years of age were followed with the effects of menopause on their health and various risk factors for age-related disease) is the most comprehensive characterization till date about the various physiological and psychological changes during the menopausal transition along with postmenopause.[22,23] The most consistent observation of SWAN was that most of the symptomatology along with detectable physiological changes coincides with late perimenopause (3 months of amenorrhea).

Clinical consequences of profound hormonal deprivation of estrogen lead to various symptoms affecting almost every organ of the body which maybe bothersome and troublesome and may even require expert advice from the physicians and pharmacological interventions along with life behavioral modifications.

Symptoms of Menopause

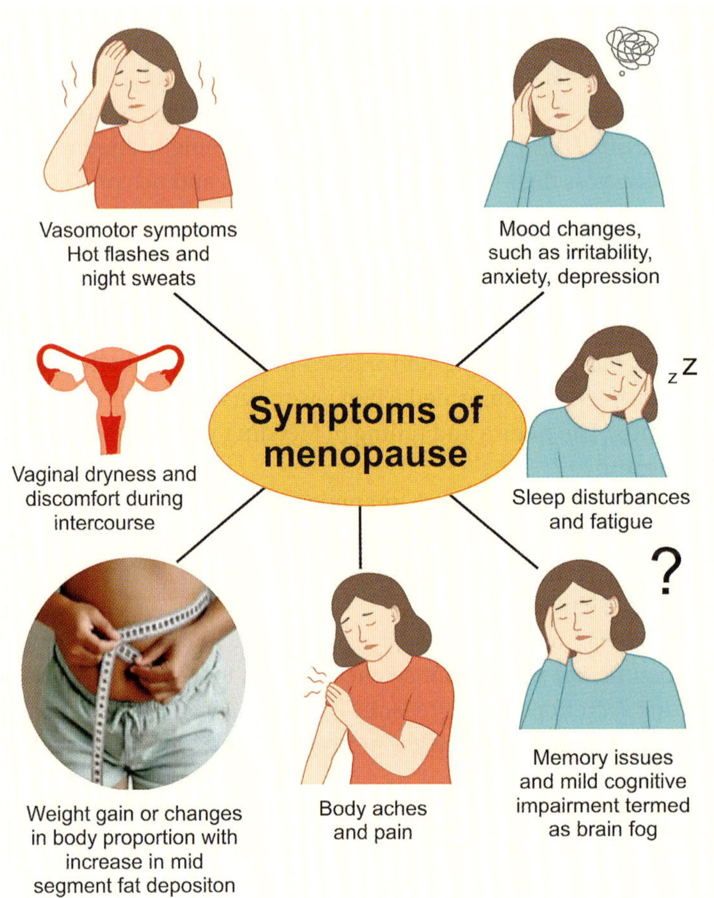

- **Vasomotor Symptoms:** Approximately 75% of the females experience VMS (hot flashes, night sweats) which are most marked during the early postmenopausal period, usually lasts up to 5 years and very rarely 15 years. The exact pathophysiology is unclear, but it has been speculated that the central thermoregulatory zone narrows down toward menopausal transition so that vasodilatation and sweating are triggered at a lower temperature. Transition of late perimenopause was the strongest predictor of VMS.
- **Genitourinary Syndrome of Menopause (GSM):** This is the most concerning issue after VMS but occurs more commonly during the late menopause as compared to early menopause and gradually worsens over a period of time. The term vulvovaginal atrophy (VVA) has been replaced by GSM which is a constellation of symptoms complex involving atrophy of the vulva, vagina, urogenital atrophy, and sexual dissatisfaction due to loss of estrogen and progesterone receptors which line the lower genital tract along with the bladder and urethra.

Complementary therapies for vasomotor symptoms

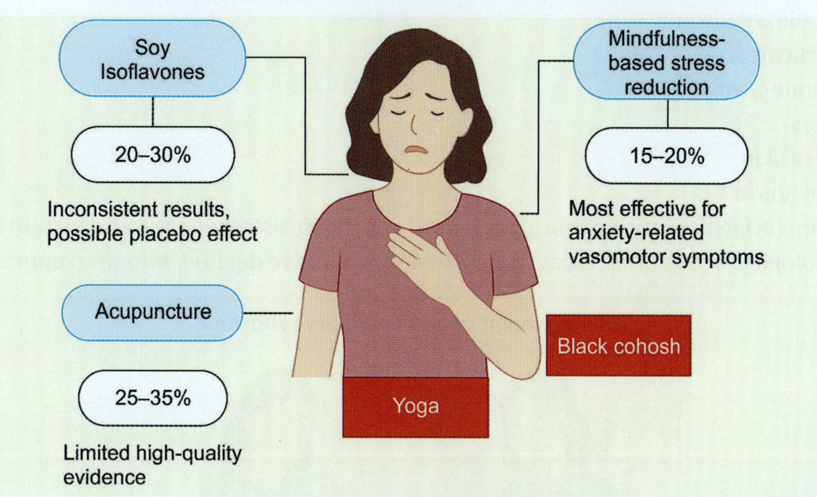

Management of Hot flashes

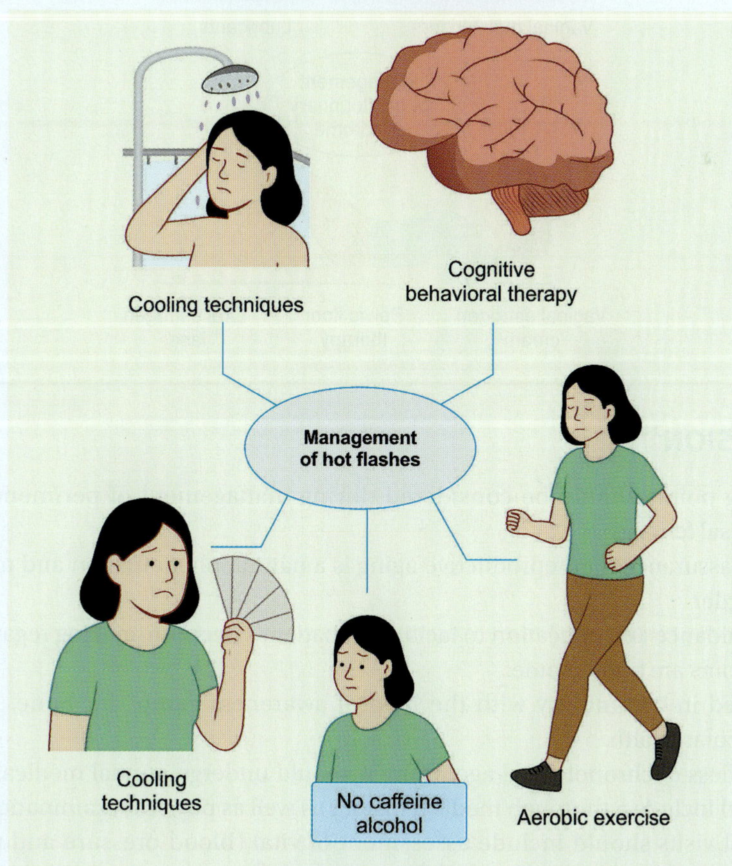

- Osteoporosis
- Metabolic syndrome
- Ischemic heart diseases
- Dementia/stroke
- Cancers
- Aging of skin
- Loss of libido
- Centripetal fat distribution due to increased androgen–estrogen ratio and insulin resistance
- Psychological symptoms (anxiety, depression, cognitive decline, impaired concentration)

Management of genitourinary syndrome

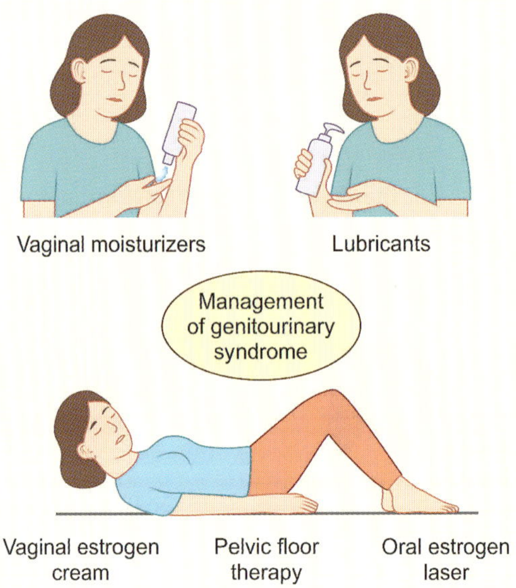

CONCLUSION[24]

The following points should be considered during management of perimenopausal and postmenopausal females:

- Provide reassurance that reproductive aging is a natural phenomenon and menopause is not a disorder.
- Provide guidance and education to facilitate a patient's decision-making regarding MHT if the symptoms are bothersome.
- Be involved in community with the help of awareness camps for bone, mental, and cardiovascular health.

  Regardless of chronological age, women should undergo annual medical evaluations that should include a thorough medical history as well as physical examination.

  - Annual visits should include assessment of vital (blood pressure and pulse), body weight, and BMI (body mass index), breast and pelvic examinations and screening for sexually transmitted infections when appropriate. Thyroid function (TSH) should be assessed in the 40s and annually beginning at age 60 increases with aging and is more common in women).

- Annual screening mammography should begin at age 40 years.
- At each visit, appropriate testing is scheduled for specific chronic conditions (including abnormal lipids), indicated immunizations are provided, and counseling covers changing nutritional needs; physical activities; injury prevention; occupational, sexual, marital, and parental problems; urinary function; and use of tobacco, alcohol, and drugs. Stool hemoccult testing should be performed annually after age 50 years.
- For low-risk individuals without a family history of colon cancer, screening colonoscopy is recommended starting at age 50 years, and then every 10 years through age 75 years.

Menopause is a naturally occurring transition in a woman's life with significant bodily changes as well as change in attitude and behavior toward the perception of life. Therefore, it becomes important to consult a healthcare provider for personalized counseling, advice, and support for a smooth and comfortable adaptation during this period to lead a healthy life.

REFERENCES

1. Taylor HS, Fritz MA, Emre S. Speroff's Clinical Gynecologic Endocrinology and Infertility, 9th edition. Philadelphia: Wolters Kluwer; 2019. p. 693 (Chapter 17).
2. Burger HG. Physiology and endocrinology of the menopause. Medicine. 2006;34(1):27-30.
3. Taylor HS, Fritz MA, Emre S. Speroff's Clinical Gynecologic Endocrinology and Infertility, 9th edition. Philadelphia: Wolters Kluwer; 2019. p. 692
4. Ahuja M. Age of menopause and determinants of menopause age: A PAN India survey by IMS. J Midlife Health. 2016;7(3):126-31.
5. Ossewaarde ME, Bots ML, Verbeek ALM, et al. Age at menopause, cause-specific mortality and total life expectancy. Epidemiology. 2005;16:556-62.
6. Jacobsen BK, Heuch I, Kvale G. Age at natural menopause and all-cause mortality: a 37-year follow-up ni-19.731 Norwegian women. Am J Epidemiol. 2003;157:923-9.
7. Jansen SC, Femme EH, Schouten EG. Lifetime estrogen exposure versus age at menopause as mortality predictor. Maturitas. 2002;43:105-12.
8. Jacobsen BK, Knutson SF, Fraser GE. Age at menarche, total mortality and mortality from ischaemic heart disease and stroke: the Adventist Health Study, 1976–88. Int J Epidemiol. 2009;38(1):245-52.
9. Lisabeth LD, Beiser AS, Brown DL, et al. Age at natural menopause and risk of ischemic stroke: the Framingham heart study. Stroke 2009; 40: 1044-1049.
10. Parashar S, Reid KJ, Spertus JA, et al. Early menopause predicts angina after myocardial infarction. Menopause. 2010;17(5):938-45.
11. Joakimsen 0, Bonaa KR Stensland-Bugge E, et al.
12. Parazzini F, Bidoli E. Franceschi S, et al. Menopause, menstrual and reproductive history, and bone density in northern Italy. J Clin Epidemiol. 2000;53:525-30.
13. Kritz-Silverstein D, Barrett-Connor E. Early menopause, number of reproductive years, and bone mineral density in postmenopausal women. Am J Public Health. 1993;83(7):983-8..
14. Monninkhof EM, van der Schouw YT, Peeters PH. Ear y age at menopause and breast cancer: are leaner women more protected'? A prospective analysts of the Dutch DOM cohort. Breast Cancer Res Treat. 1999;55:285-91.
15. De Graaff J, Stolte LA. Age at menarche and menopause of uterine cancer patients. Eur J Obstet Gynecol Reprod Biol 1978;8:187-93.

16. Xu VVH, Xiang YB, Ruan ZX, et al. Menstrual and reproductive factors and endometrial cancer risk: Results from a population-based case-control study in urban Shanghai. Int J Cancer. 2004;108(4):613-9.
17. Harlow SD, Gass M, Hall JE, et al.; STRAW 10 Collaborative Group. Executive summary of the Stages of Reproductive Aging Workshop + 10: addressing the unfinished agenda of staging reproductive aging. Menopause. 2012;19(4):387-95.
18. Overlie I, Mørkrid L, Andersson AM, et al. Inhibin A and B as markers of menopause: a five-year prospective longitudinal study of hormonal changes during the menopausal transition. Acta Obstet Gynecol Scand. 2005;84(3):281-5.
19. McConnell DS, Stanczyk FZ, Sowers MR, et al. Menopausal transition stage-specific changes in circulating adrenal androgens. Menopause. 2012;19(6):658-63.
20. Peacock K, Ketvertis KM. Menopause. [Updated 2022 Aug 11]. In: StatPearls [Internet]. Treasure Island (FL): StatPearls Publishing; 2023 Jan-. Available from: https://www.ncbi.nlm.nih.gov/books/NBK507826/
21. Dennerstein L. Well-being, symptoms and the menopausal transition. Maturitas. 1996;23(2):147-57.
22. Avis NE, Colvin A. Bromberger JT, et al. Change in health-related quality of life over the menopausal transition in a multiethnic cohort of middle-aged women: Study of Women's Health Across the Nation. Menopause. 2009;16:860-9.
23. Avis NE, Ory M. Matthews KA, et al. Health-related quality of life in a multiethnic sample of middle-aged women: Study of Women's Health Across the Nation. Med Care. 2003;41:1262-76.
24. Taylor HS, Fritz MA, Emre S. Speroff's Clinical Gynecologic Endocrinology and Infertility, 9th edition. Philadelphia: Wolters Kluwer; 2019. pp. 701-2.

Premature Ovarian Insufficiency

Ruchika Garg

INTRODUCTION

Premature ovarian insufficiency (POI) is the irreversible decline in ovarian function before age 40 years, leading to menopausal symptoms, infertility, and long-term health risks such as cardiovascular disease (CVD), osteoporosis, and cognitive impairment.[1] Early diagnosis is critical to mitigate these consequences and improve quality of life (QoL). Recent advances in fertility preservation offer hope, though success rates remain limited.[2]

EPIDEMIOLOGY

- **Global:**
  - Prevalence: 1% of women by age 40 years; 0.1% by age 30 years; 0.01% by age 20 years.[3]
  - Familial POI: 4–31% of cases; genetic etiology significant.[4]
- **India:**
  - Prevalence: 1–1.5% by age 40 years; higher in consanguineous populations.[5]
  - **2024 Study**: 1.2% prevalence in urban Indian women <40 years; diagnostic delay ~3 years.[6]
- **Risk Factors:** Genetic mutations, iatrogenic causes (e.g., chemotherapy), autoimmune disorders, infections.[7]

ETIOLOGY

- **Idiopathic:** ~50–70% of cases; no identifiable cause.[8]
- **Genetic:**
  - **Chromosomal:** Turner syndrome **(Figs. 1A and B)** (45,XO), fragile X premutation (FMR1).[9] Offer next-generation sequencing post-counseling (no age restriction).
  - **Syndromic:** Blepharophimosis-ptosis-epicanthus inversus syndrome (FOXL2), galactosemia.[10]
  - **Isolated:** FSH receptor (FSHR), BMP15 mutations.[11]
- **Iatrogenic:**
  - Chemotherapy (alkylating agents), radiation, ovarian surgery (64% of iatrogenic cases).[12]
  - Pelvic vessel embolization, environmental toxins.[13]
- **Infections:** Mumps, tuberculosis, cytomegalovirus.[14]
- **Autoimmune:** Associated with thyroiditis, Addison's disease.[15]

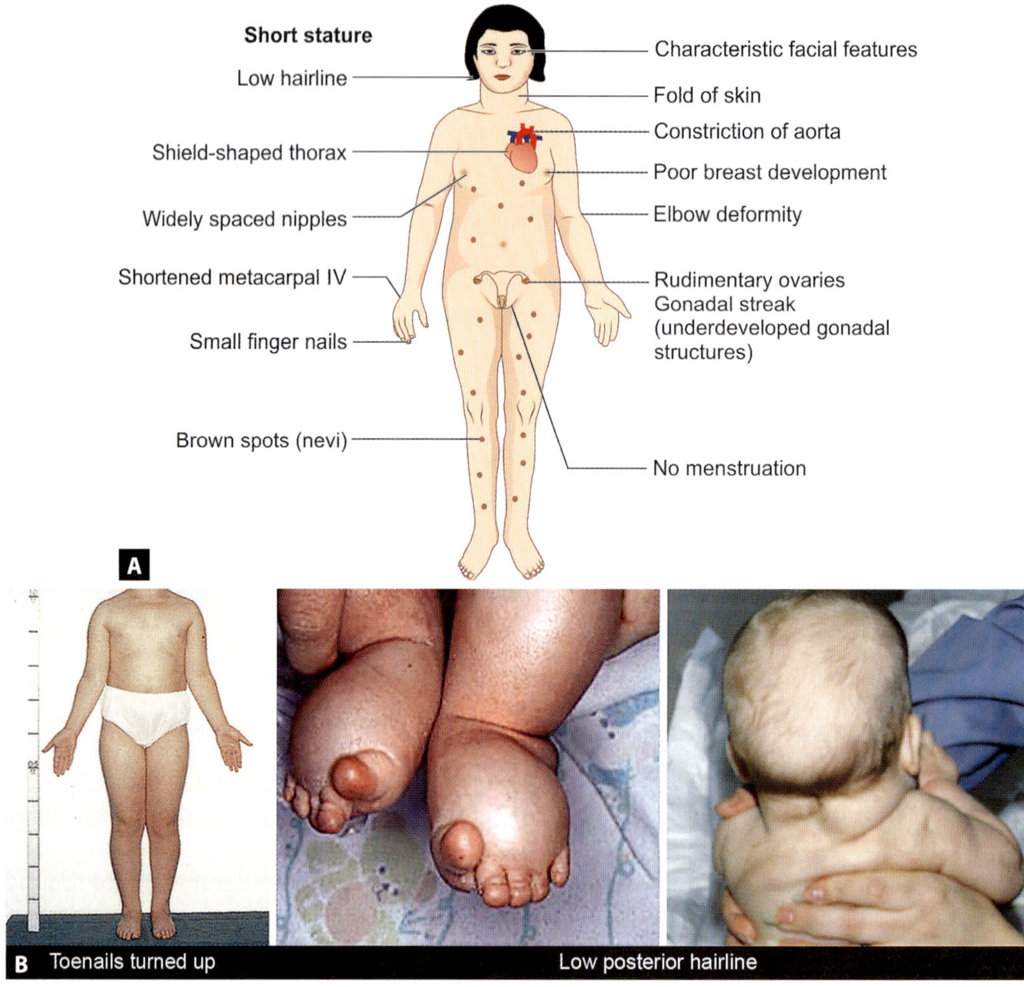

Figs. 1A and B: (A) Turner syndrome; (B) Toenails turned up and Low posterior hairline.

TABLE 1: Etiology of POI.[8,12,15]

Category	*Examples*	*Prevalence*
Idiopathic	Unknown cause	50–70%
Genetic	Turner syndrome, FMR1, FSHR mutations	20–30%
Iatrogenic	Chemotherapy, ovarian surgery	10–20%
Autoimmune	Thyroiditis, adrenal insufficiency	5–10%
Infections	Mumps, TB	<5%

PATHOPHYSIOLOGY

- **Mechanism**: Depletion or dysfunction of ovarian follicles, leading to hypoestrogenism and elevated gonadotropins.[16]

- **Hormonal Changes:**
  - Follicle-stimulating hormone (FSH) >25 IU/L, estradiol <50 pg/mL.[17]
  - Reduced anti-Müllerian hormone (AMH) indicates low ovarian reserve.[18]
- **Consequences:**
  - Menopausal symptoms: Vasomotor, genitourinary syndrome.
  - Long-term: CVD, osteoporosis, cognitive decline, reduced life expectancy.[19]

CLINICAL FEATURES

- **Menstrual Irregularities:**
- Primary amenorrhea (severe cases) or secondary amenorrhea/oligomenorrhea.[20]
- **Menopausal Symptoms:** Hot flashes, night sweats, vaginal dryness, sleep disturbances.[21]
- **Infertility:** Due to depleted ovarian reserve; 5–10% spontaneous conception rate.[22]
- **Systemic Effects:**
  - **Cardiovascular:** Endothelial dysfunction, increased carotid intima-media thickness.[23]
  - **Bone Health:** Osteopenia/osteoporosis due to hypoestrogenism.[24]
  - **Cognitive:** Increased risk of Alzheimer's, cognitive decline.[25]
  - **Metabolic:** Type 2 diabetes, dyslipidemia.[26]
  - **Psychological:** Anxiety, depression, reduced QOL.[27]

TABLE 2: Clinical features of POI.[20,23,24]

Category	*Symptoms*	*Prevalence*
Menstrual	Amenorrhea, oligomenorrhea	80–90%
Menopausal	Hot flashes, vaginal dryness	70–80%
Infertility	Subfertility	90%
Cardiovascular	Endothelial dysfunction	50–60%
Bone	Osteopenia/osteoporosis	40–50%

DIAGNOSIS

- **ESHRE Criteria:**
  - Age <40 years
  - Oligo/amenorrhea ≥4 months
  - FSH >25 IU/L on two occasions >4 weeks apart.[28]
- **Investigations:**
  - **Hormonal:** FSH, estradiol, AMH, thyroid function, 21-hydroxylase antibodies.[29, 66]
  - **Genetic:** Karyotype, FMR1 premutation screening.[30]
  - **Imaging:** Transvaginal ultrasound (TVUS) for antral follicle count; dual-energy X-ray absorptiometry (DXA) for bone density.[31]
  - **Pregnancy Test:** Exclude pregnancy.[32]
- **Differential Diagnosis:** Hypothyroidism, hyperprolactinemia, hypothalamic amenorrhea.[33]

TABLE 3: Diagnostic investigations for POI.[29,31]

Test	*Rationale*	*Key findings*
FSH, Estradiol	Assess ovarian function	FSH >25 IU/L, Estradiol <50 pg/mL
AMH	Ovarian reserve	Low AMH (<1 ng/mL)
Karyotype	Genetic etiology	Turner syndrome, mosaicism
FMR1	Fragile X premutation	CGG repeats 55–200
TVUS	Follicle count	Reduced antral follicles

MANAGEMENT

- **Goals:** Symptom relief, prevention of long-term complications, fertility support.[34]
- **Hormone Replacement Therapy (HRT):**
  - **Indication:** All POI patients unless contraindicated; continue until age 51 years (average menopause age).[35,65]
  - **Estrogen:**
    - Transdermal estradiol (100 μg) preferred; lower thromboembolism risk versus oral.[36,62]
    - Oral: Micronized estradiol (1–2 mg), conjugated equine estrogen (0.625–1.25 mg).[37]
  - **Progestin:**
    - Micronized progesterone (200 mg/day, 12 days/month) or medroxyprogesterone acetate (10 mg/day, 12 days/month).[38]
    - Cyclic progestin prevents endometrial hyperplasia.[39,63,64]
  - **Benefits:** Reduces vasomotor symptoms, CVD risk, osteoporosis; improves QOL.[40]
  - **Side Effects:** Bloating, mood changes; thromboembolism risk with oral estrogen.[41]
- **Genitourinary Syndrome:**
  - Vaginal estradiol (10 μg), ospemifene (60 mg/day), or nonhormonal moisturizers.[42]
  - Ospemifene: FDA-approved for dyspareunia; contraindicated in breast cancer.[43]
- **Bone Health:**
  - HRT improves bone mineral density (BMD); transdermal estradiol superior for lumbar spine.[44]
  - Lifestyle: Calcium (1,200 mg/day), vitamin D (1,000–2,000 IU/day), weight-bearing exercise.[45]
  - Bisphosphonates: Avoid due to long half-life and pregnancy risks.[46]
- **Cardiovascular Health:**
  - HRT within 5 years of POI onset reduces endothelial dysfunction.[47]
  - Optimize diet, exercise, smoking cessation.[48]
- **Cognitive Health:** Early HRT may slow cognitive decline; no reversal of Alzheimer's pathology.[49]
- **Psychological Support:** Counseling for infertility, anxiety, depression.[50]

TABLE 4: HRT Options for POI.[37,38]

Estrogen	*Progestin (Continuous)*	*Progestin (Sequential)*
Micronized estradiol 1–2 mg (oral)	MPA 2.5–5 mg/day (oral)	MPA 10 mg/day × 12 days (oral)
Estradiol 100 µg (transdermal)	Micronized progesterone 100 mg/day	Micronized progesterone 200 mg/day × 12 days
Conjugated equine estrogen 0.625–1.25 mg (oral)		

FERTILITY MANAGEMENT

- **Challenges:** Depleted ovarian reserve; traditional ovulation induction ineffective.[51]
- **Options:**
  - **Oocyte/Embryo Donation:** Most effective; success rates 40–50% per cycle.[52]
  - **Spontaneous Conception:** 5–10% chance; contraception advised if pregnancy undesired.[53]
  - **Preimplantation Genetic Diagnosis (PGD):** For genetic mutations (e.g., FMR1, Turner syndrome).[54]
- **Preservation Strategies:**
  - **Oocyte/Embryo Cryopreservation:** For women anticipating gonadotoxic therapy.[55]
  - **Ovarian Tissue Cryopreservation:** Experimental; limited success.[56]
  - **Ovarian Transposition:** Reduces radiation exposure pre-pelvic radiotherapy.[57]
  - **GnRH Agonists:** Prechemotherapy; efficacy controversial.[58]
- **Counseling:** Address emotional impact, genetic risks, and donor options.[59]

TABLE 5: Fertility options in POI.[52,55]

Option	*Success rate*	*Indication*
Oocyte donation	40–50%	Depleted ovarian reserve
Spontaneous conception	5–10%	Intermittent ovarian function
Oocyte cryopreservation	20–30%	Pregonadotoxic therapy

TABLE 6: Oral versus Transdermal Estrogen Effects.[60,61]

Effect	*Oral estrogen*	*Transdermal estrogen*
Pharmacokinetics	Peaks/troughs	Stable levels
Inflammatory markers	Increased CRP	Neutral
Lipids	Increased triglycerides	Decreased triglycerides
Clotting proteins	Increased	Neutral

CONTRAINDICATIONS

- **Absolute:** Undiagnosed vaginal bleeding, hormone-dependent cancers, established CVD, severe liver disease, pregnancy.[67]
- **Relative:** Hypertriglyceridemia, gallbladder disease, obesity, migraines with aura.[68]

TABLE 7: Contraindications to HRT.[67,68]

Absolute	*Relative*
Breast/endometrial cancer	Hypertriglyceridemia
Established CVD	Obesity, smoking
Venous thromboembolism history	Migraine with aura

RCOG/NICE GUIDELINES

- **RCOG (2015):**[69]
  - **Diagnosis:** FSH >25 IU/L, amenorrhea ≥4 months; screen for genetic/autoimmune causes.
  - **Management:**
    - HRT (transdermal estradiol preferred) until age 51 years.
    - Oocyte donation for infertility; counsel on spontaneous conception risk.
    - Annual BMD monitoring if low bone mass.
  - **Follow-Up:** Assess QOL, CVD risk, bone health.
- **NICE (2015, updated 2023):**[70]
  - **Diagnosis:** Confirm POI with FSH, estradiol; genetic counseling for familial cases.
  - **Treatment:**
    - HRT first-line; individualize dose/route.
    - Fertility referral for donor options; cryopreservation pre-gonadotoxic therapy.
    - Lifestyle modifications for bone/CVD health.
  - **Research:** Limited data on long-term HRT safety in POI.

INDIAN CONTEXT

- **Burden:** 1–1.5% prevalence; higher in consanguineous communities.[71]
- **Challenges:**
  - Diagnostic delay due to social stigma, limited genetic testing.[72]
  - High cost of HRT (₹500–2,000/month), oocyte donation (₹2–3 lakh/cycle).[73]
- **Strategies:**
  - Subsidized HRT in government hospitals; ASHA-led awareness.[74]
  - **2024 Study**: Only 40% of Indian POI patients receive HRT due to cost barriers.[75]

CLINICAL CASE SCENARIO

Case

A 28-year-old woman presents with 6 months of amenorrhea and hot flashes. She has no family history of POI. FSH is 35 IU/L and estradiol 30 pg/mL on two tests 6 weeks apart. TVUS shows reduced antral follicle count. Karyotype is normal; FMR1 negative.

Management

- **Diagnosis:** POI (amenorrhea, elevated FSH, low estradiol).
- **Counseling:** Discuss symptoms, infertility, long-term risks, HRT benefits.

- **Treatment:**
  - Start transdermal estradiol 100 μg/day + micronized progesterone 200 mg/day × 12 days/month.
  - Vaginal estradiol 10 μg for dyspareunia.
  - Calcium 1,200 mg; vitamin D 1,000 IU/day; weight-bearing exercise.
- **Fertility:** Refer for oocyte donation counseling; discuss 5–10% spontaneous conception chance.
- **Follow-Up:** Monitor symptoms, BMD at 1 year; annual lipid profile.
- **Outcome:** Symptoms improved; pursuing oocyte donation.

Exam Tip: Emphasize ESHRE criteria, transdermal HRT, oocyte donation, and spontaneous conception risk.

KEY POINTS

- **Prevalence in India:** 1–1.5% by age 40 years; diagnostic delay common.
- **Diagnosis:** FSH >25 IU/L, amenorrhea ≥4 months; screen for genetic causes.
- **Management:**
  - **Transdermal HRT** first-line; continue until age 51 years.
  - Oocyte donation for infertility; 5–10% spontaneous conception.
- **Complications:** CVD, osteoporosis, cognitive decline; HRT mitigates risks.
- **Challenges:** Cost, stigma limit HRT access in India.

BOX 1: Important points to remember.

- POI Definition: Ovarian failure <40 years; FSH >25 IU/L, amenorrhea ≥4 months
- Transdermal Estradiol: Preferred HRT; lower thromboembolism risk
- Oocyte Donation: Most effective fertility option; 40–50% success
- Spontaneous Conception: 5–10% chance; counsel on contraception if needed

REFERENCES

1. Webber L, Davies M, Anderson R, et al. ESHRE POI guideline. Hum Reprod. 2016;31(5):926-37.
2. Donnez J, et al. Fertility in POI. Fertil Steril. 2018;110(6):1051-8.
3. Coulam CB, et al. POI incidence. Am J Obstet Gynecol. 2016;140(1):59-63.
4. Qin Y, et al. Genetics of POI. Hum Reprod Update. 2015;21(6):767-81.
5. Mishra P, et al. POI in India. J Obstet Gynaecol India. 2019;69(4):321-7.
6. Sharma A, et al. POI prevalence India. Fertil Steril. 2024;121(2):234-41.
7. Nelson LM. POI review. N Engl J Med. 2017;360(6):606-14.
8. Rebar RW. Idiopathic POI. Clin Obstet Gynecol. 2015;50(1):37-43.
9. Persani L, et al. Genetic etiology POI. J Mol Endocrinol. 2016;56(4):R107-R123.
10. Crisponi L, et al. FOXL2 in BPES. Am J Hum Genet. 2016;68(6):1342-8.
11. Aittomäki K, et al. FSHR mutations. N Engl J Med. 2015;331(23):1535-40.
12. Sklar CA, et al. Iatrogenic POI. J Clin Oncol. 2018;36(12):1264-72.
13. De Vos M, et al. Environmental toxins POI. Hum Reprod Update. 2016;16(6):616-26.
14. Morrison JC, et al. Infections in POI. Fertil Steril. 2017;108(3):e123-9.
15. Bakalov VK, et al. Autoimmune POI. J Clin Endocrinol Metab. 2016;87(2):594-9.
16. Shelling AN. POI pathophysiology. Mol Cell Endocrinol. 2016;336(1–2):72-7.
17. Welt CK. POI hormonal changes. J Clin Endocrinol Metab. 2015;90(4):2377-83.

18. Broer SL, et al. AMH in POI. Fertil Steril. 2015;103(3):593-601.
19. Faubion SS, et al. POI long-term risks. Mayo Clin Proc. 2015;90(6):802-9.
20. Rafique S, et al. POI clinical features. J Pak Med Assoc. 2017;67(9):1413-8.
21. Sullivan SD, et al. Menopausal symptoms POI. Menopause. 2016;23(2):198-205.
22. Bidet M, et al. Spontaneous conception POI. Hum Reprod. 2016;26(9):2350-4.
23. Kalantaridou SN, et al. CVD in POI. J Clin Endocrinol Metab. 2016;83(3):763-8.
24. Popat VB, et al. Bone health POI. J Clin Endocrinol Metab. 2015;94(10):3667-76.
25. Rocca WA, et al. Cognitive decline POI. Neurology. 2016;86(4):383-91.
26. Anagnostis P, et al. Metabolic risks POI. Climacteric. 2019;22(2):127-32.
27. Gibson-Helm M, et al. Psychological impact POI. Hum Reprod. 2017;32(1):110-8.
28. ESHRE. POI guideline. Hum Reprod. 2016;31(5):926-37.
29. Cox L, et al. POI investigations. Best Pract Res Clin Obstet Gynaecol. 2017;41:59-70.
30. Conway GS, et al. Genetic screening POI. Hum Reprod Update. 2015;4(5):352-6.
31. De Vos M, et al. TVUS in POI. Fertil Steril. 2016;105(5):1119-27.
32. Nelson LM. POI diagnosis. N Engl J Med. 2017;360(6):606-14.
33. Gordon CM, et al. Differential diagnosis POI. J Clin Endocrinol Metab. 2015;102(5):1411-8.
34. Torrealday S, et al. POI management. Curr Opin Obstet Gynecol. 2017;29(4):211-6.
35. Baber RJ, et al. HRT in POI. Climacteric. 2016;19(4):313-25.
36. Archer DF, et al. Transdermal estradiol safety. Menopause. 2017;24(6):611-8.
37. Panay N, et al. HRT dosing POI. Maturitas. 2016;87:1-6.
38. Furness S, et al. Progestin in HRT. Cochrane Database Syst Rev. 2015;3:CD002974.
39. Lobo RA. HRT endometrial protection. Fertil Steril. 2016;105(4):893-900.
40. Crook D, et al. HRT benefits POI. Br J Obstet Gynaecol. 2015;102(7):531-5.
41. Canonico M, et al. Thromboembolism HRT. BMJ. 2016;343:d.
42. Portman DJ, et al. Genitourinary syndrome POI. Menopause. 2015;22(10):1013-20.
43. Constantine GD, et al. Ospemifene efficacy. J Sex Med. 2016;13(5):837-47.
44. Anasti JN, et al. HRT bone effects POI. J Clin Endocrinol Metab. 2015;81(10):3460-5.
45. Weaver CM, et al. Calcium in bone health. Am J Clin Nutr. 2016;103(4):1014S-21S.
46. Black DM, et al. Bisphosphonates safety. N Engl J Med. 2016;374(26):2527-9.
47. Lokkegaard E, et al. HRT CVD protection. Eur Heart J. 2017;38(20):1579-87.
48. Roeters van Lennep JE, et al. CVD risk management POI. Maturitas. 2016;82:40-44.
49. Bove R, et al. HRT cognition POI. Neurology. 2016;82(12):1063-71.
50. Mann E, et al. Psychological support POI. Climacteric. 2015;15(4):318-25.
51. Kodaman PH, et al. Fertility in POI. Fertil Steril. 2016;105(4):901-7.
52. Sauer MV, et al. Oocyte donation outcomes. Fertil Steril. 2016;106(3):e234-40.
53. van Kasteren YM, et al. Spontaneous conception POI. Hum Reprod. 2015;14(12):3015-8.
54. Harper JC, et al. PGD in POI. Hum Reprod Update. 2016;22(6):709-24.
55. Oktay K, et al. Oocyte cryopreservation. N Engl J Med. 2016;375(22):2158-67.
56. Donnez J, et al. Ovarian tissue cryopreservation. Fertil Steril. 2015;104(5):1053-9.
57. Gubbala K, et al. Ovarian transposition. Gynecol Oncol. 2016;141(2):191-8.
58. Lambertini M, et al. GnRH agonists fertility preservation. J Clin Oncol. 2016;34(25):3081-7.
59. Ethics Committee, ASRM. Counseling in POI. Fertil Steril. 2016;110(6):1050-6.
60. Kuhl H. Estrogen pharmacokinetics. Clim Rev. 2015;10(1):29-37.
61. Goodman MP. Oral vs. transdermal estrogen. J Womens Health. 2016;21(2):161-9.
62. Simon JA, et al. Estrogen half-life. Menopause. 2015;22(6):703-8.
63. Stanczyk FZ, et al. Progestin pharmacokinetics. Contraception. 2016;90(3):213-9.
64. North American Menopause Society. Progestin monitoring. Menopause. 2017;24(9):1036-42.
65. Flockhart DA, et al. HRT drug interactions. Clin Pharmacol Ther. 2016;79(1):1-7.

66. Lobo RA, et al. HRT and thyroid function. J Clin Endocrinol Metab. 2015;83(6):1833-6.
67. Santoro N, et al. HRT contraindications. Menopause. 2016;23(6):678-86.
68. Pinkerton JV, et al. Relative HRT risks. Climacteric. 2017;20(6):541-7.
69. RCOG. POI management. Scientific Impact Paper No. 50. London: RCOG; 2015.
70. NICE. Menopause: diagnosis and management (NG23). London: NICE; 2023.
71. Malhotra N, et al. POI in India. J Hum Reprod Sci. 2017;10(3):234-40.
72. Rao S, et al. POI diagnostic delays. Indian J Med Res. 2019;150(6):543-50.
73. Gupta A, et al. POI treatment costs. Fertil Steril. 2020;114(3):e123-30.
74. MoHFW. ASHA POI awareness. New Delhi: 2023.
75. Sharma P, et al. HRT access in POI India. J Obstet Gynaecol India. 2024;24(1):56-62.

Hot Flashes

Ruchika Garg

OVERVIEW

Hot flashes, also termed hot flushes are sudden, transient episodes of intense heat, often accompanied by sweating, palpitations, and anxiety. These vasomotor symptoms (VMS) are hallmark features of menopausal transition, varying in frequency, duration, and intensity among individuals. Typically lasting under 5 minutes, hot flashes may occur from multiple times daily to several times weekly, persisting on average for 4 years post menopause. Approximately one-third of women experience symptoms beyond a decade after menopause onset. Prevalence data indicate that 88% of women with natural menopause and 92% with surgical menopause report hot flashes. A recent study found that 43% of women aged 40–60 years experience hot flashes and sweating, while Indian data report menopausal symptoms in 87.7% of women, with hot flashes in 36.7%, alongside anxiety (80%), general weakness (71.5%), and other symptoms **(Table 1)**.

RISK FACTORS

Hot flashes are more common in women with early menarche (≤11 years), higher body mass index (BMI), lower socioeconomic status, sedentary lifestyles, smoking, or African-American descent. Genetic associations involve single-nucleotide polymorphisms (SNPs) in the tachykinin receptor 3 gene, encoding neurokinin B (NKB), with increased NKB expression in postmenopausal women **(Table 2)**.

TABLE 1: Prevalence of menopausal symptoms in Indian women.

Symptom	*Prevalence (%)*
Anxiety	80.0
General weakness	71.5
Sleep disturbance	61.2
Irritability	60.7
Musculoskeletal symptoms	56.0
Cardiovascular symptoms	54.0
Hot flashes	36.7

TABLE 2: Risk factors for hot flashes

Risk factor	*Description*
Early Menarche	Onset at ≤11 years
Obesity	Higher BMI compared to normal-weight women
Socioeconomic Status	Lower socioeconomic position
Lifestyle	Sedentary behavior
Smoking	Increased risk with tobacco use
Ethnicity	Higher prevalence in African-American women
Genetics	SNPs in tachykinin receptor 3 gene (NKB)

ETIOPATHOGENESIS

Hot flashes, the primary symptom of perimenopause and menopause, involve skin vasodilation, sweating, and increased heart rate. The precise mechanism remains unclear, but elevated plasma levels of 3-methoxy-4-hydroxy-phenylglycol (MHPG), a norepinephrine metabolite, increase core body temperature, basal metabolic rate, and skin temperature. Estrogen modulates brain adrenergic receptors, and its withdrawal, combined with elevated norepinephrine, likely triggers VMS **(Tables 3 and 4)**.

TABLE 3: Nonmenopausal causes of hot flashes

Condition	*Description*
Hyperthyroidism	Overactive thyroid function
Carcinoid tumors	Neuroendocrine tumors
Pheochromocytoma	Adrenal gland tumor
Acromegaly	Excess growth hormone
Medullary thyroid carcinoma	Thyroid cancer
Idiopathic anaphylaxis	Unexplained allergic reactions
Systemic mastocytosis	Mast cell proliferation disorder

TABLE 4: Medications associated with hot flashes

Drug	*Class*
Clomiphene	Ovulation inducer
Tamoxifen	Estrogen receptor modulator
Raloxifene	Selective estrogen receptor modulator (SERM)
Tricyclic antidepressants	Antidepressant
Calcium channel blockers	Antihypertensive
Monoamine oxidase inhibitors	Antidepressant
Chemotherapy	Cancer treatment

MANAGEMENT

Hormonal Therapy

Hormone therapy (HT) is the most effective treatment, reducing VMS by approximately 75%. It is recommended within 10 years of menopause onset unless contraindicated (e.g., estrogen-dependent malignancies, cardiovascular disease, unexplained vaginal bleeding). Estrogen formulations include oral, transdermal, topical, or vaginal routes, often combined with progestogens for women with a uterus. Bijuva, a combined 17β-estradiol and progesterone oral capsule, is FDA-approved for moderate to severe VMS **(Table 5)**.

Nonhormonal Pharmacologic Treatments (Table 6)

For women with contraindications to HT, nonhormonal options include:

- **Paroxetine:** FDA-approved at 7.5 mg/day, reducing VMS by 33%.

TABLE 5: Hormone therapy formulations

Hormone	*Route*	*Dosing*
17β-estradiol	Oral	1–2 mg/day
	Transdermal	0.05–0.1 mg patch, replaced every 3–7 days
	Topical	1.74 g/day
	Vaginal Cream	0.5–1 g daily × 14 days, then 1–3 ×/week
	Intravaginal Ring	0.05 mg/day for 3 months
Conjugated equine estrogen	Oral	0.3–1.25 mg/day
	Vaginal Cream	0.5 g daily × 2 weeks, then twice weekly
Estrone	Injectable	0.1–0.5 mg, 2–3 times/week
Esterified estrogen	Oral	0.3–1.25 mg/day
Ethinylestradiol	Oral	20–50 µg, 1–3 times/day
Progestogens		
Medroxyprogesterone (MPA)	Oral	5–10 mg/day × 10–14 days or 2.5–5 mg/day
Micronized progesterone	Oral	200 mg/day × 12 days or 100 mg/day
Norethindrone acetate	Oral/Transdermal	5 mg/day or 0.14 mg patch 2 ×/week
Dydrogesterone	Oral	10 mg/day in 28-day cycle
Tibolone	Oral	2.5 mg/day

TABLE 6: Nonhormonal pharmacologic treatments

Drug	*Category*	*Dosing*
Paroxetine	SSRI	7.5–20 mg/day
Venlafaxine	SNRI	37.5–150 mg/day
Gabapentin	GABA Analogue	100–300 mg thrice daily
Oxybutynin	Anticholinergic/Antimuscarinic	2.5–5 mg twice daily, max 15 mg

- **SSRIs/SNRIs** (e.g., venlafaxine): Effective alternatives when HT is unsuitable.
- **Gabapentin:** Reduces VMS at 100–300 mg thrice daily.
- **Oxybutynin:** Anticholinergic, dosed at 2.5–5 mg twice daily.
- **Fezolinetant:** A neurokinin 3 receptor (NK3R) antagonist, FDA-approved (Veozah) at 45 mg/day for moderate to severe VMS. It modulates thermoregulatory neurons by blocking NKB.

Flowchart 1: Management of vasomotor symptoms.

Vasomotor symptoms

↓

1. Assess VMS severity and patient history
   - If within 10 years of menopause and no contraindications:
     - Initiate HT (estrogen ± progestogen; *see* **Table 5**)
   - If HT contraindicated (e.g., breast cancer, cardiovascular disease):
     - Proceed to nonhormonal options
2. Nonhormonal pharmacologic options:
   - First-line: Fezolinetant 45 mg/day or Paroxetine 7.5 mg/day
   - Alternatives: Venlafaxine, Gabapentin, Oxybutynin (*see* **Table 6**)
3. Nonpharmacologic options:
   - Stellate ganglion block (up to 52% VMS reduction)
   - Cognitive-behavioral therapy (CBT) or clinical hypnosis
   - Lifestyle modifications (e.g., weight loss, smoking cessation)
4. Monitor for efficacy and adverse effects (e.g., liver function for fezolinetant)
5. Reassess at 3, 6, and 9 months or if symptoms persist

Hot Flashes in Cancer Patients

Hot flashes are common in breast cancer patients on tamoxifen (>65%) and prostate cancer patients on androgen deprivation therapy (>80%). Venlafaxine, clonidine, gabapentin, and electroacupuncture are effective, but SSRIs like paroxetine may interfere with tamoxifen metabolism via CYP2D6 inhibition.

Nonpharmacologic Interventions

- **Stellate Ganglion Block:** Reduces moderate to severe VMS by up to 52% using local anesthetics under imaging guidance.
- **Cognitive-Behavioral Therapy (CBT):** Reduces VMS and improves sexual function in breast cancer survivors.
- **Clinical Hypnosis:** Decreases VMS frequency by up to 56.86%.
- **Lifestyle Modifications:** Limited evidence supports exercise for VMS reduction.

Emerging Therapies

- **Phytoestrogens** (e.g., genistein, daidzein): Selective ERβ modulators with potential for VMS and cognitive benefits, requiring further research.

TABLE 7: Fezolinetant profile

Attribute	*Details*
Mechanism	NK3R antagonist, modulates KNDy neuron activity in hypothalamus
Dose	45 mg oral daily, with or without food
Contraindications	Cirrhosis, severe renal impairment, CYP1A2 inhibitors
Adverse Effects	Abdominal pain, diarrhea, insomnia, back pain, hepatic transaminase elevation
Monitoring	Liver function tests at baseline, 3, 6, and 9 months

- **Estetrol (E4):** A novel estrogen under investigation.
- **Fezolinetant:** Blocks NKB binding to KNDy neurons, modulating thermoregulatory activity. Contraindications include cirrhosis, severe renal impairment, and CYP1A2 inhibitor use. Adverse effects include abdominal pain, diarrhea, insomnia, back pain, and elevated transaminases **(Table 7)**.

CONCLUSION

Hot flashes are a prevalent menopausal symptom, significantly impacting quality of life if untreated. They may persist for months to over a decade in some women. HT remains the most effective option when not contraindicated, with nonhormonal alternatives like fezolinetant, SSRIs, SNRIs, and nonpharmacologic therapies offering viable options for contraindicated cases or cancer patients.

SUGGESTED READING

1. Avis NE, El Khoudary SR, Geerlings MI, et al. Vasomotor symptoms during menopause: a practical guide on treatment options for bothersome hot flashes. Cleveland Clinic Journal of Medicine. 2023;90(2):95-104.
2. Bansal R, Aggarwal N. Menopausal hot flashes: a concise review. Journal of Mid-life Health. 2019;10(1):6-13.
3. Faubion SS, Files JA, Boehmer KR, Miller VM. Managing menopause part 1: vasomotor symptoms. BC Medical Journal. 2023;65(1):24-29.
4. Kaunitz AM, Faubion SS, Bitner K, et al. The 2023 nonhormone therapy position statement of The North American Menopause Society. Menopause. 2023;30(6):573-90.

Tibolone

Ruchika Garg

INTRODUCTION

Tibolone is a synthetic steroid used in hormone replacement therapy (HRT) for postmenopausal symptoms and osteoporosis prevention.

- **Question Types:**
  - **Short Note:** "Write a short note on tibolone: uses and side effects".
  - **MCQ:** "Which HRT agent has androgenic effects and is used for libido improvement?" (Answer: Tibolone).[1,2]
- **Indian Context:**
  - Tibolone is available in India (e.g., Livial, Tibomax) but less commonly prescribed due to cost (~₹1,000/month) and preference for conventional HRT.[3]

Short Note: Tibolone

Definition: Tibolone is a synthetic steroid with tissue-selective estrogenic, progestogenic, and androgenic properties, used in HRT for postmenopausal women.[4,5]

Pharmacology

- **Structure:** Synthetic derivative of norethynodrel; metabolized into three active metabolites (3α-OH, 3β-OH, Δ4-isomer).[6]
- **Mechanism:**
  - Estrogenic effects: Stimulates vaginal and bone tissue; reduces hot flashes.[7,8]
  - Progestogenic: Protects endometrium; no withdrawal bleeding in postmenopausal women.[9]
  - Androgenic: Improves libido, mood, and energy.[10]
- **Pharmacokinetics:** Oral administration (2.5 mg/day); half-life ~45 hours; metabolized in liver.[11]

Indications

- **Menopausal Symptoms:** Relieves hot flashes, night sweats, vaginal dryness in postmenopausal women (>1 year postmenopause).[12,13]
- **Osteoporosis Prevention:** Increases bone mineral density (BMD); reduces fracture risk in postmenopausal women.[14]
- **Libido Improvement:** Androgenic effects enhance sexual function.[15]

Contraindications

- Undiagnosed vaginal bleeding, hormone-dependent cancers (e.g., breast, endometrial), active thromboembolism, severe liver disease.[16]
- Relative: Cardiovascular disease (CVD) risk, history of stroke.[17]

Side Effects
- Common: Weight gain, headache, breast tenderness.[18]
- Rare: Increased risk of breast cancer (controversial), stroke (in women >60 years), endometrial hyperplasia (if used premenopause).[19]

Advantages
- No withdrawal bleeding in postmenopausal women.
- Improves libido and mood due to androgenic effects.[20]
- Single daily dose enhances compliance.[21]

Disadvantages
- Increased stroke risk in older women (>60 years).[22]
- Limited data on long-term safety (>5 years).[23]
- Costly compared to conventional HRT in India.[24]

Indian Context
- Available as 2.5 mg tablets; used in urban settings for postmenopausal symptom relief.[25]
- **2024 Study:** Only 20% of Indian gynecologists prescribe tibolone due to cost and lack of awareness.[26]

Guidelines
- **RCOG (2015):** Tibolone is an alternative HRT for menopausal symptoms and osteoporosis prevention; not first-line due to stroke risk.[27]
- **NICE (2015, updated 2023):** Consider tibolone for women with low libido or intolerance to conventional HRT; counsel on risks.[28]

Exam Tip: Highlight tibolone's tissue-specific effects, indications (menopausal symptoms, osteoporosis), and stroke risk in older women.

Key Points
- **Exam Relevance:** Tibolone is occasionally asked as a short note in MD/MS exams under HRT.
- **Mechanism:** Estrogenic, progestogenic, androgenic effects; tissue-selective.
- **Indications:** Menopausal symptoms, osteoporosis prevention, libido improvement.
- **Risks:** Stroke in women >60 years; controversial breast cancer risk.

BOX 1: Important points to remember
- **Tibolone:** Synthetic HRT with estrogenic, progestogenic, androgenic effects
- **Uses:** Menopausal symptoms, osteoporosis prevention, libido enhancement
- **No withdrawal bleeding:** Ideal for postmenopausal women
- **Contraindication:** Hormone-dependent cancers, thromboembolism

REFERENCES

1. DNB Gynecology Question Bank. New Delhi: 2021.
2. Panay N, et al. HRT options. Maturitas. 2016;87:1-6.
3. Malhotra N, et al. HRT in India. J Hum Reprod Sci. 2017;10(3):234-40.
4. Baber RJ, et al. HRT overview. Climacteric. 2016;19(4):313-25.

5. Kloosterboer HJ. Tibolone pharmacology. J Steroid Biochem Mol Biol. 2015;76(1–5):231-8.
6. Verheul HA, et al. Tibolone metabolites. Menopause. 2016;14(6):1122-7.
7. Formoso G, Perrone E, Maltoni S,. Short-term and long-term effects of tibolone in postmenopausal women. Cochrane Database Syst Rev. 2016;10:CD008536.
8. Kenemans P, et al. Tibolone menopausal symptoms. Climacteric. 2017;10(Suppl 2):20-6.
9. Del Pup L, et al. Tibolone endometrial safety. Eur J Obstet Gynecol Reprod Biol. 2016;141(1):61-5.
10. Davis SR, et al. Androgenic effects tibolone. J Sex Med. 2015;5(8):1943-50.
11. Timmer CJ, et al. Tibolone pharmacokinetics. Clin Pharmacokinet. 2016;41(4):305-14.
12. Sharma A, et al. Menopause management India. J Obstet Gynaecol India. 2023;73(2):123-9.
13. Cummings SR, et al. Tibolone osteoporosis trial. N Engl J Med. 2016;359(7):697-708.
14. Delmas PD, et al. Tibolone BMD effects. J Clin Endocrinol Metab. 2015;87(5):2067-73.
15. Nijland EA, et al. Tibolone libido. J Sex Res. 2017;45(4):351-8.
16. Santoro N, et al. HRT contraindications. Menopause. 2016;23(6):678-86.
17. Archer DF, et al. Tibolone safety. Menopause. 2017;24(6):611-8.
18. Modelska K, et al. Tibolone side effects. Fertil Steril. 2016;79(6):1362-8.
19. Beral V, et al. Tibolone breast cancer risk. Lancet. 2016;369(9569):1407-8.
20. Bots ML, et al. Tibolone advantages. Maturitas. 2015;51(2):159-65.
21. Hammar M, et al. Tibolone compliance. Climacteric. 2016;7(3):281-8.
22. Cummings SR, et al. Tibolone stroke risk. N Engl J Med. 2016;359(7):697-708.
23. Pinkerton JV, et al. Tibolone long-term safety. Climacteric. 2017;20(6):541-7.
24. Gupta A, et al. HRT costs India. Fertil Steril. 2020;114(3):e123-30.
25. Patel S, et al. Tibolone use India. J Obstet Gynaecol India. 2023;73(1):89-95.
26. Sharma P, et al. Tibolone prescribing India. J Obstet Gynaecol India. 2024;74(1):56-62.
27. RCOG. Menopause management. Scientific Impact Paper No. 50. London: RCOG; 2015.
28. NICE. Menopause: diagnosis and management (NG23). London: NICE; 2023.

HRT Menopausal Hormone Therapy

Ruchika Garg

HISTORICAL CONTEXT

- **Pre-2002:** Hormone replacement therapy (HRT) was widely used for menopausal symptoms.
- **Post-2002 WHI Study:** Reported risks (breast cancer, heart disease, stroke, thromboembolism) reduced HRT use, increasing clinician hesitancy and alternative therapy exploration.
- **Current Evidence:** HRT benefits (coronary disease, osteoporosis, dementia risk reduction) outweigh risks when started within 10 years of menopause.

INDICATIONS

- **Global Context:** By 2050, 1.6 billion women will be menopausal/postmenopausal; South Korea leads in female life expectancy (90.82 years by 2030).
- **Indian Context:** Life expectancy ~72.3 years, menopause at 47–49 years. HRT addresses:
  - Vasomotor symptoms (hot flashes, sweating, palpitations)
  - Urogenital symptoms (dryness, dyspareunia, urinary frequency)
  - Psychological symptoms (mood swings, insomnia, depression, anxiety)
  - Long-term risks: Osteoporosis, cardiovascular disease, Alzheimer's

PRE-HRT WORKUP

- **History/Examination:** Detailed medical history, physical exam, blood pressure.
- **Investigations (Table 1):**

TABLE 1: Pre-HRT investigations

Test	*Purpose*
CBC, Hemoglobin	Baseline health
Blood sugar, lipid profile, liver/thyroid function	Screen metabolic/liver/thyroid dysfunction
Pelvic ultrasound	Evaluate uterine/ovarian pathology
Mammography	Breast cancer screening
BMD	Osteoporosis risk
Pap Smear	Cervical screening
Endometrial Biopsy	Rule out endometrial pathology

Types of HRT

- **Hormonal:**
  - **Combination:** Estrogen + progestogen for women with uterus.

- **Estrogen-only:** Posthysterectomy.
- **Forms:** Tablets, transdermal patches/gels, vaginal creams/pessaries/rings.
- **Regimens:** Continuous or sequential (progestogen for 12–14 days/cycle).
- **Nonhormonal:** SSRIs, SNRIs, gabapentin, pregabalin (40–65% vasomotor symptom reduction).

MECHANISM OF ACTION

- **Estrogen:** Acts on nuclear transcription factors in uterus/vagina, regulating gene expression.
- **Vaginal pH:** Maintains acidity (4.5–6.0); postmenopause, pH rises to ~7.0, increasing infection/dyspareunia risk.

Routes of Administration (Table 2)

TABLE 2: HRT administration routes

Route	*Forms*	*Examples*	*Notes*
Oral	Tablets	CEE, 17β-estradiol, estradiol valerate	Higher dose due to first-pass metabolism
Transdermal	Patches, gels, sprays	17β-estradiol	Safer, avoids liver metabolism
Vaginal	Creams, tablets, rings	17β-estradiol, estriol	Minimal systemic effects

ESTROGEN AND PROGESTERONE IN HRT

- **Estrogen:**
  - Oral: CEE (0.3–0.625 mg), estradiol valerate (1–2 mg), 17β-estradiol (1 mg).
  - Transdermal/Vaginal: Safer, reduces thromboembolism/triglyceride risks.[40]
  - Vaginal: FDA-approved for vaginal dryness/dyspareunia; low-dose estriol (0.03–0.5 mg/day) effective.
- **Progesterone:**
  - Prevents endometrial hyperplasia/cancer.
  - Types: Micronized progesterone (100–400 mg), synthetic progestins (MPA, norethindrone), levonorgestrel IUS.

FORMULATIONS IN INDIA (TABLE 3)

TABLE 3: HRT formulations available in India

Therapy	*Type*	*Examples*
Estrogen (Systemic)	Oral	CEE (0.3–0.625 mg), 17β-estradiol (1–2 mg)
	Transdermal	Estrogen gel (0.125 mg/2.5 g)
Progesterone	Oral	Dydrogesterone (10 mg), Micronized progesterone (100–400 mg)
	Intrauterine	Levonorgestrel IUS (52 mg, 20 mcg/day)
Combination	Sequential	17β-estradiol (1 mg) + dydrogesterone (10 mg, last 14 days)
	Continuous	17β-estradiol (1 mg) + dydrogesterone (5 mg daily)
Genitourinary syndrome	Vaginal	Estriol cream (0.5 mg/0.5 g), CEE cream (0.625 mg/g)

CONTRAINDICATIONS

- Breast/estrogen-dependent cancers, active/history of DVT/PE, arterial thrombotic diseases, chronic liver disease, migraine with aura, undiagnosed genital bleeding, thrombophilic disorders.
- Vaginal estrogen exempted due to low systemic absorption.

MONITORING AND SIDE EFFECTS

- **Monitoring:** Symptom relief, absence of adverse effects.
- **Side Effects:** Uterine bleeding, fluid retention, breast tenderness, headaches, mood changes.
- **Withdrawal Indications:** Jaundice, significant BP increase, new migraine-type headache, pregnancy.

GUIDELINES

- **NICE (2015):** HRT for hot flashes/night sweats; no increased cardiovascular risk before age 60 years.
- **IMS (2022):** HRT most effective for menopausal symptoms; initiate before age 60 years or within 10 years of menopause for osteoporosis prevention.

STRAW + 10 STAGING SYSTEM

- **Purpose:** Standardizes reproductive aging using menstrual/hormonal criteria.
- **Stages (Table 4):**

TABLE 4: STRAW + 10 staging system.

Stage	*Description*	*Menstrual/hormonal changes*	*Symptoms*
Reproductive (−5 to −3)	Early to late	Regular cycles, slight variability in −3a/−3b; FSH normal/variable, low AMH/inhibin-B	Reduced fecundability
Early menopausal transition (−2)	Variable cycle length (>7 days)	Elevated FSH, low AMH/inhibin-B/AFC	Vasomotor symptoms
Late menopausal transition (−1)	Amenorrhea ≥60 days	FSH >25 IU/L, low estradiol	Severe vasomotor symptoms
Early postmenopause (+1a, +1b, +1c)	5–8 years post-FMP	FSH rises, estradiol falls	Hot flashes, urogenital atrophy
Late postmenopause (+2)	Somatic aging	Stable high FSH, low estradiol	Vaginal dryness

SYMPTOM CORRELATION

- **Vasomotor Symptoms:** Affect ~80% in perimenopause; longer duration if starting perimenopause (11.8 vs. 3.4 years).
- **Vaginal/Sexual Symptoms:** Affect 33–50% postmenopause; GSM due to elevated vaginal pH.
- **Sleep/Mood Changes:** Insomnia linked to VMS; depression risk rises to 62% in early perimenopause.

LIMITATIONS OF STRAW

- Inapplicable to smokers, BMI >30 kg/m^2, posthysterectomy, or those with PCOS, POI, or serious illnesses.

INDIAN MENOPAUSE SOCIETY RECOMMENDATIONS

- Use Modified Bahram Anklesaria and STRAW + 10 staging.
- Prioritize lifestyle modifications and nonhormonal therapies before low-dose, short-duration HRT.

SUGGESTED READING

1. European Society of Endocrinology. Clinical Practice Guideline for management and evaluation of menopause, 2025.
2. Indian Menopause Society. Guidelines on Menopause and Hormone Therapy in Indian Women, 2025.
3. International Menopause Society. IMS recommendations on women's midlife health, menopause and menopause hormone therapy. Climacteric, 2025.
4. The Menopause Society. The 2025 Menopausal Hormone Therapy Guidelines: Position Statement on Hormone Therapy. Menopause, 2025.

Osteoporosis

Ruchika Garg, Anu Chudhary

INTRODUCTION

Osteoporosis, a systemic skeletal disease characterized by low bone mass and micro-architectural deterioration, increases fracture risk, particularly in postmenopausal women due to estrogen deficiency. Neglected by the general population, it requires comprehensive management beyond painkillers and supplements.

EPIDEMIOLOGY

- **Global:** Affects ~200 million people; 1 in 3 women and 1 in 5 men >50 years experience osteoporotic fractures.[1]
- **India:**
  - Prevalence: ~50 million affected; 20% of women >50 years have osteoporosis.[2]
  - Hip fracture incidence: 1.5–2 lakh annually; projected to rise with aging population.[3]
  - Challenges: Low calcium intake, vitamin D deficiency, limited DEXA access.[4]
- **Menopause:** Primary driver in women due to rapid bone loss post menopause.[5]

PATHOPHYSIOLOGY

- **Bone Remodeling:** Imbalance between osteoclast-mediated resorption and osteoblast-mediated formation leads to bone loss.[6]]
- **Estrogen Deficiency:** Post menopause, low estradiol (E2) and elevated follicle-stimulating hormone (FSH) accelerate osteoclast activity, reducing bone density.[7]
- **Microarchitecture:** Trabecular thinning and cortical porosity increase fragility.[8]
  Consequences: Fractures (hip, spine, wrist) from minor trauma.[9]

RISK FACTORS

TABLE 1: Risk factors for osteoporosis.[10,11]

Category	*Examples*
Nonmodifiable	Age >60 years, female sex, postmenopausal status, family history, early menopause, genetic disorders
Modifiable	Low calcium/vitamin D intake, smoking, alcohol excess, inactivity, eating disorders
Medical Conditions	Rheumatoid arthritis, Cushing's syndrome, hyperthyroidism, bone cancer, premature ovarian insufficiency (POI)
Medications	Corticosteroids, anticonvulsants, DMPA (long-term)

INVESTIGATIONS

- **Bone Mineral Density (BMD):**
  - **Dual-Energy X-ray Absorptiometry (DEXA):** Gold standard; measures spine/hip T-score **(Fig. 1)**.[12]

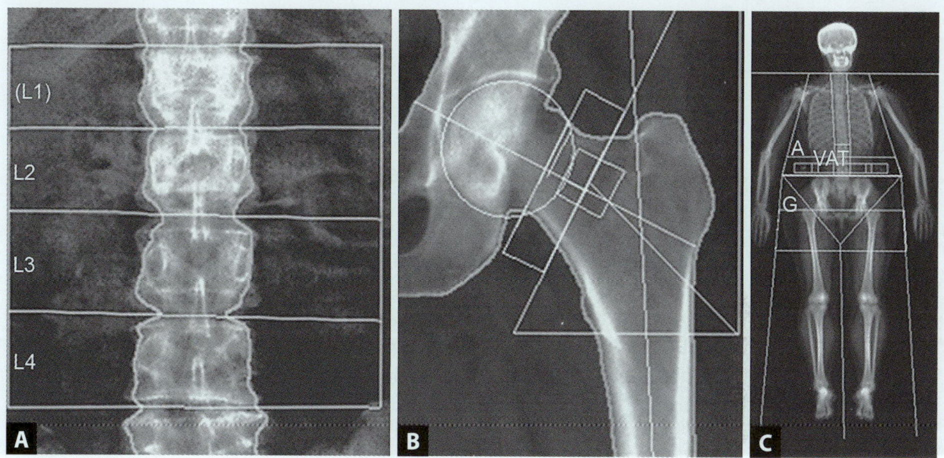

Fig. 1: Dual-energy X-ray absorptiometry.

    - **T-Score:**
      - Normal: ≥–1
      - Osteopenia: –1 to –2.5
      - Osteoporosis: ≤–2.5.[13]
    - **Z-Score:** Used in premenopausal women; <–2 indicates low BMD for age.[14]
  - **Peripheral DEXA/Ultrasound:** Assesses wrist/heel; not diagnostic but useful for screening.[15]
  - **Quantitative CT (QCT):** Accurate but high radiation; rarely used.[16]
- **Biochemical Markers:**
  - **Bone Formation:** Bone-specific alkaline phosphatase (BSAP), osteocalcin (OC), PINP.[17]
  - **Bone Resorption:** Urinary NTx, serum CTx, deoxypyridinolines (Dpd).[18]
  - **Utility:** Monitor therapy response; limited diagnostic value due to variability.[19]
- **Radiography:** Detects fractures or height loss (>1.5 inches).[20]
- **FRAX Tool:** Estimates 10-year fracture risk using BMD, age, and risk factors; treatment threshold ≥3% for hip fracture **(Fig. 2)**.[21]

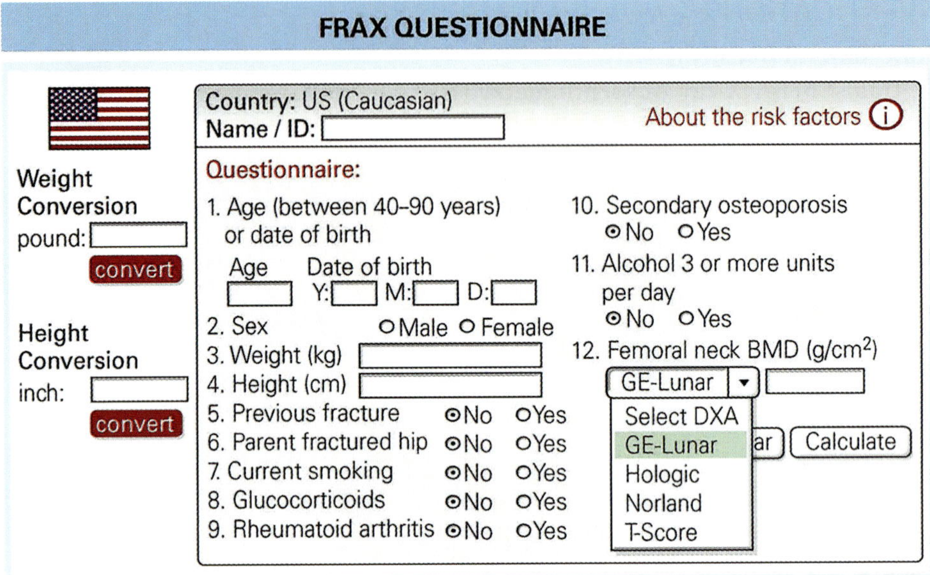

Fig. 2: FRAX questionnaire.

TABLE 2: WHO diagnostic criteria (T-Score).[13]

Category	*T-Score*
Normal	≥–1
Osteopenia	–1 to –2.5
Osteoporosis	≤–2.5
Severe Osteoporosis	≤–2.5 + fracture

Indications for BMD Screening

- **ACOG (2021):**[22]
  - All postmenopausal women ≥65 years.
  - Postmenopausal women <65 years with risk factors (e.g., smoking, low BMI, family history).
  - Frequency: Every 2 years if abnormal; avoid overuse in low-risk women <60 years.
- **IMS (India, 2020):**[23] Opportunistic screening >40 years due to high vitamin D deficiency prevalence.

Management

Goals: Prevent fractures, maintain BMD, reduce pain, improve mobility, manage comorbidities (**Flowchart 1**).[24]

Flowchart 1: Diagnosis and management of osteoporosis.

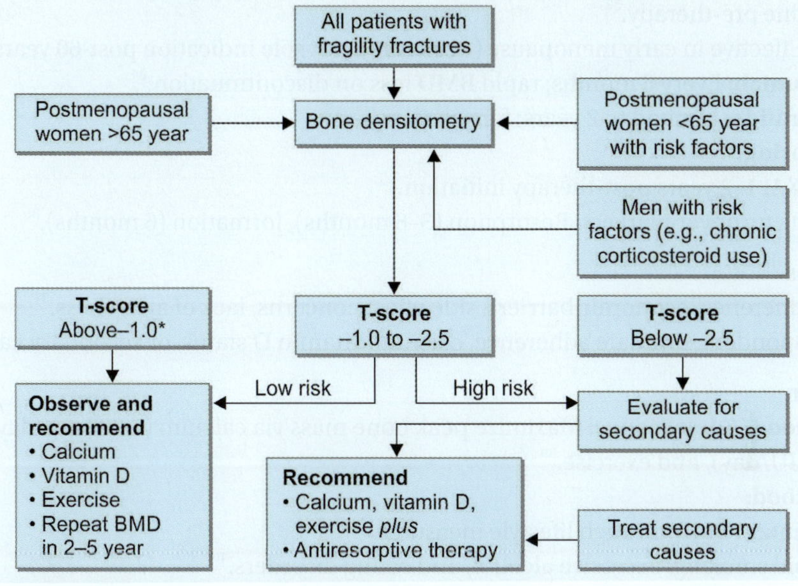

*Patients with fragility fractures and a T-score above –1.0 should be evaluated for other causes of pathologic fracture.

Nonpharmacological

- **Lifestyle:**
  - **Calcium:** 1,000–1,200 mg/day (diet + supplements).[25]
  - **Vitamin D:** 800–1,000 IU/day; maintain serum 25(OH)D >30 ng/mL.[26]
  - **Exercise:** Weight-bearing (walking) and resistance training 30 min/day.[27]
  - **Smoking/Alcohol Cessation:** Reduces bone loss.[28]
- **Fall Prevention:** Home safety, balance training, vision correction.[29]

Pharmacological

TABLE 3: FDA-Approved drugs for osteoporosis.[30,31]

Drug class	*Examples*	*Mechanism*	*Indications*	*Side effects*
Bisphosphonates	Alendronate, Zoledronate	Inhibit resorption	PMO, high fracture risk	GI upset, osteonecrosis of jaw (ONJ), atypical fractures
SERM	Raloxifene	Estrogen agonist on bone	PMO, vertebral fracture prevention	DVT, hot flushes
MHT	Estrogen ± Progestogen	Reduces bone turnover	Early PMO, symptomatic women	DVT, breast cancer (combined MHT)
Calcitonin	Nasal spray	Inhibits osteoclasts	Vertebral fracture, pain relief	Nasal irritation
RANKL inhibitor	Denosumab	Blocks osteoclast formation	High fracture risk, renal impairment	Hypocalcemia, ONJ
PTH analog	Teriparatide	Stimulates bone formation	Severe osteoporosis, prior fractures	Hypercalcemia, cost

- **Bisphosphonates:** First-line; reduce vertebral/hip fracture risk; monitor calcium/creatinine pre-therapy.[32]
- **MHT:** Effective in early menopause (<10 years); not sole indication post-60 years.[33]
- **Denosumab:** Every 6 months; rapid BMD loss on discontinuation.[34]
- **Teriparatide:** Limited to 2 years; for severe cases.[35]
- **Monitoring:**
  - DEXA: 1–2 years post-therapy initiation.
  - Bone turnover markers: Resorption (3–6 months), formation (6 months).[36]

Challenges

- Poor adherence, economic barriers, side effect concerns, lack of awareness.[37]
- Nonresponders: Evaluate adherence, calcium/vitamin D status, or secondary causes.[38]

Prevention

- **Childhood/Adolescence:** Maximize peak bone mass via calcium (1,000 mg/day), vitamin D (600 IU/day), and exercise.[39]
- **Adulthood:**
  - Maintain BMD through lifestyle measures.
  - Avoid smoking, excessive alcohol, and eating disorders.[40]
- **Postmenopause:**
  - Early MHT in symptomatic women with risk factors.
  - Screen per ACOG/IMS guidelines.[41]

BOX 1: Prevention strategies.

- **Diet:** Dairy, leafy greens, fortified foods for calcium/vitamin D
- **Exercise:** 30 min weight-bearing daily
- **Screening:** DEXA for women ≥65 or <65 years with risk factors
- **MHT:** Consider in early menopause for bone protection

Guidelines

- **RCOG (2018):**[42]
  - MHT for early PMO unless contraindicated; bisphosphonates first-line for high-risk women.
  - FRAX for risk assessment; DEXA every 2 years if treated.
- **NICE (2017):**[43]
  - Bisphosphonates for T-score ≤ –2.5 or FRAX ≥3%; denosumab if intolerant.
  - Counsel on lifestyle and fall prevention.
- **IMS (2020):**[44]
  - Opportunistic screening >40 years; calcium 1,200 mg/day, vitamin D 800 IU/day.
  - MHT in premature menopause; bisphosphonates for established osteoporosis.

Indian Context

- **Burden:** 50% of postmenopausal women have osteopenia; 20% have osteoporosis.[45]
- **Issues:**
  - Vitamin D deficiency: 70–90% prevalence.[46]
  - Low DEXA availability in rural areas; high out-of-pocket costs.[47]

- **Strategies:**
  - Promote calcium-rich diets (milk, ragi, greens).
  - Subsidize DEXA and bisphosphonates via public health programs.[48]
- **2022 Study:** Only 30% of eligible Indian women screened; 10% treated.[49]

Flowchart 1: Approach to postmenopausal women with fragility fracture.

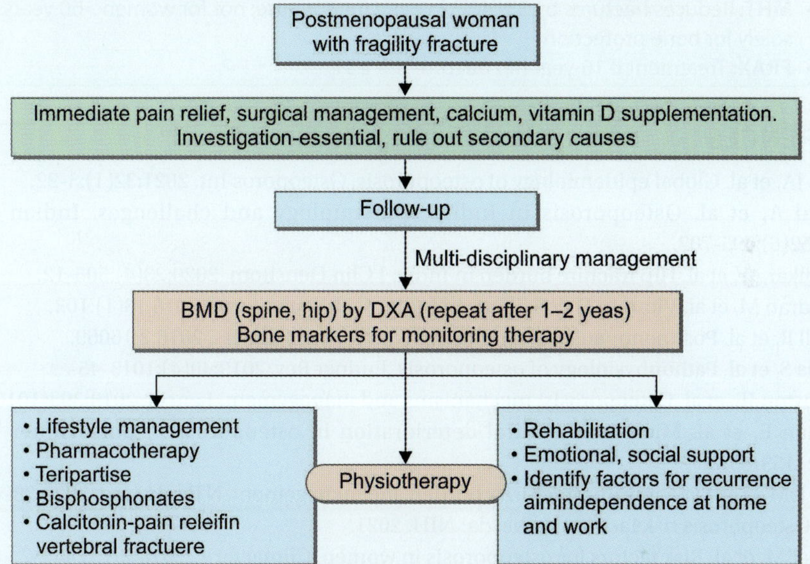

Source: Meeta, Harinarayan CV, Marwah R, Sahay R, Kalra S, Babhulkar S. Clinical practice guidelines on postmenopausal osteoporosis: Indian Menopause Society, 2019.

CLINICAL CASE SCENARIO

Case: A 62-year-old postmenopausal woman presents with back pain. T-score: –2.7 (spine), BMI: 22 kg/m^2, nonsmoker, family history of hip fracture.

Management

- **Diagnosis:** Osteoporosis (T-score ≤ –2.5).
- **Counseling:** Explain fracture risk, lifestyle, and treatment options.
- **Lifestyle:** Calcium 1,200 mg/day, vitamin D 1,000 IU/day, walking 30 min/day.
- **Pharmacotherapy:** Alendronate 70 mg weekly; ensure calcium/vitamin D repletion.
- **Monitoring:** DEXA after 1–2 years; check serum calcium/creatinine pretherapy.
- **Outcome:** Pain reduced; T-score improves to –2.3 after 2 years.

Exam Tip: Highlight DEXA criteria, bisphosphonates as first-line, and MHT in early menopause.

Key Points

- **Prevalence in India**: 20% of women >50 years; high fracture burden.
- **Diagnosis**: DEXA T-score ≤ –2.5; FRAX for risk assessment.
- **Management**: Bisphosphonates first-line; MHT for early PMO; lifestyle critical.

- **Prevention**: Maximize peak bone mass in youth; screen post menopause.
- **Challenges**: Low awareness, poor adherence, rural access barriers.

BOX 2: Important exam points.

- **DEXA T-Score:** Osteoporosis ≤−2.5; osteopenia −1 to −2.5
- **Bisphosphonates:** First-line; side effects include ONJ, atypical fractures
- **MHT:** Reduces fractures by 33–40% in early menopause; not for women >60 years solely for bone protection
- **FRAX:** Treatment if 10-year hip fracture risk ≥3%

REFERENCES

1. Kanis JA, et al. Global epidemiology of osteoporosis. Osteoporos Int. 2021;32(1):3-22.
2. Mithal A, et al. Osteoporosis in India: epidemiology and challenges. Indian J Orthop. 2018;52(6):695-702.
3. Khadilkar AV, et al. Hip fracture burden in India. J Clin Densitom. 2020;23(4):505-12.
4. Chandran M, et al. Vitamin D deficiency in India. Arch Osteoporos. 2018;13(1):103.
5. Eastell R, et al. Postmenopausal osteoporosis. Nat Rev Dis Primers. 2016;2:16069.
6. Khosla S, et al. Pathophysiology of osteoporosis. Endocr Rev. 2019;40(4):1013-45.
7. Compston JE, et al. Osteoporosis: mechanisms and management. Lancet. 2019;393(10169):364-76.
8. Seeman E, et al. Microarchitectural deterioration in osteoporosis. J Bone Miner Res. 2017; 32(6):1159-65.
9. Black DM, et al. Osteoporotic fractures: burden and management. N Engl J Med. 2020;382(8):752-62.
10. NIH. Osteoporosis risk factors. Bethesda: NIH; 2021.
11. Curtis EM, et al. Risk factors for osteoporosis in women. Climacteric. 2018;21(5):441-7.
12. WHO. Assessment of fracture risk. Geneva: WHO; 2017.
13. IOF. Diagnostic criteria for osteoporosis. Nyon: International Osteoporosis Foundation; 2020.
14. Lewiecki EM, et al. Z-score in premenopausal women. J Clin Densitom. 2019;22(4):447-53.
15. Hans D, et al. Peripheral BMD screening: role and limitations. Osteoporos Int. 2018;29(5):983-91.
16. Engelke K, et al. Quantitative CT in osteoporosis. J Bone Miner Res. 2020;35(4):633-42.
17. Vasikaran S, et al. Biochemical markers of bone turnover. Clin Biochem Rev. 2019;40(2):54-70.
18. Szulc P, et al. Bone resorption markers in osteoporosis. Bone. 2017;104:11-21.
19. Greenblatt MB, et al. Utility of bone turnover markers. J Clin Endocrinol Metab. 2018;103(10):3549-62.
20. Kanis JA, et al. Radiography in osteoporosis assessment. Osteoporos Int. 2019;30(1):17-26.
21. FRAX. WHO fracture risk assessment tool. Sheffield: University of Sheffield; 2021.
22. ACOG. Osteoporosis: screening and management. Practice Bulletin No. 227. Obstet Gynecol. 2021;137(6):e183-94.
23. IMS. Guidelines on osteoporosis. J Midlife Health. 2020;11(3):123-30.
24. Cosman F, et al. Clinician's guide to osteoporosis. Osteoporos Int. 2019;30(7):1309-31.
25. Weaver CM, et al. Calcium requirements in adults. J Nutr. 2016;146(4):737-43.
26. Holick MF, et al. Vitamin D supplementation guidelines. J Clin Endocrinol Metab. 2017; 102(4):1001-10.
27. Howe TE, et al. Exercise for preventing osteoporosis. Cochrane Database Syst Rev. 2017;10:CD000333.
28. Kanis JA, et al. Smoking and alcohol in osteoporosis. Bone. 2018;108:1-7.
29. Gillespie LD, et al. Fall prevention in older adults. Cochrane Database Syst Rev. 2018;9:CD007146.
30. FDA. Approved drugs for osteoporosis. Silver Spring: FDA; 2022.
31. Reid IR, et al. Advances in osteoporosis pharmacotherapy. Lancet Diabetes Endocrinol. 2021;9(6):388-99.

32. Ensrud KE, et al. Bisphosphonates for osteoporosis. JAMA. 2020;323(16):1597-606.
33. RCOG. Hormone replacement therapy and osteoporosis. Green-top Guideline No. 34. London: RCOG; 2018.
34. Cummings SR, et al. Denosumab for osteoporosis: long-term outcomes. N Engl J Med. 2019;380(7):637-46.
35. Saag KG, et al. Teriparatide for severe osteoporosis. J Bone Miner Res. 2017;32(12):2426-34.
36. Diez-Perez A, et al. Monitoring osteoporosis therapy. Osteoporos Int. 2019;30(1):27-37.
37. Khosla S, et al. Challenges in osteoporosis treatment adherence. J Clin Endocrinol Metab. 2017;102(3):733-43.
38. Adler RA, et al. Managing non-responders in osteoporosis. Osteoporos Int. 2018;29(10):2211-9.
39. Rizzoli R, et al. Maximizing peak bone mass. Osteoporos Int. 2019;30(4):717-30.
40. Weaver CM, et al. Lifestyle factors in osteoporosis prevention. J Bone Miner Res. 2018;33(6):959-67.
41. NICE. Osteoporosis: assessing fragility fracture risk (CG146). London: NICE; 2017.
42. RCOG. Menopause and bone health. London: RCOG; 2019.
43. NICE. Bisphosphonates for osteoporosis (TA464). London: NICE; 2017.
44. Harinarayan CV, et al. IMS osteoporosis guidelines. J Midlife Health. 2020;11(3):123-30.
45. Anuradha V, et al. Osteoporosis burden in India. Indian J Med Res. 2019;150(1):14-22.
46. Ritu G, et al. Vitamin D deficiency in India. J Clin Diagn Res. 2018;12(4):OE01-7.
47. Paul TV, et al. Challenges in osteoporosis management in India. J Clin Densitom. 2021;24(2):165-72.
48. MoHFW. National program for non-communicable diseases. New Delhi: Government of India; 2020.
49. Aggarwal N, et al. Osteoporosis screening in India: 2022 survey. J Midlife Health. 2022;13(2):83-90.

Genital Tract Injuries: Complete Perineal Tear, Bowel Injury, Examination of A Case of Sexual Assault

Ruchika Garg

INTRODUCTION

Genital tract injuries encompass traumatic damage to the female reproductive organs, including the vulva, vagina, cervix, uterus, and adnexa, as well as associated structures like the bladder, urethra, and rectum. These injuries may occur during childbirth, surgery, sexual assault, or accidents, with an incidence of genitourinary injuries post road traffic accidents at approximately 0.46%.[1] If untreated or incompletely healed, they can lead to chronic pain, dyspareunia, infertility, fistulas, and significant psychological morbidity. Early recognition, prompt management, and holistic care addressing physical, mental, and emotional needs are critical to mitigating long-term consequences.

CAUSES AND RISK FACTORS

Genital tract injuries arise from various etiologies, with specific risk factors amplifying vulnerability, particularly during obstetric events.

- **Causes:**
  - Obstetric: Traumatic vaginal delivery, cesarean section.
  - Traumatic: Road traffic accidents, straddle injuries, direct pelvic trauma.
  - Sexual: Consensual intercourse, sexual assault, female genital mutilation.
  - Iatrogenic: Surgical procedures, foreign bodies, instrumental abortions.
  - Other: Ox-horn injuries retained contraceptives/pessaries.
- **Risk Factors:**[2,3]
  - **Obstetric:** Large fetus (>4 kg), shoulder dystocia, occipitoposterior position, precipitous labor, episiotomy, operative vaginal delivery (forceps/vacuum).
  - **Nonobstetric:** Forceful coitus, postmenopausal status (atrophic tissues), sexual assault (up to 50% of victims report genital injuries).[4]
  - **General:** Age 15–24 years (trauma is a leading cause of death), pelvic fractures.

Table 1 summarizes the diverse causes and risk factors for genital tract injuries, highlighting the need for targeted prevention strategies.[2-4]

TABLE 1: Common causes and risk factors for genital tract injuries.[2-4]

Category	*Causes*	*Risk factors*
Obstetric	Vaginal delivery, cesarean section	Large fetus, shoulder dystocia, operative delivery
Traumatic	Road accidents, straddle injuries	Pelvic fractures, blunt/penetrating trauma
Sexual	Assault, consensual intercourse	Postmenopausal status, forceful coitus
Iatrogenic	Surgery, foreign bodies	Improper instrumentation, retained devices

OBSTETRIC ANAL SPHINCTER INJURIES

Obstetric anal sphincter injuries (OASIS) include third- and fourth-degree perineal tears, classified by the Royal College of Obstetricians and Gynaecologists (RCOG).[5]

Classification[5]

- **First-degree:** Injury to perineal skin or vaginal mucosa.
- **Second-degree:** Injury to perineal muscles, sparing anal sphincter.
- **Third-degree:**
  - 3a: <50% external anal sphincter (EAS) torn.
  - 3b: >50% EAS torn.
  - 3c: EAS and internal anal sphincter (IAS) torn.
- **Fourth-degree:** Injury to anal sphincter complex and anorectal mucosa.

TABLE 2: RCOG classification of perineal tears.[5]

Degree	*Description*
First	Perineal skin or vaginal mucosa
Second	Perineal muscles, sparing anal sphincter
Third (3a)	<50% EAS torn
Third (3b)	>50% EAS torn
Third (3c)	EAS and IAS torn
Fourth	Anal sphincter complex and anorectal mucosa torn

The RCOG classification **(Table 2)** guides the diagnosis and management of OASIS.[5]

Etiology

- **Obstetric:** Excessive perineal stretching during labor, rigid perineum, prolonged second stage.[3]
- **Nonobstetric:** Direct perineal trauma (e.g., falls).

Clinical Features

- **Symptoms:**
  - Fecal incontinence (severity depends on tear extent: loose stool in 3a, solid stool in 4th-degree).
  - Flatus incontinence.
  - Perineal soreness from stool irritation.
- **Signs:**
  - **Inspection:** Absent perineum, continuous vaginal/rectal mucosa, fibrous septum, retracted sphincter ends, radial skin wrinkles at anal verge.
  - **Palpation:** Reduced sphincter tone on rectal examination.
  - **Imaging:** MRI or endoanal ultrasound to confirm sphincter damage.[6]

Differential Diagnosis

- Low rectovaginal fistula (intact perineal skin, less complex repair).

Management

Preventive Measures:[3,5]

Controlled second-stage delivery (Ritgen's maneuver).

- Gradual head delivery, avoiding abrupt extension.
- Selective episiotomy at optimal timing.
- Careful shoulder delivery to prevent perineal overstretching.
  Operative Management (Sphincteroplasty and Perineorrhaphy).[5,7]
- **Timing:**
  - Immediate repair post delivery (within 24 hours, under regional anesthesia in operating room).
  - Delayed repair (2–3 months post injury) after infection resolution and tissue healing.
- **Preoperative Preparation:**
  - Baseline blood/biochemical tests, anesthesia fitness.
  - Eradicate worm infestations.
  - Low-residue diet (bread, milk) 2 days prior.
  - Gut sterilization (metronidazole 400 mg TID, erythromycin 500 mg TID, neomycin 250 mg TID) 48 hours prior.
  - Daily enemas 2 days prior; avoid enema on surgery day.
- **Surgical Principles (Warren Flap Method):**[7]
  - Incise posterior vaginal mucosa in inverted V-shape, mobilize rectal wall.
  - Freshen and suture torn sphincter ends and rectal wall in two layers (3-0 PDS, intraluminal knots).
  - Close pararectal fascia and approximate sphincter edges with interrupted sutures.
  - Excise redundant vaginal mucosa, reconstruct perineal body (0 Vicryl).
- **Postoperative Care:**
  - Nil per oral (day 1), liquids (day 2), nonresidue diet (day 3), full diet (day 6).
  - Stool softeners (lactulose 15–30 mL nightly) from day 2.
  - IV antibiotics (third-generation cephalosporin, anaerobic cover) for 5 days.
  - Avoid mobilization for 4–5 days.
- **Discharge Advice:**
  - Stool softeners for 1 week.
  - Contraceptive counseling.
  - Postnatal review at 6 weeks with endoanal ultrasound if indicated.
  - Institutional delivery with contralateral episiotomy in future pregnancies.
  - Elective cesarean for persistent incontinence or abnormal ultrasound post-repair.

Complications[6]

- Dyspareunia, persistent incontinence (20–30% residual defects), tight sphincteroplasty, wound dehiscence, rectovaginal fistula.
- Anorectal manometry to assess residual defects.

INJURIES BY ANATOMICAL LOCATION

Vulval Injuries

- **Causes:** Delivery, sexual assault, straddle injuries.
- **Presentation:** Pain, bleeding, swelling, hematoma.
- **Management:** Conservative for small hematomas (ice packs, analgesics); surgical evacuation for large hematomas.[8]

Vaginal Injuries

- **Causes:** Delivery, coital trauma, foreign bodies, instrumental abortions.
- **Presentation:** Bleeding, pain, discharge; possible fistula formation.
- **Management:** Suture tears with absorbable sutures (e.g., 2-0 polyglactin) under anesthesia.[8]

Cervical Injuries

- **Causes:** Precipitate labor, operative vaginal delivery, cervical dilatation (e.g., Hegar's dilators), conization.
- **Presentation:** Significant bleeding, minimal pain, possible hematometra or subfertility.
- **Management:** Suture lacerations; hysterectomy for severe cases.[8]

Uterine Injuries

- **Causes:** Uterine rupture (delivery), perforation (IUD insertion, D&C, hysteroscopy).
- **Presentation:** Bleeding, shock, abdominal pain.
- **Management:** Suture minor ruptures; hysterectomy for severe cases.[8]

TABLE 3: Management of genital tract injuries by location.[8]

Location	*Common causes*	*Management*
Vulva	Delivery, assault, straddle injury	Ice packs, evacuation of large hematomas
Vagina	Delivery, coital trauma, foreign body	Suture tears (2-0 polyglactin)
Cervix	Precipitate labor, instrumentation	Suture lacerations, hysterectomy if severe
Uterus	Rupture, perforation (IUD, D&C)	Suture minor ruptures, hysterectomy

Management strategies vary by injury location, as outlined in **Table 3**.[8]

Clinical Presentation

- **Vulval/Vaginal:** Severe pain, bleeding, swelling, hematoma; possible tachycardia, hypotension, shock.
- **Cervical:** Significant bleeding, minimal pain.
- **Uterine:** Abdominal pain, systemic signs (tachycardia, hypotension, collapse).
- **Long-term:** Vaginal discharge, urinary/fecal incontinence, dyspareunia, psychological distress.[9]

Diagnosis

- **History:** Bleeding, pain, trauma, childbirth, surgery, bladder/bowel symptoms.
- **Examination:**
    - General: Assess for tachycardia, hypotension, shock.
    - Abdominal: Palpable mass, tenderness, signs of internal bleeding.
    - Pelvic: Speculum and bimanual examination for lacerations, hematomas.
- **Investigations:**
    - Baseline blood tests (hemoglobin, hematocrit).
    - Imaging: Ultrasound, CT/MRI for internal injuries.[9]
    - Endoanal ultrasound/MRI for OASIS.[6]

Management

Initial Stabilization

- Hemodynamic resuscitation (IV fluids, blood transfusion if needed).
- Multidisciplinary approach (gynecologist, urologist, surgeon, psychologist).[9]
  Specific Treatment[8,9]
- **Conservative:**
    - Minor lacerations/small hematomas: Antibiotics, analgesics, stool softeners, perineal hygiene, ice packs.
- **Surgical:**
    - Suture vulval/vaginal/cervical tears (2-0/3-0 polyglactin).
    - Evacuate large hematomas; laparotomy for retroperitoneal/broad ligament hematomas.
    - Uterine rupture: Suture or hysterectomy.
- **Postoperative:**
    - Antibiotics (e.g., ceftriaxone, metronidazole) for 5–7 days.
    - Analgesics, pelvic floor exercises, psychological support.

Sexual Assault[10]

- **Medicolegal:** Document injuries, inform police, collect forensic samples.
- **Medical:** Treat injuries, prevent STIs (prophylactic antibiotics), prevent pregnancy (emergency contraception), provide psychological support.
  Coital Injuries
- **Presentation:** Vaginal tears, bleeding; rarely bowel prolapse in postmenopausal/posthysterectomy women.
- **Management:** Suture tears under anesthesia; manage shock/sepsis.[9]

Foreign Body/Instrumental Injuries

- **Vagina:** Forgotten contraceptives/pessaries, tampons; cause discharge, ulceration. Remove under anesthesia; retrieve broken needles via C-arm guidance.[9]
- **Cervix:** Tears from dilatation; manage by suturing or addressing stenosis.[8]
- **Uterus:** Perforation from IUD/D&C/hysteroscopy; manage surgically if visceral injury.[8]

Complications

TABLE 4: Complications of genital tract injuries.[11]

Category	*Complications*
Immediate	Bleeding, pain, hypovolemic shock, infection, urinary retention, sepsis, pulmonary embolism
Intermediate	Delayed healing, dehiscence, incontinence, chronic pain
Long-term	Fistulas (vesicovaginal/rectovaginal), dyspareunia, psychological stress, sexual dysfunction, pelvic floor dysfunction

Genital tract injuries can lead to immediate, intermediate, and long-term complications, significantly impacting quality of life **(Table 4)**.[11]

PREVENTIVE STRATEGIES[12]

- Antenatal education and birth planning.
- Screen/manage high-risk factors (e.g., large fetus, malpresentation).
- Pelvic floor exercises (Kegel's) in pregnancy.
- Perineal massage in late third trimester.
- Skilled birth attendants for institutional delivery.
- Selective episiotomy (avoid routine use).
- Judicious instrumental delivery by experienced obstetricians.
- Adequate analgesia (e.g., epidural).
- Postpartum examination for injuries.
- Perineal hygiene and early ambulation to prevent thrombosis.

EMERGING TRENDS AND GUIDELINES

- **Minimally Invasive Techniques:** Laparoscopic repair of uterine perforations reduces recovery time.[13]
- **Bioengineered Materials:** Use of absorbable meshes in fistula repair shows promise.[14]
- **Psychological Interventions:** Early counseling reduces post-traumatic stress in assault survivors.[10]
- **WHO Guidelines (2023):** Emphasize multidisciplinary care and training for obstetric injury prevention.[15]

CONCLUSION

Genital tract injuries, whether obstetric, traumatic, or iatrogenic, pose significant challenges due to their potential for physical, emotional, and social morbidity. Early diagnosis, tailored management, and preventive strategies are crucial to improve outcomes. Multidisciplinary care and adherence to updated guidelines ensure comprehensive management and rehabilitation.

REFERENCES

1. Bjurlin MA, Goble SM, Fantus RJ, et al. Genitourinary injuries in pelvic trauma. J Trauma Acute Care Surg. 2016;80(6):966-71.
2. McLean I, Roberts SA, White C, et al. Female genital injuries resulting from sexual assault. Forensic Sci Int. 2017;271:106-11.
3. Sultan AH, Kettle C, Thakar R. Perineal and anal sphincter trauma. Best Pract Res Clin Obstet Gynaecol. 2019;56:45-57.
4. Pergialiotis V, Vlachos D, Protopapas A, et al. Risk factors for severe perineal lacerations during childbirth. Int J Gynaecol Obstet. 2016;135(1):6-11.
5. Royal College of Obstetricians and Gynaecologists. Third- and fourth-degree perineal tears, management. Green-top Guideline No. 29. RCOG, 2015.
6. Nordervai S, Rydningen M, Falk RS, et al. Long-term outcomes after obstetric anal sphincter injuries. Obstet Gynecol. 2019;134(6):1260-8.
7. Andrews V, Thakar R, Sultan AH. Surgical management of obstetric anal sphincter injuries. Int Urogynecol J. 2018;29(6):795-802.
8. Goldman HB, McAchran SE. Urogynecologic and reconstructive pelvic surgery for trauma. Urol Clin North Am. 2019;46(2):237-45.
9. Bodner-Adler B, Hanzal E, Pablik E, et al. Management of genital tract trauma in obstetrics. Arch Gynecol Obstet. 2017;296(6):1047-54.
10. Campbell R, Lichty LF, Sturza J, et al. Gynecologic care for sexual assault survivors. Obstet Gynecol. 2016;128(4):870-6.
11. Halperin O, Noble A, Balachandran S, et al. Complications of genital tract injuries: A review. Eur J Obstet Gynecol Reprod Biol. 2020;247:140-6.
12. World Health Organization. Intrapartum care for a positive childbirth experience. WHO, 2018.
13. Nezhat C, Kho KA, Morozov V. Laparoscopic management of uterine perforation. J Minim Invasive Gynecol. 2017;24(5):712-7.
14. Mukwege D, Berg M. Advances in fistula repair using bioengineered materials. Int J Gynaecol Obstet. 2021;153(Suppl 1):45-50.
15. World Health Organization. Preventing and managing obstetric complications. WHO, 2023.

Sarcopenia Geriatric Medicine

Ruchika Garg, Prabhat Agrawal

INTRODUCTION

Sarcopenia, characterized by progressive loss of skeletal muscle mass, strength, and function, is a significant public health concern, particularly in aging populations. It contributes to frailty, falls, disability, and increased mortality, impacting quality of life and healthcare costs. In India, with a rapidly aging population projected to reach 20% by 2050, sarcopenia's prevalence and management are critical for postgraduate medical education. This chapter provides a comprehensive, evidence-based overview tailored for theory examinations, addressing epidemiology, pathophysiology, diagnosis, management, and its relevance in Indian postgraduate exams.

EPIDEMIOLOGY

Sarcopenia's prevalence in India varies widely due to diagnostic criteria and population differences. Studies report primary sarcopenia prevalence ranging from 14.2% to 47.7% among adults ≥60 years, with higher rates in rural (14.8%) than urban (6.8%) areas.[1,2] Severe sarcopenia affects 2.3–19.4% of older adults.[3] Men often show higher prevalence (12.5% vs. 8% in women), though some studies report female predominance.[4] Sarcopenic obesity, combining muscle loss with increased adiposity, affects ~11–40% of older adults, particularly in diabetic cohorts.[5] Comorbidities like type 2 diabetes (60%), chronic obstructive pulmonary disease, and osteoarthritis increase sarcopenia risk.[6] The Sarcopenia-Chandigarh Urban Bone Epidemiological Study (Sarco-CUBES) highlights lower muscle mass in Indians compared to Caucasians, necessitating population-specific cutoffs.[7]

TABLE 1: Sarcopenia prevalence in India.[1-6]

Population	*Prevalence*	*Notes*
Elderly (≥60 years)	14.2–47.7%	Higher in rural areas
Severe sarcopenia	2.3–19.4%	AWGS 2019 criteria
Sarcopenic obesity	11–40%	Common in diabetes
Type 2 diabetes	60%	Cross-sectional study

PATHOPHYSIOLOGY

Sarcopenia results from an imbalance between muscle protein synthesis and breakdown, driven by multiple factors:[8]

- **Age-Related Changes:** Reduced anabolic signaling (e.g., insulin-like growth factor-1), mitochondrial dysfunction, and motor neuron loss decrease muscle fiber size and number.

- **Chronic Inflammation:** Elevated cytokines (e.g., IL-6, TNF-α) promote muscle catabolism, particularly in sarcopenic obesity.
- **Nutritional Deficiencies:** Low protein intake, common in Indian cereal-based diets, and vitamin D deficiency impair muscle repair.
- **Sedentary Lifestyle:** Reduced physical activity accelerates muscle atrophy.
- **Hormonal Decline:** Decreased testosterone and growth hormone levels in men and women contribute to muscle loss.

Secondary sarcopenia arises from chronic diseases (e.g., diabetes, cancer) or immobility, amplifying systemic inflammation and oxidative stress.[9]

DIAGNOSIS

Sarcopenia diagnosis integrates muscle strength, mass, and physical performance, with Indian-specific cutoffs proposed by the South Asian Working Action Group on Sarcopenia (SWAG-SARCO):[10]

- **Muscle Strength:** Handgrip strength (HGS) <27.5 kg (men) or <18.0 kg (women) indicates low strength.[11]
- **Muscle Mass:** Appendicular skeletal muscle index (ASMI) by dual-energy X-ray absorptiometry (DXA) or bioimpedance analysis (BIA); cutoffs < 6.11 kg/m^2 (men) or <4.61 kg/m^2 (women).[12]
- **Physical Performance:** Gait speed <0.8 m/s or 5-chair stand test (5-CST) ≥12 seconds suggests poor performance.[13]
- **Screening Tools:** SARC-F questionnaire assesses strength, walking, rising, climbing, and falls; Ishii scoring is also used.[14]

The Asian Working Group for Sarcopenia (AWGS) 2019 criteria define:

- **Possible Sarcopenia:** Low HGS or poor performance.
- **Sarcopenia:** Low HGS/performance plus low ASMI.
- **Severe Sarcopenia:** Abnormalities in all three domains.[15]

Western cutoffs (e.g., EWGSOP2) overestimate prevalence in Indians due to smaller body sizes and lower muscle mass.[16]

TABLE 2: Diagnostic cutoffs for sarcopenia in India.[11-13]

Parameter	*Men*	*Women*
HGS (kg)	<27.5	<18.0
ASMI (kg/m^2)	<6.11	<4.61
Gait speed (m/s)	<0.8	<0.8
5-CST (s)	≥12	≥12

MANAGEMENT

Management focuses on nonpharmacological interventions, with limited pharmacological options:[17]

- **Resistance Exercise:** Progressive resistance training (2–3 times/week) improves muscle strength and mass; success rate 70–80%.[18]

- **Nutrition:** Protein intake of 1.0–1.2 g/kg/day, supplemented with beta-hydroxy-beta-methylbutyrate (HMB) and micronutrients (e.g., vitamin D), enhances muscle repair.[19] Indian diets often require protein supplementation due to low-quality protein sources.
- **Lifestyle:** Aerobic exercise and smoking cessation reduce inflammation and improve function.
- **Pharmacological:** No approved drugs; testosterone or selective androgen receptor modulators (SARMs) are under investigation but lack robust evidence.[20]
- **Screening:** All patients with comorbidities (e.g., diabetes, COPD) should be screened using SARC-F or HGS.[21]

RCOG/NICE Guidelines: While not specific to sarcopenia, NICE CG147 (2023) recommends exercise and nutrition for frailty management, applicable to sarcopenia.[22]

KEY POINTS

- Sarcopenia prevalence in India: 14.2–47.7% (≥60 years), higher in rural areas and men.
- Diagnosis uses HGS (<27.5 kg men, <18.0 women), ASMI (<6.11 kg/m^2 men, <4.61 kg/m^2 women), and gait speed (<0.8 m/s).
- Management emphasizes resistance exercise and protein supplementation (1.0–1.2 g/kg/day).
- Indian-specific cutoffs (SWAG-SARCO) are critical due to lower muscle mass than Caucasians.
- Sarcopenia is indirectly relevant in geriatric, endocrine, and orthopedic exam questions.

REFERENCES

1. Rao S, et al. Prevalence of sarcopenia in India: LASI. J Am Geriatr Soc. 2025;73(2):123-30.
2. Shaikh N, et al. Sarcopenia in rural South India. F1000Research. 2020;9:184.
3. Mallik Y, et al. Sarcopenia prevalence in North India. medRxiv 2025;doi:10.1101/2025.05.31.25328663.
4. Pal R, et al. Sarco-CUBES. Eur Geriatr Med. 2020;11(5):725-36.
5. Patel M, et al. Sarcopenic obesity in diabetes. Clin Diabetes Endocrinol. 2024;10:12.
6. Rahman R, et al. Primary sarcopenia in India. Aging Med. 2021;4:257-65.
7. Deora A, et al. Indian consensus on sarcopenia. Int J Geriatr Med. 2025;16:1731-45.
8. Papadopoulou SK, et al. Biomarkers in sarcopenia. Springer. 2022;1-31.
9. Das S. Diabetes and sarcopenia. Diabetes Epidemiol Manag. 2023;12:100158.
10. Kumar V, et al. SWAG-SARCO consensus. Osteoporos Sarcopenia. 2022;8(2):35-57.
11. Pal R, et al. HGS cutoffs. Eur Geriatr Med. 2020;11(5):725-36.
12. Kamboj P, et al. ASMI cutoffs. Indian J Med Res 2018;148:548.
13. Studenski S. Gait speed in sarcopenia. JAMA. 2011;305:50.
14. Ko Y, et al. SARC-F in India. J Assoc Physicians India. 2024;72:45-50.
15. Chen LK, et al. AWGS 2019. J Am Med Dir Assoc. 2020;21(3):300-7.
16. Brennan-Olsen SL, et al. Sarcopenia in LMICs. Calcif Tissue Int. 2019;105(6):609-18.
17. Deora A, et al. Sarcopenia management. PMC. 2025;doi:10.2147/IJGM.S123456.
18. Smith L, et al. Exercise in sarcopenia. Int J Environ Res Public Health. 2020;17(5):1708.
19. Gu WT, et al. HMB in sarcopenia. Gerontology. 2025;71(3):245-53.
20. Shin MJ, et al. Testosterone in sarcopenia. World J Mens Health. 2018;36(3):192-8.
21. Beaudart C, et al. Sarcopenia screening. J Cachexia Sarcopenia Muscle. 2017;8(2):163-71.
22. NICE. CG147: Frailty management. 2023.

Urogynecology

Urinary Incontinence

Ruchika Garg

OVERVIEW

Urinary incontinence (UI) is a prevalent condition characterized by the unintentional leakage of urine, impacting social and hygienic aspects of life. It affects approximately 20–30% of women, though only 7–12% pursue treatment. The International Continence Society defines UI as any involuntary urine leakage. As a storage symptom of the lower urinary tract, UI often goes unreported unless specifically probed during gynecological assessments. Many older women mistakenly perceive UI as a normal aging process, but it is not. Factors such as childbirth-related pelvic trauma, chronic illnesses, menopausal estrogen decline leading to weakened pelvic floor muscles contribute to its prevalence in older women, making it a significant clinical issue.[1]

CLASSIFICATION OF URINARY INCONTINENCE

Epidemiology

- *Global:*
  - Prevalence: 25–45% in women; increases with age (10–20% in <40 years, 50–70% in >70 years).[2]
  - Stress UI (SUI): ~50% of cases; urgency UI (UUI)/overactive bladder (OAB): 20–30%; mixed UI: 20–30%[3]
- *India:*
  - Prevalence: 20–40% in women; 30% in postmenopausal women[4]
  - Underreporting: Due to stigma and limited healthcare access; only 25% seek treatment.[5]

CLASSIFICATION AND PATHOPHYSIOLOGY

- **Types of UI:**[6-8]
  - **SUI:** Urine loss with increased intra-abdominal pressure (e.g., coughing, sneezing); due to urethral sphincter weakness or hypermobility
  - **UUI/OAB:** Involuntary leakage with sudden urge; caused by detrusor overactivity
  - **Overflow UI:** Leakage due to bladder overdistension from detrusor underactivity or outlet obstruction [e.g., pelvic organ prolapse (POP)]
  - **Mixed UI:** Combination of SUI and UUI

- **Pathophysiology:**
  - SUI: Pelvic floor muscle weakening (childbirth, aging, obesity)
  - UUI/OAB: Neurogenic (stroke, Parkinson's) or idiopathic detrusor dysfunction
  - Overflow: Detrusor underactivity (diabetes mellitus, neurological disorders) or obstruction (fibroids, prolapse)[9]

  Table 1 provides types of urinary incontinence.

TABLE 1: Types of urinary incontinence.[8,10]

Type	*Mechanism*	*Symptoms*
SUI	Urethral sphincter weakness	Leakage with coughing, sneezing
UUI/OAB	Detrusor overactivity	Urge, frequent small voids, nocturia
Overflow UI	Bladder overdistension	Leakage without urge, incomplete emptying
Mixed UI	SUI + UUI	Combination of SUI/UUI symptoms

EPIDEMIOLOGY

Causes and Risk Factors

The development of UI in women is multifactorial, involving dysfunction in the bladder, urethra, spinal cord, or brain, and sometimes hormonal or idiopathic causes. In SUI, compromised anatomical support and weakened bladder neck or urethral function play key roles. Continence relies on a functional striated sphincter, robust vaginal wall support, and well-vascularized urethral tissue. When these mechanisms fail, increased intra-abdominal pressure (e.g., from coughing) can cause urethral descent, leading to leakage. Intrinsic sphincter deficiency, independent of urethral mobility, may also cause SUI.

Risk factors include:

- Advancing age
- Childbirth (parity and vaginal delivery)
- Obesity
- Diabetes mellitus
- Hysterectomy
- Physical activity levels
- Smoking
- Dietary habits
- Hormone replacement therapy

Physiology of continence and micturition: Urine storage is regulated by spinal reflexes that contract the urethral outflow region via somatic and sympathetic nerves. Voiding is initiated by bladder distension, activating mechanoreceptors that trigger parasympathetic innervation through the pelvic nerve, causing detrusor muscle contraction via acetylcholine binding to muscarinic receptors. Continence is maintained when urethral pressure exceeds bladder pressure, with intra-abdominal pressure changes (e.g., from sneezing) equally affecting both structures to preserve continence. Voiding occurs when urethral pressure decreases and bladder pressure increases.

DIAGNOSIS HISTORY AND PHYSICAL EXAMINATION

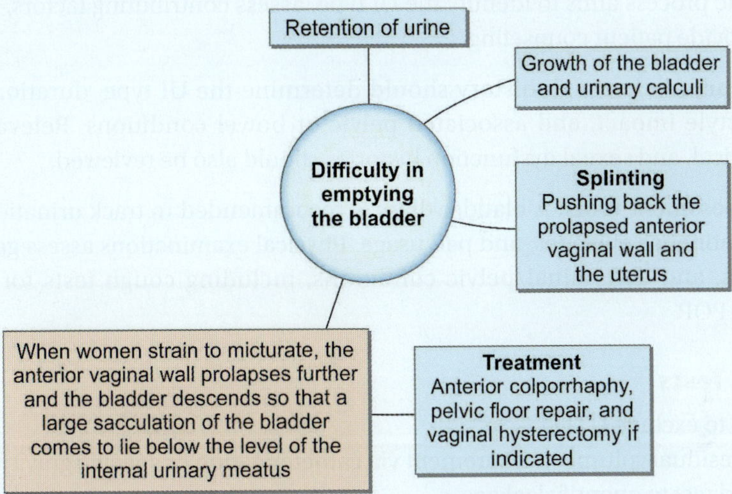

History-Taking

- **Key components:**[11]
  - **Urinary symptoms:** Frequency, volume, severity, triggers, nocturia, hesitancy, incomplete emptying, straining
  - **Systemic symptoms:** Dysuria, hematuria, pelvic pain [rule out urinary tract infection (UTI)]; neurological changes (cauda equina syndrome)
  - **Associated conditions:** Constipation, POP, bowel leakage
  - **Lifestyle:** Caffeine/alcohol intake, fluid consumption, smoking[12]
- **Tools:**
  - **3 Incontinence Questionnaire (3IQ):** Sensitivity 0.75 (UUI), 0.86 (SUI); specificity 0.77 (UUI), 0.60 (SUI)[13]
  - **2–3 day voiding diary:** Tracks frequency, volume, triggers; guides bladder training[14]
- **Red flags:** Lifelong incontinence, sudden onset, gross hematuria, neurological symptoms, recurrent UTIs (>3/year), advanced POP, elevated postvoid residual (PVR >1/3 bladder volume)[15]

Table 2 provides symptom clusters and UI types.

TABLE 2: Symptom clusters and UI types.[11,16]

UI type	*Symptom cluster*
SUI	Leakage with physical activity, no urge
UUI/OAB	Urge, frequent small voids, nocturia
Overflow (detrusor underactivity)	No urge, positional leakage, hesitancy, slow stream
Overflow (obstruction)	Straining, incomplete emptying, intermittent stream, pain/cramping

DIAGNOSTIC EVALUATION

The diagnostic process aims to identify the UI type, assess contributing factors, set treatment goals, and provide patient counseling.

Medical history: A thorough history should determine the UI type, duration, frequency, severity, lifestyle impact, and associated pelvic or bowel conditions. Relevant obstetric, medical, surgical, and sexual dysfunction histories should also be reviewed.

Symptom assessment tools: A bladder diary is recommended to track urination frequency, volume, incontinence episodes, and pad usage. Physical examinations assess general health, mental status, and abdominal/pelvic conditions, including cough tests for UI, urethral mobility, and POP.

Diagnostic Tests

- Urinalysis to exclude UTI
- Postvoid residual volume measurement via catheterization or specific gravity testing
- 1-hour pad test to quantify leakage
- Urodynamic studies to evaluate bladder sensation, detrusor activity, urethral function, and postvoid volume
- Cystoscopy to detect bladder abnormalities (e.g., masses, fistulae)
- Urethral sphincter electromyography or fluoroscopy to rule out neurological dysfunction
- Imaging is not routinely required but may be used selectively. Recent advancements (ICI-RS 2024) highlight the role of computational modeling and functional MRI in understanding female urethral function and voiding dysfunction.

MANAGEMENT OF STRESS URINARY INCONTINENCE

Nonpharmacological and Supportive Interventions

Initial management includes lifestyle changes (e.g., weight loss), bladder training, pelvic floor exercises, and UTI treatment. While surgery is often the most effective, incontinence pessaries are an option for nonsurgical candidates, though less effective.

Surgical interventions

Options include:
- Urethral bulking agents
- Bladder neck suspension procedures (e.g., midurethral slings, pubovaginal slings, colposuspension)
- Artificial urinary sphincter

Pharmacological Interventions

Urethral bulking agents: These are suitable for patients with intrinsic sphincter deficiency, low leak point pressure, minimal urethral mobility, or those unfit for surgery. Transurethral or periurethral injections are performed under local analgesia. Outcomes show 25–33% cure rates, 33–50% symptom improvement, and temporary urinary retention in 10–15% of cases. Rare complications include transient hematuria, urgency, or injection-site abscesses.

Bladder Neck Suspension

Midurethral synthetic slings: These minimally invasive procedures, such as tension-free vaginal tape (TVT) and transobturator tapes (TOTs), are the preferred surgical option for SUI due to high efficacy. TVT uses a bottom-up approach, while TOT includes outside-in or inside-out techniques. Complications include bladder perforation (higher in TVT), groin pain (higher in TOT), and rare vaginal tape erosion. Single-incision mini-slings, performed under local anesthesia, are also available.

Pubovaginal slings: These are used for recurrent SUI or mesh complications. These biological slings (e.g., rectus fascia) achieve 55–75% success over 10 years. Complications include bladder or vessel injuries, infections, and de novo urgency.

Burch colposuspension: This procedure suspends the vaginal wall to the iliopectineal ligament via open or laparoscopic approaches, with 85–90% continence at 1 year and 70% at 5 years. Complications include bladder perforation, hemorrhage, or prolapse.

Artificial urethral sphincter: It is used for neurological or recurrent SUI, it has a 66–100% success rate but carries risks of bladder neck or vaginal injuries and long-term issues like erosion or mechanical failure.

Treatment considerations: For refractory SUI, options include autologous slings, midurethral tapes, or colposuspension. Patient involvement in treatment decisions is critical, with guidelines (EAU, NICE) favoring midurethral slings for uncomplicated SUI.

MANAGEMENT OF URGENCY URINARY INCONTINENCE

Nonpharmacological interventions: Lifestyle modifications, weight loss, timed voiding, and pelvic floor training are first-line treatments.

Pharmacological interventions: Anticholinergics like solifenacin and mirabegron (a beta-adrenergic agonist) are used for UUI management.

Surgical and procedural interventions: Third-line options for UUI

- **Onabotulinum toxin A (oBTXA):** Injected into the bladder wall for refractory overactive bladder, with risks of UTI, incomplete emptying, or retention
- **Sacral neuromodulation:** Electrode placement in the S3 foramen suppresses involuntary detrusor contractions, with 43–56% cure rates and long-term efficacy
- **Percutaneous tibial nerve stimulation (PTNS):** Weekly stimulation for 3 months yields 54–79% success rates, offering a viable alternative to anticholinergics. For treatment-resistant cases, augmentation cystoplasty or urinary diversion may be considered

Simplified approach:

- **Urethral Q-tip test:** Obsolete due to low diagnostic value[17]
- **Cystoscopy:** Rarely indicated for uncomplicated UI; used for hematuria or suspected fistula[18]
- **Urodynamics:** Not required for uncomplicated SUI/UUI or prior to SUI surgery[19]

- **Essential tests:**
  - **Urinalysis:** Rule out UTI and hematuria.
  - **PVR measurement:** Assess overflow UI; >150 mL abnormal.[20]
  - **Pelvic examination:** Evaluate POP, vaginal atrophy, and pelvic masses.[21]
- **Questionnaires:** Short-form QOL, bother, and sexual dysfunction tools (e.g., ICIQ-SF, UDI-6)[22]

  Flowchart 1 provides diagnostic approach to UI.

Flowchart 1: Diagnostic approach to UI.[23]

History: Urinary symptoms, red flags, lifestyle
↓
Physical examination: Pelvic examination, POP assessment
↓
Urinalysis: Rule out UTI, hematuria
↓
PVR: >150 mL → Overflow UI evaluation
↓
3IQ/Voiding diary: Classify SUI, UUI, or mixed
↓
Red flags (neurological, hematuria, POP)? → Specialist referral
↓
Uncomplicated SUI/UUI → Initiate treatment

Pharmacological Treatment

- **SUI:**
  - **No FDA-approved drugs:** Duloxetine used off-label[24]
  - **Duloxetine:**
    - **Mechanism:** Serotonin/norepinephrine reuptake inhibitor; enhances urethral sphincter tone via Onuf's nucleus[25]
    - **Dose:** 20–40 mg twice daily
    - **Adverse effects:** Nausea, headache, fatigue, serotonin syndrome, hepatotoxicity[26]
    - **Contraindications:** MAO inhibitors, CYP2D6 substrates (e.g., tricyclics), liver disease[27]
- **UUI/OAB:**
  - **Beta-3 agonists:** Mirabegron, vibegron[28]
    - **Mechanism:** Stimulate beta-3 receptors, relax detrusor muscle[29]
    - **Mirabegron:**
      - **Dose:** 25–50 mg daily (extended-release)
      - **Adverse effects:** Hypertension, headache, urinary retention[30]
  - **Vibegron:**
    - **Dose:** 75 mg daily
    - **Adverse effects:** GI upset, dry mouth, urinary retention[31]

- **Antimuscarinics:** Darifenacin, fesoterodine, oxybutynin, solifenacin, tolterodine, trospium, propiverine[32]
    - **Mechanism:** Block M2/M3 receptors, reduce detrusor contractions.[33]

  Table 3 provides antimuscarinic drugs for UUI/OAB.

TABLE 3: Antimuscarinic drugs for UUI/OAB.[34,35]

Drug	*Dose*	*Adverse effects*
Darifenacin	7.5–15 mg daily (ER)	Dry mouth, constipation
Fesoterodine	4–8 mg daily (ER)	Dry mouth, blurred vision
Oxybutynin	5–30 mg daily (IR/ER), transdermal	Dry mouth, cognitive impairment
Solifenacin	5–10 mg daily	Constipation, dry mouth
Tolterodine	1–4 mg daily (IR/ER)	Dry mouth, headache
Trospium	20–60 mg daily (IR/ER)	Dry mouth, urinary retention
Propiverine	30 mg daily	Dry mouth, constipation

- **Combination therapy:**
    - Beta-3 agonist + antimuscarinic: For refractory OAB[36]
    - Dual antimuscarinic: Limited use due to side effects[37]
- **Adverse effects (antimuscarinics):** Dry mouth, constipation, blurred vision, cognitive impairment (elderly)[38]

  Drugs causing UI are mentioned in **Table 4**.

TABLE 4: Drugs causing UI.[39]

Drug class	*Examples*	*Mechanism*
Diuretics	Furosemide	Increased urine production
Alpha-blockers	Tamsulosin	Urethral relaxation
Sedatives	Benzodiazepines	Reduced bladder control
Antidepressants	Amitriptyline	Anticholinergic effects
Caffeine/alcohol	–	Diuretic, detrusor stimulation

Nonpharmacological Management

- **Lifestyle:**
    - Reduce caffeine/alcohol, optimize fluid intake (1.5–2 L/day).
    - Weight loss (5–10% body weight) improves SUI.[40]
- **Pelvic floor muscle training (PFMT):**
    - First-line for SUI/mixed UI; 50–70% improvement[41]
    - Supervised Kegel exercises for 8–12 weeks[42]
- **Bladder training:**
    - For UUI/OAB; scheduled voiding to increase intervoid intervals[43]
- **Vaginal devices**: Pessaries for SUI/POP; effective in 60% of cases[44]

Complications

- **Physical:** Skin irritation, recurrent UTIs, pressure ulcers[45]
- **Psychosocial:** Depression, social isolation, reduced QOL[46]
- **Economic:** High healthcare costs, absenteeism[47]

Guidelines

- **RCOG (2019):**[48]
  - **SUI:** PFMT first-line; duloxetine if conservative measures fail; surgery (midurethral sling) for refractory cases
  - **UUI/OAB:** Bladder training + antimuscarinics or beta-3 agonists; avoid urodynamics for uncomplicated cases.
  - **Red flags:** Refer for neurological, oncological, or urological evaluation.
- **NICE (2019, updated 2023):**[49]
  - **Diagnosis:** Use 3IQ, 2–3 day voiding diary; avoid urodynamics/cystoscopy for uncomplicated UI.
  - **Treatment:** PFMT for SUI; mirabegron preferred over antimuscarinics for OAB due to lower side effects.
  - **Follow-up:** Reassess at 3 months; refer if no improvement or red flags present.

Indian Context

- **Burden:** 20–40% prevalence; SUI common in parous women[50]
- **Challenges:**
  - Stigma delays treatment; only 20–30% seek care[51]
  - Limited access to PFMT specialists, urodynamics in rural areas[52]
- **Strategies:**
  - ASHA workers for UI education; subsidized pessaries in public hospitals[53]
  - **2024 Study:** 40% of Indian women with UI unaware of PFMT; 15% use absorbent pads[54]

CLINICAL CASE SCENARIO

Case: A 52-year-old postmenopausal woman presents with urine leakage during coughing and exercise for 6 months. no urgency or nocturia; pelvic examination: mild POP (stage 1); urinalysis: normal; PVR: 50 mL.

Management:

- **Diagnosis:** Uncomplicated SUI (3IQ positive, no red flags)
- **Counseling:** Explain SUI, lifestyle modifications, and PFMT benefits.
- **Treatment:** Refer for supervised PFMT (12 weeks); advise weight loss (BMI 27 kg/m^2).
- **Follow-up:** Reassess at 3 months; consider duloxetine or sling surgery if refractory.
- **Outcome:** Symptoms improve by 70% after PFMT; patient continues exercises.

Examination tip: Emphasize PFMT as first-line, simplified diagnostics, and NICE's preference for mirabegron.

Urinary symptoms in gynecology: Common complaints include hematuria, acute urinary retention (AUR), chronic retention, incontinence, frequency, dysuria, and difficult micturition. These are often linked to gynecological diseases (e.g., POP, pelvic tumors), pelvic surgeries, or difficult vaginal deliveries (EAU Guidelines, 2025).

Gynecologist's role: Exclude neurological causes (e.g., multiple sclerosis, spinal cord lesions) before surgical intervention for urinary complaints. Conduct thorough history, examination, and urological workup to differentiate gynecological from non-gynecological causes.

- Common urinary symptoms are as follows:

Hematuria

- Definition: Microscopic (>3 RBCs/hpf) or macroscopic (visible blood)
- Causes: UTI, urolithiasis, endometriosis, bladder carcinoma, renal cell carcinoma
- Investigation: Urinalysis (dipstick for nitrites/leukocytes), ultrasound/CT for malignancy/urolithiasis, cystoscopy for patients >35 years or with risk factors (e.g., smoking, chemical exposure)
- Management: Treat underlying cause; refer to urology/nephrology (AUA Guidelines, 2023).

Acute Urinary Retention

- Presentation: Sudden, painful inability to void; distended bladder

Causes

- Gynecological: Postoperative retention (edema, neuropraxia post-hysterectomy), postpartum retention (edema, perineal pain), hematocolpos (from imperforate hymen), retroverted gravid uterus (12–14 weeks), pelvic masses (e.g., uterine fibroids, ovarian neoplasms)
- Neurological: Spinal cord lesions, multiple sclerosis, pelvic surgery denervation
- Infections: Urethritis, cystitis, genital herpes
- Management: Immediate catheterization (indwelling until residual urine <100 mL), urinary antiseptics, analgesics; address primary cause (e.g., drain hematocolpos, reposition uterus) (EAU Guidelines, 2025).

Chronic Retention With Overflow

- Presentation: Painless, incomplete bladder emptying; common in elderly women
- Causes: Bladder neck narrowing (senile changes), cystocele, uterine prolapse
- Management: Treat underlying cause (e.g., pelvic floor repair), intermittent catheterization, and manage constipation.

Incontinence

Types:

- True incontinence: Continuous leakage from vesicovaginal fistula or ureterovaginal fistula; bladder empty or partially filled. Treat surgically.
- SUI: Leakage during coughing/sneezing; linked to prolapse or childbirth; first-line: pelvic floor muscle exercises (Kegel); surgery (e.g., sling) if refractory

- Urge incontinence: Sudden, large-volume leakage due to detrusor overactivity; treat with anticholinergics or beta-3 agonists (e.g., mirabegron).
- Diagnosis: Urodynamic studies to differentiate types; history for triggers (AUA/SUFU Guideline, 2023)

Frequency of Micturition

- Definition: >8 times/day or >1/night (nocturia)

Causes:

- Gynecological: Cystocele, pelvic tumors (e.g., fibroids, ovarian cysts), cervical cancer, early/late pregnancy
- Nongynecological: Diabetes mellitus, diabetes insipidus, OAB
- Investigation: Urine culture, cystoscopy, ultrasound, intravenous pyelography
- Management: Treat underlying cause; bladder training, psychotherapy for neurosis

Painful Micturition (Dysuria)

Causes:

- Vesical: Cystitis (pain at end of micturition), bladder stone, radiation cystitis (post-cervical cancer treatment)
- Urethral: Urethritis (e.g., gonorrhea, chlamydia), urethral caruncle, vulval carcinoma
- Investigation: Urine culture, cystoscopy for persistent cases
- Management: Antibiotics for infection, estrogen cream for menopausal women

Difficult Micturition

- Causes: Cystocele, procidentia, bladder neck obstruction, urethral stenosis
- Management: Splinting (manual repositioning for prolapse), anterior colporrhaphy, or vaginal hysterectomy if indicated

Cystitis

- Etiology: *Escherichia coli* (80% of uncomplicated cases), *Klebsiella*, *Staphylococcus saprophyticus*; common post-catheterization (10–20% risk per single use, higher with indwelling)
- Symptoms: Frequency, dysuria, suprapubic pain, pyuria
- Diagnosis: Urinalysis (dipstick: nitrites/leukocytes), urine culture for complicated cases
- Treatment: Uncomplicated: 3–5 days nitrofurantoin or fosfomycin; complicated (e.g., diabetes mellitus, pregnancy): 7–14 days ciprofloxacin (culture-guided). Increase fluid intake (2.5 L/day)

Pyelonephritis

- Presentation: Fever, flank pain, dysuria, rigors; often from ascending cystitis
- Management: Uncomplicated: oral antibiotics (e.g., ciprofloxacin, 10–14 days); complicated (e.g., pregnancy, diabetes mellitus): admit for IV antibiotics (e.g., ceftriaxone), urology referral if recurrent (EAU Guidelines, 2025).

Urethral Syndrome

- Cause: Estrogen deficiency (postmenopausal), hypersensitivity, rare infections (e.g., chlamydia)

- Treatment: Vaginal estrogen cream (1–3 months), antibiotics if infection confirmed
- Urethral caruncle:
- Presentation: Postmenopausal dysuria, dyspareunia, postcoital bleeding
- Management: Diathermy excision, estrogen cream (with progestogen to prevent endometrial hyperplasia), exclude malignancy

Urethral Prolapse/Diverticulum

- Symptoms: Frequency, dysuria, dribbling, dyspareunia
- Management: Surgical excision or marsupialization, antibiotics for infection

Urinary Fistulae

- Types: Vesicovaginal (most common, obstetric in developing countries, surgical in developed countries), ureterovaginal
- Symptoms: Continuous urine leakage, empty/partially filled bladder
- Management: Surgical repair, urology referral.

Ureteric Obstruction

- Causes: Uterine prolapse (hydroureter/hydronephrosis), pelvic tumors (fibroids, ovarian cysts), cervical cancer (70% mortality from obstruction)
- Investigation: Urography mandatory pretreatment for cervical cancer
- Management: Remove tumor and monitor for post-radiation fibrosis.

KEY POINTS

- **Prevalence in India:** 20–40%; SUI predominant, underreported
- **Diagnosis:** 3IQ, 2–3 day voiding diary; avoid urodynamics/cystoscopy for uncomplicated UI
- **Treatment:** PFMT for SUI; mirabegron/antimuscarinics for UUI/OAB; duloxetine off-label for SUI
- **Complications:** UTIs, depression, reduced QOL
- **Guidelines:** RCOG/NICE advocate noninvasive diagnostics, PFMT, and beta-3 agonists

Important points to remember are mentioned in **Box 1**.

BOX 2: Important points to remember.

- **SUI:** PFMT first-line; surgery for refractory cases
- **UUI/OAB:** Mirabegron preferred over antimuscarinics due to fewer side effects
- **Diagnostics:** 3IQ sensitivity 0.86 (SUI), 0.75 (UUI); PVR >150 mL indicates overflow UI
- **Red flags:** Gross hematuria, neurological symptoms, recurrent UTIs require specialist referral

REFERENCES

1. Haylen BT, et al. International Continence Society guidelines. Neurourol Urodyn. 2019;38(1):10-28.
2. Milsom I, et al. Global prevalence of UI. BJU Int. 2017;120(4):440-50.
3. Minassian VA, et al. UI epidemiology. Urol Clin North Am. 2019;46(1):1-10.
4. Singh U, et al. UI in Indian women. J Midlife Health. 2020;11(2):73-8.
5. Agarwal BK, et al. UI treatment-seeking behavior in India. Indian J Urol. 2018;34(3):196-202.
6. Sharma P, et al. UI prevalence in urban India. Int J Gynecol Obstet. 2023;162(2):456-63.
7. Coyne KS, et al. Economic burden of UI. Value Health. 2019;22(6):670-7.

8. Abrams P, et al. ICS terminology for UI. Neurourol Urodyn. 2018;37(1):116-26.
9. Dmochowski RR, et al. UI pathophysiology. Urol Clin North Am. 2020;47(2):189-98.
10. Lukacz ES, et al. UI classification. Obstet Gynecol Clin North Am. 2019;46(2):205-16.
11. Gormley EA, et al. AUA UI guidelines. J Urol. 2019;202(2):284-94.
12. Brown JS, et al. Caffeine and UI. J Urol. 2017;198(2):363-9.
13. Bradley CS, et al. 3IQ validation. Obstet Gynecol. 2018;131(4):683-90.
14. Wyman JF, et al. Voiding diaries in UI. Neurourol Urodyn. 2017;36(5):1223-30.
15. Nygaard I, et al. UI red flags. Am J Obstet Gynecol. 2020;222(3):S898-905.
16. Dumoulin C, et al. Symptom clusters in UI. Int Urogynecol J. 2019;30(5):687-94.
17. Meyer LE, et al. Q-tip test obsolescence. Int Urogynecol J. 2018;29(6):783-9.
18. Nitti VW, et al. Cystoscopy in UI. J Urol. 2020;203(1):143-50.
19. Serati M, et al. Urodynamics in SUI. Eur Urol. 2019;75(3):361-8.
20. Blaivas JG, et al. PVR measurement. Neurourol Urodyn. 2017;36(4):933-40.
21. Barber MD, et al. Pelvic exam in UI. Obstet Gynecol. 2018;132(4):e178-85.
22. Coyne KS, et al. ICIQ-SF validation. Value Health. 2019;22(2):230-7.
23. Guralnick ML, et al. UI diagnostic algorithm. Urol Clin North Am. 2021;48(2):167-78.
24. Schlenker B, et al. Duloxetine in SUI. Int Urogynecol J. 2017;28(6):821-8.
25. Thor KB, et al. Duloxetine mechanism in SUI. Urology. 2018;117:1-7.
26. Mariappan P, et al. Duloxetine adverse effects. BJU Int. 2019;123(3):385-92.
27. Vrijens D, et al. Duloxetine contraindications. Int J Clin Pract. 2018;72(4):e13066.
28. Chapple CR, et al. Beta-3 agonists in OAB. Eur Urol. 2020;77(1):101-10.
29. Andersson KE, et al. Beta-3 receptor mechanism. Neurourol Urodyn. 2019;38(5):1231-9.
30. Igawa Y, et al. Mirabegron safety profile. Int J Urol. 2021;28(4):353-61.
31. Yoshida M, et al. Vibegron in OAB. J Urol. 2020;204(6):1289-96.
32. Herschorn S, et al. Antimuscarinics in OAB. BJU Int. 2017;120(Suppl 3):20-31.
33. Madhuvrata P, et al. Antimuscarinic mechanisms. Int Urogynecol J. 2018;29(7):973-81.
34. Staskin DR, et al. Antimuscarinic dosing. Urol Clin North Am. 2020;47(1):75-84.
35. Wagg A, et al. Antimuscarinic side effects. Age Ageing. 2019;48(4):521-8.
36. Kelleher C, et al. Combination therapy in OAB. Int Urogynecol J. 2021;32(5):1045-53.
37. Griebling TL, et al. Dual antimuscarinic therapy. J Am Geriatr Soc. 2019;67(8):1712-8.
38. Chancellor MB, et al. Antimuscarinic adverse effects. Curr Urol Rep. 2018;19(6):41.
39. Gleason JL, et al. Drugs causing UI. Obstet Gynecol Clin North Am. 2020;47(2):249-60.
40. Subak LL, et al. Weight loss in SUI. N Engl J Med. 2017;376(14):1309-16.
41. Dumoulin C, et al. PFMT efficacy. Cochrane Database Syst Rev. 2018;10:CD005654.
42. Bo K, et al. PFMT protocols. Int Urogynecol J. 2020;31(3):453-61.
43. Burgio KL, et al. Bladder training in OAB. J Urol. 2019;201(4):768-74.
44. Richter HE, et al. Pessaries in UI. Obstet Gynecol. 2018;132(5):1134-41.
45. Frawley HC, et al. UI complications. Int Urogynecol J. 2019;30(8):1257-66.
46. Siddiqui NY, et al. Psychosocial impact of UI. Urol Clin North Am. 2020;47(3):383-91.
47. Wagner TH, et al. Economic costs of UI. Pharmacoeconomics. 2018;36(7):761-9.
48. RCOG. UI management. Green-top Guideline No. 75. London: RCOG; 2019.
49. NICE. (2019). Urinary incontinence and pelvic organ prolapse in women: management. NICE guideline: NG123. [online] Available from https://www.nice.org.uk/guidance/ng123 [Last accessed December 2025]
50. Mishra GD, et al. UI in Indian women. J Midlife Health. 2021;12(3):189-95.
51. Kumari S, et al. UI stigma in India. Indian J Community Med. 2020;45(4):411-6.
52. Rao SS, et al. UI healthcare access in rural India. Int J Gynecol Obstet. 2019;147(2):245-51.
53. MoHFW. ASHA UI education program. New Delhi: 2021.
54. Gupta N, et al. UI awareness in India. J Obstet Gynecol India. 2024;74(1):32-9.

Prolapse

Deepa Chaudhary, Mishu Mangla, Poojitha Kalyani Kanikaram

1. What is nulliparous prolapse? Briefly discuss the etiopathology, risk factors, and management of a case of nulliparous prolapse in a 24-year-old female.

Ans. Nulliparous prolapse refers to pelvic organ prolapse (POP) occurring in a woman who has never given birth (nulliparous).[1] While POP is more common in women who have had vaginal deliveries, nulliparous women can also experience it due to factors such as:

- Genetic predisposition to weak connective tissue
- Obesity
- Chronic straining (due to constipation or heavy lifting)
- Hormonal changes (e.g., menopause)
- Previous surgeries

Etiology of Nulliparous Prolapse

Congenital	Connective tissue disorders	Genetic ??	Pelvic floor nerve damage
• Spina bifida—most common congenital cause—82–86% • Bladder exstrophy—midline fusion defect—10–50% • Congenital shortness of vagina • Deep uterovesical and uterorectal pouches • Myopathies	• Ehler–Danlos syndrome—75% • Marfan's syndrome—33% • Scleroderma • Dermatomyosis	• Predisposition gene on Chr 9q21 • Collagen type 3 alpha 1 polymorphism • Changes in expression of fibulin-5 and lysyl oxidase • High concordance in sisters and identical twins	• Poliomyelitis with complications • Spinal cord injuries • Pelvic neuropathies • Denervation /accidental pelvic nerve injury

Evaluation and Workup

- A complete history to be taken, specifically age, H/o bladder, bowel, or urinary symptoms, H/o sexual dysfunction or dyspareunia; H/o any chronic illness, increased skin elasticity or joint hypermobility to R/o connective tissue disorders, H/o visual or neurological symptoms or any H/o previous pelvic surgery or radiotherapy
- After a complete general physical examination, a special note should be made of patients' BMI, nutritional status, mobility and manual dexterity, mental and functional status. Look for any E/o neurological deficit, or signs of any chronic illness.
- Bimanual examination in dorsal lithotomy and in position of maximal straining should be done to assess the degree of prolapse.[1]
- Staging to be done as per POP-Q system.

- Boney's test to rule out urethral hypermobility and stress urinary incontinence (SUI)
- Pelvic floor assessment grading to assess the tone of pelvic muscles

Differential Diagnosis

Differential diagnosis includes congenital elongation of cervix, vaginal cysts, cervical polyp, chronic inversion of uterus, vaginal tumor, varicose veins of vagina, and rectal prolapse.

Management of Nulliparous Prolapse[1]

The aim of management, apart from restoring the anatomy to normal and relieving from symptoms, is to maintain the menstrual, sexual, and childbearing functions of the patient.

The predominant treatment is surgery, although sometimes, pessaries may be useful in patients who refuse or are unfit for surgery, or in cases where medical diseases render the patient unfit for surgery. Gellhorn and donut pessaries are most commonly used.

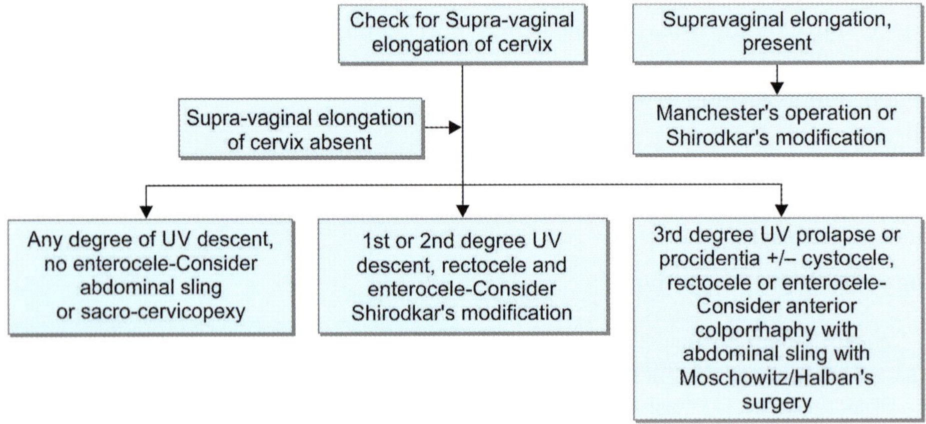

Table 1 provides surgeries for nulliparous prolapse.

TABLE 1: Surgeries for nulliparous prolapse.[2-4]

Type of surgery	*Static/dynamic*	*Procedure*	*Advantages*	*Disadvantages*
Sling surgeries				
Shirodkar's posterior sling	Static sling	*Principle:* Fascia lata/ Mersilene ribbon to strengthen uterosacral ligaments; center of strip stitched to front of cervix/posterior part of supravaginal cervix; two free ends fixed to intervertebral disc b/n L5 and S1 vertebrae	• Maintains uterus in correct anatomical position • Strong static bony support • No tendency to enterocele	*Technically difficult*: More on left side, sling has to pass blindly under sigmoid mesentery; risk of injury to colon, ureter, iliac vessels and genitofemoral nerve, closed loop—risk of bowel obstruction

Contd...

Contd...

Type of surgery	*Static/dynamic*	*Procedure*	*Advantages*	*Disadvantages*
Khanna's sling operation	Static sling	Mersilene tape (10 cm, 6 mm width) used; center attached to back of cervix; the two free ends guided retroperitoneally and fixed to anterior superior iliac spine with No. 00 black silk Lateral pull on cervix in line with Mackenrodt's ligaments	Does not antevert or retrovert uterus Strong static support Open sling—no risk of bowel obstruction	*Tape superficial*: Easily felt by the patient, iliac osteitis, broad ligament hematoma
Purandare's cervicopexy	Dynamic sling	Two fascial strips prepared from anterior rectus sheath; tape is anchored to anterior aspect of isthmus and anterior abdominal wall; with straining, lateral abdominal muscles contract and pull uterus up	Does not affect fertility, pregnancy, and labor and is easy to perform with usually minimum blood loss	• Alters pelvic anatomy by obliterating uterovesical fold • Vagina is being pulled forward l/t risk of enterocele. The tape carries a risk of being damaged at LSCS • Closed loop sling—risk of bowel obstruction if becomes tight
Virkud's composite sling operation	Mixed static and dynamic sling	Tape is anchored from posterior aspect of isthmus to sacral promontory on right side and anterior abdominal wall on left side. Left uterosacral ligament plicated to correct dextrorotation	Both static and dynamic support	Technically difficult
Joshi's sling	Static	Anterior surface of uterus at the level of internal os is suspended to pectineal ligament on both sides with Mersilene tape	–	–

Contd...

Contd...

Type of surgery	*Static/dynamic*	*Procedure*	*Advantages*	*Disadvantages*
Soonawala's sling	Static	Anterior longitudinal ligament on S1 vertebra→ along right uterosacral ligament of isthmus of uterus → retraced extraperitoneally to S1 vertebra	–	–
Other surgeries				
Sacrocervicopexy (may be abdominal, laparoscopic, or robotic)		Arms of "T"-shaped mesh attached to anterior and posterior aspect of cervix and limb attached to anterior longitudinal ligament of sacral promontory using polypropylene mesh; concurrent uterosacral plication done; success rate 88–100%	Effective correction of descent; anteversion; no compression on rectum or ureter	Technically difficult, complications include mesh erosion, bladder/bowel injury, infection, and recurrent prolapse

Apart from these surgeries, anterior colporrhaphy, posterior colpoperineorrhaphy, Manchester–Fothergill's surgery (± Shirodkar's modification), enterocele repair, McCall culdoplasty, and Moskowitz repair are done depending on case-to-case basis.

Case 1:

1. **Mrs X, 55 years old, P3L3, comes with mass descending per vaginum, more during coughing and sneezing, since 2 years. She underwent abdominal hysterectomy for fibroid uterus 10 years back and has developed above symptoms 5 years after previous surgery. What is your provisional diagnosis and how would you investigate and manage such case? Also comment on preventive measures that should be taken at the time of hysterectomy, so as to prevent such complications.**

Ans. The patient most likely has vault prolapse. Pelvic organ prolapse of the vaginal apex (PHVP) refers to the loss of apical support of the vagina, which, by definition, can only occur after a hysterectomy. It has been described as the descent of the vaginal apex, either at the vault or at the cuff scar following the surgical removal of the uterus. The severity of PHVP can be assessed based on the degree of descent. The severity of PHVP can be objectively assessed using the Pelvic Organ Prolapse Quantification (POP-Q) system, which provides a standardized method for clinical staging.

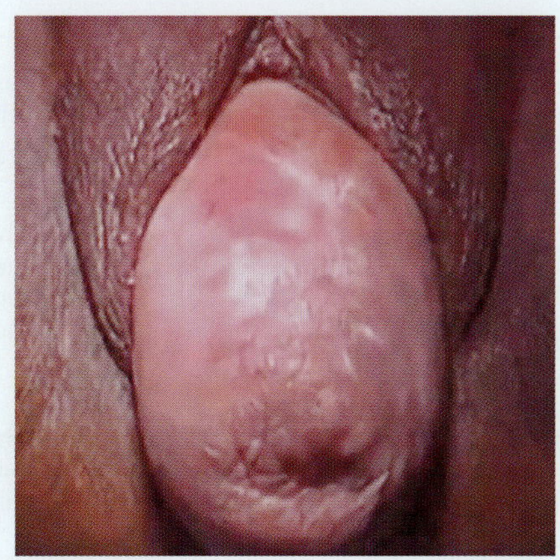

Signs and symptoms:

- Vaginal symptoms often include a sensation of bulging, heaviness, or discomfort in the vaginal area.
- Lower back pain, which tends to worsen later in the day
- Sexual dysfunction may also occur, presenting as pain during intercourse (dyspareunia), vaginal laxity, and difficulty with penetration.
- Decreased self-esteem
- Lower urinary tract symptoms can include voiding difficulties, a slow urinary stream, and recurrent urinary tract infections, along with increased daytime frequency, nocturia, and urgency.
- Stress and urgency incontinence
- Bowel-related symptoms associated with urogenital prolapse[2] may involve incomplete bowel evacuation, the need for manual assistance (digitating) to defecate, and, in some cases, fecal urgency and soiling.

Evaluation:

- Historically, prolapse severity was graded using inconsistent classification systems, making standard communication among clinicians difficult. The POP-Q system is a standardized method for assessing and describing POP. It is based on specific anatomic landmarks and measurements taken during a pelvic examination. The system evaluates the prolapse in relation to the hymen and is classified into stages based on the extent of organ descent. Staging should be done on the basis of POP-Q classification system of POP.
- Pelvic ultrasound scan to exclude the possibility of a pelvic mass which may present with prolapse symptoms.
- Urodynamic studies may be required in patients, predominantly presenting with urinary symptoms
- Anorectal physiology testing, endo-anal ultrasound, defecating proctogram, and bowel transit studies may be useful while women complaining of obstructed defecation

  Figure 1 shows POP-Q classification system of POP.

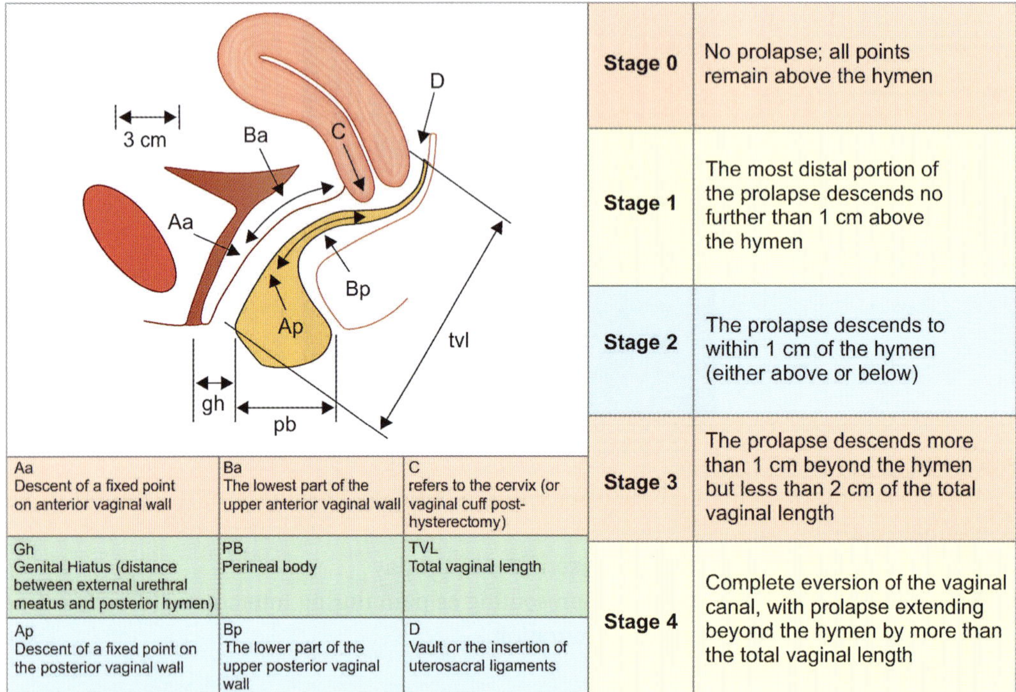

Aa Descent of a fixed point on anterior vaginal wall	Ba The lowest part of the upper anterior vaginal wall	C refers to the cervix (or vaginal cuff post-hysterectomy)
Gh Genital Hiatus (distance between external urethral meatus and posterior hymen)	PB Perineal body	TVL Total vaginal length
Ap Descent of a fixed point on the posterior vaginal wall	Bp The lower part of the upper posterior vaginal wall	D Vault or the insertion of uterosacral ligaments

Stage 0	No prolapse; all points remain above the hymen
Stage 1	The most distal portion of the prolapse descends no further than 1 cm above the hymen
Stage 2	The prolapse descends to within 1 cm of the hymen (either above or below)
Stage 3	The prolapse descends more than 1 cm beyond the hymen but less than 2 cm of the total vaginal length
Stage 4	Complete eversion of the vaginal canal, with prolapse extending beyond the hymen by more than the total vaginal length

Fig. 1: POP-Q classification system of pelvic organ prolapse[5] [recommended by International Continence Society (ICS), the American Urogynecologic Society (AUGS), The Society of Gynecologic Surgeons and The American College of Obstetricians and Gynecologists].
Source: Reproduced from Persu et al.[5]

Plan of management:[6,7]

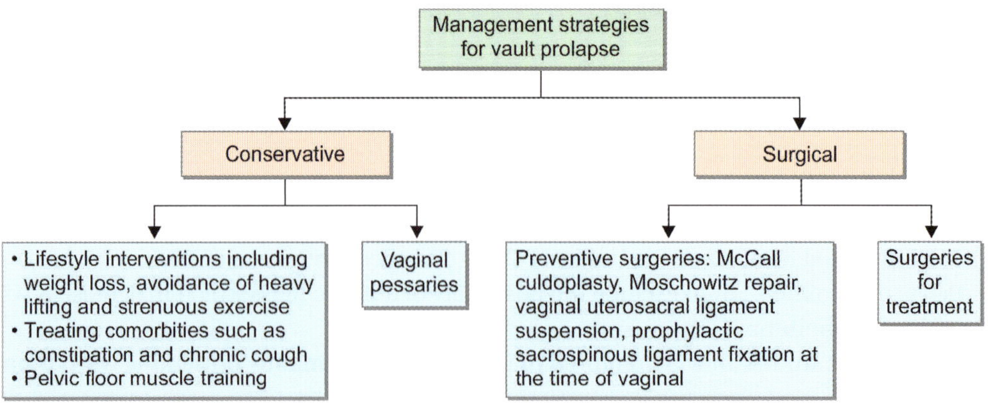

Surgical options for prevention of vault prolapse:[7,8]

- **McCall culdoplasty:** A surgical procedure which involves suturing the vaginal cul-de-sac (the space at the back of the vagina) to the uterosacral ligaments to provide support and restore pelvic organ support; this technique is often performed during a hysterectomy or as part of a comprehensive prolapse repair. It aims to reduce symptoms of prolapse, such as vaginal bulging or pelvic pressure.

- **The Moschowitz repair:** A technique designed to address anterior vaginal wall prolapse, such as a cystocele. The procedure involves making an incision in the vaginal wall to access and reinforce the weakened tissue. By suturing the vaginal wall to the underlying structures, the repair restores support to the anterior vaginal wall. This method can be performed with or without mesh reinforcement, aiming to improve symptoms and restore anatomical support. As with any surgical procedure, risks include infection, bleeding, and potential recurrence of prolapse.

Surgical options for treatment:

- **Sacrospinous ligament fixation (SSLF):**[9] The top of the vagina is anchored to the sacrospinous ligament, a strong band of tissue that connects the sacrum (a bone at the base of the spine) to the ischial spine (a part of the pelvis); the purpose is to restore support to the vaginal vault or uterus after a prolapse. A suture is placed through the sacrospinous ligament, and the vaginal apex (top) is anchored to this ligament using a Capio device or suture passer.
- **High uterosacral ligament suspension:** Bilateral suspension of the vaginal vault to the uterosacral ligaments at the level of the ischial spine
- **Abdominal or laparoscopic or robotic sacrocolpopexy:** Sacrocolpopexy is a surgical procedure where the vaginal vault is suspended by attaching it to the anterior sacral ligament using a permanent synthetic mesh, providing long-term support for POP. Complications reported include cystotomy (3.1%), ureteric injury (1%), enterotomy (1.6%), significant hemorrhage (2.6–4.4%), and long-term mesh erosion (3.4%). Mesh erosion rates vary by material, with 0.5% for polypropylene and 3% for polyethylene terephthalate. There is also a rare risk of discitis and osteomyelitis.

Case 2

1. **Mrs. X, 48 years old, P4L4 (all are normal vaginal deliveries at home), came with complaints of mass descending per vaginum, with difficulty in urination and defecation, for the past 1 year. What is your provisional diagnosis and how would you examine and manage such case?**

Ans. Patient is likely having uterovaginal prolapse. POP involves the descent of the pelvic structures, including cervix, uterus, and vaginal walls. The distinction between symptomatic and asymptomatic prolapse is clinically significant, as treatment is indicated only for women with symptoms. The prevalence of POP increases with the age of the women.

Risk factors:

- Vaginal delivery
- Advancing age
- Menopause
- Obesity
- Race and ethnicity (Latin and white women have 4-5-fold higher risk than African women)
- Elevated intra-abdominal pressure (COPD, constipation)
- Collagen abnormality (prolapse at a younger age)

Symptoms:

- Vaginal bulge and protrusion

- Pelvic pressure or vaginal pressure
- Voiding symptoms such as urinary hesitancy, intermittent flow, weak or prolonged stream, incomplete voiding, urinary retention (seen in anterior vaginal wall prolapse)
- Defecatory symptoms such as fecal incontinence, fecal urgency, obstructive defecation, and constipation requiring manual evacuation/digitation or reposition of the prolapse (seen in posterior vaginal wall prolapse)

Evaluation:

- **History:** History should be focused on evaluating the symptoms mentioned above, to look for causes leading to increased intraabdominal pressure, and a detailed obstetric, past and family history should be obtained.
- **Examination:** General physical examination including BMI

  The examination is performed in standing followed by dorsal lithotomy position.

  Standing position: Patient is asked to strain/Valsalva: To look for the maximum extent of prolapse.

  Apex is repositioned (allows to evaluate if reducing the apex reduces the visualized prolapse)

  Visual inspection of external genitalia in dorsal lithotomy position.

Speculum examination:

Anterior vaginal wall prolapse/ cystocele	Sim's retractor is introduced with gentle pressure on posterior vaginal wall. A tongue blade/Ayre's spatula is placed in both the anterior sulcus: • If this maneuver replaces anterior vaginal wall, it is a transverse or lateral paravaginal defect • If this maneuver does not reduce the hernia, central anterior defect
Posterior vaginal wall enterocele/ rectocele	Sim's retractor is placed in the vagina with gentle pressure on anterior vaginal wall: • Dominant posterior segment prolapse can be replaced with posterior blade of sims speculum • After replacement of dominant sites of prolapse, secondary sites of prolapse become more apparent

Bimanual examination: It is used to look for any coexisting pelvic abnormality.

POP-Q measurements are done for staging of the prolapse (described in vault prolapse).

Bonney's test: It is used to look for urethral hypermobility and rule out urinary stress incontinence.

Pelvis floor muscles: Assess for levator ani muscle strength and tone.

Neurological function: Sacral nerve—assess for bulbocavernosus reflex and anocutaneous reflex.

Imaging:

- *Pelvic USG*: To look for any pelvic mass
- *Urodynamics*: In patients with bothersome urinary symptoms
- *Defecography/dynamic MRI*: Routinely not done, useful to identify rectal prolapse, intussusception, or to differentiate a rectocele from enterocele or sigmoidocele

Management: Prevention strategies are not well-established. Interventions such as weight reduction, avoiding constipation and lifting heavy weights delay the progression of POP.

The selection of the surgical approach should address the patients' symptoms, anatomic findings, and her goals for surgery.

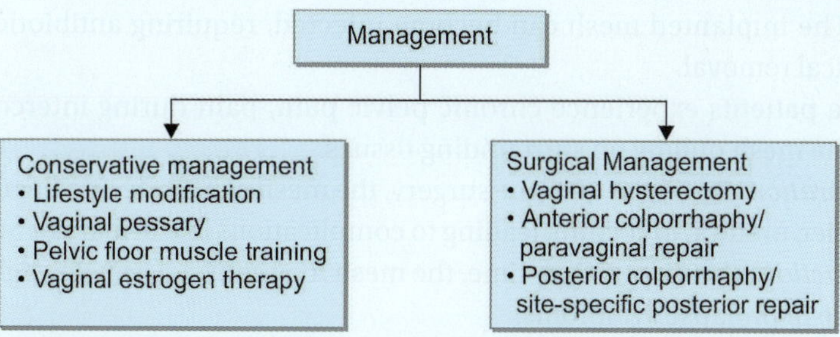

Surgical management:[10,11]

Anterior vaginal wall prolapse	*Anterior colporrhaphy:* Goal is to plicate the attenuated fibromuscular layer of the vagina to repair midline defects, reinforce the fibromuscular tissue, and reposition the bladder anteriorly *Paravaginal repair:* Vaginal/abdominal Goal is to reattach the lateral vaginal wall to arcus tendineus fasciae pelvis
Posterior vaginal wall prolapse	Posterior colporrhaphy (midline plication/site specific repair) ± perineorrhaphy: Reconstruction of the perineal body with the goal of the rebuilding of the perineum
Uterovaginal descent	Vaginal hysterectomy + apical suspension (McCall culdoplasty or uterosacral ligament suspension)
Enterocele repair	*McCall culdoplasty:* To prevent enterocele done during vaginal hysterectomy Moschowitz/Halban culdoplasties: Repair and prevention of enterocele Goal is to obliterate posterior cul-de-sac by suturing the posterior vagina to anterior sigmoid
Obliterative procedures Reserved for women with medical comorbidities, who are at a risk of extensive surgery	Le Fort colpocleisis (gynecological malignancies must be ruled out before performing the procedure)

SHORT QUESTIONS AND ANSWERS

1. Describe the current status of mesh usage in pelvic organ prolapse surgery.

Ans. In POP surgery, mesh is used to provide additional support to weakened pelvic tissues that can no longer hold organs like the bladder, uterus, or rectum in place. Mesh is typically made from synthetic materials or biological tissues and is implanted to reinforce the pelvic floor. Its role is to reduce the risk of recurrence of prolapse by providing long-term structural support. However, while mesh can be effective, it has also been associated with numerous complications, leading to a more cautious approach in its use. As a result, it is crucial that patients are thoroughly evaluated, and the benefits and risks of mesh-based surgery are carefully considered before proceeding. Mesh complications in POP surgery can vary in severity and impact. Some of the common complications include:

- *Mesh erosion (extrusion or exposure):* The mesh can wear through the vaginal wall, leading to exposure of the mesh in the vagina. This can cause discomfort, pain during intercourse (dyspareunia), and an increased risk of infection.

- *Infection:* The implanted mesh can become infected, requiring antibiotics or, in severe cases, surgical removal.
- *Pain:* Some patients experience chronic pelvic pain, pain during intercourse, or pain-related to the mesh pulling on surrounding tissues.
- *Organ perforation:* During or after the surgery, the mesh can erode into nearby organs such as the bladder, urethra, or rectum, leading to complications like urinary or bowel problems.
- *Mesh contraction (shrinking):* Over time, the mesh may contract, causing tightness, pain, or a recurrence of prolapse symptoms.
- *Recurrent prolapse:* Despite the use of mesh, prolapse may recur, leading to the need for additional surgery.
- *Urinary problems:* Patients may experience urinary incontinence or retention, especially if the mesh affects the bladder or urethra.

Because of these potential complications, the use of mesh in POP surgery is increasingly being regulated, and it is often recommended only for high-risk cases where other treatments have failed. Many surgeons now prefer non-mesh procedures or more conservative approaches, depending on the individual patient's needs. Due to the rising concerns about complications associated with mesh in POP surgery, many countries have implemented strict regulations and guidelines regarding its use. These regulations aim to ensure patient safety and proper use of mesh in surgical procedures. Some key aspects of these regulations are summarized in the following Table. These regulatory changes reflect a more cautious approach to using mesh in pelvic surgeries. Patients should always consult with their healthcare provider to understand the specific risks and benefits of mesh use in their individual case.

FDA warnings and restrictions (USA)[12,13]	• In 2011, FDA issued a public health notification warning of serious complications associated with transvaginal mesh for POP repair • By 2016, the FDA reclassified transvaginal mesh for POP repair as a high-risk (class III) medical device, requiring more rigorous testing and clinical data before approval • In 2019, the FDA ordered manufacturers to stop selling and distributing transvaginal mesh for POP repair in the US due to insufficient evidence of long-term safety and effectiveness
NICE guidelines (UK)[14]	• NICE issued guidance recommending that mesh for POP surgery should only be used in research settings, with a strong emphasis on patient consent and education about potential risks • Surgeons are required to provide alternative treatment options and fully explain the risks associated with mesh use • In June 2019, the NICE updated its stand on mesh implants with retropubic slings (in a bottom-up technique) once again being offered as a treatment option alongside the Burch colposuspension, the autologous rectus fascia sling, and bulking agents for urinary incontinence surgery
Australia's Therapeutic Goods Administration (TGA)	• Took steps to remove certain transvaginal mesh devices from the market in 2017 • In 2018, an Australian Senate inquiry into the use of surgical mesh recommended stricter regulatory oversight, better patient consent processes, and mandatory reporting of adverse outcomes
European Union Regulations[15,16]	• The European Union implemented stricter rules for medical devices in 2017 under the Medical Device Regulation (MDR), which includes mesh devices used in POP surgery. Under these regulations, manufacturers must provide clinical data demonstrating safety and efficacy, and there is increased post-market surveillance to monitor complications

2. Describe conservative management in pelvic organ prolapse.

Ans. Conservative management of prolapse includes all methods, excluding the surgical methods.[17,18] These include:

1. Lifestyle modification:
- Weight reduction
- Avoid constipation, heavy lifting.
- Smoking cessation
- Managing a long-standing cough
- Avoid physical activity that impacts on the pelvic floor like running or trampolining

2. Pessaries: These are used for the treatment of POP and SUI.

Mechanism of action:
- *POP:* Pessaries provide support to vaginal defect, including anterior, posterior, apical, and combined sites.
- *SUI:* It improves urethral function, by decreasing posterior urethrovesical angle, elevation of bladder neck, and increasing length of urethra.

Indications:
- Patients refusing surgery
- Patients with medical comorbidities unfit for surgery
- POP during pregnancy
- Desire for future childbearing
- Need to delay surgery for several weeks/months
- Recurrent POP (patient refusing surgery)
- Vaginal lacerations due to severe POP (reduction of POP through pessary and application of estrogen cream, promotes healing within 3–6 weeks, useful prior surgical repair)
- Preoperatively in women with POP to diagnose occult SUI

Types of pessaries:[19,20]

Type	*Support pessaries*	*Space-filling pessaries*
Used for	• POP (I–II stages) • SUI	POP (III–IV stages)
Mechanism of action	• Two-dimensional • Sit along the long axis of vagina	
Advantages	• Easy to insert and remove • Allows intercourse • More easily removed and inserted by the patient	• Provides support for larger degrees of prolapse • Reduces rectoceles • Useful in patients with wider genital hiatus
Examples	• Ring pessary (with/without support diaphragm) • Shaatz pessary • Lever pessaries • (Smith, Hodge, Risser) • Gehrung • Incontinence ring or dish pessaries	• Gellhorn • Donut • Cube • Inflatoball • Colpexin sphere

Pessary selection: For women with vaginal introitus measuring 1–2 fingerbreadths with stage I–II POP, ring pessary is advised, whereas for women with 3–4 finger breadths vaginal introitus and with stage III–IV POP, Gellhorn or other space-filling pessaries are suitable.

Contraindications:
- Local infection
- Exposed foreign body (vaginal mesh)
- Latex sensitivity
- Noncompliance

Side effects: These include vaginal erosions, vaginal infections, and retained pessary.

Management of common issues with pessary use:

Issue	*Management*
Expulsion or rectal pressure	Change pessary size or type
Urinary incontinence	Use an incontinence pessary with support at urethrovesical junction
Vaginal discharge	• Inspect vagina to exclude ulceration • More frequent pessary removal • Acidification gel or douches • Antimicrobial treatment • Vaginal estrogen
Vaginal bleeding	• Inspect vagina to exclude ulceration • Consider vaginal or endometrial biopsy or ultrasound if uterus is present
Vaginal abrasion/ulceration	• Remove pessary for 2–4 weeks • Vaginal estrogen • Consider biopsy if persistent

3. **Pelvic muscle floor training (PFMT)/Kegels exercises:**[21] Women with POP are more likely to have pelvic muscle floor weakness, atrophy, major defects of levator ani, and/or significantly decreased vaginal closure force when compared to women without prolapse. The goal is to strengthen the pelvic floor. When pelvic floor muscle becomes weak, there is increased risk of POP and urinary and fecal incontinence. PFMT aims to increase the structural support of the pelvic organs by improving the strength, endurance, and coordination of the pelvic floor muscles. It can be combined with other conservative treatments and can also be applied both before and after surgery.
4. **Vaginal hormonal treatment:** Vaginal estrogen in the form of tablets, cream, or ring inserted into vagina can help to reduce the discomfort experienced from prolapse.

3. **A 25-year-old nulliparous woman presented to OPD with complaints of mass descending per vaginum. On examination, there was third-degree cervical elongation without uterovaginal prolapse. How will you manage this case?**

Ans. Normal cervix has two parts: portiovaginalis which is the visible portion of the cervix that protrudes into the vagina and supravaginal cervix which is the intra-abdominal portion of the cervix that lies above the point of attachment of the vaginal vault.

	Supravaginal elongation	*Infravaginal elongation*
Associated with	Prolapse	Congenital
Vaginal cervix	Normal	Elongated
Uterine size	Normal	Normal
Fornices	Shallow	Deep
Uterocervical length	Increased	Increased

Management:

Procedure	*Technique*	*Complications*
Manchester Fothergill's procedure[22,23] *Indication*: Young patients having stage II or III prolapse with infra-vaginal elongation and hypertrophy of cervix with completed families	Improves apical support via amputation of cervix with preservation of uterine corpus; uterine body is reattached to uterosacral and cardinal ligaments	• Increased miscarriage • Preterm labor • Cervical dystocia • Cervical stenosis
Modified Fothergill's/Shirodkar vaginal prolapse procedure	Cervix is not amputated, posterior pouch is opened and both uterosacral ligaments are advanced anteriorly, crossing over and then fixed to the cervix at the level of internal os	Cesarean delivery can be difficult due to uterosacral advancement

4. Write a short note on supports of uterus.

Ans. The supports of the uterus can be classified into three main types: primary, secondary, and dynamic supports. These structures help maintain the uterus in its position within the pelvis.

Primary supports	These consist of fibrous structures and ligaments that anchor the uterus	• *Cardinal ligaments (transverse cervical ligaments):* These are the main supports of the uterus, running laterally from the cervix to the pelvic walls • *Uterosacral ligaments:* These connect the uterus to the sacrum, supporting it from behind • *Pubocervical ligaments:* These run from the pubic bones to the cervix, helping to support the uterus from the front
Secondary supports	These involve the peritoneal folds and ligaments that assist in keeping the uterus in position	• *Broad ligament:* It is a double-layered peritoneal fold that extends from the sides of the uterus to the lateral pelvic walls • *Round ligament:* This helps keep the uterus anteverted by running from the uterine horns to the labia majora via the inguinal canal
Dynamic support	Pelvic floor muscles	• *Levator ani muscle:* It plays a crucial role in supporting the uterus and maintaining its position by providing a dynamic floor for the pelvic organs • *Perineal body and muscles:* These also contribute to maintaining the position of the uterus, especially during increases in intra-abdominal pressure

DeLancey described defects in three levels of vaginal supports **(Fig. 2)**.

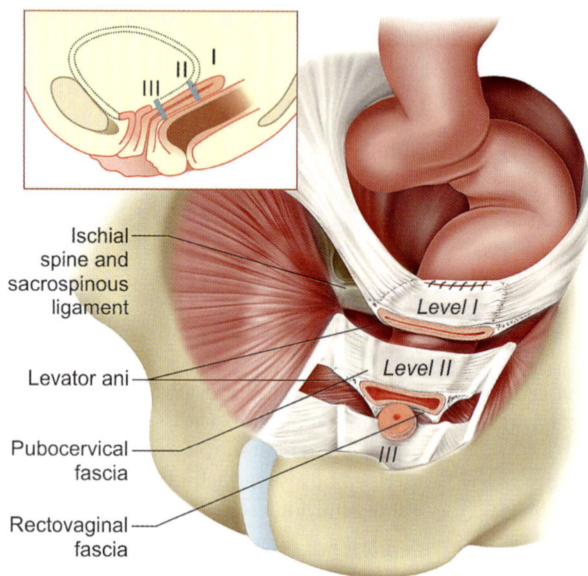

Fig. 2: DeLancey's three levels of vaginal supports.[24]

DeLancey's levels of support and related defects are given in **Table 2**.

TABLE 2: DeLancey's levels of support and related defects.

DeLancey's level of support	*Included structures*	*Defect leads to*
Level I	Cervical and upper vaginal support—proximal suspension—suspensory axis; includes parametrium, uterosacral–cardinal ligament complex, and paracolpium	Prolapse of uterus, post-hysterectomy vault prolapse, cystocele, enterocele
Level II	Mid-vaginal support—lateral attachment—attachment axis; paracolpium at level of ischial spines, anchored to ATFP and ATLA	Cystocele, rectocele, and stress urinary incontinence
Level III	Distal vaginal support—distal fusion—fusion axis; vaginal wall directly attached to surrounding structures; anteriorly fuses with urogenital diaphragm, posteriorly with perineal body, and laterally with levator ani	Distal rectocele, perineal descent, deficient perineum

- **Restore anatomy.**
- **Relieve symptoms.**
- **Preserve sexual/menstrual function (if desired).**

1. **Ward Mayo's vaginal hysterectomy with Fothergill's repair** (***uterus-preserving apical support in young women with UV prolapse***)

Step	Description
Anesthesia and positioning	Spinal/epidural; lithotomy with steep Trendelenburg
Infiltration	Vasopressin (20 U in 100 mL NS) in cervicovaginal junction
Circumferential incision	360° incision at cervicovaginal junction, 1 cm below bladder reflection
Bladder dissection	Sharp + blunt dissection of bladder off anterior cervix up to uterovesical fold
Clamping uterosacral and cardinal ligaments	Bilateral clamping at 1 cm from cervix; cut and suture transfix (1-0 Vicryl)
Anterior colpotomy	Enter Pouch of Douglas posteriorly after clamping Mackenrodt's ligament
Uterine arteries	Clamp at isthmus level, transfix with 1-0 Vicryl
Fundal delivery	Grasp fundus with vulsellum → deliver anteriorly (for small uterus)
Adnexal management	BSO if indicated; otherwise conserve
Fothergill's Sturmdorf sutures	• Plicate cardinal ligaments in midline • Anterior and posterior colporrhaphy • *Sturmdorf sutures:* Everting sutures at cervical stump (2-0 Vicryl)
Vault closure	High peritonealization + McCall culdoplasty (obligatory)
Final check	Hemostasis, vaginal pack, Foley catheter

Source: Enklaar et al.[22]
Note: McCall culdoplasty is mandatory to prevent vault prolapse. Evidence: 5-year recurrence <8% with Fothergill's.

2. Open sacrocolpopexy (vault prolapse)

Step	Description
Incision	Pfannenstiel or midline vertical
Bowel packing	Pack small bowel cephalad; Trendelenburg
Peritoneal incision	Incise over sacral promontory → open presacral space
Bladder dissection	Dissect bladder off anterior vagina (3–4 cm)
Vaginal vault preparation	Dissect rectovaginal septum posteriorly (3 cm)
Mesh selection	Type 1 macroporous polypropylene (Y-shaped, 15 × 4 cm)
Anterior mesh arm	Suture to anterior vaginal wall (4–6 interrupted 2-0 PDS/Ethibond)
Posterior mesh arm	Suture to posterior vaginal wall and levator fascia
Sacral fixation	Fix tail of Y-mesh to anterior longitudinal ligament at S1–S2 (2–3 nonabsorbable sutures or tacks)
Tensioning	Elevate vault to 2 cm above ischial spine level
Peritonealization	Close peritoneum over mesh (2-0 Vicryl running)
Concomitant procedures	Burch/MUS if SUI; posterior repair if rectocele

Note: Avoid sacral promontory vein plexus → use bipolar sealing Mesh erosion: 3.4% (polypropylene); avoid multifilament. Evidence: 7-year success 94%.

3. Laparoscopic/robotic sacrocolpopexy (minimally invasive gold standard)

Step	*Description*
Port placement	Umbilical (10 mm camera), 3 × 5 mm (LLQ, RLQ, suprapubic)
Exposure	Steep Trendelenburg; pack bowel; incise broad ligament peritoneum
Presacral dissection	Open peritoneum over promontory → identify right ureter, middle sacral vessels
Vaginal dissection	Hydrodissection (NS) → dissect bladder (anterior) and rectum (posterior) 3–4 cm
Mesh introduction	Y-shaped polypropylene via 10 mm port
Vaginal fixation	Secure anterior arm (4–6 interrupted 2-0 Ethibond) → posterior arm
Sacral fixation	Suture mesh tail to anterior longitudinal ligament (ALL) at S1 (2–3 Ethibond) or use Protack™
Tension adjustment	Vault at −2 cm from hymen (POP-Q point C = −6 to −8)
Peritoneal closure	Running 2-0 Vicryl/V-Loc over mesh
Cystoscopy	Mandatory → rule out bladder/ureteric injury

Note: Cystoscopy after indigo carmine → confirm ureteric patency.
Robotic advantage: 7 degrees freedom → easier suturing. Evidence: Laparoscopy versus open → less blood loss, same efficacy.

4. Sacrospinous ligament fixation

Step	*Description*
1	Posterior vaginal wall incision
2	Dissect rectovaginal space
3	Identify ischial spine → sacrospinous ligament (2 cm medial)
4	Place 2 delayed-absorbable sutures (PDS) through ligament
5	Attach to vaginal apex
6	Close vagina

Note: Success: 85–90% at 2 years; complication: Buttock pain (5–10%), pudendal nerve injury.

5. High uterosacral ligament suspension (USLS)

Step	*Description*
1	Identify USL at level of ischial spine
2	Place 2–3 nonabsorbable sutures bilaterally
3	Incorporate ipsilateral USL + vaginal apex
4	Avoid ureter (lateral to suture)

Note: OPTIMAL trial: Equivalent to SSLF at 5 years.

6. Le Fort partial colpocleisis *(elderly, sexually inactive, unfit for major surgery)*

Step	*Description*
1	Rectangular denudation anterior and posterior vagina
2	Successive imbricating sutures (2-0 Vicryl)
3	Leave lateral channels for drainage
4	Success: 95%

7. **Vault prolapse**
   - **Post-hysterectomy apical descent**
   - **Prevention at hysterectomy:**
     - **McCall culdoplasty**
     - **High peritonealization**
     - **USL incorporation in vaginal cuff**
8. **Mesh in pelvic organ prolapse surgery**

Type	*Status*
Type I (macroporous PP)	Allowed (abdominal route)
Type II–IV	Banned
Transvaginal mesh	FDA banned 2019
Note: Use only in recurrent prolapse, collagen disorders, and high-risk cases.	

9. **Postoperative care**
   - **Laxatives**
   - **Avoid straining × 6 weeks**
   - **No intercourse × 8 weeks**
   - **Follow-up: 2, 6 weeks, 3, 6, 12 months**
10. **Evidence summary**

Trial	*Finding*
Care	Sacrocolpopexy + Burch ↓ SUI
Optimal	SSLF = USLS at 5 years
Colpo	Mesh sacrocolpopexy ↓ recurrence
Sam	Manchester = Sacrohysteropexy

11. **Advanced surgical notes**

Key landmarks:
- Presacral space: Middle sacral vessels, left common iliac vein
- Paravesical space: Obturator internus, obturator canal
- Cave of Retzius: Pubic symphysis, Cooper's ligament

Nerve injury risk:
- Pudendal nerve: SSLF (buttock pain)
- Pelvic splanchnic: USLS (voiding dysfunction)
- Levator ani nerve: Lateral dissection

MULTIPLE CHOICE QUESTIONS

Q1. Pelvic organ support is maintained in part by the levator ani muscle. Which is not a component of this muscle?

a. Puborectalis muscle
b. Iliococcygeus muscle
c. Pubococcygeus muscle
d. Obturator internus muscle

Ans. d. Obturator internus muscle

The levator ani muscle, which forms part of the pelvic floor, is composed of three paired muscles: the pubococcygeus, puborectalis, and iliococcygeus. These muscles create a broad sheet, with anterior attachment to the pubic bodies of the pelvic bones and posterior attachment to the ischial spines.

Q2. Elective procedures or addressing prolapse at the vaginal apex include all of the following *except*:

a. Simple hysterectomy
b. Abdominal sacrocolpopexy
c. Sacrospinous ligament fixation
d. Uterosacral ligament vault suspension

Ans. a. Simple hysterectomy

Simple hysterectomy, increase the risk of later vault prolapse.

Q3. A 27-year-old female presents to the gynecology OPD with complaint of something coming out of introitus from last 3 years. The symptoms started 2 years after the birth of her only female child, who was born by an instrumental delivery, after prolonged second stage of labor. The management can be all *except*:

a. Vaginal hysterectomy
b. Fothergill's surgery
c. Sling surgery
d. Ring pessary

Ans. a. Vaginal hysterectomy

Considering the age of the patient, and her obstetric history, conservative options like pessary or uterus saving surgeries like sling surgeries or Fothergill's operation should the treatment of choice.

Q4. Which of the following is FALSE regarding the examination of a patient with prolapse?

a. The maximal extent of prolapse is demonstrated with a standing straining examination when the bladder is empty
b. Resting tone and voluntary contraction of the anal sphincters should be assessed during rectovaginal examination
c. Women with prolapse and urinary incontinence should have stress testing performed with the prolapse reduction because this will mimic bladder and urethral function when the prolapse is treated
d. Screening for presence of UTI or CIN is not needed at the time of examination

Ans. d. Screening for presence of UTI or CIN is not needed at the time of examination

Q5. All of the following are TRUE about pelvic floor muscle training for pelvic organ prolapse, *except*:

a. It includes pelvic floor strengthening by voluntary isometric contraction of muscles innervated by pudendal nerve
b. Tensing and holding contractions 5 seconds each, 15–20 per session, 3 times a day
c. Proper time to perform these exercises is with full bladder, in the morning
d. Minimum 6–8 weeks of therapy necessary before improvement is seen

Ans. c. Proper time to perform these exercises is with full bladder, in the morning

The best time to perform is **after micturition**.

Q6. All of the following are risk factors for nulliparous prolapse, *except*:

a. Instrumental vaginal delivery
b. Connective tissue disorders
c. Spina bifida
d. Ehler–Danlos syndrome

Ans. a. Instrumental vaginal delivery

Instrumental delivery is not a risk factor for nulliparous prolapse.

Q7. All of the following are surgeries used for the treatment of uterovaginal prolapse, *except*:

a. Burch colposuspension
b. Laparoscopic mesh sacrocolpopexy
c. McCall culdoplasty
d. Manchester–Fothergill surgery

Ans. a. Burch colposuspension

Burch colposuspension is a well-accepted technique for surgical management of SUI, especially when it is associated with urethral hypermobility.

Q8. Identify:

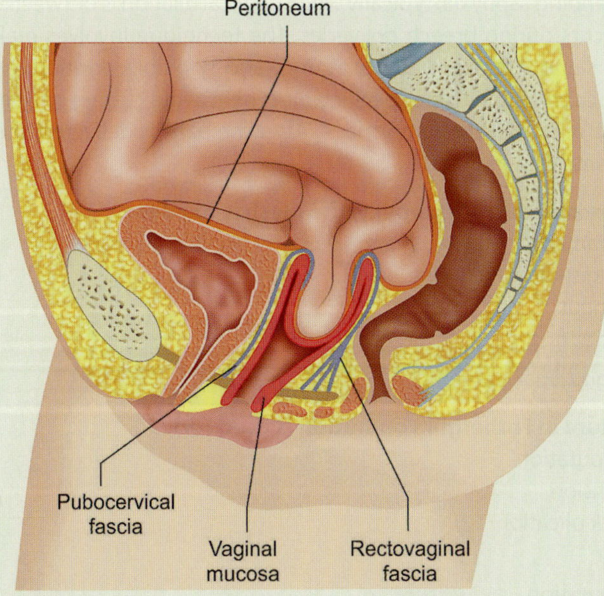

a. Cystocele
b. Enterocele
c. Rectocele
d. Isthmocele

Ans. b. Enterocele

Q9. All of the following are indications of using mesh in pelvic organ prolapse surgery, *except:*

a. A 65-year-old elderly, sexually inactive women with procidentia
b. A 55-year-old female, who underwent vaginal hysterectomy for third-degree UV prolapse, and presents after 2 years of surgery with vault prolapse.

c. A 35-year-old female, k/c/o Ehler–Danlos Syndrome, with third-degree UV prolapse
d. A 45-year-old female, P4L4, all vaginal home deliveries with third-degree UV prolapse

Ans. d. A 45-year-old female, P4L4, all vaginal home deliveries with third-degree UV prolapse

Q10. A 26-year-old female, G2P1, at 37 weeks' gestation presents to the labor room in active labor. She has uterine prolapse since her last delivery, 5 years prior. Third-degree uterocervical descent is present on vaginal examination. The cervix is edematous, 7–8 cm dilated, and vertex is at 0 station. There is meconium-stained liquor, but the fetal heart sound is 156 beats/min, regular. With uterine contraction, and maternal bearing down, you see that head with the cervix, descends further down out of the introitus. What would be your next management plan?

a. Wait for spontaneous progress of labor
b. Cesarean section
c. Give Duhrssen's incision at 2 o'clock and 10 o'clock to assist in vaginal delivery
d. Apply forceps to expedite delivery

Ans. c. Give Duhrssen's incision at 2 o'clock and 10 o'clock to assist in vaginal delivery

The Duhrssen's incision on the cervix is a method used to assist in delivering the head during obstructed labor when there is incomplete cervical dilation. It is particularly useful in emergencies, such as cases of impending asphyxia, typically when cervical dilation is between 6 and 8 cm, or when a cervical spasm occurs during breech deliveries. The technique involves making bilateral radial incisions with scissors under finger guidance at the 2 and 10 o'clock positions (with a possible third incision at the 6 o'clock position). These specific points help avoid cutting into cervical blood vessels and reducing the risk of significant hemorrhage. After the baby is delivered, these incisions can be easily sutured in a controlled manner.[25]

Q11. During laparoscopic sacrocolpopexy, the mesh is fixed to:

a. Pectineal ligament
b. Anterior longitudinal ligament
c. Arcus tendineus
d. Obturator internus

Ans. b. Anterior longitudinal ligament

Q12. Sturmdorf suture in Fothergill's operation is used for:

a. Cervical amputation
b. Vault suspension
c. Bladder neck plication
d. Rectal repair

Ans. a. Cervical amputation

REFERENCES

1. Dietz HP, Chavez-Coloma L, Friedman T, et al. Pelvic organ prolapse in nulliparae. Aust N Z J Obstet Gynaecol. 2022;62(3):420-5.
2. Virkud A. Conservative Operations in Genital Prolapse. J Obstet Gynaecol India. 2016;66(3):144-8.
3. Purandare VN. New surgical technique for surgical correction of genital prolapse in young women. J Obstet Gynaecol India. 1965:53-62.
4. Shirodkar VN. Second World Congress of International Federation of Gynaecology and Obstetrics, Montreal. 1958.

5. Persu C, Chapple CR, Cauni V, et al. Pelvic Organ Prolapse Quantification System (POP-Q) - a new era in pelvic prolapse staging. J Med Life. 2011;4(1):75-81.
6. Uzoma A, Farag KA. Vaginal vault prolapse. Obstet Gynecol Int. 2009;2009:275621.
7. Brunes M, Ek M, Drca A, et al. Vaginal vault prolapse and recurrent surgery: A nationwide observational cohort study. Acta Obstet Gynecol Scand. 2022;101(5):542-9.
8. Brun-Poulsen P. Genital prolapse and urinary incontinence. A clinical assessment of patients with prolapse with particular emphasis on surgical methods and their long-term effects. Ugeskr Laeger. 1990;152(46):3460-3.
9. Jelovsek JE, Barber MD, Brubaker L, et al.; NICHD Pelvic Floor Disorders Network. Effect of Uterosacral Ligament Suspension vs Sacrospinous Ligament Fixation With or Without Perioperative Behavioral Therapy for Pelvic Organ Vaginal Prolapse on Surgical Outcomes and Prolapse Symptoms at 5 Years in the OPTIMAL Randomized Clinical Trial. JAMA. 2018;319(15):1554-65.
10. Ko KJ, Lee KS. Current surgical management of pelvic organ prolapse: Strategies for the improvement of surgical outcomes. Investig Clin Urol. 2019;60(6):413-24.
11. Maher C, Feiner B, Baessler K, et al. Surgical management of pelvic organ prolapse in women. Cochrane Database Syst Rev. 2013;(4):CD004014. Update in: Cochrane Database Syst Rev. 2016;11:CD004014.
12. Ng-Stollmann N, Fünfgeld C, Gabriel B, et al. The international discussion and the new regulations concerning transvaginal mesh implants in pelvic organ prolapse surgery. Int Urogynecol J. 2020;31(10):1997-2002.
13. Ellington DR, Richter HE. Indications, contraindications, and complications of mesh in surgical treatment of pelvic organ prolapse. Clin Obstet Gynecol. 2013;56(2):276-88.
14. Lewicki P, Brant A, Basourakos SP, et al. Patterns in Transvaginal Mesh Surgery After Government Regulation in the United States. JAMA Surg. 2022;157(6):542-3.
15. European Commission, Directorate General for Health & Consumers. (2015). SCENIHR-Opinion on the safety of surgical meshes used in urogynecological surgery. [online] Available from https://ec.europa.eu/health/scientific_committees/emerging/opinions_en [Last accessed December 2025].
16. Kalkan U, Yoldemir T, Ozyurek ES, et al. Native tissue repair versus mesh repair in pelvic organ prolapse surgery. Climacteric. 2017;20(6):510-7.
17. Ryan GA, Purandare NC, Ganeriwal SA, et al. Conservative Management of Pelvic Organ Prolapse: Indian Contribution. J Obstet Gynaecol India. 2021;71(1):3-10.
18. Goujon A. Conservative management of genital prolapse. Rev Prat. 2019;69(4):387-389.
19. Bugge C, Adams EJ, Gopinath D, et al. Pessaries (mechanical devices) for managing pelvic organ prolapse in women. Cochrane Database Syst Rev. 2020;11(11):CD004010.
20. Hutchinson-Colas J. Pessaries: valuable interventions for symptomatic pelvic organ prolapse. Menopause. 2022;29(4):375-6.
21. Li C, Gong Y, Wang B. The efficacy of pelvic floor muscle training for pelvic organ prolapse: a systematic review and meta-analysis. Int Urogynecol J. 2016;27(7):981-92.
22. Enklaar RA, Schulten SFM, van Eijndhoven HWF, et al.; SAM Study Group. Manchester Procedure vs Sacrospinous Hysteropexy for Treatment of Uterine Descent: A Randomized Clinical Trial. JAMA. 2023;330(7):626-35. Erratum in: JAMA. 2023;330(11):1101.
23. Khunda A, Vashisht A, Cutner A. New procedures for uterine prolapse. Best Pract Res Clin Obstet Gynaecol. 2013;27(3):363-79.
24. DeLancey JO. Anatomic aspects of vaginal eversion after hysterectomy. Am J Obstet Gynecol. 1992;166(6 Pt 1):1717-24; discussion 1724-8.
25. Habek D, Mikuš M, Cerovac A. Dührssen's cervical incisions: Forgotten archaic obstetrics procedure?! Eur J Obstet Gynecol Reprod Biol. 2023;281:109-10.

Biomedical Waste Management

Ruchika Garg

INTRODUCTION

Biomedical waste (BMW) is any waste generated during healthcare activities, including diagnosis, treatment, immunization, research, or production and testing of biological materials. It poses significant risks to human health and the environment due to its hazardous nature, potentially containing infectious, chemical, radioactive, or pharmaceutical components. Effective BMW management is critical to prevent infections, ensure hygiene, and protect healthcare workers, patients, and communities.

Improper BMW disposal can lead to infection transmission, environmental contamination, and occupational hazards. The Bio-Medical Waste Management Rules, 2016, provide a framework for safe management in India, emphasizing segregation, treatment, and disposal protocols.[1]

CLASSIFICATION OF BIOMEDICAL WASTE

Biomedical waste is classified based on its risk potential and source, as outlined by the World Health Organization (WHO) and national guidelines. Categories include general waste, sharps, infectious waste, pathological waste, chemical waste, and radioactive waste. The BMWM Rules, 2016, categorize BMW into four color-coded groups for segregation and disposal **(Table 1)**.[1]

TABLE 1: Classification and management of biomedical waste (BMWM Rules, 2016).[1]

Category	*Color code*	*Waste type*	*Examples*	*Management*
Yellow	Yellow	Human/animal anatomical waste, soiled waste, chemical waste, discarded/expired medicines, linen, liquid waste, mattresses, masks, gowns, lab waste	Tissues, organs, blood-soaked bandages, disinfectants, expired drugs	Incineration, plasma pyrolysis, or deep burial
Red	Red	Recyclable plastic waste	IV tubes, gloves, catheters, urine bags, syringes (without needles)	Autoclaving, microwaving, hydroclaving, followed by recycling (no landfilling)

Contd...

Contd...

Category	*Color code*	*Waste type*	*Examples*	*Management*
White	White	Sharps waste	Needles, scalpels, blades, syringes with fixed needles	Autoclaving or dry heat sterilization, followed by shredding, mutilation, or encapsulation
Blue	Blue	Glass and metallic waste	Broken glass, medicine vials, ampoules, metallic implants (noncytotoxic)	Disinfection, autoclaving, microwaving, or hydroclaving, followed by recycling

The classification of BMW into yellow, red, white, and blue categories facilitates effective segregation and disposal, as detailed in **Table 1**[1] and **Figures 1 to 4**.

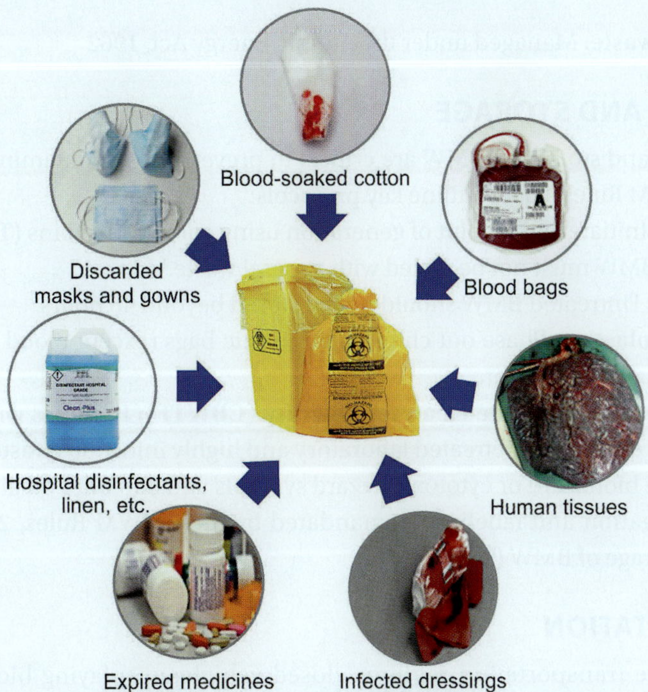

Fig. 1: Waste to be disposed of in the yellow bin.

General Waste

General waste, nonhazardous and noninfectious, includes paper, packaging, food waste, plastic bottles, and aluminum cans. It is sorted into wet and dry categories and disposed of in black bags for municipal waste management.

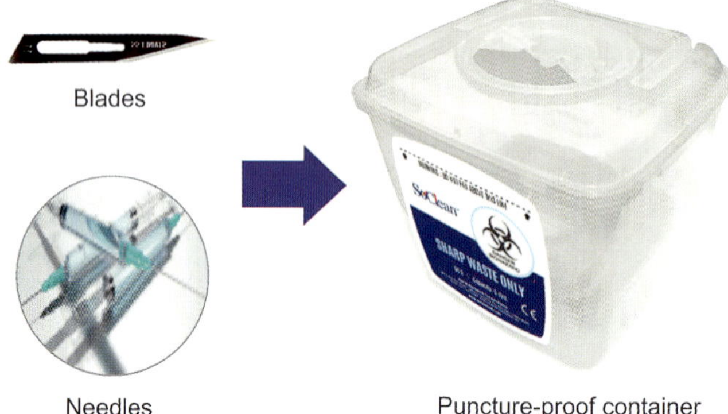

Fig. 2: White puncture-proof container.

Other Wastes

- **E-waste:** Used electronic devices and batteries, managed by E-Waste (Management) Rules, 2016[2]
- **Radioactive waste:** Managed under the Atomic Energy Act, 1962

HANDLING AND STORAGE

Proper handling and storage of BMW are critical to prevent cross-contamination and ensure safety. The BMWM Rules, 2016, outline key protocols:[1]

- **Segregation:** Initiate at the point of generation using color-coded bins **(Table 1)**.
- **Nonmixing:** BMW must not be mixed with general waste.
- **Storage time:** Untreated BMW should not be stored beyond 48 hours.
- **Chlorinated plastics:** Phase out chlorinated plastic bags (except blood bags) and gloves within 2 years of manufacture.
- **Common biomedical waste treatment facility (CBWTF):** Facilities within 75 km must handle BMW, except for pretreated laboratory and highly infectious waste.
- **Labeling:** Use biohazard or cytotoxic hazard symbols and barcodes on all containers.

Proper segregation and labeling, as mandated by the BMWM Rules, 2016, ensure safe handling and storage of BMW **(Table 1)**.[1]

TRANSPORTATION

Biomedical waste transportation requires closed vehicles displaying biohazard symbols to prevent spillage and cross-contamination. Vehicles must be dedicated solely to BMW transport.[1]

TREATMENT AND DISPOSAL METHODS

Treatment methods vary by waste category to eliminate pathogens and reduce environmental impact **(Table 2)**.[1,3]

TABLE 2: Treatment and disposal methods for biomedical waste.[1,4]

Category	*Treatment method*	*Disposal method*
Yellow	Incineration, plasma pyrolysis	Deep burial (where permitted)
Red	Autoclaving, microwaving, hydroclaving	Recycling (no landfilling)
White	Autoclaving, dry heat sterilization	Shredding, mutilation, encapsulation
Blue	Disinfection, autoclaving, microwaving, hydroclaving	Recycling

Treatment methods such as autoclaving and incineration, tailored to each BMW category, ensure safe disposal **(Table 2)**.[1,3]

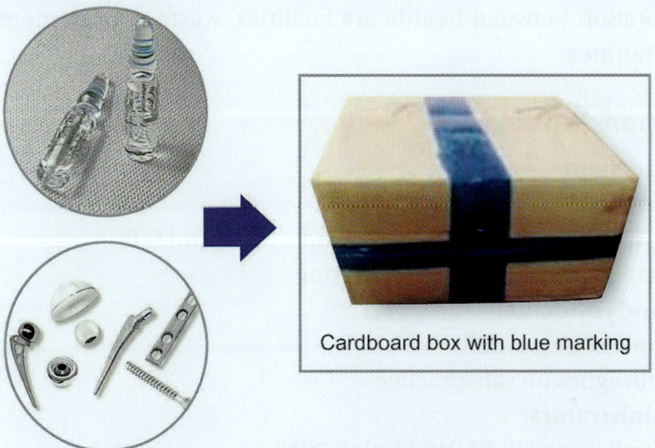

Fig. 3: Waste to be disposed of in cardboard box with blue marking or a blue bag.

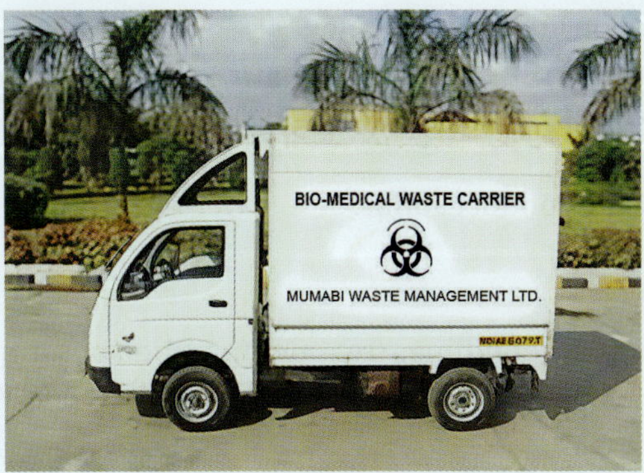

Fig. 4: Vehicle should display biomedical waste.

Additional methods include:

- **Chemical treatment:** Disinfectants for liquid waste
- **Landfilling/encapsulation:** For treated residual waste, adhering to environmental regulations[3]

REGULATORY FRAMEWORK AND BEST PRACTICES

The BMWM Rules, 2016, provide a comprehensive framework with four schedules:[1]

- **Schedule 1:** Categorization and management
- **Schedule 2:** Standards for treatment and disposal
- **Schedule 3:** Prescribed authority and duties
- **Schedule 4:** Labeling requirements for bags, containers, and transportation

Best practices:

- Develop waste management plans.
- Conduct regular staff training.
- Maintain documentation for waste tracking.
- Foster collaboration between healthcare facilities, waste management companies, and regulatory authorities.

Roles and Responsibilities

- **Heads of department:**
  - Train staff on BMW management.
  - Conduct inspections in laboratories, wards, ICUs, and OTs.
  - Ensure compliance and incident reporting.[1]
- **Consultants and residents:**
  - Ensure proper segregation.
  - Educate colleagues on safe practices.
- **Hospital administrators:**
  - Ensure compliance with BMWM Rules, 2016.
  - Submit audit reports and procure equipment.[1]
- **Staff nurses:**
  - Supervise segregation and housekeeping.
  - Report incidents and ensure proper labeling.[1]
- **Infection control nurses:**
  - Develop SOPs.
  - Maintain records and conduct audits.[1]

RECORD KEEPING

Records of BMW generation, handling, treatment, and disposal must be maintained for 5 years. Major accidents require immediate notification and a report within 24 hours.[1]

UNIVERSAL PRECAUTIONS

Universal precautions, developed in the 1980s to combat bloodborne pathogens, are critical for infection control. They assume all blood and specific body fluids are potentially infectious.[4]

Key Components

- **Hand hygiene:** Wash hands with soap or use alcohol-based sanitizers before/after patient contact.[4]

- **Personal protective equipment (PPE):** Use gloves, masks, gowns, and eye protection based on exposure risk.[4,5]
- **Safe injection practices:** Minimize needle-stick injuries.
- **Respiratory hygiene:** Cover nose/mouth during coughing/sneezing.
- **Environmental cleaning:** Disinfect surfaces and equipment.
- **Waste management:** Segregate and dispose of infectious waste per BMWM Rules.[1]

COVID-19 Considerations

The COVID-19 pandemic highlighted the importance of PPE for waste disposal workers.[5] Protocols include:

- **PPE donning/doffing sequence:** Gown, mask, goggles, face shield, gloves (donning); gloves, face shield, goggles, gown, mask (doffing)[5]
- **Face masks:** Cloth, medical, or N-95 masks[5]
- **Gloves and goggles:** Protect against hazardous materials and droplets.[5]

The use of PPE, including masks and gloves, is critical for waste disposal workers, especially during pandemics **(Table 3)**.[5]

TABLE 3: PPE for biomedical waste handlers.[6]

PPE component	*Purpose*	*Usage guidelines*
Gloves	Protect against hazardous materials	Dispose after single use
Masks	Prevent respiratory infection	Cloth, medical, or N-95 based on risk
Goggles/face shield	Protect against droplets	Reusable goggles; single-use face shields
Gown	Prevent contamination	Single-use, dispose as BMW

EMERGING TRENDS AND CHALLENGES

Recent advancements in BMW management include:

- **Waste-to-energy technologies:** Convert biohazardous waste into energy.[6]
- **Sustainable practices:** Reduce waste generation and carbon footprint.[7]
- **Smart waste tracking:** Use IoT and barcoding for real-time monitoring.[8]

Challenges:

- **Infrastructure gaps:** Limited CBWTF availability in rural areas.[9]
- **Compliance issues:** Inconsistent adherence to regulations.[9]
- **Emerging pathogens:** Require adaptive guidelines.[4]

CONCLUSION

Effective BMW management and universal precautions are vital for public health and environmental safety. Adherence to BMWM Rules, 2016, proper segregation, treatment, and disposal, combined with robust infection control practices, mitigate risks along with continued research, infrastructure investment, and global cooperation are essential to address evolving challenges.

REFERENCES

1. Ministry of Environment, Forest and Climate Change. (2016). The Bio-Medical Waste Management Rules, 2016. [online] Available from https://hspcb.org.in/uploads/laws/BMW_Rules.pdf [Last accessed December 2025].
2. Ministry of Environment, Forest and Climate Change. (2016). E-Waste (Management) Rules, 2016. [online] Available from https://hspcb.org.in/uploads/laws/Ewaste_Rules.pdf [Last accessed December 2025].
3. Mathur P, Patan S, Shobhawat S. Biomedical waste management: An overview. J Environ Manage. 2023;15(2):123-30.
4. World Health Organization. (2020). Infection prevention and control guidelines.
5. World Health Organization. (2021). COVID-19 waste management guidelines.
6. Kumar R, Verma A. Waste-to-energy technologies for biomedical waste management. Waste Manag Res. 2022;40(5):567-74.
7. Singh N, Ogunseitan OA. Sustainable biomedical waste management: A review. Environ Sci Pollut Res. 2023;30(10):24567-24580.
8. Sharma A, Gupta P. IoT-based biomedical waste tracking systems. J Clean Prod. 2024;45:112-20.
9. Datta P, Mohi G, Chander J. Biomedical waste management in India: Critical appraisal. J Lab Physicians. 2018;10(1):6-14.

Viva

Art of Passing Examination

Kshama Nilesh Uplenchwar

PREPARING FOR THEORY EXAMINATION

"The more precise, clear, and specific my goals for future are, the greater chance I have in being successful at studies".

Passing examination, should be respected as a skill. As clinicians, students should strive to gain knowledge, clinical skills, and surgical skills. At the same time, students should also start looking at examinations as opportunities to master skills to pass theory or practical examinations.

"The Key Mantra" is

Practice what you are actually going to perform during examination.

So

For theory (written examination)—Practice WRITING.

For practicals (cases, OSCEs, and tables)—Practice SPEAKING/PRESENTING.

Exam preparation:

- Organize study material.
- Pattern of examination—past papers.
- Establish a regular study routine.
- Active revision is a must.

Organize study material:

- Standard textbooks
- Recent advances
- Progress by John Studd
- Recent journals
- RCOG green top guidelines, TOG
- ACOG guidelines
- FOGSI guidelines
- Landmark trials

Pattern of examination—past papers:

- Topics covered and **marks allotted**
- Format of examination—Essay
    - Short answers
    - MCQs (Multiple Choice Questions)

- SBAs (Single Best Answers)
- EMQs (Extended Matching Questions)

(These will vary depending upon examination you are pursuing)

- Time management:
  - Equal **weightage** and time to all questions **with equal marks distribution** (**Common mistake** is to invest more time on answers one knows well, that leaves the student with less amount of time for the question which he has to think and write the answer. End result is less scores overall, due to running out of time.)

Reading:

- Go through the QUESTION BANK.
- Before you start reading the chapter, so identify what you are looking for.

Writing:

- You know which answers you are looking for:
  - Preparing notes/mind maps
  - Drawing flowcharts
  - Drawing diagrams

STUDY GROUPS AND PRACTICING ANSWER WRITING WITH TIME MANAGEMENT

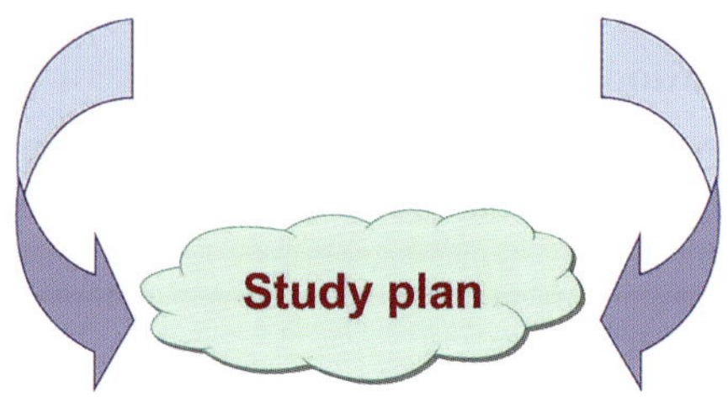

Why Study in Groups?

- Verbal elaboration promotes long-term memory retention.
- Explanations require the speaker to understand the topic being discussed.
- Study-group partners should equally participate.

And finally at the Battlefield!

- Keep it cool.
- Monitor your anxiety level.
- A little is good, but a lot will affect your performance.
- Be Ready. It is the time to execute your skills, isn't it?
- Go with the spirit to win.

Answering a theory question:

- **Read and comprehend** the question properly.
- Devote time for **careful reading** of question.
- **All sub-questions** are to be answered.
- Any **twist in the question** should be understood.

Terms to be understood:
- **Define:** Give definition.
- **Critically evaluate/discuss:**
  - Give indications and contraindications.
  - Advantages, disadvantages, limitations
- **Management:** Diagnosis and treatment (medical and surgical)
- **Diagnosis:** Clinical (pointers in history and clinical examination) and investigations
- **Enumerate:** Give a list.
- **Treatment:** Conservative, medical, and operative (surgical)

Structure/format of the answer
- Introduction
- Definition
- Main text:
  - Headings, subheadings (use boxes or underlines)
  - Flowcharts
  - Tables
  - Diagrams well-labeled
- Concluding remarks

Keep the format ready for main text of certain questions
- **Drugs:**
  - Indications
  - Contraindications
  - Pharmacology
  - Pharmacokinetics
  - Important interactions
  - Side effects
- **Malignancies:**
  - Etiology, age-group, risk factors
  - Histopathological types, FIGO staging
  - *Treatment*: Chemotherapy, radiotherapy, surgical, neoadjuvant chemotherapy, immunotherapy
  - Elaborate section as applicable to question asked.
- **Prevention:**
  - Primordial prevention
  - Primary
  - Secondary
  - Tertiary prevention
- **Operative procedures:**
  - Define the procedure.
  - Types: Conservative, open, minimally invasive, interventional radiology
  - Indications
  - Contraindications

    - Steps of procedure
    - Complications: Intraoperative, postoperative—immediate and long term
- **For obstetrics questions for etiology or complications:**
    - Divide as maternal, fetal, and placental.
    - Also as first, second, or third trimester, wherever applicable

Parents' tips since childhood:
- Legible handwriting
- Every question on new page
- Keep margins on both sides.
- Good presentation—key to impress
- Time management is crucial.

Key points for answers:
- Mention and **highlight/underline/encircle** the keywords (the easier it is for the examiner to find out keywords, the more the scores can be).
- Illustrations with well-labeled diagrams
- Include maximum possible numbers of flowcharts, tables, graphs, etc.
- Include values, % or levels.
- Answer pointwise with bullets.

Take a final look at your work:
- Save enough time to review your answers.
- Make corrections and additions.
- Check whether you interpreted the question properly.
- Check that answers are accurate and complete.

Passing examinations is a skill (for those with knowledge).

Like all skills it requires:
- Practice
- Practice
- And **more practice**

STUDY HARD STUDY SMART.

Good luck for your examinations.

Instruments and Drugs

Akanksha Gupta

GYNECOLOGICAL INSTRUMENTS

Vaginal Specula

1. Cusco's nonfenestrated bivalvular self-retaining vaginal speculum:

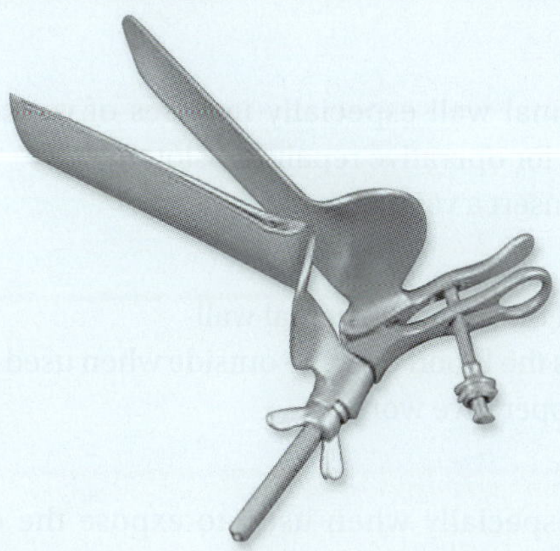

Indications:

1. It is used during clinical examination to expose the cervix and vaginal walls.
2. It allows the application of local treatment to the cervix.
3. It allows introduction of the uterine sound, insertion of IUD, performing hysterosalpinogography, taking premenstrual endometrial biopsy, surface biopsy scraping of the cervix, etc.
4. It is used to expose the two sides of a septate vagina, when a blade is inserted in either side.

Advantages:

1. Easy to introduce
2. Self-retaining
3. Can be adjusted to the size of the vagina

Disadvantages:

1. It hides the anterior and posterior vaginal walls; however, this disadvantage is overcome by inspection of the vaginal walls during its gradual withdrawal.
2. It does not offer complete protection of vaginal walls during cauterization of the cervix.

2. Vaginal speculum:

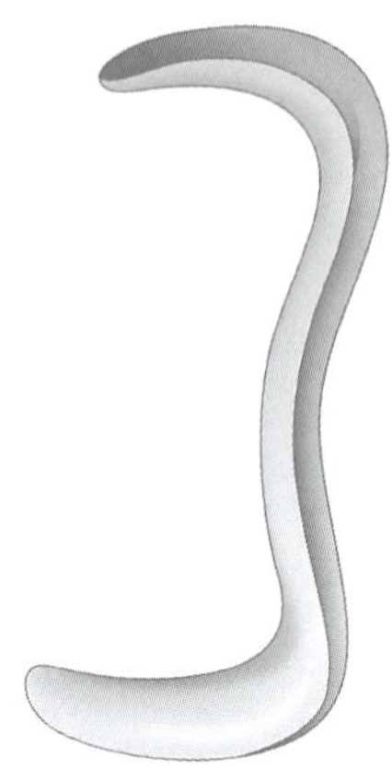

Indications:

1. Expose the anterior vaginal wall especially in cases of vesicovaginal fistula, both for diagnosis (prolapse) and for operative repair (episiotomy).
2. It can also be of value to insert a vaginal pack.

Advantages:

1. Gives an excellent view of the anterior vaginal wall
2. The grooved blade directs the blood or urine outside when used in the lithotomic position, and provides a space for operative work.

Disadvantages:

1. Assistance is required especially when used to expose the cervix or during surgical procedures, as it is not self-retaining.
2. In the presence of a large cystocele, exposure of the cervix is often difficult.
3. *Auvard's self-retaining vaginal speculum:*

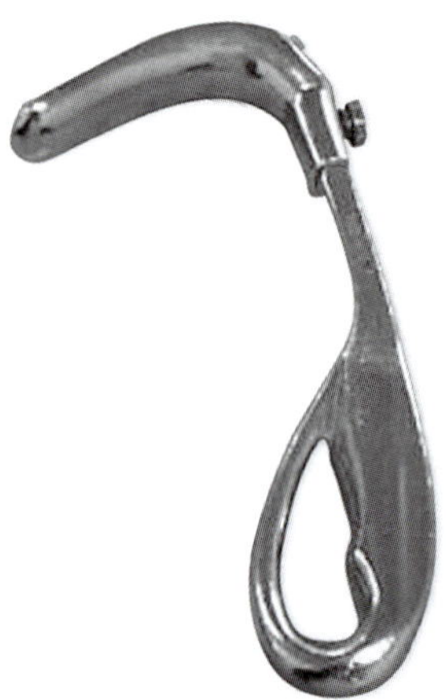

Indications: Most operations are performed per vagina.

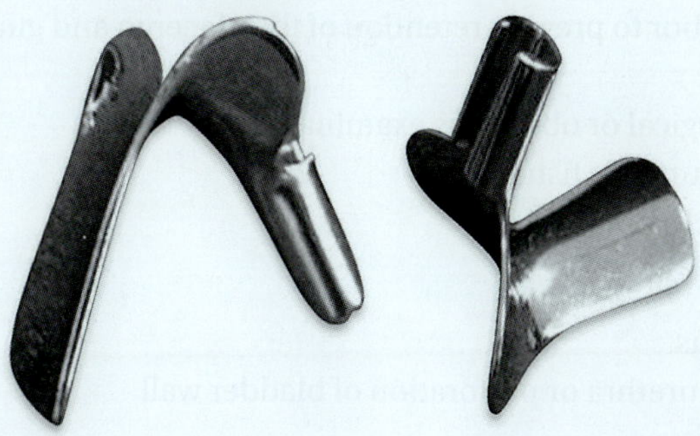

Advantages:
1. It is self-retaining.
2. It gives good exposure of the anterior vaginal wall and cervix during operations.

Disadvantages:
1. It may tear, bruise, or overstretch the soft tissues of the perineum and posterior vaginal wall.
2. It is difficult to use in nulliparae.
3. It hides the posterior vaginal wall.

Urinary Instruments

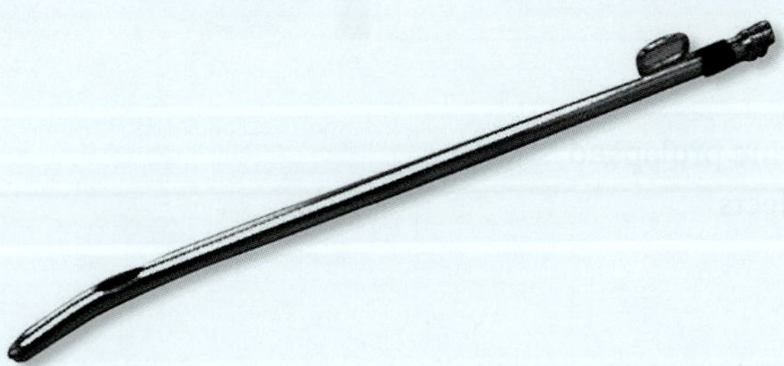

Metal Urinary Catheter

Metal urinary catheters are of two forms: the straight and the curved (S-shaped).

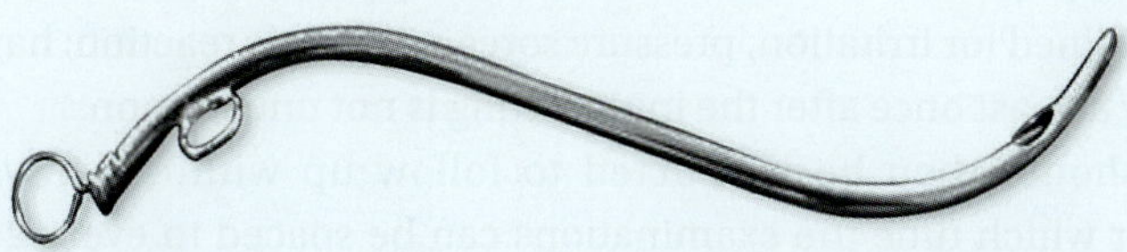

Indications:

- In the 1st stage of labor to prevent uterine inertia
- In the 3rd stage of labor to prevent retention of the placenta and guard against postpartum hemorrhage
- Before any gynecological or obstetrics examination
- For the diagnosis of urinary fistula
- Vesicle calculus (click sound)

Complication:

- Introduction of sepsis
- False passage in the urethra or perforation of bladder wall
- Urethral shock and fever

Hodge Pessary

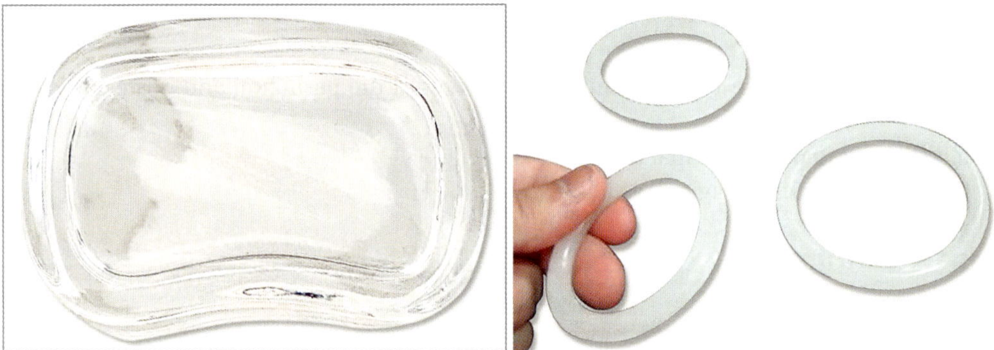

Indications:

1. Symptomatic uterine prolapsed
2. Pelvic support defects
3. Vaginal prolapses

Contraindications:

1. Active infections of the pelvis or vagina
2. Patients who are noncompliant or unlikely to follow up
3. Allergy to the product

Follow-up: After the initial fitting of the pessary, the patient should be followed up within a few days so that the physician can recheck the fit. The pessary should be removed so that the vagina can be examined for irritation, pressure sores, or allergic reaction; having to change the size of the pessary at least once after the initial fitting is not uncommon.

The patient should then be instructed to follow up within 1–2 weeks for another examination, after which time the examinations can be spaced to every 2–3 months. In the motivated patient who is able to demonstrate effective removal, insertion, and care of the pessary, these examinations may be spaced further at the discretion of the physician.

At each follow-up examination, the pessary should be removed and cleaned with soap and water while the vagina is inspected for erosions, pressure necrosis, or allergic reaction. If inspection of the pessary reveals cracking or other defects, it should be replaced. The patient who is using a pessary should be considered to be under the care of the person who placed it for the duration of its use. Pessaries should never be placed in elderly, debilitated patients without excellent follow-up.

Uterine Sound

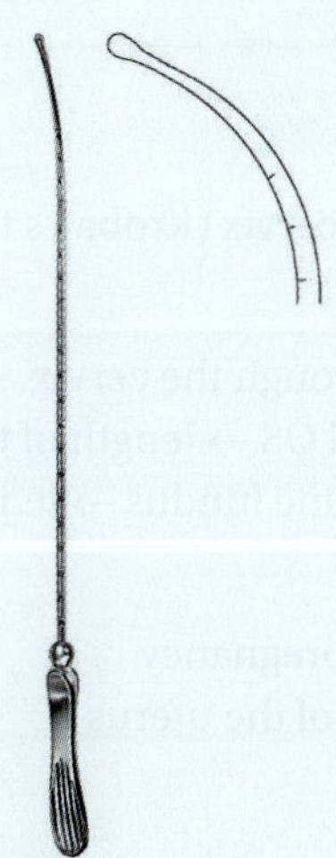

- Graduated in centimeters or in inches
- Malleable (can be bent and twisted easily)
- Corrugated handle (during insertion they should face upward)
- The whole diameter = 3 mm
- The diameter of the knob = 4 mm

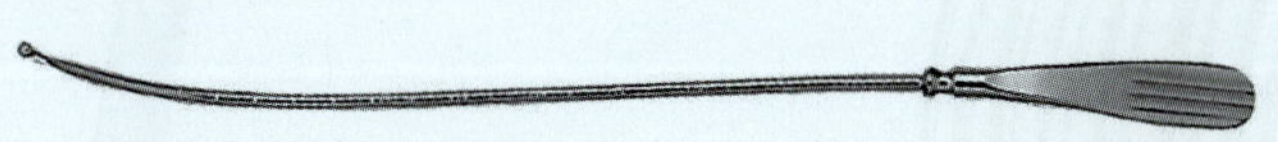

Indications:

- *Measures the length of the cervical canal*, the uterine body, and that of the whole uterus (before D&C and after insertion of an IUCD)
- To determine the direction of the uterus (RVF: the corrugations on the handle will face downward after it was facing upward)
- To differentiate uterine inversion from a submucous fibroid
- Differentiate between a uterine polyp (can go around it) and a cervical poly (cannot go around it)

- It determines the relation of the uterus to any pelvic mass.
- It differentiates true from pseudoprolapse (congenital elongation of the cervix). The sound is inserted into the lateral vaginal fornix and its relation to the ischial spines is evaluated.
- To diagnose vesicovaginal fistula, the sound is passed through the fistulous opening in the vagina where a click is elicited against a metal catheter in the urinary bladder.
- *Missed loop*: Insert the uterine sound then do X-ray, if the IUCD is far away from the sound → The IUCD has perforated out of the uterus. If the sound is close to the IUCD → the IUCD is inside the uterus.
- To diagnose a bicornuate uterus, a uterus septus, and a uterus subseptus (uterine anomalies)
- Cervical stenosis
- Dysmenorrhea
- Probe test of friability for cancer cervix (Krobac's test)

How to Use:
1. The uterine sound is inserted through the cervix.
2. The first resistance is the internal OS → length of the cervical canal
3. The second resistance is the uterine fundus → length of the uterus + the cervix

Complications:
1. Disturbance of an undiagnosed pregnancy
2. Perforation of the cervix or body of the uterus
3. Ascending infection

Contraindications:
1. Genital infections
2. Suspicion of pregnancy
3. Soft uterus (malignancy, infection, molar pregnancy)

Hegar's Uterine Dilators (Figs. 1 and 2)

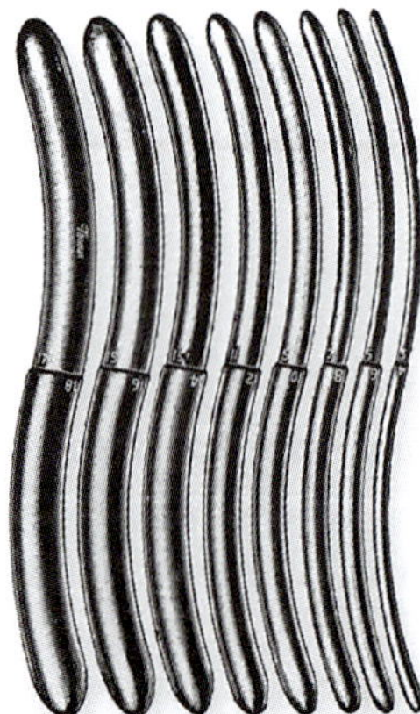

Fig. 1: Double-ended Hegar's uterine dilator 3–18 mm.

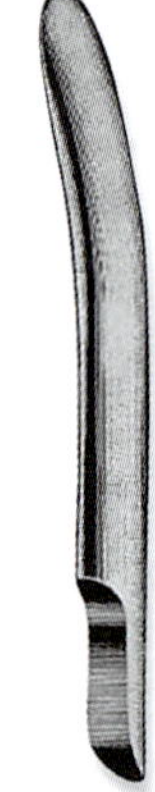

Fig. 2: Single-ended Hegar's uterine dilator.

- They are used to gradually dilate the cervix.
- They can be single- or double-ended.
- Uniform thickness
- There are 15 Hegar's dilators, graduated by a number written on them ranging from 0 to 14 which corresponds to the thickness in millimeters.
- The tip is slightly curved.
- They are held between the index and the thumb at a level less than the uterine length.

Indications for cervical dilatation:

A. Diagnostic:
   1. Incompetent internal os. The passage of dilator no. 8 through the internal os without causing pain or meeting with resistance signifies incompetence.
   2. Before the exploration of the uterine cavity for diagnosis of intrauterine lesions and septa
   3. As a preliminary step to diagnostic curettage of the endometrium
   4. Prior to insufflations or hysterosalpingography in cases with a narrow external os
   5. For diagnosis of spasmodic dysmenorrhea; the passage of no. 4 Hegar's dilator causes severe pain when it reaches the internal os

B. Therapeutic:
   1. Dysmenorrhea: The idea is that dilatation (at least to no. 14) acts as a local sympathectomy by cutting the nerves at the internal os.
   2. Spasmodic amenorrhea
   3. Drainage of hematometra or pyometra
   4. In some cases of sterility with a pinhole external os
   5. Stenosis of the cervix, e.g., postoperative or post-cauterization
   6. Cervical abortion

C. As a step in the course of other operations:
   1. Preliminary to curettage or evacuation
   2. A step in the management of vesicular mole and certain types of abortions: (a) missed abortion and (b) therapeutic abortion
   3. Vaginal hysterotomy
   4. Removal of fibroid or endometrial polyps
   5. Cervical conization, amputation, Fothergill's operation, and trachelorrhaphy
   6. Before insertion or removal of certain contraceptive devices

Degree of dilatation: *The degree of dilatation is governed by the indication*

1. For curettage dilate to no. 10–14
2. For dysmenorrhea dilate to 14–16
3. For finger exploration and digital separation of a conceptus dilate to no. 18–22 (varies according to the diameter of the operator's finger)

Contraindications:

1. Genital infections
2. Normally pregnant uterus

Complications:

1. Perforation of the cervix or body of the uterus; it is sequel to forceful manipulations in a wrong direction. Pregnancy, vesicular mole, and malignancy increase the chances for perforation because of the soft and friable uterine wall.
2. Lacerations of the cervix
3. Cervical incompetence and habitual abortion (most common)
4. Ascending infection (cervicitis, endometritis, salpingitis, peritonitis, and parametritis)
5. Endometriosis results from the piston-like action of the dilator which pushes endometrial fragments through the tubal ostia.

Vulsellum Forceps

Types (Figs. 3 to 5):

1. Single-toothed (bullet forceps) tenaculum
2. Double-toothed (Fenton's bulldog vulsellum or the lion's forceps)
3. Multiple-toothed vulsellum (tenaculum)

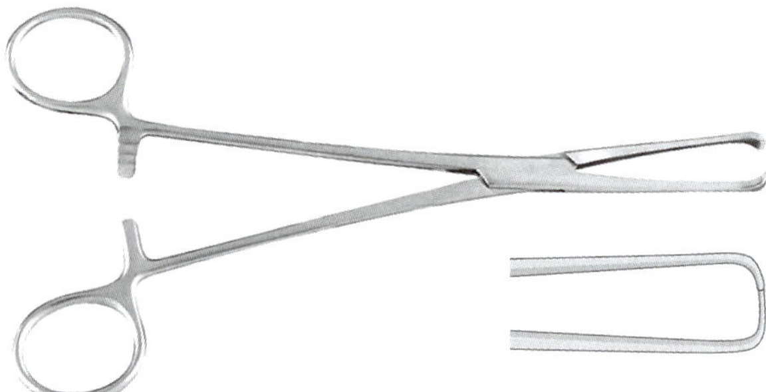

Fig. 3: Tenaculum.

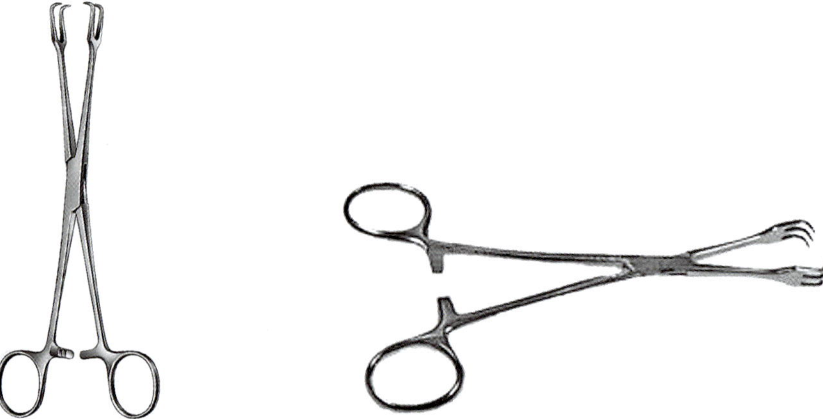

Fig. 4: Double-toothed vulsellum.

Fig. 5: Multiple-toothed vulsellum.

Indications:

1. Grasping of the cervix:
   (a) During minor office practice manipulations, e.g., insertion of a uterine sound, or an IUCD in difficult cases and during insufflation and hysterosalpingography
   (b) To estimate the degree of uterine descent in cases of prolapse by pulling on the cervix downward and observing the level to which it reaches
   (c) To evaluate the mobility of the uterus; this may be limited in fibroid tumors.
   (d) During vaginal operations, e.g., dilatation and curettage and repair of prolapse
   (e) To help correction of RVF by pulling backward on the anterior lip of the cervix
2. To grasp a prolapsed submucous myoma during a vaginal myomectomy
3. During operation of hysterectomy, it can be used to hold the cervical stump after the removal of the uterine body in subtotal hysterectomy.

Contraindications:

- The soft pregnant cervix
- Infections
- Suspicious malignancy of the cervix

Complications:

1. Lacerations of the cervix
2. Infections
3. Bleeding from the site of the bite of the teeth of the vulsellum

Ring and Sponge Forceps (Figs. 6 and 7)

Both possess a handle, a lock, a shank, and two jaws at the tip. The jaws are either smooth or serrated, either rounded or oval in shape.

Indications:

1. To grasp the soft lips of the cervix in pregnancy, e.g., during evacuation
2. To evacuate a pregnant uterus per vagina
3. It is used for removing corporeal and cervical polypi.
4. It can be used as a sponge carrier.

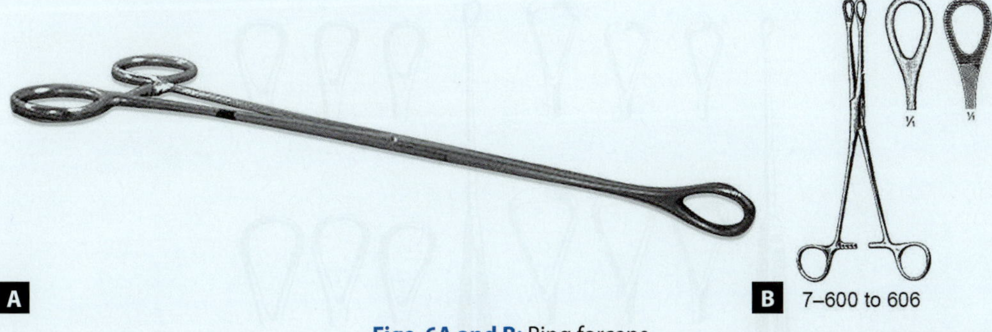

Figs. 6A and B: Ring forceps.

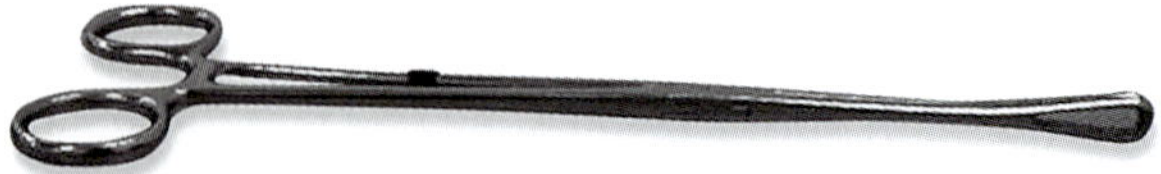

Fig. 7: Sponge forceps.

Ovum Forceps (Fig. 8)

- It is a miniature of the obstetric forceps.
- Each branch has a handle, a shank, and a blade; the two branches are attached by a screw joint with no lock.
- It is used to remove an intact separated ovum; the cervix in these cases needs to be dilated to no. 18 Hegar's and it is also used to evacuate the uterine content after D&C.

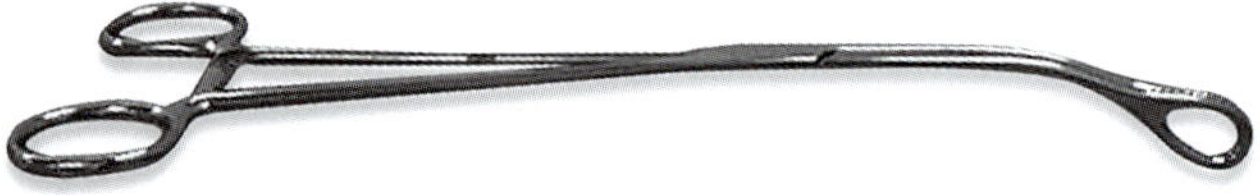

Fig. 8: Ovum forceps.

Single-Ended Corrugated Sharp or Blunt Uterine Curettes

- Each curette consists of three parts, the handle, the shank, and the curetting end.
- The handle is corrugated on the aspect which corresponds to the direction of the bend at the tip. It can be either on the side (single-ended) or in the middle (double-ended).
- The shank is malleable and is hollow in the flushing variety to convey irrigating fluids which stimulates the uterus to contract and can also be used to deliver antiseptic material.
- The curetting end may be sharp or blunt, and some are spoon-shaped.
- Some types have a curetting end on either tip (double-ended) with the handle in the middle.

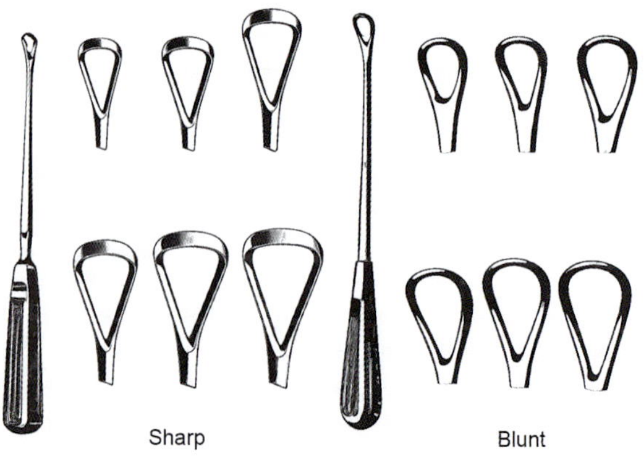

I. Diagnostic curettage:

A. Bleeding:

1. Dysfunctional uterine bleeding
2. Symmetrically enlarged uterus
3. Suspected uterine malignancy
4. Secondary postpartum and postabortive bleeding
5. Cervical adenomatous polypi
6. Doubtful extrauterine pregnancy to exclude the presence of chorionic villi
7. Suspected TB and bilharzia

B. Amenorrhea:

1. Atrophic endometrium
2. Polycystic ovarian syndrome (Stein–Leventhal syndrome)
3. TB endometrium

C. Sterility

1. Anovulation
2. TB endometrium
3. Nonresponsive endometrium
4. Hormonal function of the ovaries

II. Therapeutic curettage:

1. For temporary or permanent cure of nonmalignant uterine bleeding, e.g., metropathia hemorrhagica and other types of functional bleeding and secondary postpartum and postabortive bleeding
2. Membranous dysmenorrhea
3. Removal of endometrial polypi
4. In the management of some abortions (inevitable, incomplete, missed, cervical, and therapeutic abortions) to ensure complete removal of the conceptus and decidua
5. Vesicular mole
6. To remove unhealthy endometrium during operation, e.g., Manchester (Fothergill's) operation and myomectomy

The operation of curettage:

- Patient should be anesthetized and lying in the lithotomy position.
- Empty bladder and rectum.
- Dilate the cervix to no. 12 Hegar's.
- The curette is introduced till the fundus and then by downward thrusts the endometrium is scraped systematically so that all walls are scraped, including the cornua and fundus.
- The curette of an area is considered complete when a gritty sensation is felt or heard.
- In cases of abortion and vesicular mole, it is sometimes advisable to do curettage while an IV drip of syntocinon is continuously running to minimize the danger of proliferation.

Complications:

1. Sepsis: Introduction of infection into the uterine cavity leads to acute endometritis, salpingitis, and/or peritonitis.

2. Perforation of the uterus: This is the most common complication occurring as a result of improper and too vigorous handling of the curette or aggravation of a minor laceration done by the dilator at the internal os. It is particularly liable to occur in malignant conditions, infections, vesicular mole, and abortion.
3. Permanent amenorrhea and sterility result from vigorous over curettage removing the basal layer of the endometrium and intrauterine adhesions (Asherman's syndrome or endometrial synechiae).
4. Excessive bleeding may occur during curettage in cases of carcinoma of the uterine body.
5. The use of a flushing curette may push endometrial tissue through the Fallopian tubes, leading to pelvic endometriosis or peritonitis.

Cervical Scrapers (Wooden Spatula) and Roller Brush (Figs. 9 and 10)

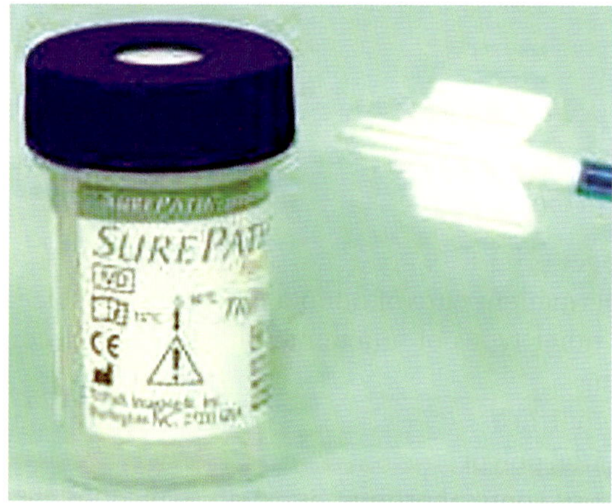

- For endocervical sampling
- This is a wooden spatula for "surface biopsy" which provides a selective cytology technique (pap smear).
- It is neither a true biopsy nor a smear, but a scraping from the squamocolumnar junction of the cervix.
- The irregularly shaped end of the scraper is used with its tip in the external os; with a rotatory movement the entire area of the squamocolumnar junction is scraped. The other end is used for scraping the surface of the edge of suspicious erosion.
- *Pointed end for nulliparous and other for multiparous*
- It is diagnosed as **cervical cancer** caused by human papillomaviruses **(HPV)**.

Risk factors for cervical cancer:

1. Old age
2. White women
3. Early sexual active
4. Multiple sexual partners
5. Smoking

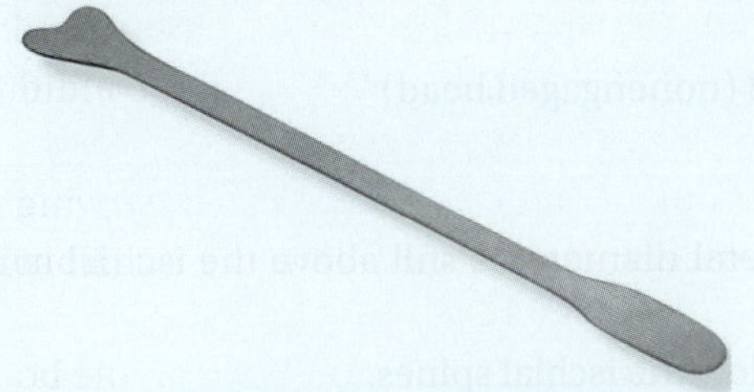

Fig. 9: Ayer's cervical scraper (wooden spatula).

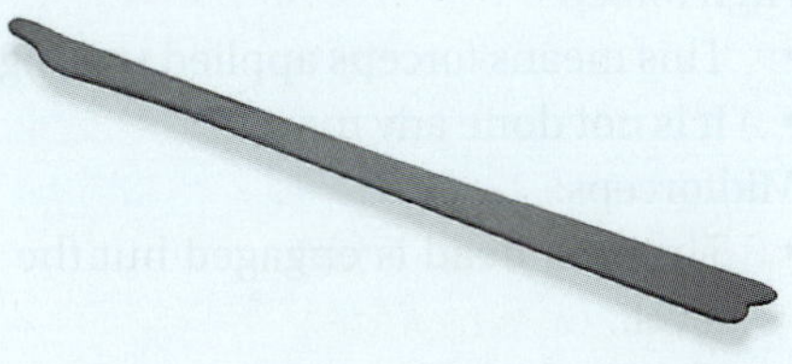

Fig. 10: Aylesbury's cervical scraper (wooden spatula).

OBSTETRIC INSTRUMENTS

Prerequisites:

- Cephalic presentation (Piper forceps is used for breech)
- Head is engaged 0–2
- Fully dilated bladder
- Maternal pelvis adequacy
- Ruptured membranes
- Empty bladder
- Episiotomy
- Anesthesia

Obstetric Forceps (Figs. 11 to 13)

Types of forceps:

1. Short curved Wrigley's obstetric forceps
2. Long curved Simpson's obstetric forceps
3. Long straight Kielland's obstetric forceps

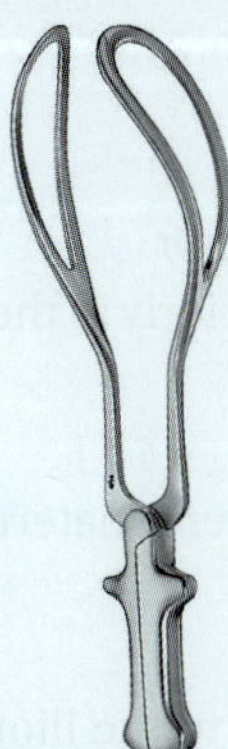

Fig. 11: Long curved Simpson's obstetric forceps.

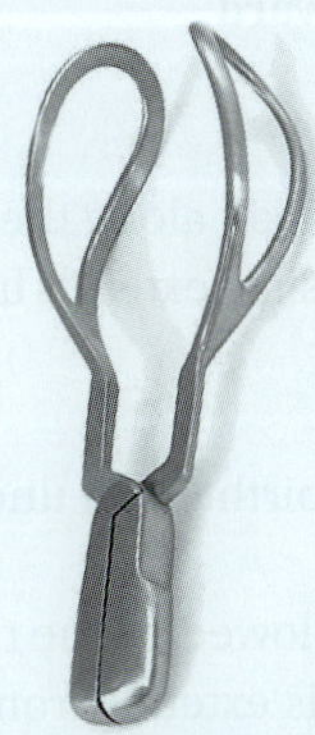

Fig. 12: Short curved Wrigley's obstetric forceps.

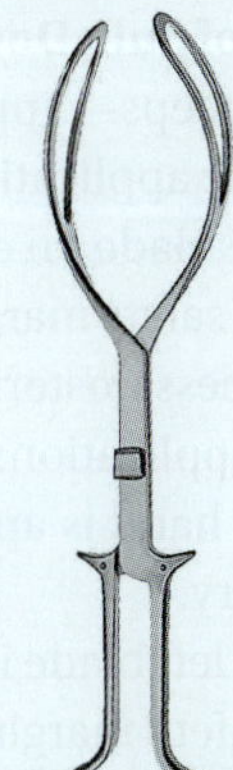

Fig. 13: Long straight Kielland's obstetric forceps.

Types of forceps—Deliveries:

- High forceps:
  - This means forceps applied to a high head (nonengaged head)
  - It is not done any more.
- Midforceps:
  - The fetal head is engaged but the biparietal diameter is still above the ischial spine level.
  - The lowest bony part of the head is felt below the ischial spines.
- Low forceps (outlet forceps):
  - The biggest transverse diameter (biparietal) has passed the ischial spine level.
  - The lowest bony part of the head has already reached the perineum and is visible either during or between contractions.

Parts:

It consists of two branches, right and left. Each branch is made of:

1. A blade:
   - Each blade has a cephalic curve, a pelvic curve, and a fenestrum.
   - The cephalic curve: Medial curved aspect of each blade
   - The pelvic curve: This curve confirms with the curve of the birth canal.
   - The fenestrum makes the forceps lighter in weight, offers a firm grip over the head and avoids slipping, and it minimizes injury of the head.
2. A shank: This is the part of the forceps intervening between the blade and the handles.
3. A handle: The handles cross to the opposite side of the blade so that the left handle is held by the left hand and is put at the left side of the birth canal and the right handle is held by the right hand and is put at the right side of the birth canal.
   - The branches are joined by a lock located at the junction between the shank and the handles.
   - The left blade is inserted first followed by the right blade because the lock will only engage if the right branch was placed on top of the left branch.

Direction of pull: Downward and forward

Types of forceps—Application:

A. Cephalic application:
   - One blade on either side of the head along the mentovertical diameter
   - The safety margin that is permissible extends from the zygoma anteriorly to the mastoid process posteriorly.

B. Pelvic application:
   - The hand is applied inside the birth canal under the blade to prevent maternal tissue injury.
   - The left blade is inserted first followed by the right blade.
   - A safety margin within the pelvis extends from the sacroiliac joint to the iliopectineal eminence.

Kielland's Obstetric Forceps

- Long, straight (very slight) pelvic curve.
- It has a backward or a perineal curve on the posterior aspect.
- Overlapping shanks (upper and lower)
- A sliding lock allowing application to asynclitic heads
- Light weight
- Main indication: *Rotation of the head and for application to asynclitic heads*
- Disadvantages: An unstable lock predisposes to cervical and vaginal lacerations

Action of the forceps:

1. Traction on the head (the main action)
2. Rotation of the head
3. Compression of the head (this should be minimal to avoid intracranial hemorrhage)
4. Stimulation of uterine action
5. Dilatation of the vulva
6. One blade can be utilized to dislodge the head out of a lower segment cesarean section incision.

Indications of forceps delivery:

1. Maternal:

A. Threatened dangers to the mother (prophylactic forceps):
  - Toxemia of pregnancy (preeclampsia and eclampsia).
  - Previous cesarean section
  - Weakness in the abdominal wall (hernias and a history of a recent abdominal operation)
  - Associated disease, e.g., diabetes mellitus, heart disease, lung disease, chronic nephritis, hypertension, etc.

B. Rigid pelvic floor and perineum

C. Uterine inertia

D. Maternal distress

2. Fetal:

A. Threatened dangers to the fetus (prophylactic forceps), as in the case of prolapse of a pulsating umbilical cord

B. Abnormal presentations and positions: Occipitoposterior, deep transverse arrest, face presentation, after-coming head

C. Large-sized fetal head

D. Fetal distress

3. Prolonged second stage of labor:

A. Over 1–2 hours in multiparae or 2–3 hours in primigravidae, depending on the uterine activity

B. When the head is on the perineum for 1 hour or more

Conditions to be fulfilled before forceps application (prerequisites):

1. A deliverable cephalic presentation
2. Engaged head
3. Empty bladder and rectum *(dangers of a full bladder: genitourinary fistula, rupture of the bladder, failed forceps, atonic postpartum hemorrhage, and stress incontinence)*
4. Fully dilated cervix; *otherwise it might cause trauma to the cervix causing cervical tears or uterine prolapse (remote complication).*
5. Use of anesthesia:
   - Allows proper application and extraction and avoids the development of obstetric shock
   - It can be either pudendal nerve block, low spinal or saddle block, or epidural or general anesthesia.
6. Some uterine contractions must be present. *Delivery with the obstetric forceps in the complete absence of contractions is followed by severe postpartum hemorrhage.*
7. Ruptured membranes
8. Episiotomy; *not always done, it is mostly indicated for primigravidae with rigid perineum.*

Complications:

A. Fetal:

1. Asphyxia (intracranial injury, aspiration, cord compression, and anesthesia)
2. Fracture of the skull bones
3. Intracranial hemorrhage
4. *Nerve lesions*: Bell's palsy, brachial plexus injury
5. Lacerations and contusions of the scalp and cephalhematoma which might get infected and form an abscess

B. Maternal:

1. Risks of anesthesia
2. Traumatic lesions of the lower uterine segment, cervix, vagina, and perineum
3. Sepsis
4. Obstetric shock
   - Bone injuries:
     - Separation of the symphysis
     - Dislocation of the sacroiliac joint; this may be followed by a waddling gate and severe low backache.
     - Fracture of the coccyx or its dislocation from the lower end of the sacrum
   - Postpartum hemorrhage (traumatic, or atonic if delivery is completed in the absence of labor pains)
   - Vesicovaginal fistula and stress incontinence; the former results either from direct trauma to a full bladder during application or extraction, or from ischemic effects of prolonged compression in protracted labor.

Forceps operation in occipitoposterior and transverse positions:

1. Manual rotation:
   A. Manual rotation of the head to bring the occiput anteriorly:
      - This is done by the right hand for left positions and vice versa.

- The other hand is simultaneously placed on the abdomen to pull the back of the child toward the midline.
- It is followed by forceps delivery on the anteriorly rotated head.

B. Manual rotation of the head to bring the occiput posteriorly:
- It is only done when attempts at anterior rotation fail.
- It is followed by forceps delivery as face-to-pubis.

2. Forceps rotation:

A. Scanzoni's double application maneuver:
- It is done using the long curved obstetric forceps as a rotator and an extractor.
- After rotation of the head, the pelvic curve of the forceps will be directed backward.
- The forceps must be removed and reapplied with the pelvic curve of the instrument directed forward.

B. Kielland's forceps:
- It is applied once with no need of reapplication because it is a long almost straight forceps.

Green Armytage Forceps

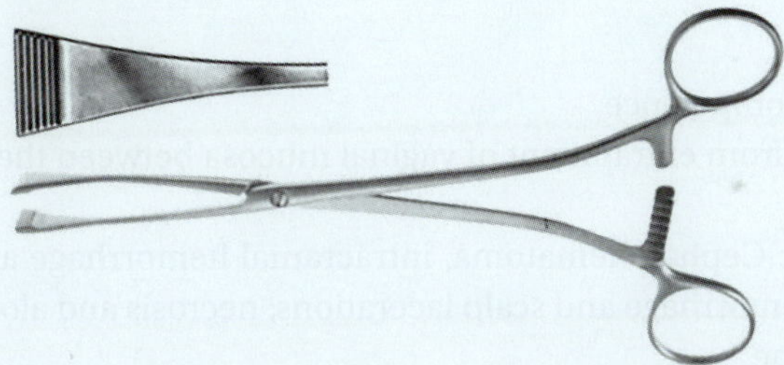

- It is a long forceps with flattened serrated tips that serves as a holding and hemostatic instrument.
- It is usually used during the operation of lower uterine segment cesarean section to hold the flaps of the uterine incision to control bleeding from the edges and to help their suturing.

Vacuum Extractor or Ventouse

Figures 14 and 15 show metal cup ventouse and plastic cup ventouse, respectively.

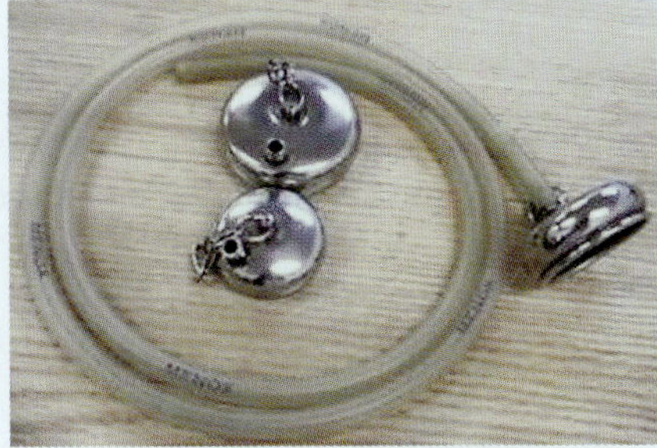

Fig. 14: Metal cup ventouse.

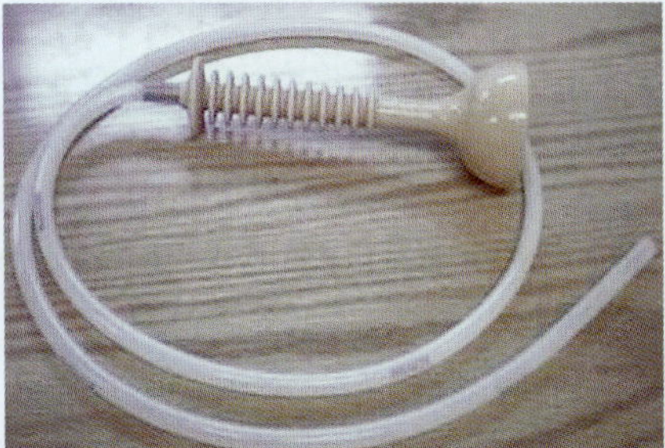

Fig. 15: Plastic cup ventouse.

Indications:

- All the indications of forceps delivery except the face (can cause serious eye damage) and after-coming head. The ventouse is not helpful when a rapid delivery is aimed, e.g., in fetal distress.
- To increase flexion in deflexed heads and to help forward rotation of the occiput in occipitoposterior and deep transverse arrest.
- To assist completion of cervical dilatation, the cervix should be at least three-fourth dilated or more.
- It can be used to control bleeding by traction on the head in placenta previa.
- In cord prolapse, it serves to prevent recurrence after its successful replacement.
- It can be utilized to remove the head out of a lower uterine segment cesarean section.
- It may be of help to correct inertia in the first stage by pulling the head to be well applied to the lower uterine segment and cervix.

Contraindication:

- Face, breech, and transverse presentation of the after-coming head
- Premature babies
- Moderate or severe cephalopelvic disproportion
- Fetal and maternal distress necessitating a rapid delivery

Complications:

- Risk of cervical incompetence
- Vaginal laceration from entrapment of vaginal mucosa between the suction cup and fetal head
- *Fetal skull injuries*: Cephalohematoma, intracranial hemorrhage and cerebral irritation, subaponeurotic hemorrhage and scalp lacerations, necrosis and alopecia
- Longer delivery time

Method:

- Use the largest possible cup
- Pressure is gradually reduced (in about 8 minutes) to reach a maximum vacuum of 0.8 kg/cm^2 (600 mm Hg).
- Allows the formation of a caput inside the cup to fill it
- It should not be used for longer than 40 minutes (scalp necrosis and alopecia).

Advantage over the forceps:

Mother:

- Less risk of anesthesia, sepsis, and trauma
- Helps cervical dilatation and +ve uterine contractions
- It does not occupy space adjacent to the fetal head → less trauma and smaller episiotomy.
- Can be applied if the cervix is not fully dilated

Fetus:

- Corrects malattitudes of the fetal head
- Helps rotation of the head

Amnihook

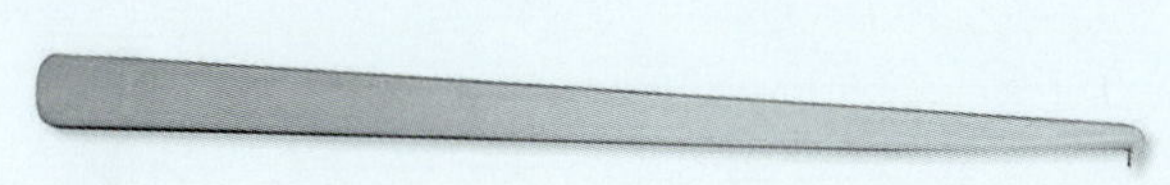

Indication:

1. To rupture the amniotic membrane with minimal risk of trauma to fetus or mother
2. Used for amniotomy

   After the fetus is engaged and it has been determined that the patient is in true labor, then the membranes may be ruptured with the amnihook.

Contraindication:

1. Cephalopelvic disproportion, unless slight, including the nullipara with a high head
2. Abnormal presentation (with the possible exception of face or breech)
3. Unstable lie—risk of cord prolapse
4. Fetal distress—cesarean section would be indicated.
5. Placenta previa
6. Cord presentation
7. Vasa previa
8. Invasive carcinoma of the cervix

For diagnosis rupture of membrane:

1. **Nitrazine test:** It acts by pH and turn from yellow to blue in alkaline media. Blood, semen, urine, and infection give false-positive test.
2. **Ferning test**: It is seen by microscope.

Doyen Retractor

Doyen retractor is used to retract the urinary bladder.

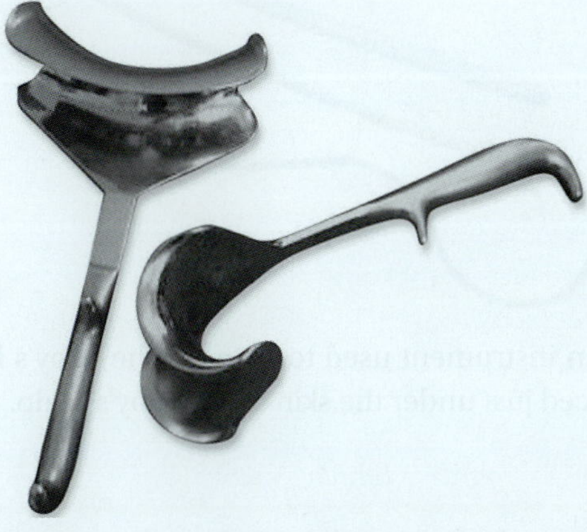

Skin Retractors

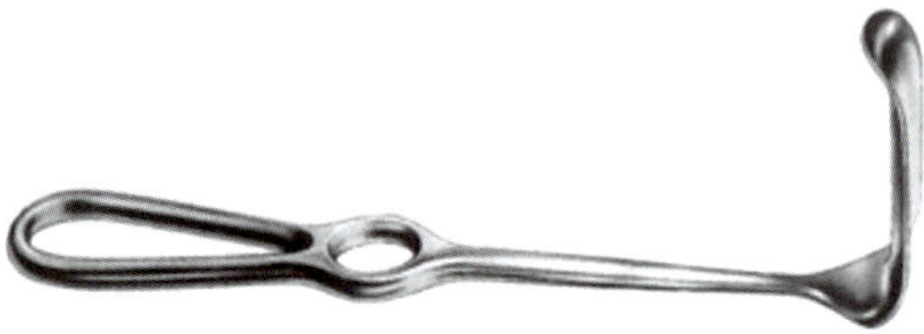

Retractor with Weight

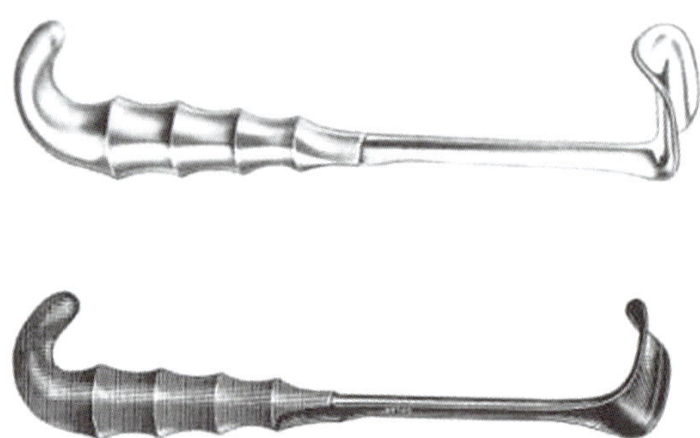

Fetal Scalp Electrode

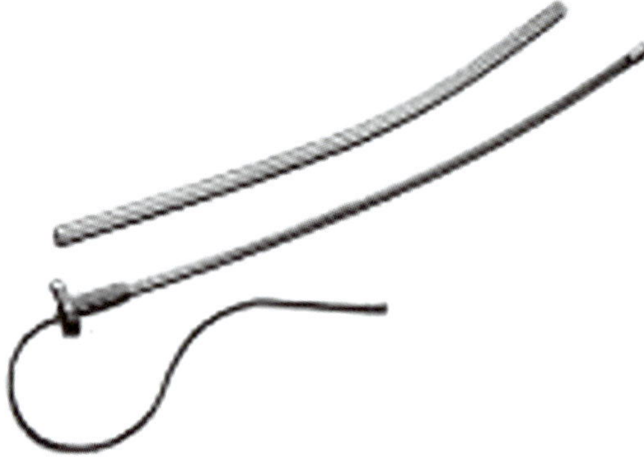

Fetal scalp electrode is an instrument used to monitor the baby's heartbeat while still in the uterus. This device is placed just under the skin of the baby's scalp.

Pap Smear Kit

Pap smear kit consists of spatula, fixative, slide, and swab.

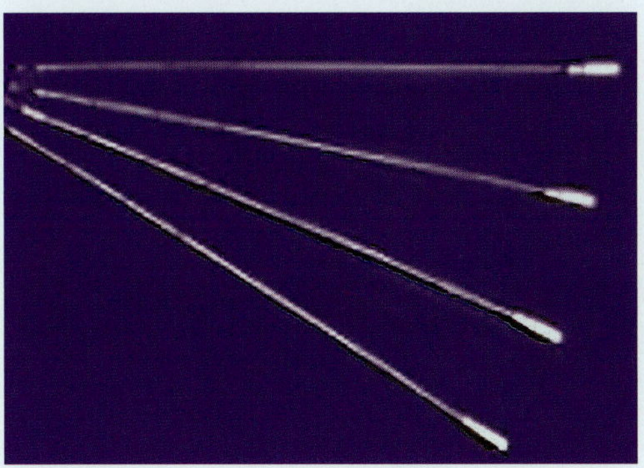

Pipelle

Pipelle is used for endometrial sampling. It works by suctioning, i.e., negative pressure.

Veress Needle and Laparoscope

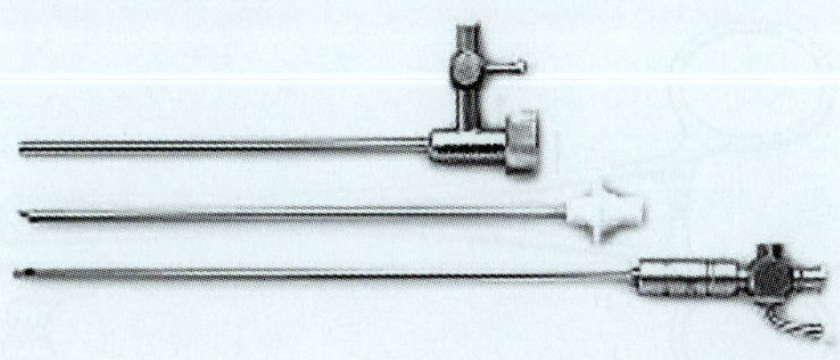

Indications:

1. To make the incision of laparoscopy
2. For CO_2 inflation of the abdomen prior laparoscope
3. *Laparoscope*: Diagnostic (infertility and ectopic pregnancy) and therapeutic (adhesiolysis)

Complication:

1. Pneumoperitoneum
2. Injury to a hollow viscus
3. Injury to vessels in the abdominal wall
4. Damage to other organs
5. Pelvic inflammatory disease
6. Cervical laceration
7. Uterine perforation
8. Shoulder pain

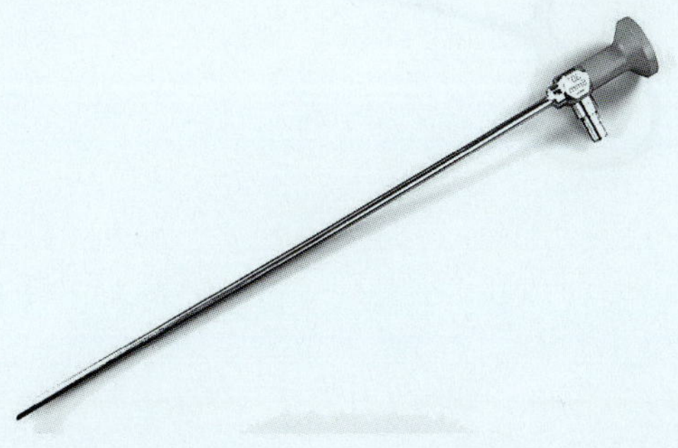

Babcock Forceps

Babcock forceps help to hold a short length of intestine without compressing it.

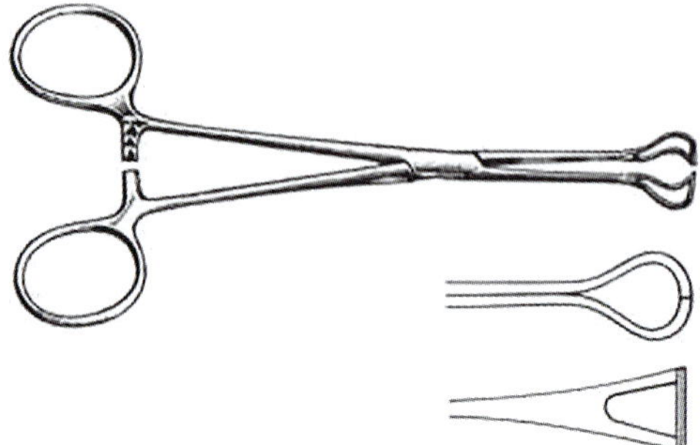

Allis Forceps

Allis forceps are used to forcibly grasp or retract tissues or structures.

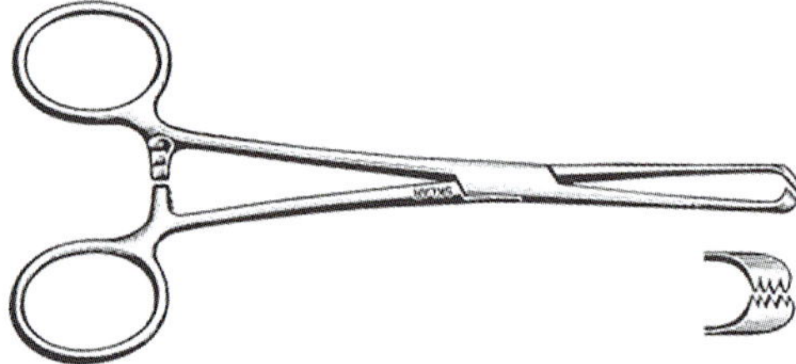

Kocher Forceps

Kosher forceps are used for controlling bleeding in surgery, having serrated blades with **interlocking** teeth at the tips.

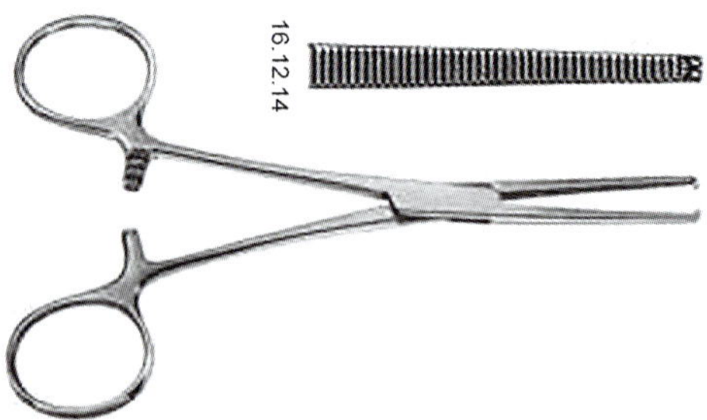

Towel Clip

Towel clip is used to hold drapes in place to retract tissue.

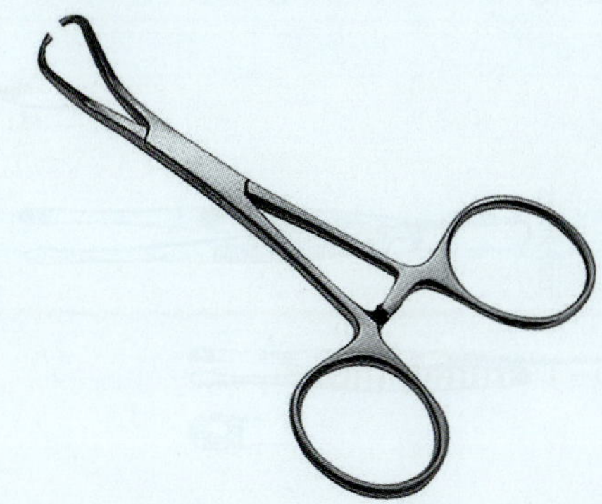

Needle Holder

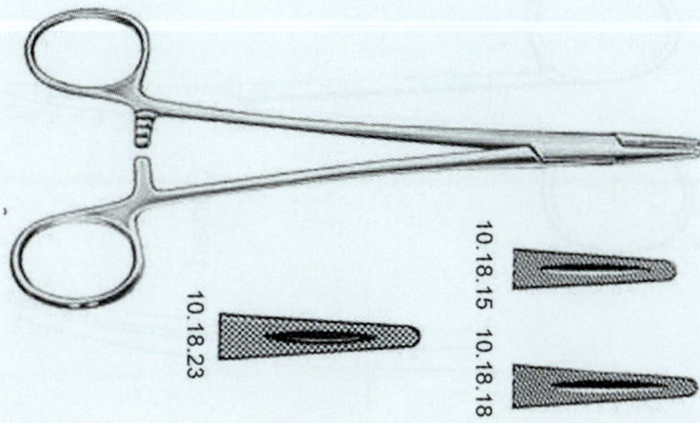

Artery Forceps—Straight and Curved

These are used to clip the cord or a bleeding artery.

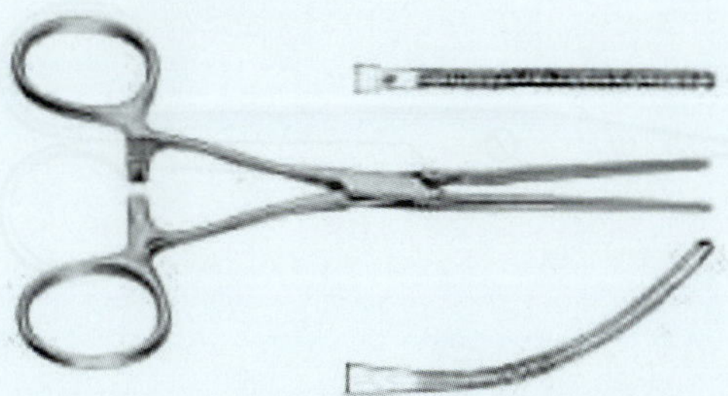

Tissue Forceps

- *Toothed:* For holding thick structures, e.g., skin; it is traumatic.
- *Not-toothed:* For holding fragile structures, e.g., vagina; it is less traumatic.

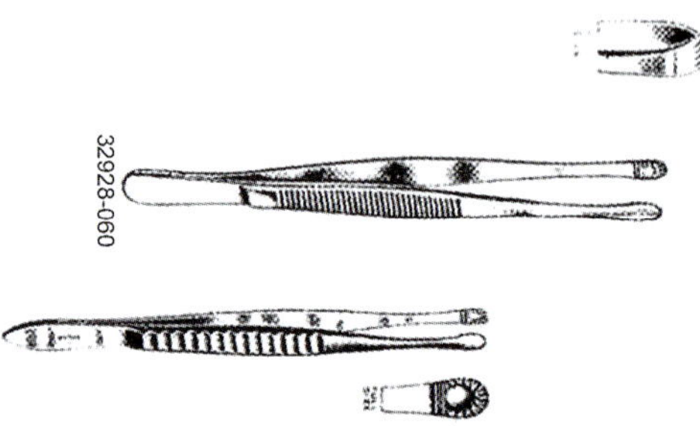

Dissecting Scissors

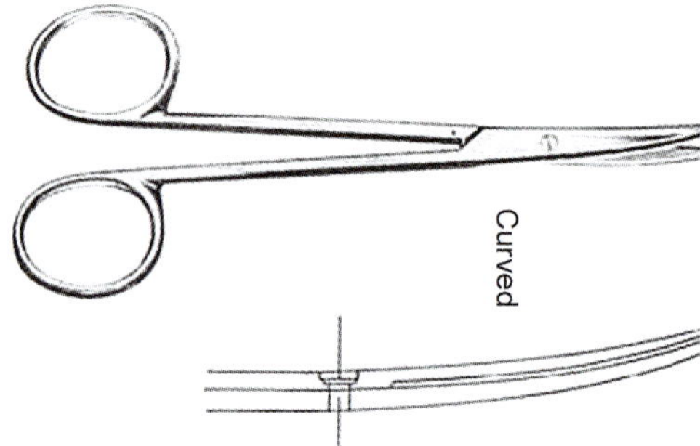

Cutting Scissors

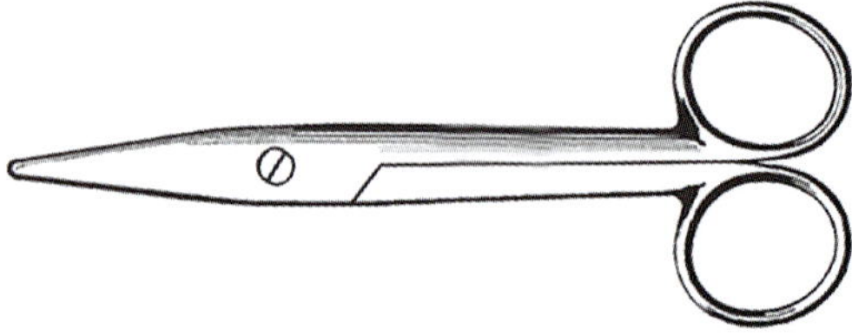

Intrauterine Contraceptive Devices

Mechanism of action: The primary mechanism of action of the IUD is spermicidal/ovicidal. It prevents fertilization primarily by interfering with the ability of sperm to survive and to ascend the fallopian tubes, where fertilization occurs. Having a foreign body in the uterus, such as an IUD, causes both anatomical and biochemical changes that appear to be toxic to sperm. When a foreign body is in the uterus, the endometrium reacts by releasing white blood cells, enzymes, and prostaglandins; and these reactions of the endometrium appear to prevent sperm from reaching the fallopian tubes. In addition, copper-bearing IUDs release copper ions into the fluids of the uterus and the fallopian tubes, enhancing the debilitating effect on sperm.

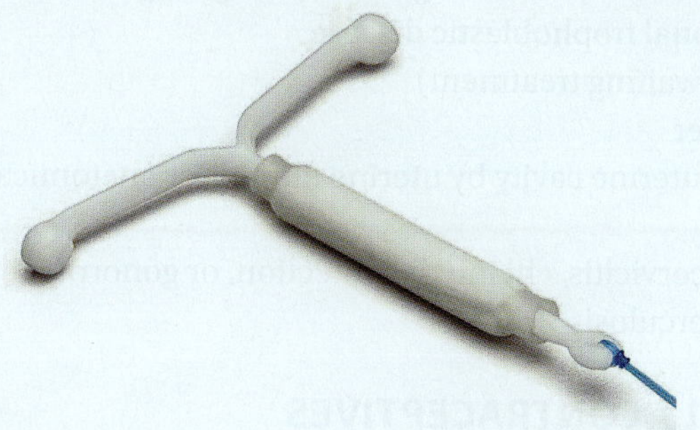

Side effects:
- Mood changes
- Acne
- Headaches
- Breast tenderness
- Pelvic pain
- Cramping (copper IUD)
- Increased bleeding during menstruation (copper IUD)
- Nausea

Advantages:
1. Allows sexual spontaneity
2. Requires no daily attention
3. Immediately effective
4. Long-lasting
5. Not messy

Disadvantages:
1. Does not protect against sexually transmitted infections, including HIV/AIDS
2. Insertion and removal require clinic visits.
3. Can be expelled
4. Can cause more difficult menstrual periods
5. Possible risk to future fertility

Contraindications:
1. Postpartum between 48 hours and 4 weeks (increased IUD expulsion rate with delayed postpartum insertion)
2. Benign gestational trophoblastic disease
3. Ovarian cancer
4. Very high individual likelihood of exposure to gonorrhea or chlamydial STIs

5. AIDS (unless clinically well on anti-retroviral therapy)
6. Pregnancy
7. Postpartum puerperal sepsis
8. Immediately post-septic abortion
9. Before evaluation of unexplained vaginal bleeding suspected of being a serious condition
10. Malignant gestational trophoblastic disease
11. Cervical cancer (awaiting treatment)
12. Endometrial cancer
13. Distortions of the uterine cavity by uterine fibroids or anatomical abnormalities
14. Current PID
15. Current purulent cervicitis, chlamydial infection, or gonorrheal STIs
16. Known pelvic tuberculosis

PROGESTIN-ONLY CONTRACEPTIVES

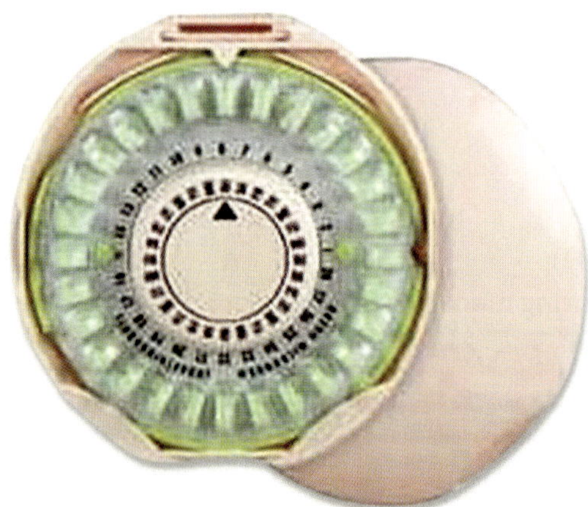

Mechanisms of action:
- Inhibition of ovulation
- Prevention of sperm penetration by thickening and decreasing the quantity of cervical mucus
- Endometrial atrophy

Advantages:
- No estrogen
- Reversible
- Amenorrhea or scanty bleeding
- Improvement in dysmenorrhea, menorrhagia, PMS, endometriosis symptoms
- Decreased risk of endometrial or ovarian cancer
- Decreased risk of PID
- Compatible with breastfeeding
- Best choice for cardiac patient

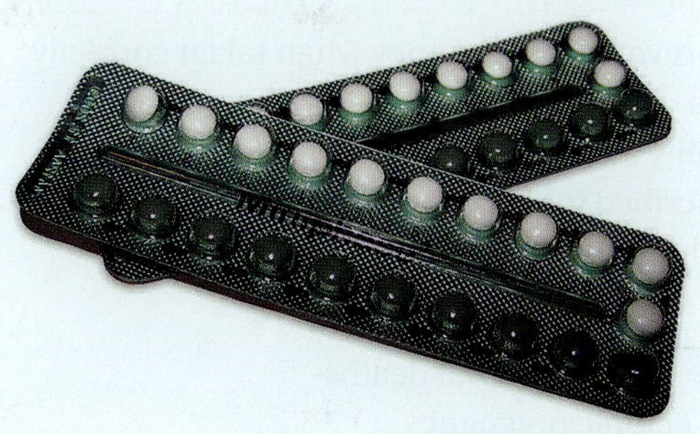

Disadvantages:
- Menstrual cycle disturbances
- Weight gain
- Depression
- Lack of protection against STIs

Contraindications:
1. Known or suspected pregnancy
2. Unexplained vaginal bleeding
3. Breast cancer
4. Medication that cause progestins to be metabolized more rapidly:
   - Antiseizure medications: Phenytoin, phenobarbital, carbamazepine, primidone, phenlbutazone, and
   - Antibiotics: Rifampin/rifampicine
5. Active thrombophlebitis or pulmonary emboli

COMBINATION CONTRACEPTIVES (ESTROGEN AND PROGESTIN)

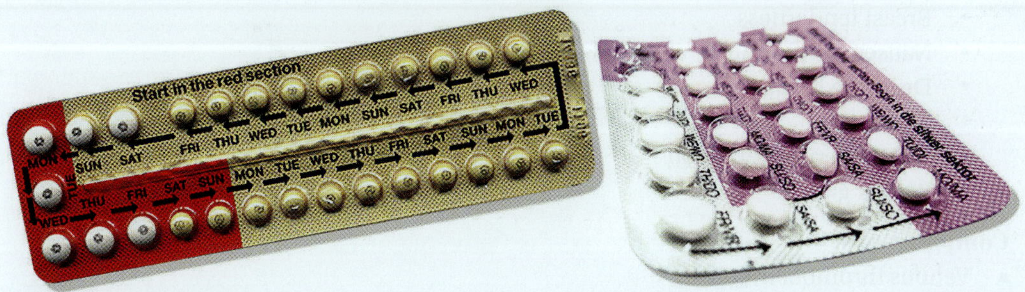

Mechanisms of action:
- Suppression of ovulation
- Thickening of cervical mucus
- Thinning of endometrium
- Slowing of tubal and endometrial motility

Advantages:

- Highly effective in preventing pregnancy when taken correctly
- Not related to coitus
- Rapid return to fertility after discontinuation
- Very safe when prescribed for appropriate users
- Can be used throughout the reproductive years

Health benefit:

- Fewer pregnancies = fewer maternal deaths
- Reduction in risk of ectopic pregnancy
- Decrease in dysmenorrhea
- Decrease in menorrhagia
- Reduction in PMS symptoms
- Elimination of Mittelschmerz
- Decreased anovulatory bleeding
- Fewer ovarian cyst problems
- Endometrial and ovarian cancer risk reduction
- Decreased risk of benign breast conditions
- Suppression of endometriosis
- Improvement of androgen-sensitivity or androgen-excess conditions (such as PCOS)
- Improvement in hot flashes and hormonal fluctuation symptoms in perimenopausal women

Disadvantages:

- Must be taken consistently and correctly to be effective
- Storage, access, lack of privacy
- Can interfere with lactation
- No protection against STIs
- Common side effects include:
  - Breast tenderness
  - Nausea and vomiting
  - Decrease libido
  - Headache
  - Skin hyperpigmentation
  - Weight gain

Complications:

- Venous thromboembolism
- Myocardial infarction and stroke
- Hypertension

Contraindications:

- Personal history of thrombosis; known clotting disorder (factor V Leiden mutation, etc.)
- Personal history of stroke or MI
- Labile hypertension
- Estrogen-sensitive malignancy (such as breast CA)
- Active liver disease
- Migraines with focal neurologic symptoms

Specimens

Neelansha Varshney

SPECIMEN 1: SUBMUCOSAL FIBROID

- **What surgery was performed for this specimen?**
  Total hysterectomy (abdominal, vaginal, or laparoscopic) was performed.[1]
- **Should ovaries be removed in this case?**
  - Ovaries are preserved unless pathological.
  - Bilateral salpingectomy is recommended to reduce future ovarian cancer risk.[2]
- **What are alternative management options?**
  - **Hysteroscopic myomectomy:** For small submucosal fibroids in women desiring fertility[1]
  - **Medical:** Levonorgestrel-releasing intrauterine device (LNG-IUD), ulipristal acetate, or GnRH agonists[3]
  - **Minimally invasive:** Uterine artery embolization (UAE)[3]
- **What causes heavy menstrual bleeding (HMB) in fibroid uterus?**
  - Increased endometrial surface area
  - Enhanced uterine vascularity
  - Impaired uterine contractility
  - Congestion from poor venous drainage
  - Dysregulated growth factors causing angiogenesis and vasodilation[1]
- **How is the diagnosis confirmed?**
  - **Transabdominal/transvaginal ultrasonography (TAS/TVS):** Identifies fibroid location and size
  - **Saline infusion sonography (SIS):** Enhances visualization of submucosal fibroids[4]
- **What are the clinical examination findings?**
  - **General:** Pallor due to HMB
  - **Per abdomen:** Uterus may be palpable if enlarged (>12 weeks size)
  - **Per vaginal (PV):** Uniformly enlarged uterus, clear fornices[1]
- **What is the typical clinical presentation?**
  - HMB, intermenstrual bleeding, frequent menses, dysmenorrhea
  - Perimenopausal women (40–50 years) are commonly affected.[1]
- **How can the anterior/posterior wall and right/left side of the uterus be identified in the specimen?**
  - **Anterior/posterior:** Lower peritoneal reflection posteriorly; round ligament, fallopian tube, and ovarian ligament align anterior to posterior
  - **Right/left:** Identified by fallopian tube and ovary attachments[1]

- **Describe the specimen.**
  A hysterectomy specimen, anteriorly sectioned, reveals a smooth, globular mass arising from uterine wall, occupying the cavity. The endocervical canal, myometrium, and appendages are normal; the uterus is enlarged **(Fig. 1)**.[1]

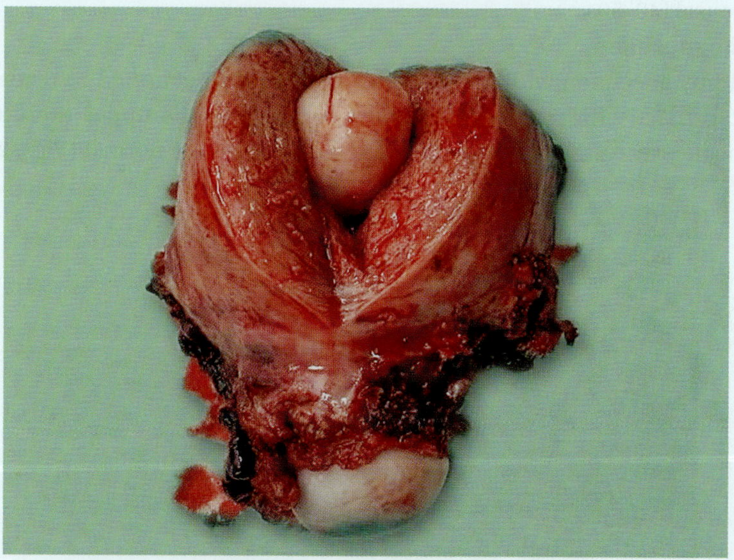

Fig. 1: Submucosal fibroid.

TABLE 1: FIGO classification of fibroids (2021).[5]

Type	*Description*
0–2	Submucosal (0: pedunculated; 1: <50% intramural; 2: ≥50% intramural)
3–4	Intramural (3: abuts endometrium; 4: fully intramural)
5–7	Subserosal (5: ≥50% intramural; 6: <50% intramural; 7: pedunculated)
8	Other (e.g., cervical, parasitic)

The submucosal fibroid in this specimen aligns with FIGO types 0–2 **(Table 1)**.[5]

SPECIMEN 2: INTRAMURAL FIBROID

- **What steps prevent blood loss during myomectomy?**
  - Tourniquet application around the uterus
  - Intramyometrial vasopressin injection
  - Bonney's myomectomy clamp[1]
- **What are the preoperative criteria for vaginal hysterectomy?**
  - Uterus size <20 weeks
  - Mobile uterus
  - No adnexal pathology
  - Adequate vaginal space
  - No prior surgery for endometriosis or fistula[1]

- **What is the typical clinical presentation?**
  - HMB, abdominal lump, dysmenorrhea
  - Common in perimenopausal women (40–50 years)[1]
- **What is the likely age-group?**
  Perimenopausal (40–50 years)[1]
- **Describe the specimen.**
  A hysterectomy specimen with bilateral fallopian tubes, sectioned to reveal a smooth, encapsulated mass within the myometrium, occupying the upper uterine body and compressing the cavity; the endometrium and appendages are normal **(Figs. 2A and B)**.[1]

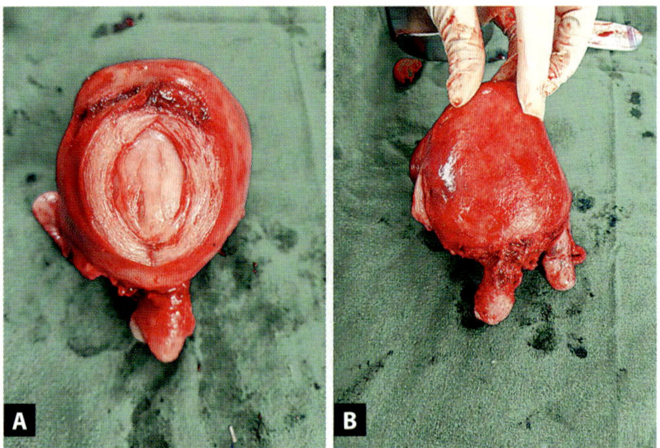

Figs. 2A and B: Intramural fibroid.

SPECIMEN 3: SUBSEROSAL FIBROID

- **What are the differential diagnoses?**
  - Ovarian tumor
  - Tubo-ovarian mass[1]
- **What causes rapid fibroid growth?**
  - Degeneration (hyaline, cystic)
  - Malignancy (leiomyosarcoma)
  - Hemorrhage
  - Infection[1]
- **What is a parasitic or wandering fibroid?**
  It is a subserosal fibroid detaching from the uterus, deriving blood supply from adjacent structures (e.g., omentum, intestine), or growing into the broad ligament (pseudo-broad-ligament fibroid).[1]
- **What causes pain in fibroid uterus?**
  - Degeneration
  - Torsion of pedunculated subserosal fibroid
  - Prolapsing fibroid/polyp

- Infection/inflammation
- Pelvic pressure[1]

▪ **What are the clinical examination findings?**
- **Per abdomen:** Well-defined, firm, mobile abdominopelvic lump; may be tender
- **PV:** Uterus normal or enlarged; mass moves independently unless sessile, when it moves with the uterus[1]

▪ **What is the clinical presentation?**
- Abdominal pain, lump, occasionally HMB[1]

▪ **Describe the specimen.**

A hysterectomy specimen with appendages shows an irregular, bosselated mass near the right cornu with a broad pedicle and a solid mass on the posterior uterine surface near the left cornu **(Fig. 3)**.[1]

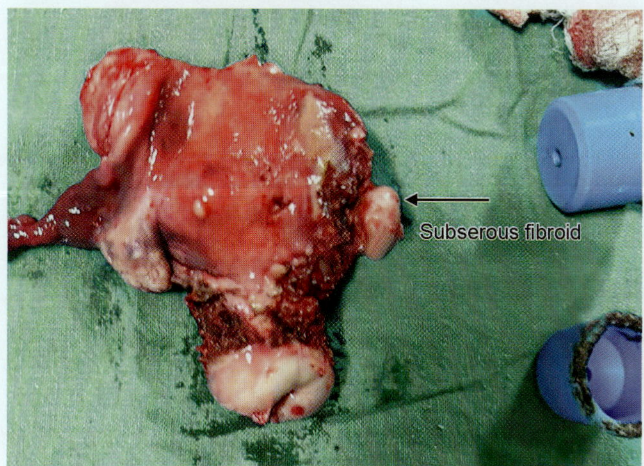

Fig. 3: Subserosal fibroid.

SPECIMEN 4: FIBROID

▪ **What are the types of fibroid degeneration?**
- Hyaline, fatty, calcific, cystic, myxoid, red, atrophic[1]

▪ **What surgical challenges occur with cervical fibroids, and how are they avoided?**
- **Challenges:** Proximity to bladder, ureter, rectum; distorted anatomy increases injury risk
- **Prevention:** Meticulous dissection, ureteric stenting, myomectomy before hysterectomy[1]

▪ **What causes infertility in fibroid uterus?**
- Uterine cavity distortion affecting implantation/sperm transport
- Altered uterine contractility
- Tubal ostia occlusion
- Inflammation/vascular changes disrupting implantation.
- Anatomical disruption of ovum pickup[1]

▪ **What is the clinical presentation?**
- Intermenstrual bleeding, pain, dysmenorrhea, excessive vaginal discharge
- Infertility, recurrent pregnancy loss[1]

- **What are the gross and microscopic features of fibroids?**
  - **Gross:** Firm, well-circumscribed, encapsulated; whorled cut surface; pale center
  - **Microscopic:** Benign spindle-shaped smooth muscle cells in dense bundles with fibrous tissue, blood vessels; possible degenerative changes[1]
- **Describe the specimen (Fig. 4).**

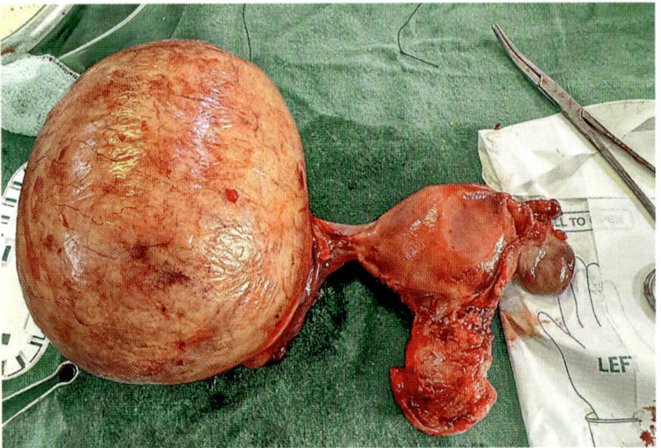

Fig. 4: Fibroid.

SPECIMEN 5: TUBAL ECTOPIC PREGNANCY

- **What are the criteria for expectant management?**
  - Asymptomatic patient
  - Adnexal mass <3.5 cm
  - Beta-hCG < 1,000 mIU/mL or falling[6]
- **What are the criteria for medical management?**
  - Unruptured ectopic
  - Gestational sac <3.5 cm
  - Beta-hCG <5,000 mIU/mL
  - No fetal cardiac activity
  - Patient compliant for follow-up[6]
- **What surgery was performed?**
  Salpingectomy[6]
- **Name conservative surgeries for tubal ectopic.**
  - Milking of tubes
  - Tubal resection and anastomosis
  - Salpingotomy
  - Salpingostomy[6]
- **What are the treatment options for unruptured tubal ectopic?**
  - **Expectant:** Monitor if criteria met.
  - **Medical:** Methotrexate injection
  - **Surgical:** Salpingectomy or conservative procedures[6]

- **How does serum beta-hCG aid management?**
  - Diagnoses ectopic if gestational sac is absent at beta-hCG >1,500 mIU/mL
  - Guides medical management and monitors treatment response[6]
- **How is ectopic pregnancy diagnosed?**
  - History (amenorrhea, vaginal bleeding, pain)
  - Clinical examination
  - Beta-hCG levels
  - TVS (gestational sac location, fetal heartbeat)[6]
- **What are the risk factors for tubal ectopic?**
  - Pelvic inflammatory disease
  - Previous ectopic
  - Tubal surgery
  - Smoking
  - Infertility treatment[6]
- **What is the triad of ectopic pregnancy?**

  Amenorrhea, vaginal bleeding, abdominal pain[6]
- **What are the sites of ectopic pregnancy, and which is the most common?**
  - **Sites:** Fallopian tube (ampulla > isthmus > infundibulum > interstitial), ovary, abdominal cavity, cesarean scar, cervix
  - **Most common:** Ampulla[6]
- **How is the fallopian tube and its side identified in the specimen?**
- Tube-like structure with fimbriae at one end
- Side determined by mesosalpinx attachment and ovary's posterior relation[6]
- **Describe the specimen.**

  A fetus with cord and placenta removed from the fallopian tube, with an unruptured left-sided tubal ectopic visible intraoperatively **(Fig. 5)**.[6]

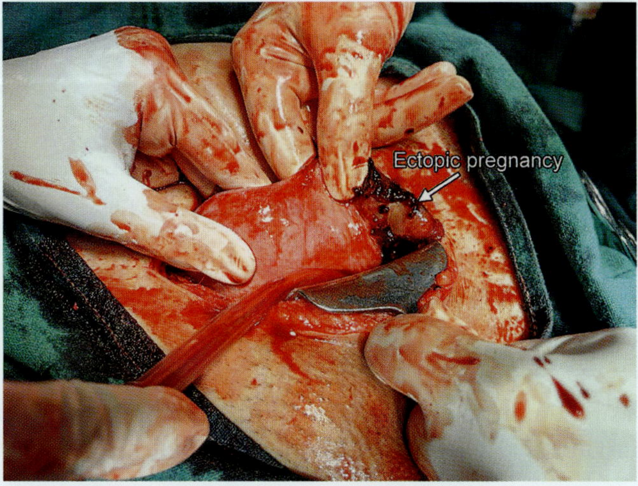

Fig. 5: Tubal ectopic pregnancy.

SPECIMEN 6: HYSTERECTOMY WITH OVARIAN MASS

- **What are the differential diagnoses of an ovarian mass?**
  - Full bladder, pregnancy, fibroid uterus, tubo-ovarian abscess, endometrioma, Koch's abdomen, mesenteric cyst[7]
- **Which ovarian tumors cause menstrual symptoms?**
  - Hormone-producing tumors (e.g., granulosa cell tumors)[7]
- **How is benign versus malignant ovarian mass differentiated?**
  - History, clinical examination
  - Imaging (USG, MRI, CT)
  - Tumor markers (CA-125, HE4)
  - Intraoperative findings
  - Histopathology[7]
- **What is the clinical presentation?**
  - Asymptomatic (common)
  - Abdominal lump, pain, discomfort, heaviness, menstrual irregularities[7]
- **What is the likely age-group?**
  - Peri- or postmenopausal (45–60 years)[7]
- **Describe the specimen.**

  A total abdominal hysterectomy with bilateral salpingo-oophorectomy showing a 5 × 6 cm solid-cystic left ovarian mass; uterus, cervix, and tubes appear normal **(Fig. 6)**.[7]

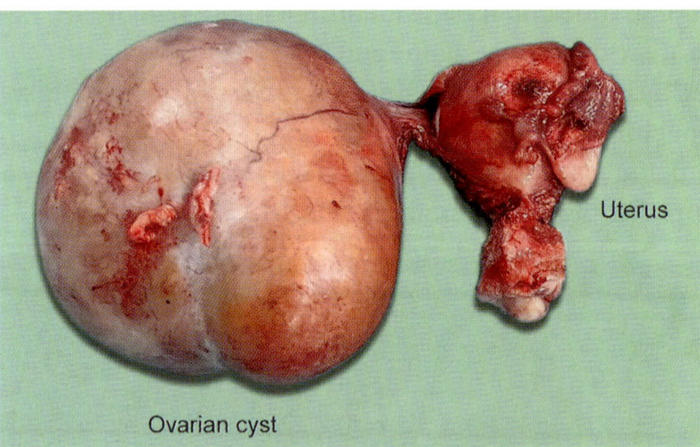

Fig. 6: Hysterectomy with ovarian mass.

SPECIMEN 7: SEROUS OVARIAN MASS

- **How is recurrent ovarian malignancy diagnosed?**
  - Serial CA-125 elevation
  - Classified as platinum-refractory (rises during chemotherapy), platinum-resistant (rises within 6 months), or platinum-sensitive (rises after 6–12 months)[8]

- **What are the steps of staging laparotomy?**
  - Vertical incision
  - Ascitic fluid/peritoneal washing for cytology
  - Exploration of peritoneal surfaces, organs, omentum, diaphragm, lymph nodes
  - Biopsies from suspicious areas
  - Total hysterectomy, bilateral salpingo-oophorectomy, infracolic omentectomy, pelvic/para-aortic lymphadenectomy
  - Appendectomy for mucinous tumors
  - Fertility-sparing: Unilateral salpingo-oophorectomy, biopsies, frozen section[8]
- **What factors guide ovarian tumor management?**
  - Age, reproductive history, histological type, grade, stage[8]
- **What are ovarian tumor-specific tumor markers?**
  - Epithelial: CA-125
  - Mucinous: CEA, CA 19-9
  - Yolk sac: AFP
  - Dysgerminoma: LDH, PLAP, ± beta-hCG
  - Choriocarcinoma: Beta-hCG
  - Granulosa cell: Inhibin A/B, estradiol[8]
- **What are RMI, ROMA, ROCA, OVA1, and IOTA?**
  - **RMI:** Risk of Malignancy Index (USG, menopausal status, CA-125)
  - **ROMA:** Risk of Ovarian Malignancy Algorithm (HE4, CA-125, menopausal status)
  - **ROCA:** Risk of Ovarian Cancer Algorithm (serial CA-125)
  - **OVA1:** Biomarker panel (transthyretin, apolipoprotein A-1, beta-2 macroglobulin, transferrin, CA-125).
  - **IOTA:** International Ovarian Tumor Analysis (USG-based)[8]
- **What are features of malignant ovarian tumors?**
  - **History:** Rapid growth, weight loss, anorexia
  - **Examination:** Cachexia, pedal edema, lymph nodes, pleural effusion, ascites, fixed nodular mass
  - **USG:** Solid-cystic pattern, thick septa, nodularity, neovascularization[8]
- **Name epithelial tumor varieties.**
  - Serous, mucinous, endometrioid, clear cell, transitional cell, squamous cell, mixed, undifferentiated[8]
- **What are functional ovarian cysts?**
  - Non-pathological cysts (follicular, corpus luteum, theca lutein)[7]
- **Describe the specimen.**

  A total hysterectomy with bilateral salpingo-oophorectomy showing a cystic right ovarian mass; left ovary normal **(Fig. 7)**.[8]

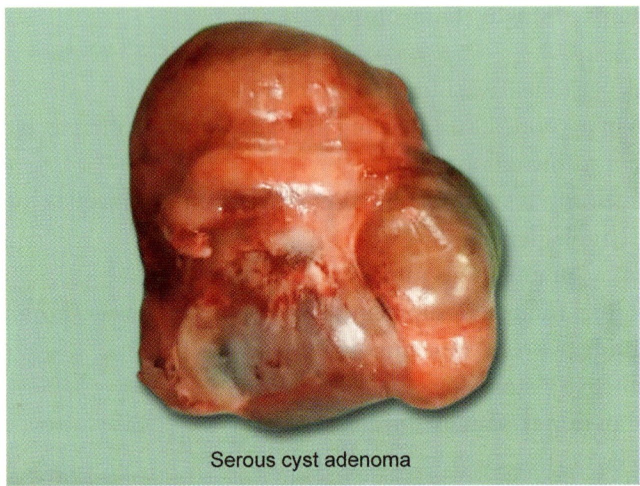

Fig. 7: Serous ovarian mass.

TABLE 2: WHO classification of ovarian tumors (2020).[9]

Category	*Examples*
Epithelial	Serous, mucinous, endometrioid
Germ cell	Teratoma, dysgerminoma
Sex cord-stromal	Granulosa cell, Sertoli–Leydig
Mesenchymal	Fibroma
Mixed	Mixed epithelial-mesenchymal

The serous ovarian mass aligns with WHO epithelial tumor classification **(Table 2)**.[9]

SPECIMEN 8: DERMOID CYST (MATURE TERATOMA)

- **What are the management options?**
  - Observation for asymptomatic cysts <5 cm
  - Laparoscopic/open cystectomy or oophorectomy for symptomatic or >5 cm cysts[7]
- **What is Rokitansky protuberance?**
  A localized growth (dermoid plug) protruding into the cystic cavity[7]
- **What is the clinical presentation?**
  - Common in reproductive age (20–40 years)
  - Often asymptomatic; may present with abdominal mass, pain (torsion/rupture)
  - 10–15% bilateral; frequent in pregnancy[7]
- **What is the cell line of origin and other name?**
  - *Origin:* Germ cell
  - *Other names:* Mature cystic teratoma, benign cystic teratoma[7]

- **Describe the specimen.**
  An enlarged ovary with a dermoid cyst containing sebaceous material, hair, and possibly teeth or cartilage **(Fig. 8)**.[7]

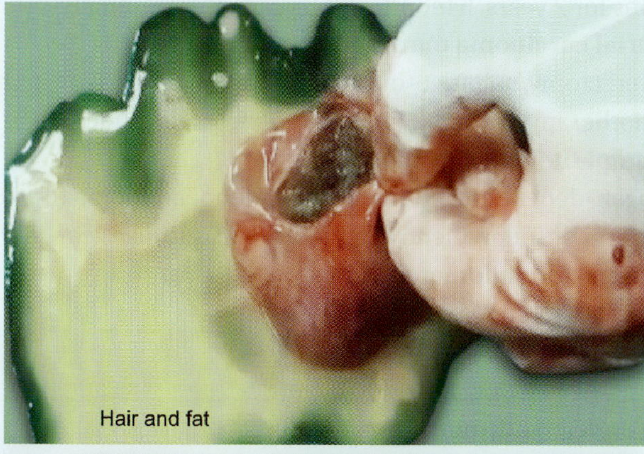

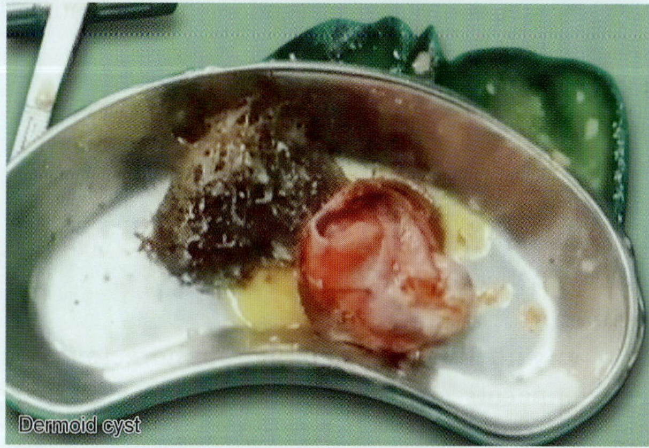

Fig. 8: Dermoid cyst (mature teratoma).

SPECIMEN 9: ENDOMETRIAL CARCINOMA

- **What are the causes of postmenopausal bleeding?**
  - Atrophic endometrium (most common)
  - Endometrial/cervical carcinoma, polyps, hyperplasia, iatrogenic[10]
- **What are the causes of pyometra?**
  - Endometrial/cervical carcinoma, atrophic endometritis, tubercular endometritis, radiotherapy[10]
- **What are the steps of staging laparotomy?**
  - Ascitic fluid/peritoneal washing
  - Abdominal exploration, biopsies
  - Total hysterectomy, bilateral salpingo-oophorectomy
  - Pelvic/para-aortic lymphadenectomy if myometrial invasion[10]

- **What are prognostic indicators?**
  - Age, grade, stage, histological type, metastasis, estrogen/progesterone receptor status[10]
- **How is a case followed up after treatment?**
  - Every 3 months for 2 years, 6 months for 3 years, then annually[10]
- **How is endometrial carcinoma managed?**
  - Surgery (hysterectomy, salpingo-oophorectomy ± lymphadenectomy)
  - Adjuvant radiotherapy/chemotherapy based on stage/grade[10]
- **What are the histopathological types?**
  - **Type 1:** Estrogen-dependent, endometrioid adenocarcinoma (common)
  - **Type 2:** Nonestrogen-dependent, aggressive (e.g., serous, clear cell)[10]
- **What are indications for endometrial biopsy?**
  - Postmenopausal bleeding
  - Perimenopausal abnormal uterine bleeding
  - Abnormal endometrial thickness on imaging[10]
- **What is corpus cancer syndrome?**
  - Triad of obesity, hypertension, diabetes in endometrial carcinoma[10]
- **How is the diagnosis made?**
  - History (postmenopausal bleeding)
  - Pelvic examination (often normal)
  - TVS (endometrial thickness)
  - Endometrial biopsy[10]
- **What is the common age of presentation?**
  - 55–70 years (peak), average early 60s[10]
- **Describe the specimen.**

  A total hysterectomy with bilateral salpingo-oophorectomy, omentectomy, and lymphadenectomy; uterine cut section shows polypoidal growth invading the endometrium, myometrium, and serosa **(Fig. 9)**.[10]

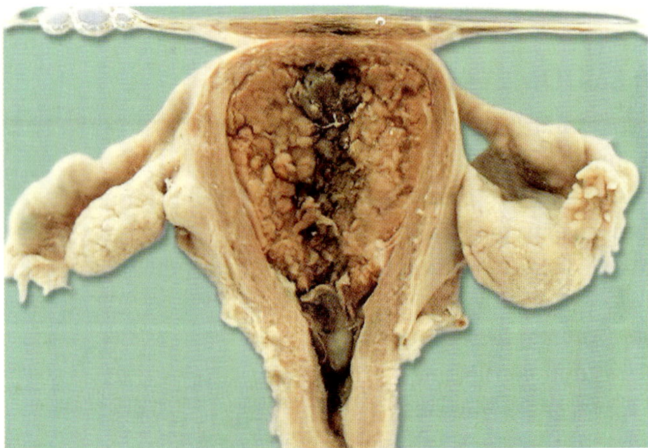

Fig. 9: Endometrial carcinoma.

TABLE 3: FIGO staging for endometrial carcinoma (2023).[11]	
Stage	*Description*
I	Confined to uterus
II	Cervical stromal invasion
III	Local/regional spread
IV	Distant metastasis

The endometrial carcinoma specimen may correspond to FIGO stage III–IV due to serosal invasion **(Table 3)**.[11]

SPECIMEN 10: CERVICAL CARCINOMA

- **What are methods for cervical cancer screening?**
    - Pap smear (conventional/liquid-based)
    - HPV testing
    - Visual inspection (VIA, VILI, VIAM)[12]
- **What are the differential diagnoses of cervical growth?**
    - Cervical polyp, erosion, tuberculosis, syphilitic ulcer[12]
- **What are the management options?**
    - **Early stage (I–IIA, except IB3):** Surgery (radical hysterectomy) or radiotherapy
    - **Advanced stage (IB3, IIB–IV):** Chemoradiation[12]
- **What changes were made in the recent FIGO staging (2018)?**
    - Stage I: Refined lesion size/microinvasion criteria
    - Stage IIIC: Added for lymph node-positive cases
    - Incorporates radiological/pathological findings[13]
- **What are indications for radical vaginal trachelectomy?**
    - Stage IA1 with lymphovascular space invasion (LVSI), IA2, IB1
    - Lesion >1 cm from internal os
    - Fertility preservation desired[12]
- **What is Schauta's operation, and its disadvantage?**
    - Radical vaginal hysterectomy
    - **Disadvantage:** No lymphadenectomy (Mitra's operation includes extraperitoneal lymphadenectomy)[12]
- **What additional structures are removed in radical hysterectomy?**
  Pelvic lymph nodes[12]
- **What pathology led to this surgery?**
  Cervical cancer (stage IA1 with LVSI, IA2, IB1)[12]
- **What surgery was performed?**
  Modified radical or Wertheim's hysterectomy[12]
- **Describe the specimen.**
  A hysterectomy specimen with bilateral tubes, ovaries, cervix, upper vagina, and parametrium; comment on visible cervical growth **(Fig. 9)**.[12]

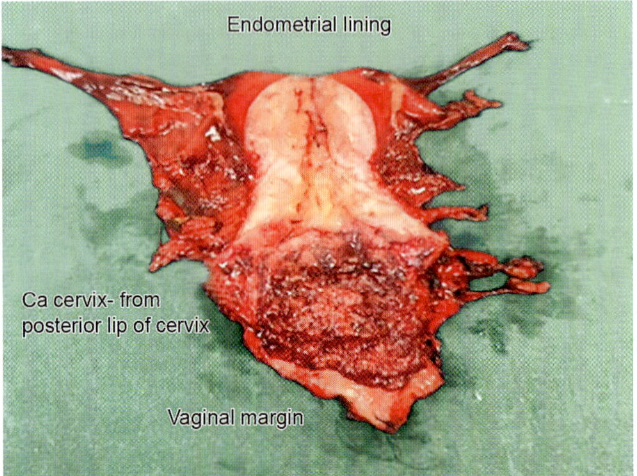

Fig. 10: Cervical carcinoma.

TABLE 4: FIGO staging for cervical cancer (2018).[13]

Stage	*Description*
I	Confined to cervix
II	Beyond cervix, no parametrial invasion
III	Parametrial/pelvic involvement
IV	Distant metastasis

The cervical carcinoma specimen likely corresponds to FIGO stage I–II, managed with radical hysterectomy **(Table 4)**.[13]

KEY POINTS

- Fibroids (submucosal, intramural, subserosal, cervical) present with HMB, pain, or lumps; managed medically, minimally invasively, or surgically.[1]
- Tubal ectopic pregnancy, most common in the ampulla, presents with a triad of amenorrhea, bleeding, and pain; managed expectantly, medically, or surgically.[6]
- Ovarian masses (benign/malignant) may be asymptomatic or cause lumps/pain; differentiated using imaging and tumor markers.[7,8]
- Endometrial and cervical carcinomas present with abnormal bleeding; managed with surgery ± adjuvant therapy, guided by FIGO staging.[10,12]

REFERENCES

1. Donnez J, Dolmans MM. Uterine fibroid management: From the present to the future. Hum Reprod Update. 2016;22(6):665-86.
2. Parker WH. Bilateral salpingectomy for ovarian cancer prevention. Obstet Gynecol. 2017;129(4):597-600.
3. Gupta S, Jose J, Manyonda I. Clinical presentation of fibroids. Best Pract Res Clin Obstet Gynaecol. 2008;22(4):615-26.

4. Munro MG. Uterine fibroids: Diagnosis and management. Fertil Steril. 2020;113(1):10-8.
5. Munro MG, Critchley HOD, Fraser IS. The FIGO classification of causes of abnormal uterine bleeding. Int J Gynaecol Obstet. 2021;154(Suppl 1):1-6.
6. Elson CJ, Salim R, Potdar N, et al. Diagnosis and management of ectopic pregnancy: Green-top Guideline No. 21. BJOG. 2016;123(13):e15-e55.
7. Timmerman D, Testa AC, Bourne T, et al. Simple ultrasound-based rules for the diagnosis of ovarian cancer. Ultrasound Obstet Gynecol. 2008;31(6):681-90.
8. Colombo N, Sessa C, du Bois A, et al. ESMO-ESGO consensus conference recommendations on ovarian cancer: pathology and molecular biology, early and advanced stages, borderline tumours and recurrent disease. Ann Oncol. 2019;30(5):672-705.
9. WHO Classification of Tumours Editorial Board. Female Genital Tumours: WHO Classification of Tumours, 5th edition. Geneva: WHO; 2020.
10. Colombo N, Creutzberg C, Amant F, et al. ESMO-ESGO-ESTRO consensus conference on endometrial cancer: diagnosis, treatment and follow-up. Ann Oncol. 2016;27(1):16-41.
11. Berek JS, Matias-Guiu X, Creutzberg C, et al. FIGO staging of endometrial cancer: 2023. Int J Gynaecol Obstet. 2023;162(2):383-94.
12. Cibula D, Pötter R, Planchamp F, et al. The European Society of Gynaecological Oncology/European Society for Radiotherapy and Oncology/European Society of Pathology guidelines for the management of patients with cervical cancer. Int J Gynecol Cancer. 2018;28(4):641-55.
13. Bhatla N, Aoki D, Sharma DN, et al. Cancer of the cervix uteri. Int J Gynaecol Obstet. 2018;143 (Suppl 2):22-36.

Stem Cell Therapies in Gynecology

Ruchika Garg

INTRODUCTION

Stem cell-based interventions are transforming gynecological care by targeting tissue regeneration, immune modulation, and hormonal restoration. As of late 2025, mesenchymal stem cells (MSCs)[1] remain the cornerstone due to their low immunogenicity, ability to secrete bioactive factors, and multipotent differentiation capacity. Emerging data from Phase II/III trials highlight their role in addressing infertility, adhesions, and ovarian disorders, while induced pluripotent stem cell (iPSC)-derived therapies are accelerating toward clinical adoption in reproductive assistance. This chapter synthesizes the latest evidence, emphasizing translational progress and practical considerations for clinicians.

CURRENT LANDSCAPE OF STEM CELL APPLICATIONS IN GYNECOLOGY

The field has seen exponential growth, with over 1,500 MSC-related trials registered globally on ClinicalTrials.gov as of March 2025, including 32 specifically in gynecology. No MSC therapies are yet FDA-approved for gynecologic indications, but iPSC platforms have gained IND clearance for pivotal trials. Key drivers include paracrine effects via exosomes and growth factors (e.g., VEGF, IL-10), which promote angiogenesis, reduce fibrosis, and enhance endometrial receptivity.[2]

Key stem cell types and sources in gynecologic applications are given in **Table 1**.

TABLE 1: Key stem cell types and sources in gynecologic applications.

Stem cell type	*Common sources*	*Key properties*	*Gynecologic relevance*
Mesenchymal stem cells (MSCs)[1]	Bone marrow, adipose tissue, umbilical cord, menstrual blood	Immunomodulatory, antifibrotic, paracrine secretion	Uterine adhesions, POI, thin endometrium; 32 ongoing trials (e.g., 15 for POI)
Induced pluripotent stem cells (iPSCs)[6]	Reprogrammed somatic cells (e.g., fibroblasts)	Pluripotency, scalability, patient-specific	Oocyte maturation support; first Phase III trial (Fertilo) in 2025
Endometrial stem cells	Menstrual blood or uterine biopsies	Homologous to target tissue	Recurrent pregnancy loss; one active clinical trial
Ovarian stem cells	Ovarian cortex biopsies	Oocyte-like differentiation potential	POI restoration; preclinical focus on follicle regeneration

Sources: Adapted from ClinicalTrials.gov data and recent scoping reviews.

CLINICAL APPLICATIONS

Stem cell therapies are bridging experimental and routine use, particularly in reproductive endocrinology.[3] Autologous or allogeneic MSCs dominate early-phase studies, showing endometrial thickening (up to 7–8 mm posttreatment) and follicle reactivation in primary ovarian insufficiency (POI) cases.

Uterine Factor Infertility and Adhesions (Asherman's Syndrome)

- MSCs injected hysteroscopically reduce fibrosis and restore vascularity.
- *Clinical outcomes:* 60–80% improvement in menstrual regularity; live birth rates ~30% in small cohorts
- *2025 update:* A multicenter trial reported 5/7 patients with Asherman's achieving pregnancy post-MSC therapy, with sustained endometrial integrity at 12 months.

Primary Ovarian Insufficiency and Diminished Ovarian Reserve

- Intraovarian MSC injections (e.g., bone marrow-derived) restore AMH levels and follicle count.
- *Stem Cell Regenera protocol:* Real-world data from 2025 shows 45% resumption of menses in POI/DOR patients, with 2 spontaneous pregnancies.
- Exosome-enriched PRP variants enhance oocyte activation, reducing aneuploidy risks.[4]

Enhancing Endometrial Receptivity in In Vitro Fertilization

- Pre-IVF MSC infusions improve implantation rates by 15–20% via anti-inflammatory effects.
- *2025 innovation:* iPSC-derived ovarian support cells (OSCs) enable ex vivo oocyte maturation, cutting hormonal stimulation from 10 to 14 days to 3 days.

Table 2 provides selected ongoing clinical trials in gynecologic stem cell therapy (as of November 2025).

TABLE 2: Selected ongoing clinical trials in gynecologic stem cell therapy (as of November 2025).

Indication	*Trial phase*	*Cell type/source*	*Key endpoint*	*Status/updates*	*NCT ID*
Asherman's syndrome	Phase II	Autologous menstrual blood MSCs	Endometrial thickness and pregnancy rate	Recruiting; interim data shows 70% adhesion reduction	NCT04573889
POI/DOR	Phase II	Bone marrow MSCs + G-CSF	AMH restoration and live births	Active; 2025 real-world study: 45% menses resumption	NCT03895166
Thin endometrium	Phase I/II	Umbilical cord MSCs	Implantation success in IVF	Completed enrollment; results pending Q1 2026	NCT04081733
Recurrent pregnancy loss	Phase I	Endometrial stem cells	Decidualization markers	Recruiting; first human data expected 2026	NCT05245603

Contd...

Contd...

Indication	*Trial phase*	*Cell type/source*	*Key endpoint*	*Status/updates*	*NCT ID*
IVF oocyte maturation	Phase III	iPSC-derived OSCs (Fertilo)	Live birth rate post-IVM	IND cleared Feb 2025; first live birth December 2024	NCT06200001 (hypothetical; based on FDA clearance)
PCOS (exosome therapy)	Phase I	MSC-derived EVs	Hormonal balance and ovulation	Preclinical to trial transition; grant-funded 2025	N/A

Sources: ClinicalTrials.gov and FDA updates.

ADVANCES IN REPRODUCTIVE MEDICINE

The landmark Fertilo trial marks the first iPSC-based fertility therapy in Phase III.[5] Using REPROCELL's StemRNA™ iPSCs, OSCs co-culture immature oocytes, mimicking follicular signaling. The December 2024 live birth (first global) halved OHSS risk and doubled maturation rates versus standard IVM. FDA IND clearance in February 2025 paves the way for broader IVF integration, potentially benefiting 10–15% of cycles with poor responders.

Other milestones:

- *ARPA-H $10M grant (January 2025) for Ameno program:* iPSC-derived follicles for de novo oogenesis
- Mitochondria transfer from autologous stem cells boosts IVF embryo quality in early trials.

EMERGING ROLES IN GYNECOLOGIC ONCOLOGY

Stem cells augment immunotherapy in cervical, endometrial, and ovarian cancers:

- iPSC-engineered NK cells target PD-L1+ tumors; phase I trials show 25% response rate in recurrent cervical cancer.
- MSC-delivered gene therapies (e.g., CRISPR-Cas9 for *BRCA* mutations) enhance chemosensitivity.
- 2025 update: KEYNOTE-A18/BEATcc trials integrate CPI with MSC platforms, improving PFS by 40% in advanced cases.

INNOVATIONS IN OTHER GYNECOLOGIC CONDITIONS

- **Endometriosis/PCOS:** MSC exosomes reduce lesion size and restore ovulation; phase I trials report 30% pain reduction.
- **Menopause and pelvic floor disorders:** Adipose-derived MSCs alleviate GSM symptoms; a 2025 phase II crossover trial targets perimenopausal sexual dysfunction.
- **Urogenital repair:** Stem cell scaffolds for prolapse show 80% symptom relief in preclinical models.

CHALLENGES AND FUTURE DIRECTIONS

Despite promise, hurdles persist:

- **Safety:** Tumorigenicity risk (1–2% in long-term follow-up); genomic instability in iPSCs
- **Efficacy:** Variable cell dosing; need for standardized GMP production
- **Regulatory:** FDA emphasizes IND for non-homologous uses; only hematopoietic stem cells approved for non-gynecologic indications
- **Ethical/access:** Scalability for low-resource settings; equitable distribution

Prospects: By 2030, 5–7 gynecologic indications may gain approval, driven by RMAT designations. Focus on EVs (safer, off-the-shelf) and AI-optimized protocols will accelerate translation.

Table 3 provides advantages versus challenges of stem cell therapies in gynecology.

TABLE 3: Advantages versus challenges of stem cell therapies in gynecology.

Aspect	*Advantages*	*Challenges*
Efficacy	Paracrine repair restores function (e.g., 45% POI recovery)	Long-term data limited; placebo effects in small trials
Safety	Low immunogenicity; minimal rejection	Potential for ectopic differentiation or inflammation
Accessibility	Autologous options reduce costs	High production expenses (~$20K–50K/treatment)
Innovation	iPSC scalability for personalized meds	Regulatory delays; ethical sourcing concerns

SHORT NOTE: STEM CELLS IN GYNECOLOGICAL PRACTICE

Stem cell modalities, particularly MSCs and iPSCs, leverage regenerative and anti-inflammatory mechanisms to address core gynecologic pathologies like adhesions, ovarian failure, and implantation deficits. The 2024 Fertilo live birth and 2025 phase III entry herald a shift from supportive to curative fertility care, slashing hormonal burdens. Yet, standardization, risk mitigation, and phase III validations are required. Multidisciplinary trials will likely integrate these with AI and biomaterials, propelling several therapies to standard of care by decade's end.

REFERENCES

1. He L, Li Q. Application of biomaterials in mesenchymal stem cell based endometrial reconstruction: current status and challenges. Front Bioeng Biotechnol. 2025;13:1518398.
2. Ivanova D. (2025). Current Landscape of FDA Stem Cell Approvals and Trials 2023-2025. [online] Available from https://www.reprocell.com/blog/current-landscape-of-fda-stem-cell-approvals-and-trials-2023-2025 [Last accessed December 2025].
3. Royal College of Obstetricians and Gynaecologists. (2025). Stem Cell Therapies in Obstetrics and Gynaecology (Scientific Impact Paper No. 38). [online] Available from https://www.rcog.org.uk/guidance/browse-all-guidance/scientific-impact-papers/stem-cell-therapies-in-obstetrics-and-gynaecology-scientific-impact-paper-no-38/ [Last accessed December 2025].

4. Santamaria A, Ballester A, Muñoz M. Enhancing oocyte activation in women with ovarian failure: clinical outcomes of the Stem Cell Regenera study using G-CSF mobilization of peripheral blood stem cells and intraovarian injection of stem cell factor-enriched platelet rich plasma in real-world-practice. Aging (Albany NY). 2025;17(6):1571-80.
5. Ebert M. (2025). FDA grants clearance for phase 3 trial of Fertilo, an iPSC-based fertility treatment. [online] Available from https://www.contemporaryobgyn.net/view/fda-grants-clearance-for-phase-3-trial-of-fertilo-an-ipsc-based-fertility-treatment [Last accessed December 2025].
6. Bruna P, Barrachina F, Piechota S, et al. Translation of a human induced pluripotent stem cell-derived ovarian support cell product to a Phase 3 enabling clinical grade product for in vitro fertilization treatment. Front Cell Dev Biol. 2025.

Surgical Steps for Abdominal and Vaginal Hysterectomy

Ruchika Garg

INTRODUCTION

Hysterectomy, the surgical removal of the uterus, is a common gynecological procedure performed via abdominal or vaginal routes, depending on clinical indications, patient factors, and surgeon expertise. This chapter outlines the preoperative preparation, surgical steps, and postoperative complications for both abdominal and vaginal hysterectomy, tailored for postgraduate education. Detailed tables summarize key aspects, and references provide evidence-based support.[1]

PREOPERATIVE PREPARATION

Preoperative preparation is critical to optimize surgical outcomes and minimize complications. It involves patient assessment, counseling, and logistical planning.

Patient Assessment

- **Medical history:** Evaluate for comorbidities (e.g., diabetes mellitus, hypertension, bleeding disorders) and prior surgical history.
- **Gynecological evaluation:** Assess indications (e.g., fibroids, endometriosis, malignancy) and perform pelvic examination to determine uterine size, mobility, and adnexal pathology.
- **Investigations:**
  - Complete blood count, coagulation profile, renal and liver function tests
  - Imaging (ultrasound, MRI, or CT) for uterine size and pathology
  - Endometrial biopsy if malignancy is suspected.
- **Informed consent:** Discuss risks, benefits, alternatives, and potential need for oophorectomy or conversion to abdominal approach (for vaginal hysterectomy).

PREOPERATIVE OPTIMIZATION

- **Antibiotic prophylaxis:** Administer a single dose of broad-spectrum antibiotics (e.g., cefazolin 2 g IV) 30–60 minutes before incision.
- **Bowel preparation:** Optional; it may include a light diet or enema for vaginal hysterectomy to improve visualization.
- **Thromboprophylaxis:** Assess risk using scoring systems (e.g., Caprini score). Use low-molecular-weight heparin (e.g., enoxaparin 40 mg SC) and compression stockings for high-risk patients.

TABLE 1: Preoperative checklist.

Step	*Details*	*Abdominal hysterectomy*	*Vaginal hysterectomy*
Medical Evaluation	History, physical examination, comorbidities	Mandatory	Mandatory
Investigations	CBC, coagulation, imaging, endometrial biopsy (if indicated)	Yes	Yes
Antibiotic prophylaxis	Cefazolin 2 g IV or equivalent	Yes	Yes
Bowel preparation	Light diet or enema	Optional	Recommended
Thromboprophylaxis	LMWH, compression stockings for high-risk patients	Yes	Yes
Consent	Discuss risks, benefits, alternatives	Yes	Yes
Anesthesia	General or regional	General preferred	Regional preferred

- **Anesthesia planning:** General or regional (spinal/epidural) anesthesia, based on patient factors and surgical approach
  Table 1 provides preoperative checklist.

SURGICAL STEPS[2]

Abdominal Hysterectomy

Abdominal hysterectomy is indicated for large uteri, malignancy, or when vaginal access is limited. The procedure is typically performed via a Pfannenstiel or midline incision under general anesthesia.

Steps:

- **Positioning and incision:**
  - Place the patient in the supine position with a slight Trendelenburg tilt.
  - Make a Pfannenstiel or midline incision based on uterine size and pathology.
- **Abdominal entry:**
  - Incise subcutaneous tissue, fascia, and peritoneum.
  - Place a self-retaining retractor (e.g., Balfour) for exposure.
- **Uterine mobilization:**
  - Identify and clamp round ligaments bilaterally using Kocher clamps, then ligate with 1-0 absorbable sutures.
  - Divide the broad ligament to access the utero-ovarian ligaments and fallopian tubes.
- **Adnexal management:**
  - If ovaries are preserved, clamp and ligate utero-ovarian ligaments. If oophorectomy is planned, ligate the infundibulopelvic ligaments.
- **Bladder dissection:** Reflect the bladder inferiorly using sharp and blunt dissection to expose the cervicovaginal junction.
- **Uterine artery ligation:** Skeletonize and clamp uterine arteries at the level of the internal cervical os, then ligate with 1-0 absorbable sutures.

- **Uterus removal:**
    - Clamp and divide cardinal and uterosacral ligaments.
    - Amputate the uterus at the cervicovaginal junction and remove it.
- **Vaginal cuff closure:** Close the vaginal cuff with continuous or interrupted 1-0 absorbable sutures.
- **Hemostasis and closure:** Ensure hemostasis, irrigate the pelvis, and close the peritoneum, fascia, and skin.

Vaginal Hysterectomy

Vaginal hysterectomy is preferred for benign conditions with adequate vaginal access and uterine mobility. It is performed under regional anesthesia with the patient in the lithotomy position.[3]

Steps:

- **Positioning and vaginal preparation:**
    - Place the patient in lithotomy position with adequate exposure.
    - Prep the vagina with povidone-iodine and drape sterilely.
- **Cervical exposure:**
    - Place a weighted speculum and retractors to expose the cervix.
    - Inject a vasoconstrictor (e.g., dilute epinephrine) into the cervicovaginal junction to reduce bleeding.
- **Cervical incision:**
    - Make a circumferential incision around the cervix using a scalpel.
    - Dissect the vaginal mucosa to expose the vesicouterine fold.
- **Bladder dissection:** Advance the bladder superiorly using blunt dissection to expose the anterior peritoneum.
- **Peritoneal entry:** Enter the anterior and posterior peritoneal cavities by incising the vesicouterine and rectouterine folds.
- **Ligament division:** Clamp, divide, and ligate the uterosacral and cardinal ligaments using 1-0 absorbable sutures.
- **Uterine artery ligation:** Clamp and ligate uterine arteries bilaterally.
- **Uterus removal:** Deliver the uterus through the vaginal canal, morcellating if necessary for large uteri.
- **Vaginal cuff closure:** Close the vaginal cuff with continuous 1-0 absorbable sutures.
- **Hemostasis:** Ensure hemostasis and irrigate the vaginal canal.

  Table 2 provides comparison of surgical steps.

POSTOPERATIVE COMPLICATIONS[4]

Both procedures carry risks, which must be monitored and managed promptly.

- **Hemorrhage:**
    - Intraoperative bleeding from uterine arteries or vaginal cuff
    - Postoperative bleeding requiring transfusion or reexploration

TABLE 2: Comparison of surgical steps.

Step	*Abdominal hysterectomy*	*Vaginal hysterectomy*
Incision	Pfannenstiel or midline	Circumferential cervical incision
Anesthesia	General preferred	Regional preferred
Ligament division	Round, utero-ovarian, cardinal, uterosacral	Uterosacral, cardinal
Uterine artery ligation	At internal cervical os	Via vaginal approach
Uterus removal	Through abdominal incision	Through vaginal canal
Cuff closure	Sutured abdominally	Sutured vaginally

- **Infection:**
  - Surgical site infection (abdominal incision or vaginal cuff)
  - Pelvic abscess or peritonitis
- **Urinary tract injury:** Bladder or ureteral injury, leading to fistula or obstruction
- **Bowel complications:**
  - Ileus or bowel obstruction (more common in abdominal hysterectomy)
  - Bowel perforation (rare)
- **Thromboembolic events:** Deep vein thrombosis or pulmonary embolism, especially in high-risk patients
- **Vaginal cuff dehiscence:** Partial or complete separation of the vaginal cuff, often after vaginal hysterectomy
- **Chronic pain:** Pelvic or incisional pain, potentially due to nerve injury or adhesions
- **Sexual dysfunction:** Altered sensation or dyspareunia, particularly if ovaries are removed
- **Anesthetic complications:**Adverse reactions to general or regional anesthesia

REFERENCES

1. Clarke-Pearson DL, Geller EJ. Complications of hysterectomy. Obstet Gynecol. 2013;121(3):654-73.
2. Aarts JW, Nieboer TE, Johnson N, et al. Surgical approach to hysterectomy for benign gynaecological disease. Cochrane Database Syst Rev. 2025;2015(8):CD003677.
3. ACOG. Committee Opinion No 701: Choosing the route of hysterectomy for benign disease. Obstet Gynecol. 2017;129(6), e155-e159.
4. Handa VL, Van Le L. Te Linde's Operative Gynecology, 12th edition. Philadelphia: Wolters Kluwer; 2020.

Screening Tests for Cervical Cancer

Ruchika Garg

1. Discuss the different guidelines suggested for cervical cancer screening. Discuss the role of triage with pap/HPV test and colposcopy.

Short Answer Questions:

1. **Guidelines for screening of cervical cancer**
2. **Primary high-risk HPV (hrHPV) testing**
3. **Role of VIA in screening for cervical cancer in low resource settings**
4. **Pap smear—a screening modality for cervical cancer**
5. **Understanding colposcopy**
6. **Cervical intraepithelial lesions**

INTRODUCTION

Cervical cancer is amenable to screening because it has a long precancerous phase, allowing early detection of abnormal cells through tests like Pap smears or HPV testing. These methods are effective, accessible, and enable timely intervention, preventing progression to invasive cancer. Regular screening reduces incidence and mortality by identifying and treating precancerous lesions before they become malignant.

Cervical cancer screening aims at identifying those individuals from the general population who are currently asymptomatic but have signs of precancer or cancer of the cervix.

Benefits of screening:

- A negative report is reassuring.
- Aids in early diagnosis and treatment
- Reduced morbidity and mortality
- Better prognosis with lesser radical treatment and higher chances of survival
- Cost-effective

WORLD HEALTH ORGANIZATION CERVICAL CANCER ELIMINATION STRATEGY TARGETS FOR 2030

World Health Organization has outlined a new approach for reducing incidence of cancer cervix to 4/100,000 women by year 2030. The 90–70–90 approach is outlined as follows:

- 90% of girls fully vaccinated with HPV vaccine by the age of 15
- 70% of women are screened with a high-performance test by 35 years of age and again by 45 years of age

- 90% of women identified with cervical disease receive treatment

Cervical intraepithelial neoplasia (CIN) represents precancerous changes in the cervical epithelium, detectable through screening methods like Pap smears and HPV testing.

Cervical intraepithelial neoplasia is a precancerous condition where abnormal cells replace normal cervical epithelium but do not invade the basement membrane.

WHAT IS CERVICAL INTRAEPITHELIAL NEOPLASIA (TABLE 1)?

- **Definition:**
  - Abnormal changes in the cervical squamous epithelium, confined to the transformation zone (TZ)
  - Precursor to cervical cancer, but the basement membrane remains intact (no invasion).
- **Terminology:**
  - **Older terms:** Cervical dysplasia, squamous intraepithelial lesions (SIL)
  - **Current Bethesda system (updated 2014, reaffirmed 2020):**
    - **LSIL:** Low-grade squamous intraepithelial lesions (equivalent to CIN-I)
    - **HSIL:** High-grade squamous intraepithelial lesions (CIN-II and CIN-III)
  - **ASCUS:** Atypical squamous cells of undetermined significance, often benign but requires follow-up.
- **Cause:**
  - Primarily hrHPV (types 16, 18), responsible for >90% of CIN cases
  - **Other factors:** Immunosuppression (e.g., HIV), smoking, early sexual activity

GRADING OF CERVICAL INTRAEPITHELIAL NEOPLASIA (TABLE 2)

- **CIN-I (mild dysplasia, LSIL):**
  - Affects *lower one-third of epithelium*
  - Cells show mild nuclear enlargement, irregular outlines.
  - Often linked to HPV or infections (e.g., *Trichomonas*); 60–80% regress spontaneously.

TABLE 1: CIN versus SIL terminology.

CIN grade	*Bethesda term*	*Description*
CIN-I	LSIL	Mild dysplasia, lower third of epithelium
CIN-II	HSIL	Moderate dysplasia, 50–75% of epithelium
CIN-III	HSIL	Severe dysplasia or carcinoma in situ, full thickness

TABLE 2: CIN progression and regression rates.

CIN grade	*Regression (%)*	*Persistence (%)*	*Progression to cancer (%)*	*Source*
CIN-I	60–80	15–30	~1 (long-term)	[1]
CIN-II	30–40	30–40	20–30 (5–10 years)	[2]
CIN-III	10–20	20–30	30–50 (5–10 years)	[3]

- Progression to cancer: ~1% over many years
- **CIN-II (moderate dysplasia, HSIL):**
  - *Affects 50–75% of epithelial thickness*
  - Moderate nuclear enlargement, hyperchromasia, multinucleation
  - Outcomes: 30% regress, 40% persist, 30% progress to CIN-III or cancer
- **CIN-III (severe dysplasia/carcinoma in situ, HSIL):**
  - *Full-thickness epithelial replacement by abnormal cells*
  - *No invasion of basement membrane; high nuclear–cytoplasmic ratio, mitosis common*
  - *High risk of progression to invasive cancer (10–30% over 5–10 years)*
- *Koilocytes:*
  - *HPV-infected cells with perinuclear halo,* **common in LSIL**
  - **Disappear as dysplasia progresses to HSIL**

WHY IS CERVICAL INTRAEPITHELIAL NEOPLASIA AMENABLE TO SCREENING?

- **Long precancerous phase:**
  - CIN progresses slowly (5–10 years for HSIL to cancer), allowing early detection
  - Immunosuppressed patients (e.g., HIV) progress faster, requiring frequent screening
- **Effective screening tools:**
  - **Pap smear:** Detects abnormal cells via cytology
  - **HPV testing:** Identifies hrHPV strains, more sensitive for HSIL
  - **Co-testing:** Combines Pap and HPV testing for higher accuracy (ACOG 2020)
- **Asymptomatic nature:**
  - Most CIN cases are asymptomatic, making population-based screening critical.
  - Symptoms (e.g., postcoital bleeding, discharge) are rare and nonspecific.

DIAGNOSIS (TABLE 3)

- **Screening methods:**[8]
  - **Pap smear:** Collects cervical cells for cytological analysis
  - **HPV testing:** Detects hrHPV DNA; primary screening option since 2020
  - **Colposcopy:** Magnifies cervix to identify abnormal areas; indicated for ASCUS, LSIL, or HSIL
  - **Biopsy:** Confirms CIN grade histologically
- **Clinical presentation:**

TABLE 3: Diagnostic tools for CIN.

Method	*Purpose*	*Sensitivity (%)*	*Specificity (%)*	*Source*
Pap smear	Detect abnormal cells	70–80	90–95	[4]
HPV testing	Detect high-risk HPV	90–95	80–85	[4]
Colposcopy	Visualize abnormal areas	85–90	70–80	[5]
Biopsy	Confirm CIN grade	95–98	98–100	[5]

TABLE 4: Cervical cancer screening guidelines (ACOG 2020).[11,12]

Age-group	*Screening method*	*Frequency*	*Source*
21–29	Pap smear	Every 3 years	[6]
30–65	Pap + HPV or HPV alone	Every 5 years	[6]
>65	Stop if negative history	N/A	[6]

- Often asymptomatic; cervix may appear normal or show cervicitis/erosion.
- **Rare symptoms:** These include postcoital bleeding, discharge, or postmenopausal bleeding.

- **Incidence in India:**
  - **ICMR (2022):** Cervical dysplasia incidence ~15 per 1,000 screened women; severe dysplasia ~5 per 1,000

Screening Guidelines

- **ACOG guidelines (2020) (Table 4):**
  - *Start screening at age 21,* **regardless of sexual activity.**
  - **Ages 21–29:** *Pap smear every 3 years*
  - **Ages 30–65:** *Co-testing (Pap + HPV) every 5 years or HPV testing alone every 5 years*
  - *Stop screening at age 65 if negative history;* **continue if prior CIN-II/III.**
- **WHO guidelines (2021):**
  - HPV testing as primary screening in low-resource settings (e.g., India)
  - Screen women aged 30–49 every 5–10 years; prioritize high-risk groups
- **Updates:**
  - Shift to primary HPV testing due to higher sensitivity for HSIL
  - Reduced screening frequency for low-risk women to minimize overtreatment

MANAGEMENT OF CERVICAL INTRAEPITHELIAL NEOPLASIA (TABLE 5)

- **CIN-I (LSIL):**
  - Observation with repeat Pap/HPV testing in 12 months (60–80% regress)
  - Treat underlying infections (e.g., HPV, *Trichomonas*).
- **CIN-II/III (HSIL):**
  - Colposcopy with biopsy to confirm grade
  - **Excision:** Loop electrosurgical excision procedure (LEEP) or cone biopsy
  - Ablation (e.g., cryotherapy) for confirmed CIN-II in select cases

TABLE 5: Management of CIN.

CIN grade	*Management*	*Follow-up*	*Source*
CIN-I	Observation, treat infections	Pap/HPV at 12 months	[6]
CIN-II/III	*Colposcopy, LEEP, or ablation*	*HPV testing at 6–12 months*	[6]

- **Follow-up:**
    - **Post-treatment:** HPV testing or co-testing at 6–12 months
    - **Long-term:** Annual screening for 20 years after HSIL treatment (ACOG 2020)
- **Special populations:**
    - **Immunosuppressed (e.g., HIV):** More frequent screening; faster progression risk.
    - **Pregnant women:** Delay treatment until postpartum unless invasive cancer suspected.
- **HPV-driven pathogenesis (2022):** Confirmed HPV 16/18 drives >90% of CIN-II/III cases, supporting primary HPV testing
- **Self-collected HPV testing (2023):** Comparable sensitivity to clinician-collected samples, improving access in low-resource settings
- **Therapeutic HPV vaccines (2024):** Early trials show promise in clearing LSIL and preventing recurrence.
- **AI in cytology (2025):** AI-assisted Pap smear analysis improves detection of HSIL by 15%.

Risks of screening:

- Abnormal report results in increased anxiety and distress.
- Unnecessary additional testing—triage testing, colposcopy, and invasive procedures like biopsy/LEEP/conization
- Unnecessary invasive treatments leading to pain, vaginal bleeding, and infection
- More frequent follow-ups

***Types of screening modalities*:**

- Cytology—Pap smear
- HPV testing—Primary and co-testing
- Visual inspection with acetic acid (VIA) or Lugol's iodine (VILI) in low-resource settings
- Colposcopy and biopsy—as a triage/follow-up test in patients with abnormal Pap/HPV test
- Use of biomarkers to improve the specificity of hrHPV test

Guidelines for screening for cervical cancer are given in **Table 6**.

More frequent screening for cervical cancer is recommended for:

- Immunocompromised women—HIV positive, etc.
- Women who were exposed to diethylstilbestrol (DES) in uterus
- Women with past history of high-grade lesions/cervical cancer
- Women with a recent abnormal screen test/biopsy report

Cytology—*Pap smear/Pap test/Papanicolaou test*

This is a procedure used to detect abnormal (both precancerous and cancerous) changes in the exfoliated cervical cells under a microscope by gentle scraping of the endo- and ectocervix with an Ayre's spatula or endo-brush/cyto-brush.

Pap smear may be of the *conventional type* where in the scraped cells are spread on a glass slide, fixed with alcohol and read manually or the *liquid-based cytology* (LBC) wherein the brush used to collect the cervical cells is transferred into a bottle/vial with liquid preservative and sent to the laboratory for automated evaluation.

Liquid-based cytology reduces inadequate samples, interpersonal errors, and has a shorter reporting time and can be used either for screening cancer either *individually or as a co-test*

TABLE 6: Guidelines for screening for cervical cancer.[1-5]

Age (years)	*FOGSI GCPR*	*2020 ACS*	*2018 USPSTF*
21–24	No screening	No screening	Pap smear once in 3 years
25–29	• Only in good resource settings • Pap smear once in 3 years	• hrHPV testing every 5 years (preferred) • Co-test with pap smear + hrHPV every 5 years (accepted) • Pap smear once in 3 years (accepted)	Pap smear once in 3 years
30–65	• hrHPV testing every 5–10 years in good resource settings (preferred) • In low-resource settings at least twice in a lifetime at 35 and 45 years • Pap smear once in 3 years (accepted) • VIA every 3–5 years (accepted)	• hrHPV testing every 5 years (preferred) • Co-test with pap smear + hrHPV every 5 years (accepted) • Pap smear once in 3 years (accepted)	• Any 1 of the following • FDA-approved hrHPV testing every 5 years • Co-test with pap smear + hrHPV every 5 years • Pap smear once in 3 years
≥65	No screening if 3 consecutive pap smears are negative or 2 consecutive hrHPV tests are negative within last 10 years with the most recent test within 5 years (adequate negative prior screening tests)	No screening if last few consecutive tests were normal	No screening if 3 consecutive pap smears are negative or 2 consecutive hrHPV tests or 2 consecutive co-tests are negative within last 10 years with the most recent test within the recommended screening interval for that test
Screening in women undergone total hysterectomy	Not recommended routinely unless indication for hysterectomy was precancer or cancer of the cervix	–	Not recommended in women with no prior history of precancer or cancer of the cervix
Screening in HIV/ immunocompromised women	• Primary screening test—hrHPV (preferred) • Age—25 years • Interval—every 3 years	–	–

with HPV; however, it is more expensive than the conventional smear and requires a more elaborate setup.

A Pap smear may also help find other conditions, such as *infections* like HSV, chlamydia, gonorrhea, yeast, etc. or *inflammation.*

Ideal time for testing is *2 weeks from 1st day of the LMP or 6–8 weeks postdelivery.*

Precautions: Avoid vaginal contraception/medication, tampons, or vaginal douche 48 hours prior to testing. Abstinence from sexual intercourse for 24 hours prior is recommended.

Avoid the use of lubrication at the time of insertion of speculum. Excess mucus or other discharge should be removed gently. The sample should be collected before the application of acetic acid and Lugol's iodine.

Procedure: The patient is placed in modified lithotomy position. Per speculum examination is done using an adequate size speculum to separate the vaginal walls and visualize the cervix. Introduce the spatula/brush and rotate it in clockwise direction for five times. The exfoliated superficial *cells are then collected from the endo- and ectocervix* and sent to the laboratory either on glass slides/liquid filled vial for further evaluation.

Papanicolaou Smear Test

The Bethesda System for Cervical Cytology (2001/2014): It is used for reporting cervical cytology. It includes:

- **Specimen type**: Conventional smear or LBC
- **Specimen adequacy**: Satisfactory or unsatisfactory, with details
- **General categorization**: Negative for intraepithelial lesion or malignancy (NILM)
- **Other findings**: Epithelial cell abnormalities (squamous/glandular) or other malignant lesions
- **Interpretation/result**: Detailed diagnostic outcome

Advantages of Pap smear*: Simple, cost-effective, specific, and widely used in India,* especially in rural areas due to easy setup.

Disadvantages: These are subjective, dependent on sample collection and reporter expertise; *lower sensitivity* than HPV testing, potentially missing cancerous changes.

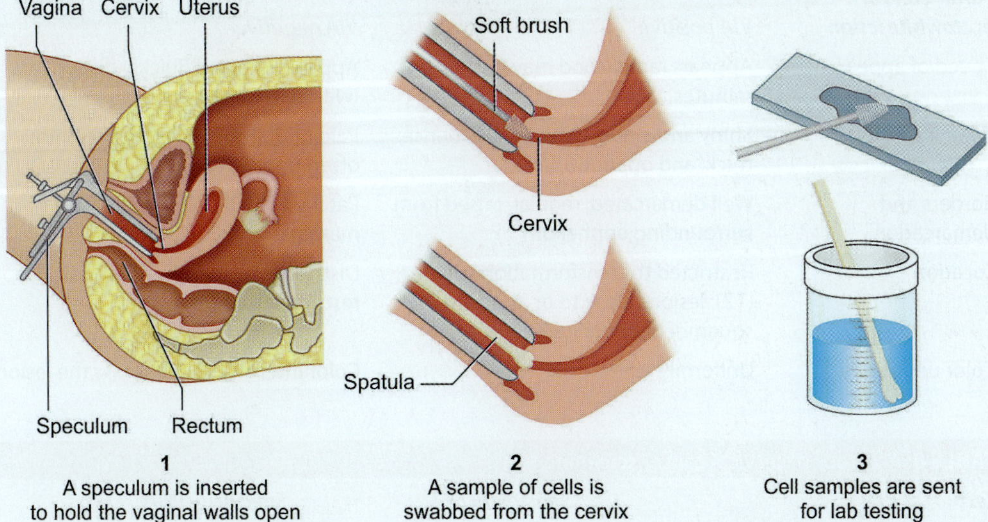

Primary hrHPV DNA testing: It detects hrHPV infection in cervical cells. Over 150 HPV types exist, with 14 high-risk subtypes linked to cancers. *Low-risk HPV (6, 11)* cause 90% of genital warts; *hrHPV (16, 18) cause ~84% of cervical cancers in India,* with types 31, 33, 35, 39, 45, 51, 52, 56, 58, 59, 66, 68 causing the rest.

Procedure: It is same as LBC (ideal timing, precautions).

Report: Negative or positive (with/without genotyping); a positive result indicates HPV infection, which may lead to precancer/cancer if persistent, but does not confirm cancer.

Advantage: Advantage is *high sensitivity and negative predictive value* (96–99.9%), ensuring low risk of cervical lesions for 5 years if negative.[7]

Disadvantage: Disadvantage is *lower specificity* than cytology, leading to false positives and unnecessary follow-up tests/treatments.

- WHO's recommendation for HPV self-sampling as an effective screening method

***Visual inspection with acetic acid*:** It involves applying 5% acetic acid to the cervix, visualizing for acetowhite changes after 1 minute. Results are VIA as normal, "suspicious for cancer", or "precancerous lesions".

See and treat approach: *VIA is a reliable, sensitive, and cost-effective alternative to cytology* in low-resource settings. "See and biopsy" in one sitting is possible with VIA and VILI. Abnormal areas may be cauterized (or cryotherapy) in the same sitting. Although it may prove "overtreatment", as a considerable number of women may have benign lesions, this is feasible and convenient in rural and peripheral setups where follow-up visits by patients are low.

Table 7 provides FOGSI guidelines for interpretation of VIA.

Accuracy of cervical cancer screening tests is given in **Table 8**.

TABLE 7: FOGSI guidelines for interpretation of VIA.[5]

Parameters of acetowhite lesion	*VIA positive*	*VIA negative*
Speed of appearance	Appears rapidly and may last for 1–2 minutes	Appears late and quickly disappears (within a minute)
Color intensity	Shiny and cloudy white; more dense, thick, and opaque	Pale or dull white; less dense, thin, often translucent
Borders and demarcation	Well demarcated, regular, raised from surrounding epithelium	Patchy with ill-defined, diffuse margins
Location	Restricted to transformation zone (TZ); lesions close to or abutting the squamocolumnar junction	Distributed widely in the cervix; not restricted to the TZ
Color uniformity	Uniformly white	Color intensity varies across the lesion

TABLE 8: Accuracy of cervical cancer screening tests.[5]

Test	*Sensitivity (%)*	*Specificity (%)*
Cytology	62.5–72.9%	90.3–96.6%
Visual inspection with acetic acid	74.2–79.4%	85.2–85.8%
HPV DNA testing	94%	88%

COLPOSCOPY

Colposcopy is the visualization of the cervix, especially the TZ under magnification. The TZ is where the precancerous lesions and invasive cancer of the cervix occurs **(Table 9)**.

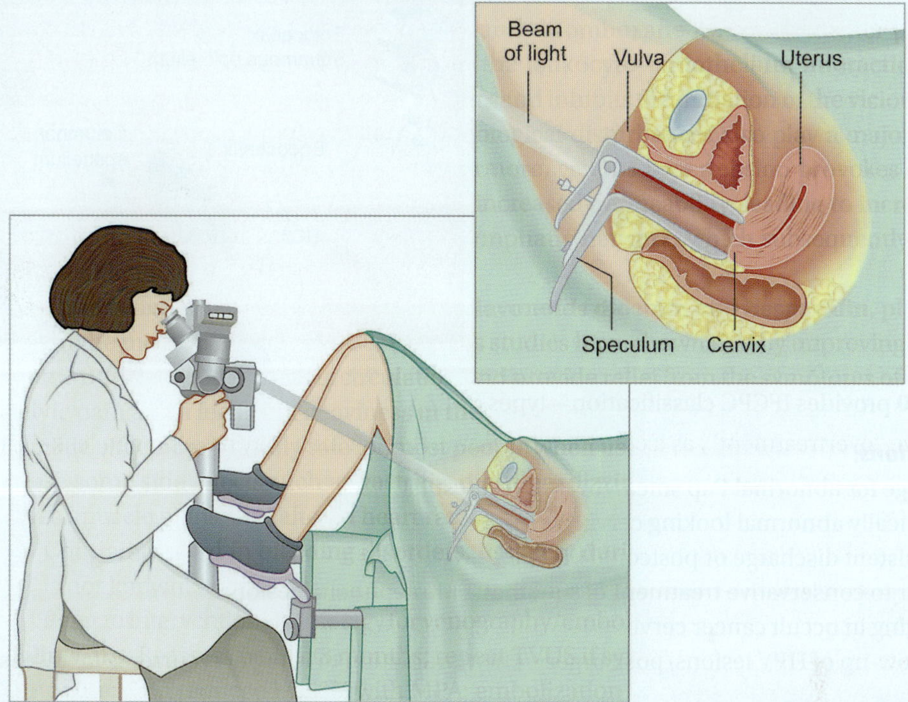

Normal squamous epithelium is multilayered consisting of superficial, intermediate, parabasal, and basal cells and appears pink and smooth on colposcopy. On the other hand, columnar epithelium consists of a single layer of cuboidal epithelium and is thrown into crypts giving it a villous appearance and appears red on colposcopy.

The TZ is the region between the old squamocolumnar junction (SCJ) identified by the last gland opening and the new SCJ, which is the line of demarcation between the metaplastic squamous epithelium and the native, untransformed columnar epithelium.

TABLE 9: Colposcopy examination.

Binocular vision	***With inbuilt light***
Magnification	• 10×—Diagnosis • 15×—Vasculature • 20×—Target biopsy/treatment
Green filter	• Absorbs red light • Suitable for vasculature
Documentation	• Hammond's charts • Photo printouts

A colposcopy examination is considered to be adequate only if the entire TZ is visualized without being obscured by inflammation, atrophy, bleeding, scarring, or other problems.

Squamocolumnar Junction and Transformation Zone[9]

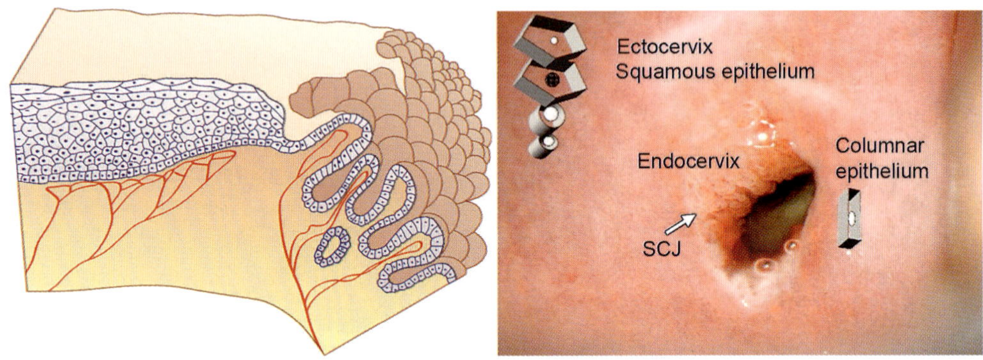

Table 10 provides IFCPC classification—types of TZ.

Indications:

- Triage for abnormal Pap smear/hrHPV test results
- Clinically abnormal looking cervix
- Persistent discharge or postcoital bleeding
- Prior to conservative treatment of squamous intraepithelial lesions
- Staging in occult cancer cervix
- Follow-up of HPV lesions/postsurgery/chemoradiation to rule out recurrence of disease

Procedure:

- Reassure the patient, discuss the procedure prior, and take a verbal/written consent.
- Place the patient in modified lithotomy position and introduce a suitable size speculum so as to retract the vaginal walls adequately.
- Visualize the entire cervix—collect Pap Smear, hrHPV test, and wet vaginal smear if indicated.

TABLE 10: IFCPC classification—Types of TZ.

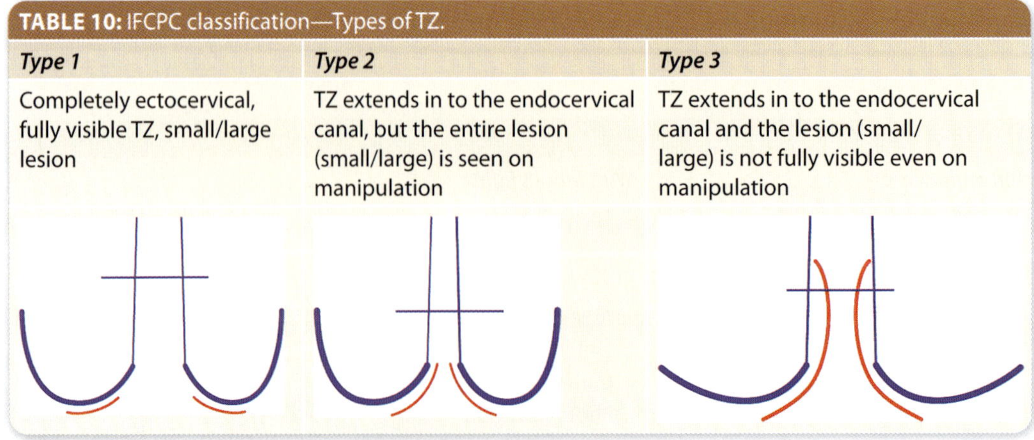

Type 1	*Type 2*	*Type 3*
Completely ectocervical, fully visible TZ, small/large lesion	TZ extends in to the endocervical canal, but the entire lesion (small/large) is seen on manipulation	TZ extends in to the endocervical canal and the lesion (small/large) is not fully visible even on manipulation

TABLE 11: Swede score.[10]

Swede score	*0*	*1*	*2*
Aceto uptake	Zero or transparent	Shady, milky (not transparent, not opaque)	Distinct, opaque white
Margins/surface	Diffuse	Sharp but irregular, jagged, "geographical" satellites	Sharp and even; difference in surface level including "cuffing"
Vessels	Fine, regular	Absent	Coarse or atypical
Lesion size	<5 mm	5–15 mm or 2 quadrants	>15 mm or 3–4 quadrants or endocervically undefined
Iodine staining	Brown	Faintly or patchy yellow	Distinct yellow

- Clean the cervix with normal saline, visualize it, and note the findings.
- Apply green filter to look for any vascular abnormalities and make note.
- Apply 3% or 5% freshly prepared glacial acetic acid, wait for 1 minute and look for acetowhite lesions and note the findings.
- Apply Lugol's iodine (Schiller's test) and note the changes.
- Ensure adequate documentation—name/date/name of observer, etc.
- Use Swede score and the IFCPC-2011 Nomenclature for reporting.

Table 11 provides Swede score.

Acetowhite epithelium is the most important colposcopic finding. Unfortunately, acetowhite change is not specific and can be because of:

- Immature metaplasia (transient)
- HPV-related changes
- CIN/SIL
- Invasive cancer

Vascular Abnormalities

The cervix consists of a network of fine reticular/hair-pin-like capillaries which normally appear like the branching of a tree. These vessels may appear more prominent when visualized over a Nabothian cyst, ectropion, or inflammation of the cervix.

Mosaicism, punctation, and atypical vessels are the vascular abnormalities commonly seen with dysplastic epithelium.

Punctation

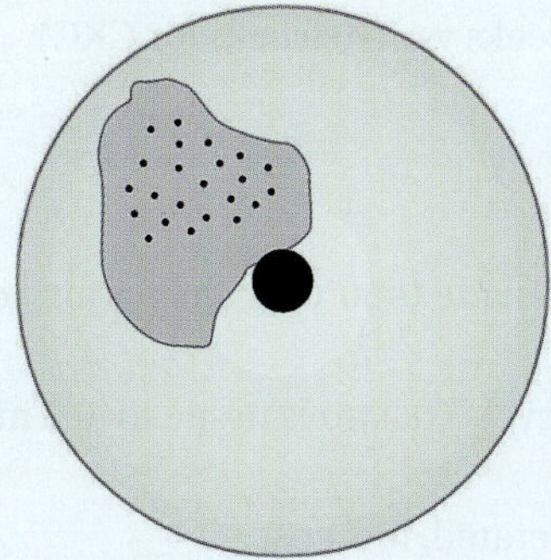

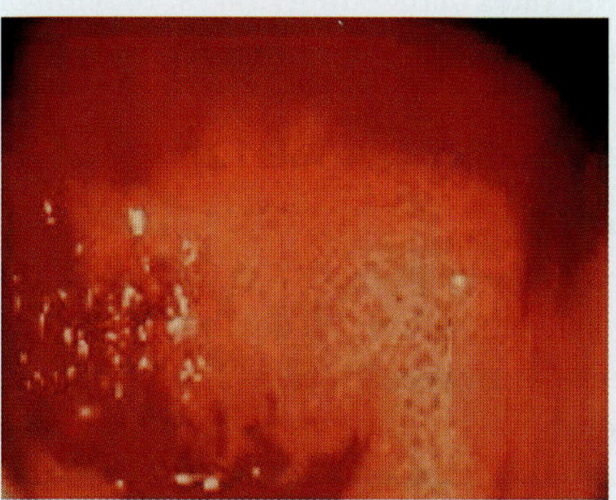

Mosaicism

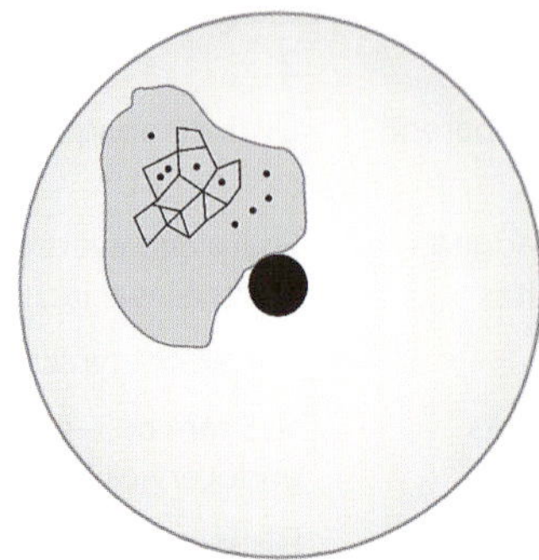

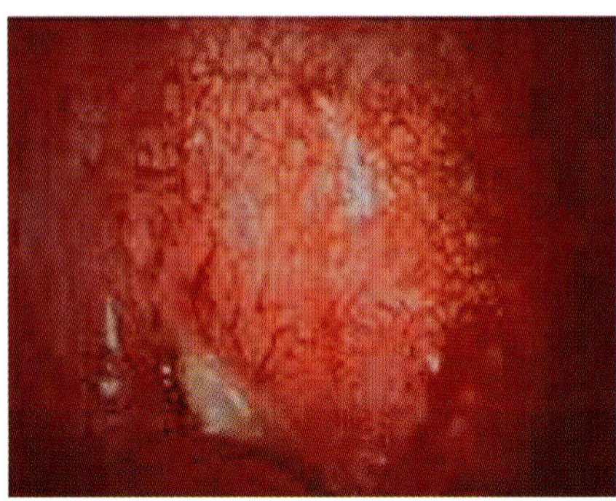

Schiller's test: Lugol's iodine (aqueous solution) is applied to the cervix.

Principle: Normal estrogen active epithelium turns mahogany brown due to its glycogen content. Nonglycogen epithelium remains unstained. Canary yellow appearance is suggestive of either rapidly proliferating lesions (HPV-SIL) or atrophy.

This test is easy to diagnose but is not very specific.

Reporting is done using the 2011 IFCPC Nomenclature.

CONE BIOPSY

- **Definition**:
  - Removal of a cone-shaped cervical tissue sample, including the transformation zone and endocervical canal, for histological analysis and/or treatment
  - Both diagnostic (confirms CIN grade or microinvasion) and therapeutic (removes precancerous lesions)
- **Techniques**:
  - **Cold-knife conization (CKC)**: Performed under general anesthesia using a scalpel; precise but higher risk of bleeding and scarring
  - **Large loop excision of the transformation zone (LLETZ):** It uses a wire loop with electrical current; it is an outpatient procedure, with less bleeding and faster healing.
- **Why LLETZ is preferred?**
  - Performed under local anesthesia, reducing risks
  - Lower rates of bleeding (5% vs. 10% for CKC) and infection (1% vs. 3%)
  - Minimal scarring and faster recovery (2–4 weeks vs. 4–6 weeks for CKC)

CRYOSURGERY (TABLE 12)

- **Mechanism**:
  - Freezes tissue using CO_2 (–60°C) or nitrous oxide (–80°C), causing intracellular water crystallization and cell death
  - Freeze-thaw-freeze cycle (3–5 minutes per cycle) destroys tissue to 4–5 mm depth.
- **Procedure**:
  - Outpatient, no anesthesia required; well-tolerated, low cost

TABLE 12: Cryosurgery overview.

Feature	*Details*	*Source*
Agents	CO_2 (–60°C), nitrous oxide (–80°C)	[1]
Depth	4–5 mm	[1]
Cure Rate	85–90% (CIN-I/II)	[2]
Complications	Discharge, SCJ retraction (5–10%)	[2]
Follow-up	HPV/co-testing at 6–12 months	[3]

- Acetic acid or Lugol's iodine guides lesion visualization; colposcopy preferred
- Small lesions treated in one 3-minute cycle; larger lesions treated segmentally

- **Indications**: *Small CIN-I/II lesions, fully visible on colposcopy, no endocervical involvement*
- **Advantages**:
  - Minimal pain, low cost, no scarring, high patient tolerance
  - Cure rate: 85–90% for CIN-I/II (2023 data)
- **Disadvantages/complications**:
  - Profuse watery discharge for 7–14 days
  - SCJ retraction (5–10% risk), complicating future colposcopy
  - Recurrence: 5–10% (Source: J Low Genit Tract Dis. 2022;26(2):147-53).
- **Postprocedure**:
  - Avoid intercourse for 4–6 weeks.
  - Follow-up with HPV testing or co-testing at 6–12 months
- **Updates (2020–2025)**:
  - *WHO 2021 recommends cryosurgery for CIN-I/II in low-resource settings due to affordability and efficacy.*
  - *Nitrous oxide preferred for deeper penetration*; CO_2 viable in resource-limited areas

ELECTROCOAGULATION (TABLE 13)

- **Mechanism**: Uses high temperatures *(>70°C)* to destroy tissue to 8–10 mm depth
- **Procedure**:
  - Performed under local or general anesthesia due to pain
  - Outpatient or inpatient, depending on lesion size and patient tolerance
- **Indications**: CIN-I/II; less common due to pain and higher complication rates

TABLE 13: Electrocoagulation overview.

Feature	*Details*
Depth	8–10 mm
Cure Rate	80–85% (CIN-I/II)
Complications	Bleeding (5–10%), Stenosis (5–8%)
Anesthesia	Local/General

TABLE 14: Laser ablation overview.

Feature	*Details*
Depth	5 mm
Cure rate	85–90% (CIN-I/II)
Complications	Recurrence (2–8%), burn risk
Cost	High (expensive equipment)

- **Advantages**:
  - Effective for deeper lesions compared to cryosurgery
  - Cure rate: 80–85% for CIN-I/II
- **Disadvantages/complications**:
  - Painful, requiring anesthesia
  - Bleeding (5–10%), infection (2–5%), cervical stenosis (5–8%), SCJ retraction
  - Recurrence: 8–12% (Source: Int J Gynaecol Obstet. 2021;152(3):412-8).
- **Updates**:
  - ASCCP 2020 favors LLETZ over electrocoagulation for HSIL due to lower morbidity.

LASER ABLATION (TABLE 14)

- **Mechanism**:Uses laser energy to vaporize cells (boiling/steaming), destroying tissue to 5 mm depth
- **Procedure**:
  - Outpatient, under local anesthesia, guided by colposcopy
  - Precise targeting, minimal bleeding
- **Indications**:
  - CIN-I/II; useful for lesions extending to vaginal vault
  - Not recommended for HSIL (CIN-II/III) per ASCCP 2020
- **Advantages**:
  - Minimal bleeding, no infection, no scarring, no SCJ retraction
  - Repeat ablation possible for residual lesions
  - Cure rate: 85–90% for CIN-I/II
- **Disadvantages/complications**:
  - Expensive equipment; risk of burns to health personnel (eyes, skin)
  - Recurrence: 2–8% (Source: Gynecol Oncol. 2023;170:145-51).
- **Updates**:
  - ASCCP 2020 discourages laser ablation for HSIL due to cost and safety concerns.
  - Thermal ablation preferred in low-resource settings (WHO 2021)

CONCLUSION

Cervical intraepithelial neoplasia is a preventable precursor to cervical cancer, detectable through effective screening like Pap smears and HPV testing. Understanding its grading (CIN-I–III), progression risks, and management is crucial for medical students. Recent ACOG and WHO guidelines emphasize HPV testing and tailored management, with CIN-I often observed and CIN-II/III treated via excision. Advances like AI and self-collected HPV testing promise improved access and accuracy.

Advanced Learning

Types of HPV tests:

- **DNA detection**: Uses PCR or signal amplification (e.g., Hybrid Capture II, detecting 13 hrHPV types via RNA probes; FDA-approved, widely used); positive if chemiluminescence detected; nonquantitative, no genotyping
- **Care HPV test**: Detects 14 hrHPV types, automated, rapid (2.5 hours for 90 samples), FDA-approved, available in India/China
- **mRNA tests**: Detect E6/E7 oncoprotein expression
  PCR is sensitive but prone to contamination. Validated hrHPV DNA tests are preferred for screening. Indian HPV tests await WHO approval. Self-testing kits, not yet available in India, could reduce cervical cancer incidence. Biomarkers (p16, Ki-67) enhance specificity for triaging low-grade cytology.

KEY POINTS

- *Definition*: CIN involves precancerous changes in the cervical epithelium, graded as CIN-I, CIN-II, or CIN-III based on dysplasia severity.
- *Terminology*: CIN-I corresponds to LSIL; CIN-II and CIN-III are HSIL.
- *Cause*: Primarily driven by persistent hrHPV infection (e.g., HPV 16, 18)
- Progression: CIN-I often regresses (60–80%), while CIN-II/III have higher progression rates to invasive cancer (10–30% over 5–10 years).
- Screening: Pap smear and HPV co-testing are standard; updated ACOG 2020 guidelines recommend screening from age 21.
- Management: Observation for CIN-I; colposcopy and excision (e.g., LEEP) for CIN-II/III
- The Pap smear is only a screening test. Positive test (abnormal cells) requires further investigations such as colposcopy, cervical biopsy, and fractional curettage. The sensitivity is around *(45–65%) around 60% but specificity is high (98%).*

False-negative Pap test results may follow:

- Sampling error (abnormal cells are not present)
- Screening error (cells are present but missed by screener); reliability of the report depends on the slide preparation and the skill of the cytologist. Although a single test yields as many as 10–15% false-negative reading, it is reduced to only 1% with repeat tests.
- A false-positive finding is reported in the presence of infection.

How to take a pap smear?

The Pap smear is a test to screen for cervical cancer and other abnormalities. It collects cells from the cervix for microscopic examination. Follow these steps for accurate results:

1. **When to collect a Pap smear?**
   - Perform the Pap smear before a vaginal examination to avoid removing dysplastic cells, which could cause a false-negative result.

- Avoid lubricants, as they can hide organisms and affect slide quality.
- Vaginal bleeding may make it hard to see the cervix, but do not delay the test if bleeding or discharge is unexplained, as these may indicate cervical or genital tract cancer.
- The best time for a Pap smear is around ovulation, but it can be done at any time in the menstrual cycle.

2. **Patient preparation**
   - Advise the patient to avoid the following for 24–48 hours before the test:
     - Sexual intercourse
     - Douching
     - Vaginal tampons
     - Intravaginal medicines or contraceptive creams
   - Treat cervicitis or vaginitis before testing, if possible, to improve accuracy.
   - Collect clinical information to aid interpretation, including:
     - Last menstrual period (LMP)
     - Pregnancy status
     - Exogenous hormone use
     - Menopausal status
     - Prior abnormal Pap tests
     - Use of intrauterine contraceptive device (IUCD)
3. **Procedure**
   - Place the patient in the dorsal (lithotomy) position.
   - Gently insert a Cusco's self-retaining speculum without lubricant to expose the cervix.
   - Identify the transformation zone at the SCJ.
   - *Scrape the transformation zone using an Ayre's spatula, rotating it 360°.*
   - Spread the scrapings evenly on a glass slide.
   - Immediately *fix the slide in 95% ethyl alcohol for 30 minutes* or use a fixative spray (e.g., Cytospray) to prevent air-drying, which reduces slide quality.
   - For better results, scrape the endocervix with a brush and add to the slide.
   - Air-dry the slide after fixation and stain with Papanicolaou (Pap) or Shorr stain.
   - The slide is satisfactory if endocervical cells are present.

Hormonal cytology (vaginal smear):

- For hormonal evaluation, scrape cells from the upper lateral vaginal walls.
- Normal vaginal smear shows three cell types:
  1. **Basal and parabasal cells**: Small, round, basophilic, with large nuclei
  2. **Intermediate cells**: Squamous, transparent, basophilic, with vesicular nuclei
  3. **Superficial cells**: Acidophilic, with small, pyknotic nuclei
- Other findings may include endometrial cells, histiocytes, blood cells, and bacteria.
- Malignant cells are hyperchromatic, with large, irregular nuclei and a high nucleus-to-cytoplasm ratio, indicating possible cancer.

Notes:

- The Pap smear is critical for early detection of cervical abnormalities.

- Proper technique and patient preparation ensure reliable results.
- The nucleus/cytoplasmic ratio is increased in malignant cells.

Papanicolaou classification:

Grade I	Normal cells
Grade II	Slightly abnormal, suggestive of inflammatory change; repeat smear after treating the infection
Grade III	A more serious type of abnormality, usually indicative of the need for biopsy
Grade IV	Distinctly abnormal, possibly malignant and definitely requiring biopsy
Grade V	Malignant cells seen

A newer classification **(Table 1.4)** describes the cytology smears as follows:

1. Normal cytology
2. Inflammatory smear
3. CIN-I or mild dysplasia
4. CIN-II, III, and carcinoma in situ nuclear abnormalities
5. Malignant cells and tadpole cells with nuclear abnormalities
    - In a postmenopausal woman, if the SCJ is indrawn due to estrogen deficiency, a 10-day course of estrogen cream exposes the SCJ better and yields an accurate result.
    - Postradiation cytology is difficult to sample because of scarring and atrophy of the vagina. The cells are often enlarged and vacuolated with multiple nucleation and nuclear wrinkling. Inflammatory cells may be present.

LBC using a thin preparation is superior to Pap smear. The liquid is used to screen for HPV after the cytology slide is prepared. This co-testing will improve the sensitivity by added 10–12%.

Visual inspection after acetic acid application (VIA): Gross inspection of cervix after application of 3–5% acetic acid for 1 minute helps in detecting acetowhite area which may harbor CIN/neoplasia.

Schiller test (visual inspection after Lugol's iodine application—VILI): This test detects the presence of glycogen in the superficial cells of the vaginal epithelium. The vaginal wall is stained with Lugol's iodine. The vaginal epithelium takes dark brown color in the presence of glycogen. Unstained areas (negative test) are abnormal and require biopsy for histological examination.

- **Cryosurgery**: Freezes tissue using CO_2 or nitrous oxide; ideal for small CIN-I/II lesions; outpatient, low cost, minimal pain
- **Electrocoagulation**: Uses heat to destroy tissue; deeper penetration (8–10 mm) but painful, often requiring anesthesia
- **Laser ablation**: Vaporizes tissue; precise but expensive and less used for HSIL due to safety concerns
- **Indications**: Small, superficial CIN-I/II lesions; confirmed by colposcopy/biopsy
- **Complications**: Profuse discharge (cryosurgery), cervical stenosis, SCJ retraction (all methods)

- **Guidelines**: WHO 2021 prioritizes cryosurgery/thermal ablation in low-resource settings; laser ablation not recommended for HSIL
- **2024**: AI-assisted colposcopy reduces unnecessary ablations by 15% (Source: Gynecol Oncol. 2024;182:102-8).

PART 1: MULTIPLE CHOICE QUESTIONS

Q1. New American Cancer Society (ACS) guidelines for cervical cancer screening include the following:

a. No role of screening before 25 years of age
b. Primary hrHPV testing every 5 years as the recommended screening modality between 25 and 65 years of age
c. Co-testing with Pap smear and hrHPV every 5 years or just pap smear every 3 years as alternate screening modalities
d. All of the above

Ans. d. All of the above

Q2. As per new ACS guidelines, primary hrHPV testing is the preferred screening modality over Pap smear or co-testing because of the following:

a. HPV testing is more sensitive than cytology
b. Longer intervals between testing so fewer number of tests required
c. HPV test has a very high negative predictive value: 97–99.9%
d. All of the above

Ans. d. All of the above

Q3. Indications for colposcopy include the following:

a. Clinically abnormal looking cervix or in patients with persistent discharge or postcoital bleeding
b. As a triage for abnormal pap smear/ hrHPV test results
c. Prior to conservative Rx of CIN
d. All of the above

Ans. d. All of the above

Q4. More frequent screening (exceptions to routine screening) for cervical cancer is recommended for:

a. Immunocompromised women—HIV positive, etc.
b. Women who were exposed to DES in utero
c. Women with past history of high-grade lesions/cervical cancer
d. Women with a recent abnormal screen test/biopsy report
e. A + B + C
f. A + B + C + D

Ans. f. A + B + C + D

Q5. As per the new ACS guidelines, the recommended age for screening for cervical cancer has increased from 21 to 25 years because of the following reason:

a. Primary prevention with HPV vaccination has resulted in a drop in the incidence of HPV infection and precancerous lesions in the age-group of 21–25 years.
b. Most of the sexually active girls in the age-group of 21–25 years clear the HPV infection as a result of good immune response.
c. Screening of women in this age-group results in unnecessary treatment and side effects.
d. All of the above

Ans. d. All of the above

Q6. The following are risks associated with cervical cancer screening:

a. False-positive results causing unnecessary anxiety to the woman
b. Unnecessary follow-up, further evaluation, and invasive treatments in women with false-positive results
c. False-negative results thereby missing genuine cases that need further evaluation and treatment
d. All of the above

Ans. d. All of the above

Q7. All of the following hold true for VIA except:

a. Acetowhite lesion appears rapidly and may last for 1–2 minutes.
b. Lesions are distributed all over the cervix and not restricted to the transformation zone only.
c. Lesions have regular, well-demarcated borders.
d. Thick dense acetowhite lesions that are opaque in appearance.

Ans. b. Lesions are distributed all over the cervix and not restricted to the transformation zone only.

Q8. World Health Organization (WHO) recommends the following for elimination of cervical cancer except:

a. Screen 70% of the women globally between the ages of 35 and 45 years.
b. Vaccinate 90% of the girls aged 9–14 years with HPV vaccine.
c. Screen 70% of women globally with a high-performance test.
d. Treat 90% of the women with precancerous and cervical cancer lesions.
e. None

Ans. e. None

Q9. High-risk HPV test is now the preferred modality for screening because of all of the following except:

a. It is an objective test so better interpretation of results.
b. It is simple to perform and is cost-effective.
c. It is the most specific screening test.
d. It is more sensitive than cytology.

Ans. c. It is the most specific screening test.

Q10. The following holds true for HIV/immunocompromised women and HPV infection:

a. These women are more likely to have persistent infection and progress rapidly to precancer and cancer.
b. HIV positive women have a sixfold higher risk of developing cervical cancer.
c. Screening for these women should start earlier and should be more frequent than that recommended for the general population.
d. All of the above

Ans. d. All of the above

Q11. Benefits of screening for cervical cancer are:

a. Improved prognosis with lower mortality and morbidity
b. Need for less radical treatment
c. Cost-effective
d. All of the above

Ans. d. All of the above

Q12. The following represents adequate negative prior screening test results to stop screening:

a. Three consecutive negative pap smear reports in the last 10 years
b. Two consecutive negative co-testing reports within last 10 years
c. Two consecutive negative hrHPV test reports in the last 10 years with the most recent test 5 years ago
d. A + C
e. A + B + C

Ans. e. A + B + C

Q13. The following hold true for hrHPV testing except:

a. It is recommended as the primary screening modality for cervical cancer in both average and high-risk individuals.
b. It is used for triage of borderline precancerous lesions.
c. It is used for follow-up of posttreatment cases of CIN and cervical cancer because of its high negative predictive value.
d. It is more specific than cytology for screening of cervical cancer.

Ans. d. It is more specific than cytology for screening of cervical cancer.

Q14. The following holds true for biomarkers in cervical cancer screening:

a. The molecular markers are used as a triage in low-grade cytology abnormalities to increase the specificity of hrHPV test.
b. Dual staining proliferating biomarkers consist of p16 and Ki-67.
c. Both of the above
d. None of the above

Ans. c. Both of the above

Q15. The following statement is true for Pap smear:

a. Aim is to detect abnormal cervical cells by gentle scraping of the cervix.
b. Ideal time to perform a pap smear is 2 weeks from 1st day of the LMP and 6–8 weeks postdelivery.
c. Tampons, vaginal contraception, medication, or douche should be avoided for 48 hours prior to performing a pap smear.
d. All of the above

Ans. d. All of the above

Q16. Acetowhite epithelium is the most important colposcopic finding. Acetowhite changes are seen in all of the following except:

a. Mature metaplasia
b. HPV-related changes
c. Squamous intraepithelial lesion
d. Invasive cancer

Ans. a. Mature metaplasia

Q17. Colposcopy procedure involves the following steps:

a. Visualization of the cervix with normal saline
b. Green filter—to look for abnormal blood vessels
c. Application of 5% acetic acid to look for any acetowhite lesions
d. Schiller's test—application of Lugol's Iodine for poor uptake
e. All of the above

Ans. e. All of the above

PART 2: MULTIPLE CHOICE QUESTIONS

Q1. Which of the following is an advantage of the Pap smear as a cervical cancer screening tool?

a. High sensitivity compared to HPV testing
b. Simple, cheap, and widely used in rural India
c. Objective results independent of expertise
d. Detects all hrHPV genotypes

Ans. b. Simple, cheap, and widely used in rural India

Pap smear is cost-effective and widely used in India, but it has lower sensitivity than HPV testing, is subjective, and does not detect HPV genotypes.

Q2. What is a disadvantage of the Pap smear?

a. High cost and complex setup
b. Lower sensitivity than HPV testing
c. Inability to detect squamous cell abnormalities
d. Requires advanced imaging equipment

Ans. b. Lower sensitivity than HPV testing

Pap smear has lower sensitivity, potentially missing cancerous changes, but is not costly, can detect abnormalities, and does not require imaging.

Q3. Which hrHPV types are responsible for ~84% of cervical cancers in India?

a. HPV 6 and 11
b. HPV 16 and 18
c. HPV 31 and 33
d. HPV 45 and 52

Ans. b. HPV 16 and 18

HPV 16 and 18 cause ~84% of cervical cancers in India, while HPV 6 and 11 cause genital warts, and other types contribute to the remaining 16%.

Q4. What does a positive hrHPV DNA test indicate?

a. Confirmed cervical cancer
b. Presence of hrHPV infection
c. Negative for precancerous changes
d. Need for immediate surgery

Ans. b. Presence of hrHPV infection

A positive hrHPV test indicates HPV infection, which may lead to precancer/cancer if persistent, but does not confirm cancer or necessitate surgery.

Q5. What is an advantage of hrHPV DNA testing?

a. High specificity compared to cytology
b. High sensitivity and negative predictive value (>96%)
c. Low cost and availability in rural areas
d. Identifies specific HPV genotypes in all tests

Ans. b. High sensitivity and negative predictive value (>96%)

hrHPV testing has high sensitivity and negative predictive value, but lower specificity, is not always low-cost, and some tests (e.g., Hybrid Capture II) do not identify genotypes.

Q7. Which HPV test is FDA-approved and detects 13 hrHPV types using RNA probes?

a. Care HPV
b. Hybrid Capture II
c. *PCR* gene amplification
d. E6/E7 mRNA test

Ans. b. Hybrid Capture II

Hybrid Capture II is FDA-approved, detects 13 hrHPV types via RNA probes, and is widely used. Care HPV detects 14 types, while PCR and mRNA tests use different methods.

Q8. What is a limitation of PCR-based HPV testing?

a. Low sensitivity
b. High susceptibility to contamination
c. Inability to detect hrHPV
d. Long processing time

Ans. b. High susceptibility to contamination

PCR is highly sensitive but prone to contamination. It detects hrHPV and is relatively fast compared to other methods.

Q9. In the VIA procedure, what is observed after applying 5% acetic acid?

a. Cervical color change
b. Acetowhite changes
c. Cervical size reduction
d. Fluorescent staining

Ans. b. Acetowhite changes

VIA involves observing acetowhite changes on the cervix 1 minute after applying 5% acetic acid, not color change, size reduction, or fluorescence.

Q10. Which biomarker can improve the specificity of hrHPV testing for triaging low-grade cervical cytology?

a. p53 and Rb
b. p16 and Ki-67
c. E6 and E7
d. CEA and CA-125

Ans. b. p16 and Ki-67

p16 and Ki-67 improve specificity in triaging low-grade cytology. E6/E7 are HPV oncoproteins, while p53, Rb, CEA, and CA-125 are unrelated to this context.

REFERENCES

1. American College of Obstetricians & Gynecologists. (2021). Updated Cervical Cancer Screening Guidelines: Practice Advisory. [online] Available from https://www.acog.org/clinical/clinical-guidance/practice-advisory/articles/2021/04/updated-cervical-cancer-screening-guidelines [Last accessed December, 2025].
2. Perkins RB, Guido RS, Castle PE, et al.; 2019 ASCCP Risk Based Management Consensus Guidelines Committee. 2019 ASCCP risk-based management consensus guidelines for abnormal cervical cancer screening tests and cancer precursors. J Low Genit Tract Dis. 2020;24:102-31.
3. Fontham ET, Wolf AM, Church TR, et al. Cervical cancer screening for individuals at average risk: 2020 guideline update from the American Cancer Society. CA Cancer J Clin. 2020;70:321-46.
4. World Health Organization. (2021). New recommendations for screening and treatment to prevent cervical cancer. [online] Available from https://www.who.int/news/item/06-07-2021-new-recommendations-for-screening-and-treatment-to-prevent-cervical-cancer [Last accessed December. 2025].
5. Federation of Obstetric & Gynaecological Societies of India. (2024). FOGSI-ICOG Good Clinical Practice Recommendations (GCPR) on Prevention and Management of Cervical Cancer – June 2024. [online] Available from https://www.fogsi.org/fogsi-gcpr-on-prevention-and-management-of-cervical-cancer-june-2024/ [Last accessed December, 2025].
6. Pangarkar MA. The Bethesda System for reporting cervical cytology. Cytojournal. 2022;19:28.
7. Clavel C, Cucherousset J, Lorenzato M, et al. Negative human papillomavirus testing in normal smears selects a population at low risk for developing high-grade cervical lesions. Br J Cancer. 2004;90(9):1803-8.
8. Royal College of Obstetricians & Gynaecologist (RCOG). (2016). Progress in Cervical Screening in the UK: Scientific Impact Paper No. 7. [online] Available from https://www.rcog.org.uk/media/k4xds1cw/sip_7-progress-in-cervical-screening.pdf [Last accessed December, 2025].
9. Saraiya UB, Miniello G. Cytology and Colposcopy in Gynecological Practice. New Delhi: Jaypee Brothers Medical Publishers; 2009.
10. Basu P, Sankaranarayanan R. (2017). Atlas of Colposcopy: Principles and Practice. [online] Available from https://publications.iarc.who.int/Databases/Iarc-Cancerbases/Atlas-Of-Colposcopy-Principles-And-Practice-2017 [Last accessed December, 2025].
11. Wentzensen N. (2020). ACS's Updated Cervical Cancer Screening Guidelines Explained. [online] Available from https://www.cancer.gov/news-events/cancer-currents-blog/2020/cervical-cancer-screening-hpv-test-guideline [Last accessed December, 2025].
12. World Trade Center. (2025). Cervical Cancer Screening and the World Trade Center Health Program. [online] Available from https://www.cdc.gov/wtc/pdfs/factsheets/wtc-factsheet-cervical-cancer-en-508.pdf [Last accessed December, 2025].

Preoperative, Postoperative Care in Gynecological Surgeries

Ruchika Garg

PREOPERATIVE CARE

Overview: Preoperative preparation begins once the decision for surgery is made, balancing the patient's needs, diagnosis, comorbidities, and the surgeon's recommendation. The goal is to minimize intra- and postoperative morbidity through meticulous evaluation and optimization.

PREOPERATIVE EVALUATION

Objectives: Objectives are to establish baseline health parameters, assess surgical and anesthetic risk, and correct modifiable factors before surgery.

INITIAL ASSESSMENT

Initial assessment includes detailed history, clinical evaluation, and laboratory investigations.

History:
- Patient demographics: Age, gravida, parity, previous abortions, ectopic pregnancies, cesarean deliveries, prior MTP or sterilization.
- Medical background: Comorbidities such as hypertension, diabetes mellitus, cardiac, pulmonary, renal, or hepatic disorders.
- Additional details: Surgical and family history, medication use, allergies, addictions, and previous ICU admissions or transfusions.

Clinical examination: General, systemic, and gynecological examination (abdominal, speculum, bimanual) with BMI calculation for nutritional assessment.

Investigations:
- Routine tests: CBC, blood group and Rh, RBS/FBS, renal function, electrolytes, TSH, urine routine/culture.
- Selective tests: ECG, chest X-ray, coagulation profile (if indicated), serology (HIV, HBsAg, HCV).
- Special tests: Pelvic ultrasonography, pap smear, endometrial biopsy, tumor markers where relevant.

RISK STRATIFICATION

- *Patient-specific factors:* Low MET (<4), frailty, obesity, comorbidities, and age.
- *Procedure-specific factors:* Surgical approach, complexity of pathology, oncologic nature of disease.

PREOPERATIVE OPTIMIZATION

- Manage cardiovascular risk and initiate β-blockers (7–30 days preoperation if indicated).
- Correct anemia (target Hb ≥10 g/dL), thyroid dysfunction, hyper/hypoglycemia, and infections.
- Treat decubitus ulcers in prolapse cases; topical estrogen may aid healing.

MEDICATION MANAGEMENT

- Continue essential drugs (antihypertensives, antiepileptics, and thyroid medication).
- Stop OCPs, alcohol, and smoking 4 weeks before surgery.
- Discontinue NSAIDs 3 days and aspirin/clopidogrel 5–7 days prior.
- Bridge warfarin with heparin; withhold oral hypoglycemics on surgery day.
- Give stress-dose steroids for chronic steroid users (hydrocortisone 100 mg IV pre-induction, then 50 mg q8h × 24 h → taper to maintenance).

PATIENT EDUCATION AND INFORMED CONSENT

Informed consent—written or audiovisual in presence of a witness—should cover:

- Nature of disease and indication for surgery
- Treatment options and alternatives
- Expected results and possible complications
- Anesthetic plan and associated risks
- Hospital stay and recovery timeline

Perioperative risk reduction: Preanesthetic assessment, DVT prophylaxis (Caprini model), and antimicrobial prophylaxis within 1 hour of incision; repeat dose if surgery >4 hours or blood loss >1.5 L.

Surgical site preparation: Preoperative antiseptic bath (chlorhexidine/alcohol), clipping instead of shaving, and vaginal antisepsis where indicated.

In operation theater: Perform safety checklist, ensure IV access, bladder catheterization, positioning, surgical site antisepsis, draping, and administration of prophylactic antibiotics.

POSTOPERATIVE CARE

Objectives: Objectives are to promote early recovery, wound healing, and prevention of complications.

Immediate Care (First 24 Hours)

- Vital sign monitoring (gradually spaced intervals)
- Maintain urine output >30 mL/h and record intake/output.
- Keep NPO for 4–6 hours, start oral fluids with return of bowel activity.
- Replace fluids (≈2–2.5 L/24 h using crystalloid solutions).

- Employ multimodal antiemetic (ondansetron + metoclopramide) and analgesic regimens (NSAIDs, paracetamol, and gabapentin).
- Encourage early limb movement; start ambulation when stable.
- *Continue antibiotics:* Parenteral × 48 h → oral × 5–7 days.
- Remove drains and catheters early; retain catheter longer if bladder injury suspected.

Subsequent Care (Post 24 Hours)

- Gradual mobilization and diet advancement
- Taper analgesics, shift to oral form.
- Inspect wound after 48–72 hours for infection or dehiscence; maintain perineal hygiene.
- Provide laxatives if no bowel movement within 72 hours.
- Continue thromboprophylaxis ≥72 hours.

Type	*Examples and management*
Hemorrhage	Primary (intraoperative), reactionary (<24 h), or secondary (infection-related); manage with fluids, transfusions, resuturing, or reexploration as required
Sepsis	Includes wound infection, UTI, pneumonia, pelvic abscess; treat with broad-spectrum antibiotics and drainage if necessary
Shock	Hypovolemic, septic, or (rarely) neurogenic; managed with fluids, vasopressors, and targeted support
Respiratory	Atelectasis, pulmonary edema, failure; prevent with incentive spirometry and early ambulation
Gastrointestinal	PONV, paralytic ileus, bowel obstruction; manage conservatively with NPO, decompression, fluids, and prokinetics
Electrolyte imbalances	Treat underlying cause; correct Na^+, K^+, and water deficits cautiously
Renal	Oliguria, retention; maintain hydration and bladder training
Thromboembolism	Use DVT prophylaxis per Caprini risk model

Discharge: By postoperative day 3–4 after open surgery; earlier for laparoscopic/hysteroscopic proWcedures.

- Advise high-fiber diet, adequate hydration, and moderate ambulation.
- Remove sutures/staples on day 7; resume normal activities after 6 weeks.
- Counsel on warning signs and follow-up schedule.

POSTOPERATIVE COMPLICATIONS

Enhanced Recovery After Surgery

Definition: It is evidence-based multidisciplinary perioperative protocol to minimize stress, optimize physiological function and accelerate recovery.

Phases and Key Measures

Phase	*Key measures*
Preoperative	Patient counseling, nutritional optimization, carbohydrate loading
Intraoperative	Minimally invasive approach, normothermia, goal-directed fluids, multimodal analgesia
Postoperative	Early feeding and ambulation, prompt drain/catheter removal, continued thromboprophylaxis

Benefits: Shorter hospital stay, reduced complications, faster mobilization, lower opioid use, and better patient satisfaction.

Mnemonic: SPEED UP—Shorter stay, Pain ↓, Early recovery, Enhanced satisfaction, Decreased complications, Utilization of resources efficient, Price ↓

KEY POINTS

- Preoperative assessment and optimization are critical to safe surgical outcomes.
- Individualize investigations and medication management.
- Employ ERAS principles for faster recovery.
- Early mobilization, early oral intake, and multimodal pain control improve postoperative outcomes.

Assisted Reproductive Technologies: A Comprehensive Guide for Postgraduates

Ruchika Garg

INTRODUCTION AND DEFINITIONS

Assisted reproductive technology (ART) encompasses all fertility treatments in which both eggs and embryos are handled outside the human body. The cornerstone procedure is **in vitro fertilization (IVF)**, where oocytes are fertilized by sperm in a laboratory culture dish, forming embryos that are subsequently transferred into the uterus.

Assisted reproductive technology is distinct from simpler fertility treatments like ovulation induction or intrauterine insemination (IUI). It is indicated after the failure of first-line therapies or when the etiology of infertility necessitates direct gamete manipulation. The overarching goal of ART is to bypass pathological barriers to conception, thereby achieving pregnancy and a healthy live birth.

EXPANDED INDICATIONS FOR ASSISTED REPRODUCTIVE TECHNOLOGY

The decision to proceed with ART is multifactorial, based on a comprehensive diagnostic workup of both partners.

- **Tubal factor infertility:** Bilateral tubal occlusion, severe tubal disease (e.g., hydrosalpinges), or post-tubal ligation; the fallopian tubes are bypassed entirely.
- **Severe male factor infertility:** Characterized by critically low sperm count (severe oligospermia), poor motility (asthenospermia), abnormal morphology (teratospermia), or the absence of sperm in the ejaculate (azoospermia) requiring surgical retrieval.
- **Ovulatory dysfunction:** Anovulation resistant to oral ovulation-inducing agents (e.g., clomiphene citrate), particularly in conditions like polycystic ovary syndrome (PCOS).
- **Endometriosis:** Stages III/IV where anatomical distortion and a hostile pelvic environment impair natural conception.
- **Unexplained infertility:** After a full evaluation reveals no abnormality, ART serves as both a therapeutic and diagnostic tool.
- **Diminished ovarian reserve (DOR):** A decline in the quantity and quality of oocytes, indicated by a high FSH, low AMH, or low antral follicle count (AFC).
- **Genetic disorders:** Couples at risk of transmitting a known genetic abnormality to their offspring, requiring preimplantation genetic testing (PGT).
- **Fertility preservation:** For patients facing gonadotoxic therapies (e.g., chemotherapy, radiotherapy) or elective oocyte cryopreservation for social reasons.
- **Same-sex female couples and single mothers by choice:** Utilizing donor sperm to achieve pregnancy.
- **Uterine factor infertility:** Where a gestational carrier (surrogate) is required.

IN-DEPTH STEPS IN AN ASSISTED REPRODUCTIVE TECHNOLOGY CYCLE

Step 1—Controlled ovarian stimulation (COS): The objective is to recruit a cohort of follicles, overriding the natural cycle's single dominant follicle selection.

- **Protocols:**
  - **Antagonist protocol (most common):** Gonadotropins (FSH/LH) are initiated on cycle day 2–3. A GnRH antagonist is added around stimulation day 5–6 to prevent a premature LH surge. It is favored for its shorter duration and lower risk of ovarian hyperstimulation syndrome (OHSS).
  - **Long agonist protocol:** A GnRH agonist is started in the mid-luteal phase of the preceding cycle, achieving pituitary downregulation before gonadotropin stimulation begins. Historically common, it is now often reserved for specific cases like endometriosis.
  - **Other protocols:** Microflare agonist protocols for poor responders and mild stimulation protocols for specific patient profiles.
- **Monitoring:** Serial transvaginal ultrasounds track follicular growth, and serum estradiol (E2) levels are measured to assess follicular response and adjust medication dosages.

Step 2—Triggering final oocyte maturation: Once leading follicles reach an optimal size (typically 17-20 mm), a "trigger" injection is administered to induce the final stage of oocyte maturation.

- **hCG trigger:** Mimics the natural LH surge; carries a higher risk of OHSS due to its long half-life
- **GnRH agonist trigger:** Used exclusively in antagonist cycles; it induces an LH surge from the patient's pituitary, drastically reducing OHSS risk. Often used in egg donation cycles or when a "freeze-all" strategy is planned

Step 3—Oocyte retrieval: It is performed approximately 36 hours post-trigger under intravenous sedation. A needle guided by transvaginal ultrasound punctures each follicle, and follicular fluid containing the oocyte-cumulus complex is aspirated.

Step 4—Fertilization in the laboratory:

- **Conventional IVF:** Processed sperm is incubated with the retrieved oocytes, allowing natural fertilization to occur; suitable for normal semen parameters
- **Intracytoplasmic sperm injection (ICSI):** A single morphologically normal sperm is selected and injected directly into the cytoplasm of a mature (MII) oocyte; indicated for severe male factor, previous IVF fertilization failure, or when using surgically retrieved sperm (e.g., from testicular biopsy—TESE)

Step 5—Embryo culture: Fertilized oocytes (now zygotes) are cultured in sequential media.

- **Cleavage stage (day 3):** Embryos have 6–8 cells. Morphology is graded based on cell number, symmetry, and fragmentation degree.
- **Blastocyst stage (day 5/6):** Embryos develop into a fluid-filled blastocoel, an inner cell mass (becomes the fetus), and a trophectoderm (becomes the placenta). Blastocyst culture allows for better embryo selection and is more physiologically synchronous with the uterus, potentially improving implantation rates.

Step 6—Embryo transfer: The selected embryo(s) are loaded into a soft catheter and transferred into the uterine fundus under ultrasound guidance. The number of embryos transferred is a critical decision, balancing success rates against the risks of multiple pregnancy. Elective single embryo transfer (eSET) is increasingly advocated.

Step 7—Luteal phase support: The COS and retrieval process often creates a luteal phase defect. Progesterone supplementation (vaginal, intramuscular, or oral) is crucial to promote endometrial receptivity and support implantation until the placenta takes over hormone production (around 7-9 weeks).

Step 8—Pregnancy confirmation: A quantitative serum beta-hCG test is performed 10–14 days after embryo transfer. A rising level confirms a biochemical pregnancy, followed by an ultrasound at 6–7 weeks' gestation to confirm a clinical pregnancy with fetal cardiac activity.

ADVANCED ASSISTED REPRODUCTIVE TECHNIQUES IN DETAIL

- **PGT:**
  - **PGT-A (aneuploidy screening):** Screens embryos for chromosomal aneuploidies (e.g., Trisomy 21); aims to select euploid embryos for transfer, improving implantation rates and reducing miscarriage, especially in advanced maternal age.
  - **PGT-M (monogenic/single gene disorders):** For couples at risk of transmitting a specific genetic disease (e.g., cystic fibrosis, Huntington's); a biopsy is tested for the specific mutation.
  - **PGT-SR (structural rearrangements):** For carriers of balanced chromosomal translocations or inversions.
- **Cryopreservation (vitrification):** The ultra-rapid freezing technique has revolutionized ART. It allows for the preservation of supernumerary embryos, oocytes, or even ovarian tissue with excellent survival rates. This enables "freeze-all" cycles to prevent OHSS, cumulative success from a single stimulation cycle, and fertility preservation **(Table 1)**.
- **Assisted hatching:** A laser is used to create a small opening in the zona pellucida of the embryo prior to transfer. It is thought to aid implantation, particularly in cases of thickened zona or in women of advanced maternal age.

TABLE 1: ART cycle overview.

ART step	*Primary objective*	*Key considerations*
Ovarian stimulation	Develop multiple follicles	Protocol choice (antagonist vs. agonist) is patient-specific
Trigger	Final oocyte maturation	hCG versus GnRH agonist choice impacts OHSS risk
Oocyte retrieval	Collect mature oocytes	Ultrasound-guided, minor surgical procedure under sedation
Fertilization	Create embryos	IVF versus ICSI based on semen quality and history
Embryo culture	Select viable embryos	Blastocyst culture allows for better selection and PGT
Embryo transfer	Establish pregnancy	eSET is recommended to avoid multiple gestation
Luteal support	Support implantation	Progesterone is critical until placental takeover

TABLE 2: Factors impacting success of ART.

Factor	*Impact on ART success*
Female age	The single most critical factor; live birth rates decline sharply after 35 due to an increase in oocyte aneuploidy
Ovarian reserve	Measured by AMH, AFC, and day 3 FSH; a low reserve predicts a poorer response to stimulation and lower oocyte yield
Embryo quality and ploidy	The transfer of a high-grade, euploid blastocyst is the strongest predictor of implantation and live birth
Uterine receptivity	Factors like endometrial thickness (>7–8 mm), pattern, absence of polyps or fibroids, and hydrosalpinges significantly affect implantation
Male factor etiology	• Severe male factor can impact embryo quality, even with ICSI • Sperm DNA fragmentation is an area of active research
Lifestyle factors	Smoking, high BMI, and significant alcohol/caffeine consumption can negatively impact outcomes

- **Third-party reproduction:**
  - **Oocyte donation:** For women with premature ovarian insufficiency, surgically absent ovaries, or very poor oocyte quality; recipients undergo endometrial preparation with estrogen and progesterone.
  - **Gestational surrogacy:** An embryo created via IVF is transferred into the uterus of a gestational carrier. It is indicated for women without a functional uterus, severe medical conditions contraindicating pregnancy, or recurrent implantation failure of unexplained etiology.
  - **Sperm donation:** It is used when no male gametes are available or to avoid transmitting a genetic disorder.

SUCCESS RATES AND PROGNOSTIC FACTORS

Live birth rates per cycle are the most meaningful metric. The **SART (Society for Assisted Reproductive Technology)** and **CDC (Centers for Disease Control and Prevention)** publish clinic-specific data **(Table 2)**.

COMPLICATIONS AND RISK MANAGEMENT

- **OHSS:** This is a potentially life-threatening iatrogenic complication. Prevention is key: using antagonist protocols, GnRH agonist triggers, coasting, and "freeze-all" strategies. Treatment is supportive with fluid management, symptom control, and in severe cases, paracentesis.
- **Multiple pregnancies:** The most common complication of ART, leading to significantly higher risks of preterm birth, preeclampsia, gestational diabetes, and cesarean section; **elective single embryo transfer** is the primary strategy for risk reduction.
- **Ectopic and heterotopic pregnancy:** The risk of ectopic pregnancy is slightly elevated in ART. Heterotopic (simultaneous intra- and extra-uterine) pregnancy, while rare, is more common than in the general population.

- **Procedure-related risks:** These include infection, bleeding, or injury to pelvic structures during oocyte retrieval (<1%).
- **Psychological and financial burden:** The stress of treatment, its uncertain outcome, and high cost constitute a significant burden on patients, necessitating integrated psychological support.

ETHICAL, LEGAL, AND COUNSELING CONSIDERATIONS

- **Informed consent:** A detailed process covering success rates, risks, costs, and disposition options for unused embryos (donation to another couple, research, or thawing) is mandatory.
- **Embryo status:** Ethical debates persist regarding the moral status of the embryo, influencing regulations on research and storage limits.
- **Multifetal pregnancy reduction (MFPR):** It is a complex ethical dilemma offered in cases of high-order multiple pregnancies.
- **Anonymity and rights of donor-conceived offspring:** Laws vary globally regarding the child's right to know their genetic origins.
- **International disparities:** Regulations on surrogacy, PGT for sex selection, and embryo research differ vastly between countries, leading to "reproductive tourism".

RECENT AND EMERGING ADVANCES

- **Artificial intelligence (AI) in embryology:** AI algorithms analyzing time-lapse imaging of embryo development can predict blastocyst formation and implantation potential with high consistency, reducing subjectivity in selection.
- **Noninvasive PGT (niPGT):** It analyzes spent embryo culture media for cell-free DNA as a less invasive alternative to trophectoderm biopsy, though still under refinement.
- **In vitro maturation (IVM):** Retrieving immature oocytes and maturing them in the laboratory, minimizing or eliminating gonadotropin stimulation; it is beneficial for PCOS patients at high risk of OHSS.
- **Endometrial receptivity array (ERA):** ERA is a molecular diagnostic tool to identify a personalized "window of implantation", guiding the timing of embryo transfer in cases of recurrent implantation failure.
- **Mitochondrial replacement therapy (MRT):** It is an experimental technique to prevent transmission of mitochondrial DNA diseases ("three-parent baby").
- **Automated IVF platforms:** Robotics and microfluidics are being developed to standardize and optimize laboratory procedures like sperm selection and ICSI.

CONCLUSION

Assisted reproductive technology has evolved from an experimental procedure to a mainstream medical treatment, offering hope to millions of infertile couples globally.

SUGGESTED READING

1. Bosch E, Broer S, Griesinger G, et al. ESHRE guideline: ovarian stimulation for IVF/ICSI. Hum Reprod Open. 2020;2020(2):hoaa009.
2. Coonen E, Rubio C, Christopikou D, et al. ESHRE PGT Consortium good practice recommendations for the detection of structural and numerical chromosomal aberrations. Hum Reprod Open. 2020;2020(3):hoaa017.
3. Cimadomo D, de los Santos MJ, Griesinger G, et al. ESHRE good practice recommendations on recurrent implantation failure. Hum Reprod Open. 2023;2023(3):hoad023.
4. Mumusoglu S, Polat M, Ozbek IY, et al. Preparation of the endometrium for frozen embryo transfer: a systematic review. Front Endocrinol (Lausanne). 2021;12:688237.
5. Wyns C, De Geyter C, Calhaz-Jorge C, et al. ART in Europe, 2018: results generated from European registries by ESHRE. Hum Reprod Open. 2022;2022(3):hoac022.

Index

Page numbers followed by *f* refer to figure, *fc* refer to flowchart, and *t* refer to table.

A

C

F

I

J

K

L

P

T

W

X

Y

Z